FUNDAMENTALS OF NURSING

Fifth Edition

FUNDAMENTALS

OF

NURSING

The Humanities and The Sciences in Nursing

ELINOR V. FUERST, R.N., M.A.

Formerly Educational Consultant,
Muhlenberg Hospital School of
Nursing, Plainfield, N. J.; Assistant
Professor of Nursing, Cornell
University—New York Hospital School
of Nursing, New York.

LuVERNE WOLFF, R.N., M.A.

Formerly Consultant, College of
Nursing, Arizona State University, Tempe, Arizona;
Research Associate, Institute of Research
and Service in Nursing Education, Teachers
College, Columbia University, New York.

MARLENE H. WEITZEL, R.N., M.S.N.

Assistant Professor, College of
Nursing, Arizona State University, Tempe, Arizona;
formerly Assistant Professor, College
of Nursing, Niagara University,
Lewiston, New York.

J. B. LIPPINCOTT COMPANY

PHILADELPHIA   TORONTO

Copyright © 1974, by J. B. Lippincott Company

This book is fully protected by copyright and, with the exception of brief excerpts for review, no part of it may be reproduced in any form by print, photoprint, microfilm, or by any other means without the written permission of the publishers.

Distributed in Great Britain by
Blackwell Scientific Publications
London • Oxford • Edinburgh

ISBN 0-397-54152-X

Library of Congress Catalog Card Number 74-519

Printed in the United States of America

2 4 6 8 9 7 5 3 1

Library of Congress Cataloging in Publication Data

Fuerst, Elinor V.
    Fundamentals of nursing.

    Includes bibliographies.
    1. Nurses and nursing. I. Wolff, LuVerne, joint
author. II. Weitzel, Marlene H., joint author.
III. Title. [DNLM: 1. Nurse-patient relations.
2. Nursing care. WY100 F954f 1974]
RT41.F85   1974   610.73   74-519
ISBN 0-397-54152-X

To our parents

Preface

This book was prepared primarily for students in basic programs of education for nursing. However, it can serve well as a reference for students in other types of educational programs for nursing as well as for the practicing nurse.

The purpose of the book has been to present content fundamental to the practice of nursing. The content is not designed for any particular age group of patients nor is it concerned with the nursing care of patients with particular pathologic conditions. It is not intended for nursing practice in any one setting. However, patients with specific clinical entities, of particular ages, and in various settings are often cited in examples illustrating concepts fundamental to nursing practice.

The fifth edition represents an extensive revision. The authors have attempted to bring the content up-to-date and to reflect current practice in nursing, several examples of which will be cited.

• Beginning with the first edition, this text has emphasized the importance of identifying and using principles, rather than empirical knowledge, to guide nursing practice. This edition continues to place emphasis on the use of principles and many new ones have been added.

• Emphasis is placed on a holistic approach when offering the patient nursing services. Man cannot be separated into psychological and physiologic entities. Similarly, man's genetic endowment is constantly subjected to environmental influences, and hence, a patient is best considered in the context of the environment whence he comes. These points are emphasized in this text.

• More and more, the position is being taken that the nurse is responsible and accountable for her practice. She is becoming more actively involved in the health team, but her role is separate and distinct from the roles of other health practitioners. Using general systems theory as a basis, the nurse gathers relevant data in relation to her patient's needs for nursing care, makes a nursing assessment, plans nursing care with the patient according to his needs, and then implements appropriate nursing care. She evaluates her care and assumes responsibility and accountability for it.

• The consumer's role in health care in this country is changing. The consumer is assuming a more active role in the planning and implementation of health care services. He is demanding high quality care, and he considers health care to be his right. He looks for preventive as well as curative care. In addition, he wants and expects to be treated with respect and dignity. This text places emphasis on preventive care. It points out how the nurse can include the patient in the planning of this care and in implementing and evaluating it also. The nurse is encouraged to assist the patient in taking an active role and in assuming responsibility to the extent to which he is able in attaining and maintaining well-being. Teaching the patient is mentioned often with emphasis on involving him as a part of a team, all members of whom are concerned and care about his welfare. Emphasis continues in this edition concerning the uniqueness of man, and the nurse is asked to respect him without regard for race, religion, or social or economic status. The reader is reminded often of ways of demonstrating respect for her patient's individuality and of giving care that shows respect for those whom she serves.

• Nurses practice in a wider variety of settings. Concerted efforts were made to take this into account in the presentation of content.

• Most patients have families, and they are often cared for in their homes. This book points out ways in which the nurse can include family members while offering services to her patient in health agencies, and makes suggestions as well concerning the care of patients at home, whether this includes care by nurses or whether the family or the patient himself assumes primary responsibility.

• Many tools and much new equipment are increasingly becoming available to nurses in their practice; the computer, monitoring systems, and disposable items are examples. Also, the trend continues to use auxiliary personnel to assist the nurse in giving care. But emphasis in this text remains on the preeminence of the nurse-patient relationship and the therapeutic value of a positive relationship. This depends to a large extent on nurses and patients meeting and working together. When the use of mechanical and electronic equipment and of the services of others keeps nurses and patients apart, this book holds that an indispensable aspect of nursing has been defeated.

A considerable amount of new material has been included in this edition. Unit 2 presents the nursing process system, based on systems theory, as a frame of reference for planning and implementing nursing care. It is based on the philosophy that effective nursing care results when the nurse uses knowledge from the psychosocial and biochemical sciences to determine and provide individual care for each patient. Four subsystems are described and illustrated in the succeeding chapters in Unit 2. An example that illustrates the use of the nursing process system appears immediately following Chapter 9. The last chapter in Unit 2 describes intrahealth team and intranursing team communications, essential ingredients in the successful use of the nursing process system.

Chapter 17 discusses new material in relation to common community activities and problems, how they influence well-being and the resulting implications for nursing. Chapter 30, another new chapter, is concerned with the nurse's role in promoting optimum sensory stimulation.

Additional new material occurs in many chapters. A few examples are: the role of the nurse as the patient's advocate; hierarchy of human needs; reverse isolation; the donning of sterile gloves; perineal care; and preoperative skin preparation. Material presented in greater detail than in previous editions occurs, for example, in relation to the law and the nurse; ecology; the role of the consumer in health care; content from physiology and biochemistry important to an understanding of fluid and electrolyte balance; roles of the nurse; and definitions of health and the health-illness continuum.

One small innovation we hope will prove helpful is the inclusion of a glossary, *with definitions*, at the opening of each chapter.

We have added many new illustrations to the text that we trust will enhance its teaching value.

Additional study situations are presented, and with few exceptions, they are new to this edition. The reader is urged to use them. Some of them present new material, or material in somewhat greater depth than was possible to incorporate in the text; an example is Study Situation No. 5 in Chapter 20, concerning circadian rhythms. Some study situations present material that is under debate today; Study Situation No. 1 in Chapter 4, concerning institutional licensing of nurses, is an example. Occasionally, a study situation presents material that may be considered tangential to content in this book but which may be of particular interest to at least some readers; Study Situation No. 3 in Chapter 18, concerning a management approach to accident prevention, is an example. Study situations in many chapters help the reader to put the nursing process system to work in specific situations; Study Situation No. 3 in Chapter 23, concerning a patient experiencing pain, and No. 1 in Chapter 24, concerning preparation of a patient for surgery, are examples.

The number of references given at the end of each chapter in many cases is rather extensive. An effort was made to include references from a variety of sources. It is hoped that readers, especially those interested in exploring a subject in greater detail, will find the references useful and helpful. Articles and books referred to in study situations are not repeated in the references at the end of chapters.

There are numerous ways in which content can be arranged. A final decision often must be made arbitrarily, with the realization that every arrangement presents advantages and disadvantages. The final arrangement arrived at does not imply a suggested course outline. Rather, it is hoped that the arrangement lends itself to easy adaptation to meet the reader's needs. A particular unit may be considered as a whole, using the several chapters in the sequence offered. This may be especially appropriate, for example, in relation to Unit 2. Or, a chapter may be considered without regard to the particular unit in which it was placed. For example, Chapter 4, concerning the legal and ethical components of nursing, may easily be considered independently of other chapters in Unit 1. In Unit 5 in particular, which discusses common nursing intervention measures, the reader may wish to use chapters in various sequences. For example, Chapter 24, which discusses fluid and electrolyte balance, appears rather early since information in many of the chapters that follow may often depend on a knowledge of fluid and electrolyte balance. The chapters dealing with maintaining nutrition and promoting elimination, for example, follow Chapter 24 for that reason. On the other hand, those who wish to consider fluid and electrolyte balance at a later or earlier time in relation to other content in Unit 5 may do so without anticipated difficulty.

We recognize that there are an increasing number of men in nursing and we encourage and welcome their entering the field. However, for the sake of clarity and convenience to the reader, we have used the feminine pronoun when referring to the nurse and the masculine pronoun, whenever appropriate, when referring to the patient.

It is our sincere hope that this text will make positive contributions to educational programs in nursing and will serve the nurse in her practice in society today, the ultimate goal of the book being improved nursing care for the patient.

Acknowledgments

The authors wish to express their gratitude to these persons who made important contributions during the preparation of this edition.

Kathleen H. Chafey, Assistant Professor and Chairman of the Continuing Education Program, College of Nursing, Arizona State University, Tempe, Arizona, who read manuscript and suggested revisions for the Chapters in Unit 2.

Dorothy M. McLeod, Director of the Medical-Surgical Graduate Program, College of Nursing, Arizona State University, Tempe, Arizona, who read manuscript and suggested revisions for Chapter 24.

Eleanor G. DelPo, Assistant Professor, College of Nursing, University of Arizona, Tucson, Arizona, who read manuscript and suggested revisions for Chapter 7.

Sharon Nielsen, Faculty Associate, College of Nursing, Arizona State University, Tempe, Arizona, formerly Coordinator, Oncology Unit, Good Samaritan Hospital, Phoenix, Arizona, who read manuscript and suggested revisions for Chapter 31.

Suzanne R. Van Ort and Rose Marie Gerber, Assistant Professors, College of Nursing, University of Arizona, Tucson, Arizona, who offered suggestions of a general nature concerning certain content.

Rabbi Albert Plotkin, Temple Beth Israel, Phoenix, Arizona, and Rabbi H. Philip Berkowitz, Temple Beth Jacob, Pontiac, Michigan. Rabbi Berkowitz suggested revisions and Rabbi Plotkin read and approved manuscript on the section dealing with Judaism in Chapter 15.

The Reverend Frank J. Babbish, S.J., Chaplain, and the Reverend Russell Roide, S.J., Assistant Chaplain, St. Joseph's Hospital and Medical Center, Phoenix, Arizona. Father Roide suggested revisions and Father Babbish read and approved manuscript on the section dealing with Roman Catholicism in Chapter 15.

The Reverend Philip A. Gangsei, Prince of Peace Lutheran Church, Phoenix, Arizona, who read and approved manuscript on the section dealing with Protestantism in Chapter 15.

Barbara M. Petrosino, Assistant Professor, College of Nursing, Niagara University, Lewiston, New York, for assistance with the final preparation of references.

David T. Miller, Managing Editor, Nursing Department, J. B. Lippincott Company, Philadelphia, Pennsylvania, who offered valuable editorial assistance and guidance.

We wish to acknowledge the members of the undergraduate faculty of the College of Nursing, Arizona State University, Tempe, Arizona, who did much of the basic work on the nursing process system from which Unit 2 was developed.

Finally, to our friends who displayed patience and understanding and offered so much support during the preparation of this edition, a very special thank you.

Contents

Contents

UNIT 1

Health Services,
Health Practitioners, and the Consumer

CHAPTER 1

The Practice of Nursing

GLOSSARY

Biomedical Engineering: Engineering concerned with the use of technology in the delivery of health care services.

Clinical Nurse Specialist: A nurse who by reason of expertise in a clinical specialty (such as medicine, surgery, obstetrics, or psychiatry) assumes primary responsibility for nursing practice and its effects on health care. Synonyms include nurse-clinician and nurse-specialist.

Consumer: One who uses a service or commodity. Health care consumer is one who uses health care services.

Continuing Education: Education, formal or informal, offered to nurses who have completed basic educational programs in nursing.

Continuity of Care: A continuum of health care, whether the patient is in a state of health or illness.

Demography: The science of population statistics.

Dependent Functions: Actions of the nurse which cannot be executed without a physician's order.

Empirical Knowledge: Knowledge gained primarily from experience or observation.

Extended Family: Family that includes parents and their children and their relatives, such as aunts, uncles, grandparents, cousins.

Health Practitioner: One engaged in the practice of dispensing health care services.

Health Team: An organization of health practitioners representing various professions that work collaboratively in planning and administering health care services.

Independent Functions: Actions of the nurse which can be executed without a physician's order.

Nuclear Family: Family that includes parents and their children.

Nurse Associate: A nurse working interdependently or in a partnership arrangement with someone of another health care profession, usually a physician.

Nurse-Midwife: A nurse who is responsible for the education, health, and obstetrical management of selected, pregnant women and for early recognition of deviations from the normal. Ordinarily, the nurse-midwife works within a framework of a medically directed health service.

Nursing Team: A group of technical and professional nursing personnel under the leadership of a qualified nurse, having the goal of providing comprehensive nursing care services.

Patient: Any person, well or ill, receiving services from a health practitioner.

Patient Advocate: One who intercedes for or works on behalf of the patient.

Primary Care Nursing: Nursing practice that offers a person his first contact with health care services and assumes responsibility for continuing care either by the nurse or in cooperation with other health personnel whose services are required by the patient.

Theory: Explanation of a process, a phenomenon, or an event based on observed fact(s) but which lacks absolute or direct proof.

INTRODUCTION

Nursing today is far removed from nursing of the past which was concerned primarily with the physical care of the sick and disabled. Nursing was task-oriented and illness-oriented. It was rich on "how-to-do" but poor on the "whys" of doing. Nursing was concerned for the most part with doing something *to* or *for* the patient but rarely with the patient.

Nursing has changed. So also has all of society and at an extraordinarily rapid rate. This chapter looks at some of the changes that are playing a part in determining the nature of nursing practice and the roles of the nurse.

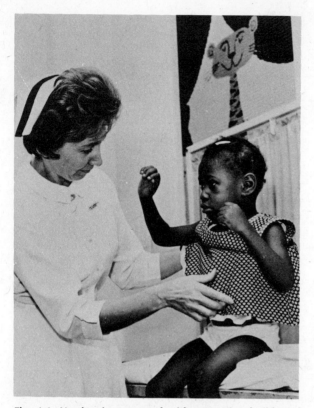

Fig. 1-1. Nursing is concerned with promoting health and early disease detection. Helping a preschooler prepare for a physical examination may be a common experience for the nurse. However, it is often a new experience for the patient who may be afraid and anxious. (Photo by Warren R. Vroom)

NURSING DESCRIBED

Nursing is concerned with services to patients. A *patient* is any person, well or ill, receiving services from a health practitioner. In some places, the word *client* is used instead of patient. In still other areas, *client* is used selectively, as for example, when speaking of persons receiving counseling services in a community setting. In this text, the word *patient* will be used throughout.

Nursing offers health services that are directed toward providing care which promotes and maintains health; prevents, detects, and treats disease and disability; and restores the highest possible level of health following illness or injury. Much factual knowledge and many techniques used to promote health are shared among all types of health practitioners. However each group of practitioners develops and uses the knowledge and techniques in a manner that will lead to attainment of its distinctive contribution to

health care. Although physicians, dentists, social workers, dietitians, sanitarians, and nurses obviously have health promotion as one of their reasons for existence, each group has its distinct area of expertise. Within each of these groups, there are specialists. The surgeon and the opthalmologist are physicians with differing specialties. The nutritionist and the therapeutic dietitian, both concerned with nutrition, offer different types of services to patients. The community health nurse meets needs that are different from those met by the intensive care nurse.

An important focus of nursing is to assist individuals to meet their daily requirements so that they can function in as satisfying a manner as possible. Nursing is based on principles developed in the physical, biological, and social sciences. The nurse uses knowledge from many disciplines to guide her in gathering pertinent information about the patient; in this way she can work with him in making decisions regarding appropriate ways to help make him more comfortable and secure, physiologically stable, knowledgeable, and independent.

Nursing is committed to personalized services for all persons without regard to color, creed, social, or economic status. It includes caring for the young and the old, the rich and the poor, the dirty and the clean. A basis for nursing is a belief in the value of every person. Competent nursing practice demonstrates this belief by seeing that a patient's health needs are met in a manner that illustrates concern for him as an individual.

Generally, nurses work directly with patients. However, in some instances, the nurse functions as the *patient advocate*; that is, she works indirectly on behalf of the patient or she intercedes for him. For example, the nurse who lobbies in the legislature in support of programs of benefit to the consumer of health services functions as a patient advocate. A few other examples are the nurse who seeks the services of other health practitioners on behalf of a patient; the nurse who intercedes for the patient by helping him obtain services from various community health agencies; and the nurse who intercedes for the patient by interpreting his needs to his family. A nurse becomes the patient advocate also as she plans his total health care while serving as a member of the health team. A study situation at the end of this chapter refers to articles that illustrate the numerous ways in which the nurse-author worked as a patient advocate.

Although hospitals are the largest single employer of nurses, they work in many other settings such as schools, industries, private homes, community health agencies, clinics, physicians' offices, convales-

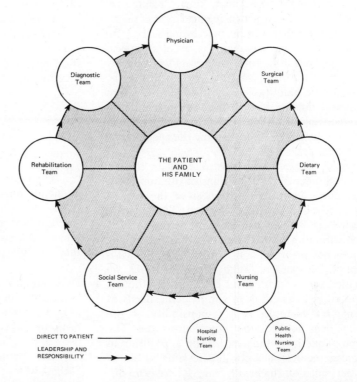

Fig. 1-2. The figure illustrates the health team whose members represent a variety of professions working collaboratively to aid in meeting the needs of the patient. Also illustrated is the nursing team whose members are responsible for planning and administering nursing care required of the patient.

cent and nursing homes, day care centers, residential treatment centers, and so on. While care of the ill and disabled remains an important part of nursing practice, promoting health and teaching and counseling the patient and his family are assuming an increasingly important role in nursing. Figure 1-1 illustrates one setting in which nurses work, Figure 1-5 illustrates still another.

THE HEALTH AND THE NURSING TEAMS

Offering society health care services requires the efforts of a variety of practitioners. The emphasis today is on comprehensive and continuing care. In order to avoid fractionated patient care, the health team has developed as a means to organize, coordinate, and dispense services.

The health team characteristically has representation from all practitioner groups, and its members work interdependently and collaboratively in offering services distinctive to its profession. For example, the physician assumes responsibility for diagnosing and prescribing therapy and in carrying out certain procedures which fall within his domain. The dietitian assumes responsibility in planning a diet appropriate for the patient's needs. Nursing is responsible for planning and administering nursing care required of the patient. Figure 1-2 illustrates the typical health team.

Each health service group represented on the health team may have, in turn, a team of persons who participate in administering the group's unique services. For example, nursing often organizes a team of personnel to help carry out nursing care. The team leader plans, supervises, and evaluates the total team effort. Characteristically, a nursing team is headed by a qualified nurse who has as her assistants other nurses as well as practical nurses, nursing assistants, nursing aides, home health aides, nursing volunteers, clerical assistants, and perhaps others. Figure 1-2 illustrates the typical nursing team also.

As Figure 1-2 shows, the focus of attention for the health team and the nursing team is the patient and *his* needs. Planning without including the patient can often lead to frustrating results, such as a plan of care he will not or cannot accept.

In some instances, a health team may lack certain services that a patient may require. For example, a dietitian may be available for consultation, but the nurse may need to assume responsibility for teaching the patient and his family about dietary matters.

Especially in remote areas, many nurses assume responsibilities that in an urban medical center might be assumed by other health practitioners. For instance, the patient may have the services of a physical therapist in a medical center; however, when he returns to his home in a rural area, the nurse may be the only health practitioner available to assist him with physical therapy he still needs. The emphasis, then, remains on providing services to the patient in the best way possible rather than on the specific role of a particular practitioner.

There are persons who have referred to the dependent and independent functions of the nurse. For example, entry 24 in the references at the end of this chapter refers to these functions. The *dependent functions* of the nurse are those which are not executed without a physician's order. For example, a nurse does not prescribe and administer drugs without a physician's order. *Independent functions* are those which can be carried out by a nurse without a physician's order. Tending to the hygienic needs of a patient, for example, is a responsibility of the nurse that does not require a physician's order. The philosophy underlying the health team is resulting in a change in the relationships and responsibilities of various personnel on the health team. There is no disputing the role of the physician who brings his high degree of scientific competence to the team in diagnosing and prescribing therapy. However, health personnel working in professions other than medicine are developing expertise and are increasingly complementing the physician's role in meeting patient needs. The independent functions of the nurse, for example, are increasing in scope, as described later in this chapter. Each year, this trend is being taken into account as nurse practice laws change. Study situations at the end of Chapter 4 illustrate efforts to change laws so that they will allow nurses to assume more independent functions. Examples of personnel other than nurses who are also assuming expanded roles that complement the physician's role include social workers, psychologists, sociologists, physical therapists, physician's assistants, and dietitians.

The following is, in part, a recommendation made by the Secretary's Committee to Study Extended Roles for Nurses, concerning the interprofessional relationships between physicians and nurses: "Collaborative efforts involving schools of medicine and nursing should be encouraged to undertake programs to demonstrate effective functional interaction of physicians and nurses in the provision of health services and the extension of those services to the widest possible range of the population. The transfer of functions and responsibilities between physicians and nurses should be sought through an orderly process recognizing the capacity and desire of both professions to participate in additional training activities intended to augment the potential scope of nursing practice." (15.7)

TRENDS INFLUENCING NURSING PRACTICE

There are strong currents in society that are influencing nursing practice. Nursing cannot remain static and continue practice that is based solely on tradition without threatening its very existence and relevance. Several trends and the manner in which they are affecting nursing are briefly discussed here.

Demographic Changes

Demography is the science of population statistics. Population statistics include life expectancy rates, mortality rates, population shifts, marriage and divorce rates, birth rates, and the like.

The population is increasing in the United States, which means more people are in need of health care services. Life expectancy has increased, resulting in more older people in our population. Also, the population under 20 years of age is presently increasing in number. Older persons and youngsters create increased demands on health practitioners since it has been observed that both these groups tend to require more health services than other age groups.

There has been a change in population patterns with more people moving to urban and suburban areas and to regions with favorable climates. The rural areas, especially those that are sparsely populated, are often isolated from adequate health care facilities or practitioners.

Family and community structures are also changing. Today's population is more mobile than in the past, resulting in weakening neighborhood and community support to family life. Divorce rates have increased, resulting in more single-parent homes. Close *extended-family* ties (that is, ties with aunts, uncles, grandparents, and cousins) that once offered assistance to the *nuclear family* of parents and children when crises arose are no longer as strong as once was the case. Changes of this nature have often required health practitioners to look to community social agencies for assistance in meeting family problems having health implications as Figure 1-3 illustrates.

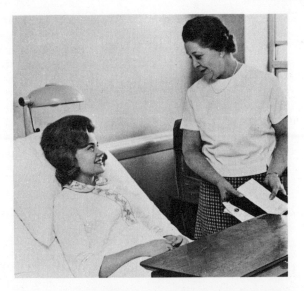

Fig. 1-3. The nurse understands this patient's problem needs the help of a social service agency person, an important member of the health team. The social service worker is helping to answer questions concerning costs of hospitalization and insurance. (Courtesy of Muhlenberg Hospital, Plainfield, New Jersey)

Nursing is responding to demographic changes in various ways. More educational offerings and programs of many varieties are evident. Recruitment is helping to attract more persons to a career in nursing. Nursing, once almost entirely limited to Caucasian women, now welcomes men and non-Caucasians to its ranks. Recruitment of inactive nurses has been on the increase. Health services, often with governmental support, are being extended to remote areas of this country, and nurses are increasingly attracted to positions in these areas. In order to utilize nurses more efficiently, careful scrutiny has resulted in delegating non-nursing tasks that once occupied much of the nurse's time to non-nursing personnel.

As responsibilities of nursing change in response to demographic changes, so too do the roles of the nurse. Nursing roles are discussed later in this chapter.

The Knowledge Explosion

Scientific research has uncovered new knowledge at a tremendously rapid pace. Also, new knowledge has been put to practical use much more rapidly today than once was the case. Consider for a moment a few relatively recent applications of new knowledge that have changed our way of living dramatically: the jet engine, television, space exploration, the computer, and communication via satellites. Or consider these examples of scientific advances more closely associated with health and illness: organ transplants, the "pill," the laser beam, and the sophisticated hardware used in electronic monitoring systems.

In the social sciences, great strides have been made in attempting to understand and predict human behavior, an important area of knowledge for health practitioners. For example, the body of knowledge in relation to values, attitudes and prejudices, social mobility, and ethnic, social, and cultural backgrounds is utilized by health practitioners in designing patient care that is appropriate and acceptable to the patient and more in accordance with his own life style.

Nurses must know more in order to function effectively, efficiently, and safely in today's world, and in more settings than previously. However, as in other areas of study, it is impossible to acquire all of the knowledge available and appropriate to nursing. Educational programs in nursing are responding to the knowledge explosion in several ways.

Educators and practitioners know that *empirical knowledge*, which is gathered primarily from experience and observation only, and the memorization of procedures and routines are no longer adequate. The result has been that educational programs are increasingly teaching scientific principles that will guide practice for all possible circumstances. For example, the nurse who has learned what equipment she will use and what steps she will take in the procedure of administering a cleansing enema to an adult patient in a particular hospital is helpless in any other setting or with other types of patients. However, the nurse who understands the scientific principles involved (introduction of a solution into the colon to stimulate peristalsis) can function anywhere, using appropriate equipment on hand.

Education for nursing places more emphasis than previously in applying knowledge from the behavioral sciences. Concern for a patient who is, first of all, a unique human being, demands a knowledge of human behavior. This approach places emphasis on the person being served.

There appears to be no evidence that the knowledge explosion is about to diminish. This requires that *continuing education*, that is, education offered to nurses who have completed basic education programs in nursing, be a part of every practitioner's life in order to be up-to-date. There is discussion today among some nurses that continuing education may have to become mandatory for maintaining licensure in the not-too-distant future. Examples of continuing education include workshops, conferences, and agency in-service education programs.

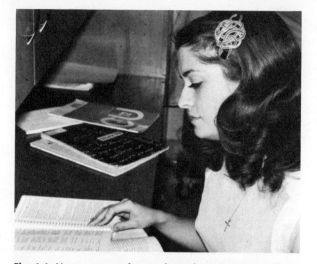

Fig. 1-4. Nurses can no longer depend on their basic education in nursing as sufficient to sustain them throughout their careers. The knowledge explosion requires frequent and continued study. Reading the latest literature is one way nurses can stay abreast of new knowledge. (Good Samaritan Hospital, Phoenix, Arizona)

The knowledge explosion has made specialization a sign of the times, and educational programs have responded accordingly. In nursing, for instance, practitioners are becoming more specialized and more learned in selected areas. This trend toward specialization has often been accomplished with greater emphasis on so-called *clinical nursing*. It is different from specialization that once was almost entirely limited to administration or teaching in nursing. There are nurses who prepare to work in cardiac and coronary units, respiratory units, hemodialysis units, community mental health centers, and well-baby and well-child clinics. Clinical practitioners in the various medical specialties, such as medicine, surgery, obstetrics, and child care, are being prepared in larger numbers today.

Many more educational programs at the graduate level are geared to prepare specialized practitioners in nursing. Those offered in institutions of higher learning grant degrees upon successful completion of master's or doctoral requirements. In addition, there are many other nondegree educational offerings, both formal and informal, with the objective of furthering the preparation of specialized clinical practitioners in nursing.

Educational programs are also increasingly developing programs that aim to prepare *primary care* nurses. These nurses offer patients their first contact with health care services and assume responsibility for continuing care of whatever nature the patient requires. A study situation at the end of this chapter refers to a report on primary care nursing in pediatrics.

With increasing emphasis on the need for a sound knowledge for practicing nursing, theories of nursing are beginning to evolve. A *theory* is an explanation of a process, a phenomenon, or an event based on observed fact(s) but which lacks absolute or direct proof. Theories are useful in predicting outcomes and in providing guidance for uncovering additional knowledge. In reference 21 at the end of this chapter, human adaptation is discussed as a theoretical base for nursing. Scholars in nursing are increasingly investigating and developing conceptual frames of references which might well serve as potential nursing theories. As more nurses become better prepared educationally, it is anticipated that the trend toward developing nursing theories will continue.

The Increasingly Knowledgeable Consumer

A better educated population, with more knowledge of health and with easy access to numerous communications media dispensing increasing amounts of health information, has resulted in a more knowledgeable consumer. At least two results are evident: the consumer is demanding more health care and he is demanding health care of higher quality. This means that nurses just like other health practitioners must prepare more and better educated nurses if consumer demands are to be satisfied. This, nursing is attempting to do, as has been pointed out earlier in this chapter. Chapter 2 will also discuss the health demands of the consumer and the implications these hold for health practitioners.

The Rise of the Social Conscience

The tendency for each person to be concerned primarily with only his own welfare is rapidly disappearing. Society today is looking closely at the moral and ethical quality of its actions and motives. This trend has resulted in a closer scrutiny of what may be considered as morally right or wrong in our relations with others. Concern for the poor, the lonely, the criminal, the alcoholic, the drug addict, the unemployed and unemployable, the neglected, and the underdog in society is evident throughout the country. Giving baskets of food to those in need on holidays is no longer deemed sufficient concern for society's poor. Isolating and forgetting the down-and-outer, the wrongdoer, or the misfit to a hopeless life of despair and frustration irritate a responsible social conscience.

Since its beginning, nursing has demonstrated interest in caring for society's unfortunates. So it is today—nursing is committed to caring for all who need care. The emphasis of that care is on compassion and understanding and in accepting the patient as he is. As one author stated, "It may be that nursing in particular, holds the key to maintenance of humane, individualistic concern for people and their health problems. And this capacity must be zealously enlarged." [1]

The Women's Liberation Movement

Nursing traces its origins to orders, often religious in nature, that expected unending service and unquestioned obedience to superiors. Nursing was a woman's occupation, and the nurse's role was that of a mother surrogate who nurtured those who were ill and helpless. A nurse would have been considered unworthy if she asked for something for herself or if she questioned authority.

Today's woman is taking steps to free herself for independent action and thought. She seeks social, economic, political, and educational equality with men. Through legislative channels she is demanding equality as a legal right, not as a privilege granted only by those who voluntarily choose to recognize her as an individual and equal. Some contemporary commentators have said that women are in the midst of a social revolution. For example, through protest, strikes, and the like, and with determination, women are progressing toward liberation.

Although men are increasingly choosing nursing as a career, most nurses are still women. These women are joining non-nurses in striving for equality in society. A study situation at the end of this chapter refers the reader to articles describing nurses who are active in the women's liberation movement, and who feel that the movement will be beneficial to nursing as well.

Increasing Professionalism in Nursing

Nursing is working toward interdependency on a partnership basis with other professional groups concerned with providing society with comprehensive health care services. The nurse seeks to define her own role in practice and asks to assume responsibility and accountability for her action. She is demanding and receiving recognition in planning and executing nursing services. The nurse is no longer primarily limited to the hospital environment but has increasingly moved out into the neighborhood and community in identifying health care needs. In addition to

[1] Lysaught, J. P.: An Abstract for Action. p. 11. New York, McGraw-Hill, 1970. Used with permission of McGraw-Hill Book Company.

effecting change, she is offering an increasing number of services to society.

Nursing is becoming more self-regulatory and self-determining. Through research, nursing is actively working to establish its own body of scientific knowledge and skill. It is progressing toward colleague equality. Also, nursing continues to work toward establishing economic security commensurate with the nurse's status and role in society.

ROLES OF THE NURSE

The literature is rich with descriptions of the changing roles of the nurse as nursing practice adapts to meet society's needs. Indeed, if nursing is to survive at all, it must be prepared not only to accept and adjust to change but to effect change as well. However, whenever change occurs, permanence remains in that the nurse continues to care for persons who need her help. Some descriptions of nursing written as long as a century ago remain valid to this day.

Early in this decade, two groups studied nursing practice and nursing education and, in their reports, focused attention on nursing in the health care system and on the roles of nurses. The National Commission for the Study of Nursing and Nursing Education presented its report in *An Abstract for Action* in 1970. The Secretary's Committee to Study Extended Roles for Nurses presented its report in *Extending the Scope of Nursing Practice* in 1971. Both reports had wide readership; both found nursing to be committed to serving the patient and helping him to meet his health needs; and both recommended changing roles for nurses as one step in improving the delivery of health care in this country.

A variety of descriptive phrases are being used to illustrate roles of the nurse that are developing or have developed in response to society's increased needs for health care services. Examples include nurse associate, clinical specialist, primary practitioner, family practitioner, community health nurse, Primex, nurse therapist, and physician's assistant.

In what ways is the nurse's role changing?

• It is expanding from one of direct and limited care of the ill patient to one involving extensive planning and coordination of total patient care. The physician diagnoses and plans a patient's medical regimen which the nurse helps to implement. But, in addition, the nurse is expected to use judgment and plan appropriate nursing care, to see to it that nursing care is properly executed and is meeting the patient's needs, and to make decisions in relation to

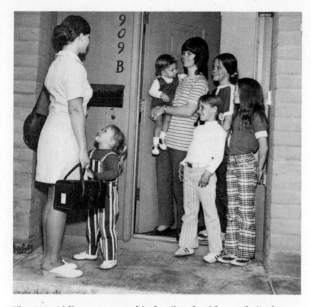

Fig. 1-5. Aiding to meet this family's health needs is the responsibility of the community health nurse. In this illustration it appears that the nurse is a welcomed caller who comes to help and support all members of the family. (Photo by Ted Hill, Arizona)

changing the nursing regimen as the patient's needs change.

• It is changing from one largely dependent on the delegation of responsibility from other health team practitioners to one that is self-regulating and self-determining.

• It is changing from one of assuming responsibility primarily in hospital settings to one of assuming responsibility in a variety of settings. Nurses practice just about any place in the country where health care services are being offered or are in demand.

• It is changing from one of limited to considerable societal responsibility. Nursing is broadening its horizons by assuming increased amounts of leadership in effecting change and in anticipating society's needs. Nurses are engaged also in a variety of innovative programs that have as their objective serving more people with better health care.

• It is shifting from one that was primarily illness-oriented to one that is health-oriented. This change of emphasis is reflected in many new responsibilities. Examples include planning for *continuity of care* through referrals among health and social agencies; observing and evaluating signs of health and illness with prevention and early detection of disease as primary goals; helping to plan for total health care regimens for families, neighborhoods, and communities, and the like. As a corollary to the shift in emphasis from illness to wellness, the nursing role that

once included a minimum of health teaching and counseling of patients and their families in relation to health maintenance now assumes a marked increase in attention. As another corollary, the nurse's role that once took limited responsibility in the rehabilitation of the ill and handicapped now implements restorative regimens extensively.

• It has changed from emphasizing doing something to or for the patient to respecting the patient's ability to collaborate in planning his care. It is also becoming generally recognized that the patient who has been consulted about his care and then encouraged to actively participate to the extent that this is possible usually experiences increased psychological as well as physical well-being from the practice.

• It is becoming enmeshed with *biomedical engineering,* a relatively new field of endeavor that is concerned with the increasing use of technology in the delivery of health care. Figure 1-6 illustrates an example. Another is the extent to which computers are being put to work. Automation is on the increase in all of society, and the nurse who fails to keep in step with the trend will soon fall short of competent practice.

• Once primarily function-oriented, it is becoming more concerned with an expressive role that assists patients to meet psychosocial needs in the nurse-patient relationship. This trend will be discussed in Chapter 11.

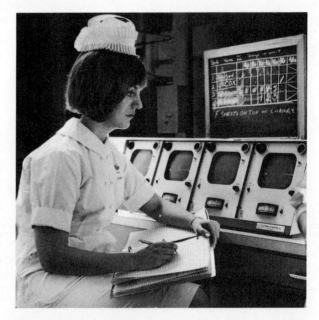

Fig. 1-6. Nursing includes the use of increasingly sophisticated equipment that aids in providing better patient care. This nurse is at a monitoring station on a coronary care unit. (Courtesy of New York Hospital—Cornell Medical Center)

• Once task-oriented, it is becoming knowledge-oriented. The change requires a sound knowledge of scientific principles and the exercise of professional judgment in the execution of competent care. This change also emphasizes the need for continuing education and for participation in research to further nursing knowledge and skill as recognized professional responsibilities.

CONCLUSION

Nurses constitute the largest single group of health personnel in the United States. In 1971, the Secretary of Health, Education, and Welfare reported that there were over one million nurses in this country. Statistics indicated that approximately 700,000 were active, the remainder being inactive. Still, with the ever-increasing need for their services, more nurses are needed. In addition, the scope and range of nursing's responsibilities in meeting the health care needs of society mean assuming increased responsibility for patient care, developing effective collaboration with other health practitioners, and supporting new and promising methods for delivering health care services more effectively.

Study Situations

1. Should nurses become involved with protests of various sorts? Opinions vary. The following article describes one point of view:
   Freeman, R. B.: Practice as protest. **Am. J. Nurs.,** 71:918–921, May, 1971.
   What three principles does the author describe that Florence Nightingale used when she worked for social change? Do you agree when the author writes on page 921, "Protest and social action must join ministration, education, and support as essential elements of nursing practice"?
2. The quote given below is taken from the following book:
   Storlie, F.: Nursing and the Social Conscience. p. 222. New York, Appleton-Century-Crofts, 1970.
   "What about nursing? Can we enlarge our concern for the hospital sick to the social sick, strive less to treat anemia and more to put meat on our children's plates? Can nursing stretch its arms to the helpless, the feeble, the aged and the infirm, the troubled and the torn, the protester, the prostitute, and the very poor? Somewhere there is a hungry child too apathetic to cry; somewhere else, a migrant family crowds into a one-room shack; a boy fifteen "rehabilitates" behind prison walls and a woman weeps for the child she does not want and the abortion

she cannot have. An old man lies restrained to his nursing-home bed. This is our land, and these are people in need." (Preface, p. ix) [2]
   How do the concerns of Freeman (referred to in Study Situation 1) and Storlie relate to content in the section "Trends Influencing Nursing Practice" in this chapter?
3. This chapter points out that present specialization in nursing is placing more emphasis on clinical practice than once was true. Also, the chapter describes nursing beginning to function on a collaborative type basis with members of the medical profession. The following reference describes how the dean of one college of nursing worked toward increasing emphasis on clinical practice and on physician-nurse collaboration:
   Brown, E. L.: Nursing Reconsidered: A Study in Change: Part 1. The Professional Role of Nursing. pp. 47–49. Philadelphia, J. B. Lippincott, 1970.
   How did the dean demonstrate that her role could serve more patients in receiving care they needed? In the same reference, read the "Quality of Nursing Care," on pages 34–38. Compare Dean Reiter's philosophy of nursing with the description of the roles of the nurse in this chapter?
4. Read the following article:
   Mussallem, H. K.: The changing role of the nurse. **Am. J. Nurs.,** 69:514–517, Mar., 1969.
   How does the author's description of the new nurse on pages 516 and 517 compare with the section "Roles of the Nurse" in this chapter?
5. Many nurses have been concerned about equal rights for women for decades. The following article relates interesting history of the efforts of nurses to obtain rights for women:
   Christy, T.: Equal rights for women: voices from the past. **Am. J. Nurs.,** 72:288–293, Feb., 1971.
   Many supporters of an equal rights amendment to the U. S. Constitution would agree that discrimination against women is not only a legal problem. In the following two articles, how do the authors describe problems which would not necessarily be eliminated by an equal rights amendment?
   Golick, T.: Equal rights for women: the amendment: do women need it? **Am. J. Nurs.,** 71:285–287, Feb., 1971.
   Edelstein, R. G.: Equal rights for women: perspectives. **Am. J. Nurs.,** 294–298, Feb., 1971.
6. In the March 1971 issue of the **Am. J. Nurs.,** pages 504–515, there is a section on the pediatric nurse practitioner which begins with a description of the growth of the concept and ends with a story showing pediatric nurse practitioners at work. Note how a concept gained acceptance as nurses assumed a primary and family-oriented type of care.
7. The author of the following articles described how she worked as a patient advocate:

2. Quote by courtesy of Appleton-Century-Crofts, Educational Division, Meredith Corporation.

Kosik, S. H.: Patient advocacy or fighting the system. **Am. J. Nurs.,** 72:694–698, Apr., 1972.

or

Henry, S.: Patient advocacy and community involvement. **Nurs. Outlook,** 19:246–248, Apr., 1971.
How did the author work to prevent the patient from becoming permanently dependent on her as she functioned on his behalf?

8. The January 1972 issue of **Nurs. Outlook** presents a number of articles under the heading, "Nursing at the Crossroads." It is recommended reading as a supplement to this chapter's discussion, "Roles of the Nurse."

9. Now read directives given to nurses by a hospital in 1887 for an interesting look at the roles of the nurse at that time:
The role of the nurse in 1887. **Nurs. Forum,** 10:31, No. 1, 1971.

References

1. Accountability: how, for what, and to whom? (Editorial). **Nurs. Outlook,** 20:315, May, 1972.

2. Alfano, G. J.: Healing or caretaking—which will it be? *In* **The Nursing Clinics of North America.** Philadelphia, W. B. Saunders, 6:273–280, June, 1971.

3. Andreoli, K. G.: A look at the physician's assistant. **Am. J. Nurs.,** 73:658–661, Apr., 1973.

4. Aradine, C. R., and Hansen, M. F.: Nursing in a primary health care setting. **Nurs. Outlook,** 18:45–46, Apr., 1970.

5. Avey, M.: Primary care for handicapped children. **Am. J. Nurs.,** 73:658–661, Apr., 1973.

6. Bennett, L. R.: This I believe . . . that nurses may become extinct. **Nurs. Outlook,** 18:28–32, Jan., 1970.

7. Biggs, B.: Nurse–clinician–practitioner–assistant–associate. **Am. J. Nurs.,** 71:1936–1937, Oct., 1971.

8. Brodt, D. E.: Excellence or obsolescence: the choice for nursing. **Nurs. Forum,** 9:19–26, No. 1, 1970.

9. Brown, E. L.: Nursing Reconsidered: A Study of Change: Part 1. The Professional Role in Institutional Nursing. Philadelphia, J. B. Lippincott, 1970.

10. ———: Nursing Reconsidered: A Study of Change: Part 2. The Professional Role in Community Nursing. Philadelphia, J. B. Lippincott, 1971.

11. Brunetto, E., and Birk, P.: The primary care nurse–the generalist in a structured health care team. **Am. J. Public Health,** 62:785–794, June, 1972.

12. Cleland, V.: Sex discrimination: nursing's most pervasive problem. **Am. J. Nurs.,** 71:1542–1547, Aug., 1971.

13. Donovan, H. M.: Toward a definition of nursing. **Supervisor Nurs.,** 1:12–15, Oct., 1970.

14. Edwards, J. A., et al.: The Cambridge-Council concept or two nurse practitioners make good. **Am. J. Nurs.,** 72:460–465, Mar., 1972.

15. Extending the Scope of Nursing Practice: A Report of the Secretary's Committee to Study Extended Roles for Nurses. Washington, D. C., U. S. Government Printing Office, 1971. (Reproduced, except for Preface and Appendix, in **Am. J. Nurs.,** 71:2346–2351, Dec., 1971.)

16. Fagin, C.: Accountability. **Nurs. Outlook,** 19:249–251, Apr., 1971.

17. Georgopoulos, B. S., and Sana, J. M.: Clinical nursing specialization and intershift report behavior. **Am. J. Nurs.,** 71:538–545, Mar., 1971.

18. Goshen, C. E.: Your automated future. **Am. J. Nurs.,** 72:62–67, Jan., 1972.

19. Greenidge, J., et al.: Community nurse practitioners—a partnership. **Nurs. Outlook,** 21:228–231, Apr., 1973.

20. Heide, W. S.: Nursing and women's liberation—a parallel. **Am. J. Nurs.,** 73:824–827, May, 1973.

21. King, I. M.: Toward a Theory for Nursing: General Concepts of Human Behavior. New York, John Wiley and Sons, 1971.

22. Lego, S.: Continuing education by mail. **Am. J. Nurs.,** 73:840–841, May, 1973.

23. Leininger, M. M., et al.: Primex. **Am. J. Nurs.,** 72:1274–1277, July, 1972.

24. Lesnik, M. J., and Anderson, B. E.: Nursing Practice and Law. ed. 2, pp. 261–282. Philadelphia, J. B. Lippincott, 1962.

25. Lysaught, J. P.: An Abstract For Action. National Commission for the Study of Nursing and Nursing Education. New York, McGraw-Hill, 1970. (Reproduced in summary report in **Am. J. Nurs.,** 70:279–294, Feb., 1970.)

26. Manthey, M.: Primary nursing is alive and well in the hospital. **Am. J. Nurs.,** 73:83–87, Jan., 1973.

27. Medicine and nursing in the 1970s—a position paper. **JAMA,** 213:1881–1883, Sept. 14, 1970.

28. Murphy, J. F., ed.: Theoretical Issues in Professional Nursing. New York, Appleton-Century-Crofts, 1971.

29. Nursing in the decade ahead. **Am. J. Nurs.,** 70:2116–2125, Oct., 1970.

30. Rafferty, R., and Carner, J.: Nursing consultants, inc.—a corporation. **Nurs. Outlook,** 21:232–235, Apr., 1973.

31. Rothberg, J. S.: Nurse and physician's assistant: issues and relationships. **Nurs. Outlook,** 21:154–158, Mar., 1973.

32. Schlotfeldt, R. M.: This I believe . . . nursing is health care. **Nurs. Outlook,** 20:245–246, Apr., 1972.

33. Schorr, T. M.: The passing of the it's smart-to-be-dumb era (Editorial). **Am. J. Nurs.,** 72:249, Feb., 1972.

34. Schutt, B. G.: Spot check on primary care nursing. **Am. J. Nurs.,** 72:1996–2003, Nov., 1972.

35. Silver, H. K., and McAtee, P. A.: Health care practice: an expanded profession of nursing for men and women. **Am. J. Nurs.,** 72:78–80, Jan., 1972.

36. Somers, A. R.: Health Care In Transition: Directions for the Future. Chicago, Hospital Research and Educational Trust, 1971.

37. Zschoche, D., and Brown, L. E.: Intensive care nursing: specialism, junior doctoring, or just nursing? **Am. J. Nurs.,** 69:2370–2374, Nov., 1969.

CHAPTER 2

Health-Illness and Implications for Health Practitioners

GLOSSARY

Continuum: A continuous whole.

Health: Optimum physical, mental and social efficiency, and well-being.

Health-Illness Continuum: States of health and illness that fluctuate within a continuum.

Health Maintenance Organization: A prepaid plan that utilizes health practitioners employed by the plan and that has as its purpose to furnish all health care services the patient requires, including services to promote health and prevent illness. Often referred to as HMO's.

High-level Wellness: A state of health that promotes functioning at the best level in relation to the individual's capabilities.

Morbidity: The incidence of disease or pathologic condition in a population.

Mortality: The ratio of deaths to a population.

INTRODUCTION

Well-being has become a generally accepted right of everyone, without regard of color, sex, age, economic or social status, or creed. Most democratic governments are pledged to promote the general welfare of the people in the belief that it belongs to everyone, not to just a privileged few.

Well-being for everyone is of international concern. World leaders are aware of the importance of health, and it has been a factor in many international relationships. The United States has interwoven health into parts of its foreign policy with considerable success. In fact, nations throughout the world are recognizing that the health of their citizens is one of their most valuable assets.

THE HEALTH-ILLNESS CONTINUUM

Professional and lay literature abounds with definitions of health, most of which in general are based on the premise that health represents physical fitness, emotional and mental stability, and social usefulness. A few examples will illustrate.

The U. S. President's Commission on the Health Needs of the Nation reported that *health* means ". . . optimum physical, mental, and social efficiency and well-being." The Commission went on to state that the first requisite for leading a full life is health, which makes possible maximum self-expression and self-development of man.

The World Health Organization, one of the specialized agencies of the United Nations, defined

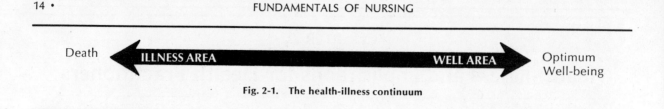

Fig. 2-1.   The health-illness continuum

health in the preamble of its constitution as "... a state of complete physical, mental and social well-being and not merely the absence of disease or infirmity." It also states that health is "... one of the fundamental rights of every human being ..."

Most persons think of themselves as being well when they are not sick. The definitions given above indicate that health is more than just the absence of illness. For example, "optimum efficiency and well-being" and a "state of well-being" are positive descriptions that indicate that health may not be necessarily constant in nature. Well-being fluctuates and at times so-called healthy people do not function or feel as well as they do at other times. A person considered healthy may have a headache and perform poorly in school that day. While he may not feel up to par, it is unlikely that he would consider himself sick. Similarly, an ill person also fluctuates in terms of his state of illness. A person so ill that he cannot care for his hygienic needs may convalesce sufficiently to meet those needs and still be ill.

A *continuum* is defined as a continuous whole. Fluctuations in health and illness can be illustrated on a health-illness continuum, as shown in Figure 2-1. There is no exact point at which health ends and illness begins. Both are relative in nature, and for each individual there is considerable range and latitude in which he may be considered ill or well.

On a continuum, health and illness may be viewed as phases related to adaptability of the human being. Adaptation is described in Chapter 3. When a person adapts and functions effectively, he can be considered in the health spectrum even though he may have, for example, a diagnosis of diabetes mellitus. Good health and well-being involve continuous adaptation. Failing adaptation eventually results in illness. When adaptation fails completely and irreversible damage to the body occurs, death results.

A physician once stated that people fall into one of four categories: those who are well and feel they are well; those who are well and feel they are ill; those who are ill and feel they are well; and those who are ill and feel they are ill. The classification may seem oversimplified, but it does illustrate the health-illness continuum from the patient's point of view. It has

been observed that a big variable in a person's state of well-being depends on the way the person sees himself. While health practitioners find the health-illness continuum helpful in viewing a person's state of health-illness, it is of limited value when the patient's opinions are ignored.

HIGH-LEVEL WELLNESS

High-level wellness may be defined as functioning at one's best. It means the potential of the individual is maximized and utilized with purpose and balance within the individual's environment.

Everyone is influenced by genetic and environmental factors. When the goal of health care services is high-level wellness, health practitioners are committed to assist persons to maximize their potential as individuals within their environment. It is no longer sufficient to consider the job well done when the "sick are made well" and discharged from a hospital. Hospital care, planned primarily for the care of the ill, is an important part of total health services, but it offers only one setting for the function of health practitioners.

A relationship between high-level wellness and the health-illness continuum can be observed. The following is an example. Consider an adult male with asthma and emphysema, two chronic conditions involving the respiratory tract. This person has permanent and irreversible damage to his respiratory tract resulting in physical limitations. He can no longer participate in sports and his exercise is limited to strolling walks; he is limited in the amount and kind of yard work he can do; and air pollution is especially troublesome to him. This man has a position demanding of his intellectual ability, but his work requires practically no physical exertion other than commuting to and from his office. His car and office are air-conditioned so that air pollution in his working environment is at a minimum. It can be observed that he is functioning at his maximum potential or at high-level wellness for him. On the health-illness continuum, he is functioning within a relatively narrow range on the continuum in terms of illness and health. It could be said that he is a sick man even when he is well. However, in this case his illnesses do not necessarily prevent him from experiencing well-being.

High-level wellness, as a national goal, involves the services of health practitioners of all types plus many other persons as well. For example, the environmental experts are crucial figures, as are engineers and architects who build the structures serving society, the social scientists who are concerned with humans and their relationships with others, and the politicians who are responsible for legislating for the promotion of well-being. Certainly, too, the consumer of health care services is an important influence. It is from him that health practitioners gain insight in relation to his problems and priorities concerning health care services. High-level wellness is everyone's concern. It requires services that are broad in scope and achieving it requires team work with representation from all groups of society.

To summarize, the consumer has rights that deserve consideration in health planning, and his uniqueness as a human being deserves respect. Health practitioners must have a sound knowledge of how the human organism functions, physically and psychologically, but their efforts to help patients attain high-level wellness may be futile if they fail to consider the environment of the individual receiving care.

COMPREHENSIVE HEALTH CARE SERVICES

Comprehensive health care services are generally considered to consist of these four services: the promotion of health, the prevention of disease, the detection and treatment of disease, and rehabilitation. To list and describe these services does not imply that any one of them is an entity unto itself; in fact, it is difficult to define exactly where one service ends and another begins since all are related in many ways. For example, in certain instances good rehabilitation practices promote health and thereby prevent disease and disability. Practices that promote health often prevent disease. Techniques that promote health and prevent disease have often improved as a result of improved methods for diagnosing and treating disease.

Nor should it be assumed that health personnel usually are concerned with only a part of these services. Many practitioners contribute to all areas of health care services. For example, each service is of major concern to nurses, and the various ways in which nurses contribute to them are discussed throughout this text.

Comprehensive health care services are sometimes further described as being primarily personal or environmental in nature. For example, a neighborhood can be thought of as a patient. The well-being of the neighborhood can be assessed and it can be offered comprehensive health services containing the same four components described above. While personal and environmental health services cannot be separated in practice, some type of distinction can be made in describing them, as the following discussion illustrates.

Promotion of Health

Science has made great progress in describing good health. The promotion of health concerns itself with advancing and encouraging individuals toward that end.

It has become common knowledge that promoting good health includes the support and development of mental as well as physical health programs. Psychologists and psychiatrists, for example, have studied individual responses to stress and strain in considerable detail. From such studies, programs that help to cope with the demands of everyday living are enabling more persons to enjoy better mental and social well-being. The numerous counseling programs are examples of a service that promotes good mental health.

An example of promotion in the area of physical health may be cited from the field of nutrition. Basic food requirements of the body have been well-established. Animal experimentation as well as scientific observation of the dietary customs of humans have illustrated the effects of both poor and good eating habits. Through intensive educational programs, nutritionists and their allied co-workers have contributed immeasurably to health promotion by helping people learn how to select proper foods.

The development of park systems throughout our country is an example of an environmental program that promotes the health of our citizens. Recreation and activity are recognized as important health factors. The regulations concerning the use of parks are designed to keep them "healthy" for persons wishing to use them.

Prevention of Disease

Despite health promotion efforts, disease still attacks man, and science is constantly at work to discover and utilize measures that will aid in illness prevention. In many instances, fortunately, the challenges of disease prevention have been well met. Certain communicable diseases that were prevalent in this country as recently as a few decades ago are now almost nonexistent, due primarily to a nationwide development of immunization programs. Examples are smallpox, diphtheria, and poliomyelitis. Certain other diseases, such as typhoid fever, have been reduced to a minimum by means of sanitation measures.

At least three trends are apparent today in preventive medicine. One is an attempt to identify early signs of chronic diseases. Preventive measures can then help to decrease the ravages of disability and physical deterioration long before they occur. For example, many of the deteriorating effects of asthma and emphysema can be decreased by early detection and medical regimens that diminish progression of these illnesses.

A second trend is increased interest in health problems of the elderly in our population. A great deal of research has been done to investigate the aging process. Some of the common occurrences in the elderly, such as dimming vision and hearing, are now being considered as normal results of aging, rather than as abnormalities or illnesses per se. Also, practitioners in preventive medicine have become increasingly interested in preparing people for those years when it may be necessary to adapt to a new way of life with different but still challenging interests.

A third trend is a marked increase in concern for environmental factors that may cause illness. The interest in pollution and its effects on health are front-page news almost daily. Legislating and lobbying to enact measures to curtail pollution are increasing throughout the country. The promotion of safe working conditions is another example of concern for environmental factors affecting the health of employees. Vacations and rest periods are recognized as important factors in industrial programs to help prevent bodily insult from unrelieved stress and strain.

Detection and Treatment of Disease

The detection and treatment of disease remain essential responsibilities of health practitioners. Traditionally the nurse's role has been one of caring for the ill, and that responsibility remains today. Through her observations and skills in carrying out and supervising nursing care, much of it being very complicated in nature, the nurse plays a critical role in the detection and treatment of disease. Also, the nurse often assists in research programs, and through her contributions it has been possible in many instances to move forward more rapidly in disease detection and treatment.

Disease detection and treatment are also noted by persons who have studied the environment of our society. For instance, a neighborhood, like an individual, may be considered to be sick. Poor housing may be one factor contributing to the illness of a neighborhood. Housing facilities that provide for privacy as well as for family sociability and that are hygienic can lead to a cure for conditions that take their toll in personal illness.

Rehabilitation

Although rehabilitation has been concerned primarily with restoring a disabled person to his best possible health, a much broader concept is accepted today: that rehabilitation is an important aspect of all health care. It is concerned with both emotional and physical disability. It encompasses all ages and occupational groups. It is not limited to that period of time when, for example, a patient may be helped with muscle reeducation in order that he may learn new skills that enable him to regain economic and social usefulness.

Rehabilitation begins with the earliest contact with any person receiving health care. It includes all elements of care and continues throughout the period of illness and thereafter until the person is restored to high-level wellness.

In previous times it was believed that nurses and other health practitioners should provide complete personal care for the patient, even though his physical condition did not necessarily warrant such care. Caring will always be important, but the best care is that which guides the patient toward independence. Rehabilitation is in progress when the patient is taught or assisted to help himself so that he loses neither the desire for self-sufficiency nor the abilities required in day-to-day living. Participation in a program of self-help provides the physical and mental stimulation that contributes to high-level wellness. Self-care also improves patient morale and dignity. Most patients experience great satisfaction and a sense of personal worth as they gradually regain their ability to care for themselves and to make whatever adjustments in living that illnesses or disabilities necessitate.

An environment can also be rehabilitated and many examples could be cited. For example, the present efforts to clean up dirty water in "dead" lakes and streams and then to restock them with plant and animal life characteristic of the natural environment are measures to rehabilitate those lakes and streams for the general good of society.

CONTINUITY OF CARE

Continuity of care, defined in Chapter 1, is implemented by the smooth transfer and follow-up among the comprehensive health care services and among health practitioners and health facilities. It means that any type of care—maintenance, preventive, curative, or rehabilitative—will be available to everyone as indicated. In far too many instances, persons may be dropped from the rosters of health practitioners or health facilities when an immediate problem has been solved. There has been a decided lack of follow-up to observe results of care given and to offer other types of needed care, either related or unrelated to the problem that initially brought the person to a health practitioner. Implicit in a philosophy of comprehensive health care for everyone is the concept of continuity in those services.

The following example will illustrate. A teacher referred a child to the school nurse because the child was having a reading problem. The school nurse examined the child and noted poor focusing of eyes with strabismus (cross-eyes). She referred the child to an eye clinic for evaluation. Surgery was recommended and the child was hospitalized for the surgical procedure. The hospital referred the child to a community health agency. A community health nurse visited the child at home, supervised his home care, and recommended his return to school at the appropriate time. Upon return to school, the nurse followed the child's progress to determine whether the surgical procedure had helped solve the reading problem. Many more people may well be involved in any one situation, but the example illustrates the continuity of the child's care. A study situation at the end of this chapter refers to an article that describes very sad results of lack of continuity of care in the case of a patient with gunshot wounds.

The example of the child who had corrective eye surgery illustrates also the importance of health team personnel working together. A health team may consist of any number of people with varying skills and educational preparation, but it needs coordination to achieve high quality care with communications carefully planned among team members. Community health facilities also need to plan together so that unnecessary duplication and gaps in services can be minimized.

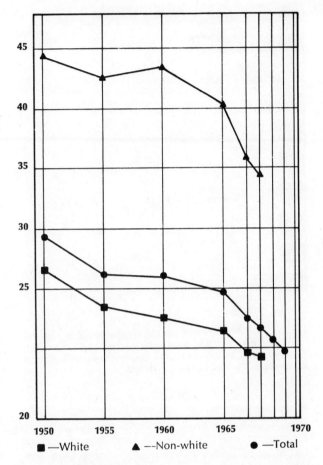

Fig. 2-2. Infant mortality rates for white, non-white and total deaths per 1,000 live births. (Data from Statistical Abstract of the U.S., 1972. U.S. Department of Commerce, Bureau of the Census.)

HEALTH-ILLNESS PROBLEMS: SOLVED AND UNSOLVED

Available statistics reflect, at least in an indirect manner, the status of health in the nation and offer guidance in health program planning.

A *mortality* rate describes the ratio of deaths to a population. The infant mortality rates reflect accomplishments, as Figure 2-2 illustrates. Yet, many other countries report even lower infant mortality rates than does the United States. While the United States ranked sixth among 15 countries with which it was compared in 1950, it ranked fifteenth in 1969. The U. S. rate had not increased during that period, as Figure 2-2 shows; rather, the rate for other countries

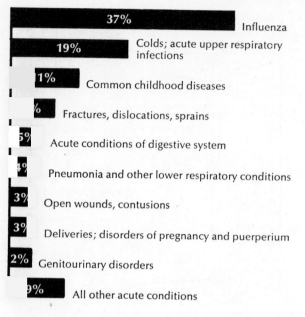

37%	Influenza
19%	Colds; acute upper respiratory infections
1%	Common childhood diseases
%	Fractures, dislocations, sprains
5%	Acute conditions of digestive system
4%	Pneumonia and other lower respiratory conditions
3%	Open wounds, contusions
3%	Deliveries; disorders of pregnancy and puerperium
2%	Genitourinary disorders
9%	All other acute conditions

Fig. 2-3. Common conditions causing bed disability among acute conditions. (Data from Facts of Life and Death. U.S. Department of Health, Education, and Welfare, revised, 1970. Percentages rounded to nearest whole.)

municable diseases. Early detection programs have been important in the control of such diseases as tuberculosis. Modern drugs and surgical procedures have added to life expectancy in many instances. Still, despite U. S. world leadership in terms of success in many areas, life expectancy in 1972 ranked twenty-fourth for men and ninth for women in the world. In Sweden, the world's leader, male life expectancy was approximately 5 years more than in the United States; life expectancy for the American woman, although greater than the American male, also lagged well behind the Swedish rate. Another statistic revealing a need for improvement is that nonwhite Americans have a life expectancy 7 to 8 years shorter than that for white Americans.

Authorities state that a primary cause for the low rank of the United States in life expectancy is due to failure to deliver health services adequately. Also, many segments of society, particularly the poor population groups, have not had adequate nutrition. Other experts point out that violent deaths in the United States, such as auto accidents, suicides, and

decreased more rapidly and eventually surpassed the United States. However, the ranking still poses interesting questions to health practitioners seeking solutions to infant mortality. Also, note that nonwhite infants died at a rate nearly double that for white infants in America, as late as 1968 when the last comparable figures were available.

A *morbidity* rate describes the incidence of disease or pathological condition in a population. Figures 2-3 and 2-4 illustrate common acute and chronic conditions resulting in limitation of activity. Much progress has been made in preventing many acute illnesses and in rehabilitating persons with chronic conditions more effectively, but as these two figures illustrate, there is much more to be done.

Figure 2-5 illustrates life expectancy in the United States. Most gains in life expectancy were made in the first half of this century when cures or methods of control for many of the greatest killers of youth and middle age were found. Safe water and food supplies have practically eliminated in some areas, and greatly reduced in others, such diseases as typhoid fever, vitamin deficiencies, and certain infant diarrheas. Vaccinations and immunizations and the use of antibiotics have served to control most com-

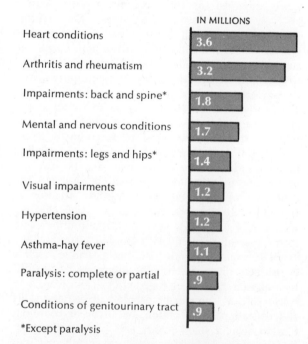

	IN MILLIONS
Heart conditions	3.6
Arthritis and rheumatism	3.2
Impairments: back and spine*	1.8
Mental and nervous conditions	1.7
Impairments: legs and hips*	1.4
Visual impairments	1.2
Hypertension	1.2
Asthma-hay fever	1.1
Paralysis: complete or partial	.9
Conditions of genitourinary tract	.9

*Except paralysis

Fig. 2-4. Ten most common chronic conditions causing limitations. (Data from Facts of Life and Death. U.S. Department of Health, Education and Welfare, revised, 1970. Rounded to nearest one-tenth of a million.)

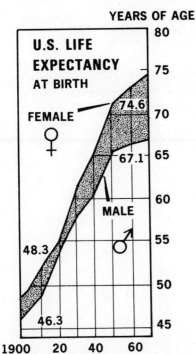

YEARS OF AGE

U.S. LIFE EXPECTANCY AT BIRTH

FEMALE ♀

74.6

67.1

MALE ♂

48.3

46.3

80
75
70
65
60
55
50
45

1900   20   40   60

Fig. 2-5. U. S. life expectancy at birth. (Reprinted by permission of TIME, The Weekly Newsmagazine. Copyright Time Inc.)

homicides, are another reason for a lower life expectancy than in many other countries.

While many diseases have been checked, many still remain unconquered. Figure 2-6 illustrates the leading causes of death and points up clearly that chronic diseases in particular require concerted attention if greater longevity is to be achieved.

The decrease in untimely deaths and the increase in life expectancy have resulted in more elders in the U. S. population, both numerically and in proportion to the rest of the population. Figure 2-7 illustrates the percentage of population in various age groups in 1940 and in 1968. Note the increase in percentage of people over 65 years of age. Only about 4 percent of the population was over 65 years of age in 1900. In 1965, there were about eight million persons over age 65. This figure is expected to reach 21 million by 1975, 25 million by 1980, and 30 million by the turn of the century. Although chronic diseases affect all age groups, invalidism and dependency due to chronic illness are particularly prevalent in the older age groups, and the public is becoming increasingly active in supporting programs leading to their solution.

The population shift from rural to urban areas

continues today, although the most marked shift occurred shortly after World War II. The social importance of this shift has sparked much interest and underlies the health needs of large sectors of people. Overcrowding, poor housing, and often inability to find work are a few examples of conditions that often exist in crowded urban areas and that result in poor health. Ironically, many of the poor, urban dwellers live almost next door to fine medical centers in large cities and yet, do not receive even minimal health care because of inability to pay for it.

The number of poor persons in our population remains distressingly high despite a continued rise in family income. As can be expected, these persons characteristically have higher morbidity and mortality rates than the more affluent. Most of our poverty-stricken population live in rural areas, but many also live in remote sections where they have been largely untouched by the rich medical resources of this country.

One disorder that, despite much public attention, still presents a particularly acute health problem is mental illness. More than one-half of hospital beds in the United States are for the mentally ill, and many more people who are not hospitalized or attending clinics are believed in need of care. There have been concerted efforts in recent years to establish programs that will promote mental health and prevent mental diseases, but the magnitude of the problem of mental illness remains largely unchanged.

Knowledge of venereal disease control and treatment is well-developed. Yet, at present, venereal diseases have reached epidemic proportions in many places in the United States. For example, the incidence of gonorrhea in the United States in 1972 was the highest recorded since the U. S. Public Health Service began keeping venereal disease statistics in 1919. The highest ranking nation (in the world) in the degree of alcoholism is the United States. Death rates from cirrhosis of the liver, a common killer of the alcoholic, have slowly increased over the past five years for both men and women across the country. As Figure 2-6 illustrates, liver diseases are now among the leading ten causes of death. Death caused by homicide is also on the rise. The rate of murder was 8.8 per 1,000 population in 1965; in 1970, the rate had increased to 13.6 per 1,000 population. As yet there is no significant abatement of drug abuse. Newly reported drug addicts numbered about 6,000 in 1965; in 1969, 14,660 were reported and known addicts increased to a total of 68,000 by December 1969. Many authorities feel

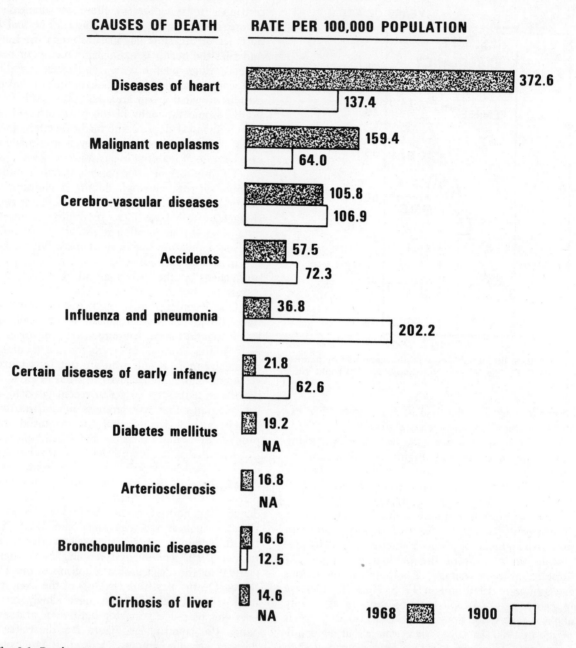

CAUSES OF DEATH   RATE PER 100,000 POPULATION

Cause of Death	1968	1900
Diseases of heart	372.6	137.4
Malignant neoplasms	159.4	64.0
Cerebro-vascular diseases	105.8	106.9
Accidents	57.5	72.3
Influenza and pneumonia	36.8	202.2
Certain diseases of early infancy	21.8	62.6
Diabetes mellitus	19.2	NA
Arteriosclerosis	16.8	NA
Bronchopulmonic diseases	16.6	12.5
Cirrhosis of liver	14.6	NA

Fig. 2-6. Death rate per 100,000 for 10 leading causes of death in 1968 and death rate for these same causes in 1900. (Data from Statistical Abstract of the U. S., 1972. U. S. Department of Commerce, Bureau of the Census.)

that pollution overshadows most other factors as a threat to health. While efforts to reduce pollution of all types are underway, much remains to be done. Suicide rates have increased in the United States, especially among the young where it ranks third in the cause of death in the 15- to 19-year-old group. Automobile fatalities are the leading cause of death for those under 25 years of age and third for those between the ages of 25 and 44. Upper respiratory infections and influenza-type illnesses have been described and studied for years, but as yet no effective methods of prevention and cure have been found. They are the most frequent causes of absence from work and school today.

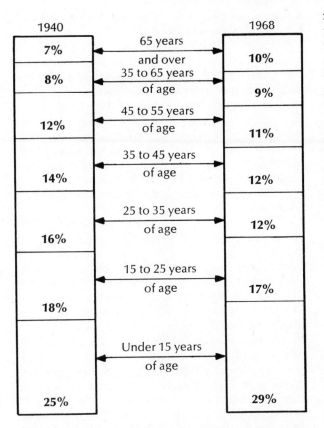

1940		1968
7%	65 years and over	10%
8%	35 to 65 years of age	9%
12%	45 to 55 years of age	11%
14%	35 to 45 years of age	12%
16%	25 to 35 years of age	12%
18%	15 to 25 years of age	17%
25%	Under 15 years of age	29%

Fig. 2-7. Percentage of population in age groups—1940 and 1968. (Data from Facts of Life and Death. U. S. Department of Health, Education, and Welfare, revised, 1970. Rounded to nearest percent.)

Retirement is a common goal among the U. S. population and is rapidly becoming a reality for many people and at earlier ages than previously. Yet, studies have illustrated that people who work after the usual retirement age tend to live longer than retirees. A possible reason is that motivated people tend to take better care of themselves than those who seem to have little reason for doing so.

The American way of life contributes little to longevity. Overeating is one factor in causes of high blood pressure and cerebral vascular accidents (strokes). Oversmoking contributes to many respiratory ailments; yet, smoking is reportedly still on the increase in this country. The stresses and strains typical of the demanding way of life of Americans underlie many heart ailments.

This has been a brief summary of solved and unsolved problems in relation to health-illness. Great credit is deserved for accomplishments, but there is

no time for relaxation of effort. Paradoxically, the toll of disease responsible for much illness and death in the United States could be reduced if we but used available skills and knowledge. What good is a service if the person needing it is unaware of its existence? Or is unable to pay for services he needs? Or refuses for one reason or another to observe health practices known to prevent certain illnesses? Or cannot have services he needs for lack of health personnel? Health problems are intertwined with social, psychologic, environmental, and economic issues. Hence, their solutions require the efforts from our entire population. But health practitioners are looked to for a leadership role in identifying problems and in seeking the support of the general population to help solve them.

THE CONSUMER SPEAKS

Until recently, the consumer of health care services has been largely ignored, although he was known to have dissatisfactions and unmet needs. He was excluded from research and planning for health care services and was offered primarily what health personnel thought he needed and wanted. But now his voice is being heard throughout the country.

The consumer may be likened to a sleeping giant who has started to awaken. Regarding health matters, he is no longer satisfied to be told what he needs and wants. He is beginning to exert what he considers to be his right to high quality health care and is demanding that he receive it at a price he can afford. Increasingly, legislators at state and federal levels are concerning themselves with finding ways to meet consumer demands and with the votes such efforts command. Labor unions have reflected consumer demands for improved health in their contracts, and these demands are being pressed for by nonunion workers as well. The news media are alert to the consumer and have expressed his voice in ever greater degrees. Very often, health practitioners have come under heavy fire by the consumer. More emphasis is now being placed on consumer consideration and from his viewpoint rather than from the sole viewpoint of the health practitioners.

The Citizens Board of Inquiry into Health Services for Americans, organized in 1969, had as its purpose to study America's health services from the viewpoint of the consumer. The Committee found the consumer to be vocal and frank. It summarized the voice of the consumer in its report, entitled *Heal Yourself*, as follows:

• "Most Americans do not have adequate health care; they have crisis care. They obtain health services only when sickness or injury forces them to muster the money and risk the obstacles and humiliations.

• Once a decision is made to seek care, many Americans have no choice of where or from whom to seek it, and those with a choice usually have available no reasonable basis for decision.

• Having decided where to go for care, the patient must still overcome a variety of obstacles before he receives services.

• On arriving at a hospital or other health care facility, the patient may discover that he must "buy a ticket" (receipt for payment) before receiving any services.

• The persistent patient who overcomes the barriers to care may find himself treated with indignity and insensitivity.

• Sometimes the line between insensitivity and poor quality care is blurred. A patient's persistent attempts to get more careful attention may have negligible or negative results.

• The patient often discovers that the medical services he has received are more expensive than he had expected, and that the insurance for which he has paid so dearly affords him only minimal coverage.

• Many of the same barriers that deterred the patient from seeking care in the first place interfere with his following through on the medical advice and recommendations he receives.

• With all the anger and the difficulties, people will still do what they feel they must to get needed health care. While there is great frustration, sometimes even desperation, there is little apathy."

The consumer has learned what constitutes quality care from many sources—education, the news media, travel, and so on. He has gained confidence to ask questions concerning the services he is receiving. He is aware of his power at the polls and his right to quality care at a price he can afford. He may well be the greatest spur to better health care that this country has ever experienced.

EFFORTS TO MEET CONSUMER DEMANDS

While efforts to respond to consumer demands are more evident today, the movement had its beginnings several decades ago. (In the 1930s, for example, the Committee on Cost of Medical Care had a wide circulation of its report entitled *Medical Care For The American People*.)

There is increased willingness to *listen* to the consumer. Work of the Citizens Board of Inquiry has been cited. Two recent White House Conferences, referred to in a study situation at the end of this chapter, had as part of their purposes to learn from consumers what they feel they need and want. The 1971 White House Conference on Youth looked to the 14- to 24-year-olds for ideas to the solution of urgent problems, many of which had health-illness implications. Local committees of every type for consumer representation are described daily in the news.

The roles of various health practitioners have come under close scrutiny within recent years. For example, better utilization of health personnel has been a subject of much study. In nursing, many tasks once performed by nurses are now being assumed by non-nurses in order to free the nurse for patient care. When the nurse was freed of what are now considered non-nursing tasks, she began assuming a role that is dramatically different from the nurse of yesteryear, as Chapter 1 describes.

Educational institutions have adopted new programs with many innovative curricula in their attempts to prepare more personnel, more adequately and in as short a time as is educationally feasible. In nursing, educational programs are gradually moving into the mainstream of general education with programs of many varieties and lengths to prepare nurses for the myriad of positions open to them in the field of health care. Continuing education programs are rapidly appearing in an effort to keep nurses on-the-job, interested and up-to-date on new knowledge in the health field.

Recruitment of persons to health service careers is national in scope. Special efforts are being exerted to attract students regardless of sex, age, ethnic origin, or social or economic status. This is especially true in nursing, with the result that statistics show an ever-increasing number of older persons, men, and nonwhite personnel selecting nursing as their occupational choice.

Demands for high quality care have resulted in statements on qualifications for practice and in improved methods of licensure for personnel and accreditation for educational and service institutions. Almost all educational programs for health practitioners are placing more emphasis than previously on the study of the behavioral sciences as the consumer demands services from personnel who will treat him with dignity, respect, sensitivity, and intelligence.

New ways of administering and organizing the delivery of health services are constantly being tried, all in an effort to provide better care for more people. Intensive care units, constant care units, day care centers, clinics, health centers, mobile health stations, convalescent facilities, cardiac and respiratory emergency services, and air ambulance services are just a few examples. Regional planning is on the increase to eliminate duplication and gaps in services. In some areas, satellite clinics and hospitals are organized around a medical center in an effort to serve more people more effectively.

The goal of high quality care for everyone may still be a dream, but efforts to reach it are numerous and commendable. Still, much has to be done and this remains one of the biggest challenges facing health practitioners today.

THE FINANCING AND DELIVERY OF HEALTH CARE SERVICES

In addition to efforts to increase the number and efficiency of health practitioners and of health facilities, two highly related factors have attracted increasing attention in recent years: the financing and the delivery of health care services. The poor cannot afford the care they need; even with increased affluence, those persons not considered at poverty levels feel that health care is rapidly becoming more elusive, more expensive, and out of their financial reach. Many people may feel they could afford at least maintenance care, but paying for crisis care is another matter. Also, health needs will continue to be poorly met if services are not available or accessible to the consumer, cost notwithstanding.

Health care is big business in the United States. It was the third largest industry in the nation in 1971 and it is predicted to be the largest by mid to late 1970s. Although statistics vary, it appears that approximately 10 to 15 billion dollars were spent in 1950 on health care. This expenditure rose to approximately 60 billion dollars in 1969, and it is estimated at as much as 70 billion dollars in 1970 and 200 billion dollars in 1980. Not only is the consumer buying more health care but the cost of services has risen sharply and at a larger rate than the general increase in prices of other-than-health-care items. In 1968, it was reported that the cost of living rose 20 percent between 1959 and 1968 while medical costs rose 45 percent and hospital costs rose 122 percent.

The traditional way of delivering health care services has been for the patient to seek out a health practitioner of his choice and then go to him for service. The practitioner selects a health facility for his patient when he feels that this is needed. The traditional method of financing has been for the patient to pay for whatever services he receives from the practitioner, a fee-for-service basis.

As pointed out, the consumer has often found the traditional way of delivering and financing health care services to be unsatisfactory. And, it is believed this dissatisfaction has played an important part in the consumer's failure to seek out health promotion and disease prevention services. The result has been health care that is primarily illness- and crisis-oriented despite campaigns to teach citizens the importance of health promotion and disease prevention.

There are numerous ways to finance and to deliver health care services. The following classifications, although based on financing, will deal with both current financing and delivery.

Donations and Bequests

Money contributed by donations and bequests (disposition of money through a will) has done much to support research, for example, the study of cancer, heart diseases, muscular dystrophy, respiratory diseases, and others. Also, money from these sources is used to support certain health facility construction and to aid in establishing innovative programs designed to finance and deliver health services in other than traditional ways.

Memorial health facilities are often largely supported through bequests and donations. Telethons and door-to-door solicitation by volunteers have raised millions of dollars to help conquer specific illnesses of various kinds. The March of Dimes is given credit for most of the research money that was used to conquer poliomyelitis. The United Fund contributes donated money to many health programs. The Rockefeller Foundation is an example of a family-endowed fund that has supported programs designed to finance and deliver health services in other than the traditional manner.

The Shriner's Hospitals for Children receive support from donations and bequests. However, a relatively small proportion of donations and bequests pay for direct health care of the nature offered by these hospitals.

Except for the support of innovative programs, donations and bequests have not changed the delivery of health care services appreciably from traditional methods.

Government Revenues

The United States supports a sizeable amount of health care with federal, state, and local tax revenues. In general, the revenues support the following types of programs:

• Programs designed to care for certain groups, such as veterans, the elderly, American Indians, merchant seamen, and the indigent.

• Programs designed to care for persons with certain illnesses, such as mental illnesses, tuberculosis, and venereal diseases.

• Public health programs designed to promote environmental and personal disease prevention.

• Specialized and often innovative programs, such as the development of health centers with money from the Office of Economic Opportunity.

Governmental revenues have also played an important role in supporting health related research, the education of health practitioners, and the construction of health facilities. The National Institutes of Health are research-oriented facilities that include some direct patient care in their research. The Hill-Burton Act supported a great deal of health facility construction. Government grants of various types have lent support to educational programs as well as to the preparation of health practitioners through loans and scholarships.

Personal Payment

The traditional method of paying for services rendered is personal payment. It is sometimes also referred to as *individual payment*. It is used for the payment of most ambulatory medical and dental care and for medications as well as for the use of health facilities such as hospitals to the extent that insurance does not cover facility use. Usually, services are rendered by solo practitioners (physicians, nurses, dentists, osteopaths, and others) although services may be offered through a group of practitioners working together on the same fee-for-service basis. As the cost of services rises, the inability to finance health care for everyone by this method is readily apparent.

The delivery of services usually is in the traditional manner.

Voluntary Insurance

Voluntary health insurance plans, or indemnity insurance, constitute a sizeable source of health care financing in the United States. About 85 percent of Americans under 65 years of age have at least some sort of insurance. About 80 percent are covered to some degree for surgical procedures. About 50 percent have some coverage for related services such as x-ray and laboratory services.

The cost of indemnity insurance varies and depends on such factors as age of the person, his health history, the amount and kind of coverage desired, deductible clauses, and so on. The costs are generally higher when purchased by individuals than by groups, the latter being a common purchasing method for employees of a particular company. Employers often contribute to the cost of health insurance. Blue Cross and Blue Shield have underwritten a great deal of group insurance although other private insurance companies are increasingly selling more group insurance.

Financing health care with voluntary insurance has not changed the traditional way of delivering health services. The insurance carrier pays the bills on a fee-for-service basis and to the extent contracted for by the patient.

Various prepaid plans provide many services by a group of health practitioners who are employed by the plan and use health facilities whose services are contracted for by the plan. The idea of these plans first originated in this country at the turn of the century in the mining and railroad industries and were known as contract practice. Two common plans that often serve as models for others today are the Kaiser-Permanente Medical Care Program in California and the Greater New York Plan in the east, often referred to as HIP, for Health Insurance Plan.

Persons eligible for prepaid group plans pay for services of both health practitioners and health facilities. Physician participants characteristically represent the common medical specialities and are employed and paid a salary by the plan in return for administering any service the membership requires. In plans in which a particular specialist may not be on the staff, the patients are referred to a nonparticipating specialist as indicated and the plan then generally pays for this service.

Prepaid group plans deliver and finance health care services differently from traditional methods. Persons enrolled are cared for by the participating health practitioners and use those health facilities contracted for use by the plan. These plans promise available personnel to their membership around the clock everyday and provide payment of services required when members are away from home as well.

Prepaid group plans sometimes are referred to as health care corporations or as *health maintenance organizations* (HMO's). By whatever name, their stated purpose is to furnish health care services that are paid for in advance on an insurancelike basis by either the member or his employer or both. The plans place emphasis on preventive care and health maintenance and offer benefits that include office

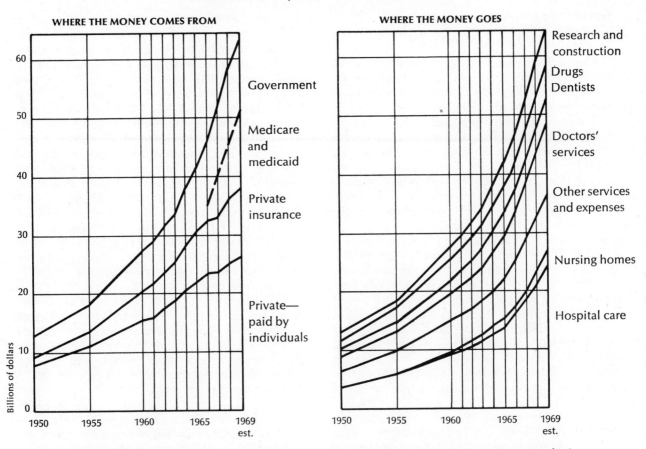

Fig. 2-8. Health care financing: sources and use of money. (Tom Cardamone Associates for Fortune Magazine.)

calls, routine health examinations, home care, prescription drugs, and others. Those that have been in existence long enough to accumulate statistics have demonstrated fewer hospital admissions and less recourse to the use of expensive facilities than, for example, persons with indemnity insurance in which admission to a hospital may be the only way to receive benefits. It has been reported that there is anywhere from 25 to 40 percent lower hospital utilization by health maintenance organization members than by people on typical indemnity insurance plans. In order to discourage needless and unreasonable requests for services, some plans charge a minimal fee for certain services; for example, two dollars for each office call requiring the services of a physician.

Social Insurance

Social insurance for the aged has been in effect since the mid 1960s through Medicare and Medicaid. Medicare provides protection for the cost of hospital and related care and covers most persons over 65 years of age. It is financed through Old Age,

Survivors and Disability Insurance (OASDI or Social Security). For those persons not covered by Social Security or by Railroad Retirement Insurance programs, the cost is met from general tax revenues.

Medicaid provides for payment of physicians' bills and certain other medical and health services after specified deductibles are paid by the patient. Participation in Medicaid is voluntary. Monthly premiums are split equally between the participant and the government which pays its share from general tax revenues. (Medicaid is also available to certain persons under 65 in some states.)

Although these programs have had problems and have not always met their original goals, they have provided improved health care with relative freedom from financial worry for a large sector of our population. The delivery of health services was not changed as a result of this social insurance legislation. The insurance carrier, in this case, the government, pays for services rendered.

Figure 2-8 summarizes the financing of health care in the United States.

LEGISLATION UNDER CONSIDERATION

Demands for changes in the delivery and financing of health care service in this country are becoming increasingly persistent. Proposed plans range from conservative to revolutionary.

Medicredit has been proposed by the American Medical Association. The plan provides for income tax credits to defray health insurance premiums with credits covering 100 percent of costs for the poor and tapering to zero for persons in high income levels.

There has been considerable interest in extending coverage similar to that now received by the elderly through Medicare and Medicaid to all citizens of the United States through legislation that would enact national health insurance. A study situation at the end of this chapter refers readers to several references on the subject. Various bills have been proposed and proponents are convinced that it is legislation necessary to provide health care services for everyone. Descriptions of these bills, as well as other proposed legislation relating to health services, are described regularly in the NEWS Section of the *American Journal of Nursing*. The House of Delegates of the American Nurses Association has called for aggressive action on national health insurance. Many argue that present bills lack plans to change the delivery of health services which they feel is necessary in order to meet the total health care needs of this country.

In 1972, a representative of the American Nurses' Association testified in Washington on health maintenance organizations and stated that what appeared to be needed ". . . is the development of integrated systems to deliver quality comprehensive health care services which are accessible and acceptable to people of all income levels and in all geographic areas of the country. The health maintenance organization is one approach for structuring delivery of comprehensive health care into such an organized system. The legislation you (the subcommittee on public health and environment) are considering would encourage this development, and we (American Nurses' Association) support its intent." (2:1200)

The final answer on how to deliver and finance quality care to everyone is still elusive. But the interest and the strong demand for change are apparent everywhere. Final solutions may well come with some sort of compromise program involving increased voluntary as well as increased government support and participation.

CONCLUSION

Comprehensive health care services with facilities and personnel to provide them for everyone is of national concern. The need for them has often been described as having reached crisis proportions. Statistics indicate that while scientific knowledge continues to grow, its incorporation into health care practices still leave much to be desired. This is particularly true in the areas of health maintenance, of the promotion of high-level wellness, of making sophisticated modern care techniques available to more people, and of reaching all persons in our population.

High-quality care is available, but few citizens are receiving it. The problem is two-sided at least. Efficient and effective methods to deliver comprehensive health care to all on a large scale have not been found. Nor has a satisfactory method of financing such care been devised.

The financing of health care services is of paramount concern and the present trend is toward more collectivization of health care financing than is presently practiced. Government support in the financing of health care services for all citizens seems to be an increasingly likely prospect, although its exact nature is still unclear at this time.

The consumer and his demands can no longer be ignored. Health practitioners who fail to listen are not meeting their obligation of providing services for all. Mankind appears to have a need in societal control and is intolerant of impediments that stand in his way. Consumers may be frustrated, but they are no longer apathetic.

Study Situations

1. In the following article, read the section entitled "The Ideal State of Health," on page 27:

   Bircher, A. U.: Mankind in crisis: an application of clinical process to population–environmental issues. **Nurs. Forum,** 11:10–33, No. 1, 1972.

   How does the author's description of health compare with the descriptions of health, the health-illness continuum and high-level wellness in this chapter?

2. Response to consumer demands is reflected in two White House conferences called by President Nixon: the White House Conference on Food, Nutrition, and Health, which met in late 1969, and the 1971 White House Conference on Aging. The following references summarize the conferences' work:

   Callahan, C. L.: A special report on . . . the White

House Conference on food, nutrition, and health. **Nurs. Outlook,** 18:58–60, Jan., 1970.

Callahan, C. L.: The 1971 White House Conference on aging. **Nurs. Outlook,** 19:96–99, Feb., 1972.

What conclusions would you draw concerning the results of these two conferences? Do you believe consumer demands were fairly considered? How do you think conference findings may influence the nursing care you give?

3. The editorial and the first five articles in **Nurs. Outlook,** 19:23–32, January, 1971, were devoted to the subject of national health insurance. The following reference also discussed the subject:

Somers, A. R.: Health Care in Transition: Directions for the Future. pp. 159–165. Chicago, Hospital Research and Educational Trust, 1971.

Discuss the advantages and disadvantages, as you see them, after reading these references on national health insurance. Now read the resolution on national health insurance passed by the House of Delegates of the American Nurses Association in 1970:

Resolution on national health insurance. **Am. J. Nurs.,** 70:1271, June, 1970.

If you had been a member of the House of Delegates, how would you have voted on the resolution on national health insurance?

4. The following article illustrates the sad results when care was given without plans for continuity:

Keller, N. S.: Care without coordination: a true story. **Nurs. Forum,** 6:280–323, No. 3, 1967.

Consider the provocative questions the author poses on page 323: "Do the health professions exist to help Carrie Jones? Or must Carrie Jones continue to exist to justify the existence of so many varied, independent health workers?"

5. In 1972, the Census Bureau released a social and economic portrait of the U.S. population. Here are some of the findings, as reported in the **Arizona Republic,** October 15, 1972:

• In 1970, 13.3 percent (about 27 million) of Americans had incomes below the government's poverty line.

• About 1.8 million Americans have never attended any school.

• About one-sixth of all children were living with only one or neither of their parents.

• About 40 percent of all women are in the labor force in this country.

• About 1 million of the 20.1 million elderly people in this country were in homes for the aged and one-fourth of all elderly people were living in what the federal government concedes as poverty.

• One-sixth of the population in 1970 was either foreign-born or born of foreign or mixed parentage.

Describe implications you find in these data that influence nursing and that influence health care in this country.

References

The statistical data used in Chapter 2 were taken from entries given in the references that follow. Most were taken from those entries numbered 1, 10, 11, and 33.

1. Americans can—and should—live longer. **Time,** 100:64–65, July 10, 1972.

2. ANA supports HMO's but asks safeguards against domination by any one group. **Am. J. Nurs.,** 72:1199–1201, July, 1972.

3. Bates, B.: Nursing in a health maintenance organization—report on the Harvard community health plan. **Am. J. Public Health,** 62:991–994, July, 1972.

4. Bill of rights for patients. **Nurs. Outlook,** 21:82, Feb., 1973.

5. Chase, H. C.: The position of the United States in international comparisons of health status. **Am. J. Public Health,** 62:581–589, Apr., 1972.

6. Cohen, W. J.: What makes an effective national health program? **Am. J. Nurs.,** 72:1828–1830, Oct., 1972.

7. Collen, F. B., et al.: Kaiser-Permanente experiment in ambulatory care. **Am. J. Nurs.,** 71:1371–1374, July, 1971.

8. Cordtz, D.: Change begins in the doctor's office. **Fortune,** 81:84–89, 130; 132; 134; Jan., 1970.

9. Dunn, H. L.: What high-level wellness means. pp. 1–7. *In* High-Level Wellness. Arlington, Va., Beatty, 1971.

10. Facts of Life and Death. Rockville, Md., U. S. Department of Health, Education, and Welfare, Public Health Service, National Center for Health Statistics, 1970.

11. Faltermayer, E. K.: Better care at less cost without miracles. **Fortune,** 81:80–83, 126; 127; 128; 130; Jan., 1970.

12. Greenberg, S. M., and Galton, R.: Nurses are key in HIP experiment to cut health care costs. **Am. J. Nurs.,** 72:272–276, Feb., 1972.

13. Heal Yourself. Report of the Citizens Board of Inquiry Into Health Services For Americans.

14. Kisch, A. I.: Planning for a sensible health care system. **Nurs. Outlook,** 20:640–642, Oct., 1972.

15. Kramer, M.: The consumer's influence on health care. **Nurs. Outlook,** 20:574–578, Sept., 1972.

16. Leininger, M.: An open health care system model. **Nurs. Outlook,** 21:171–175, Mar., 1973.

17. Levin, L. S.: Time to hear a different drum. **Am. J. Nurs.,** 72:2007–2010, Nov., 1972.

18. Lysaught, J. P.: An Abstract for Action. New York, McGraw-Hill, 1970.

19. McNerney, W. J.: Health care financing and delivery in the decade ahead. **JAMA,** 222:1150–1155, Nov. 27, 1972.

20. Magida, A. S.: The second White House Conference on aging. **Bedside Nurse,** 5:28–29, Mar., 1972.

21. Malang, J.: The difference it makes. **Am. J. Nurs.,** 72:276–279, Feb., 1972.

22. Martin, S.: How a nurse makes the difference. **Am. J. Nurs.,** 72:278–280, Feb., 1972.

23. Mecklin, J. M.: Hospitals need management even more than money. **Fortune,** 81:96–99, Jan., 1970.

24. Palmore, E., and Luikart, C.: Health and social factors related to life satisfaction. **J. Health and Social Behavior,** 13:68–80, Mar., 1972.

25. Purdom, P. W.: The shape of a national health program. **Am. J. Public Health,** 62:12–15, Jan., 1972.

26. Report of the White House Conference on Youth. Washington, D. C., U. S. Government Printing Office, 1971.

27. Richardson, J. D., and Scutchfield, F. D.: Priorities in health care: the consumer's viewpoint in an Appalachian community. **Am. J. Public Health,** 63:79–82, Jan., 1973.

28. Roemer, M. I.: Health care financing and delivery around the world. **Am. J. Nurs.,** 71:1158–1163, June, 1971.

29. Rothfeld, M. B.: Sensible surgery for swelling medical costs. **Fortune,** 87:110–114, 116; 118–119; Apr., 1973.

30. Sargent, F., II: Man-environment-problems for public health. **Am. J. Public Health,** 62:628–633, May, 1972.

31. Silver, G. A.: National health insurance, national health policy, and the national health. **Am. J. Nurs.,** 71: 1730–1734, Sept., 1971.

32. Somers, A. R.: Health Care In Transition: Directions for the Future. Chicago, Hospital Research and Educational Trust, 1971.

33. Statistical Abstract of the U. S. 1972, annual ed., 93, pp. 1–8. U. S. Department of Commerce, Bureau of the Census, 1972.

34. Storlie, F.: Nursing and the Social Conscience. New York, Appleton-Century-Crofts, 1970.

35. Terris, M.: Crisis and change in America's health system. **Am. J. Public Health,** 63:313–318, Apr., 1973.

36. The plight of the U. S. patient. **Time,** 91:54, Feb. 23, 1968.

CHAPTER 3

Principles as Guides for Health Practitioners

GLOSSARY • INTRODUCTION • PRINCIPLES, PROCEDURES, AND
POLICIES • MAN AS A UNIQUE HUMAN BEING • MAN AS AN
ORGANISM • MAN AND HIS ENVIRONMENT • CONCLUSION •
STUDY SITUATIONS • REFERENCES

GLOSSARY

Adaptation: Act of adjusting by alteration in structure or function.

Biological Environment: The aggregate of other living things surrounding man.

Ecology: Study of the relationships between organisms and their surroundings.

Environment: The aggregate of people, things, conditions, or influences surrounding man.

Law: A rule which states that a particular phenomenon always occurs when certain conditions are present.

Moral Doctrine: A teaching or advocation of behavior which is considered right or good.

Physical Environment: The aggregate of nonliving things surrounding man, such as air, water, and land.

Policy: A directive or regulation that describes a definite course of action.

Principle: A truth resulting from scientific investigations that describe a particular phenomenon.

Procedure: A mode of conducting a particular process.

Social Environment: Interpersonal relationships that exist in the environment of man.

Sociology: The study of relationships among humans.

Theory: Explanation of a process, a phenomenon, or an event based on observed fact(s) but which lacks absolute or direct proof.

INTRODUCTION

Contemporary man has concerned himself with a variety of pressing problems, the solutions to many of which he considers essential to human survival and well-being. The following questions are typical of today's concerns: How many people can the world support? Are cultures changing so rapidly that man is being overwhelmed by change? Is man destroying his life-giving environment? What results when segments of the population are denied the same rights that others enjoy in that society? Can life expectancy be further extended? How can we promote action on health maintenance and quality of life?

This chapter identifies three broad and basic principles that are considered essential guides to action in promoting man's well-being and survival in this world. They function to guide not only nurses but everyone concerned with the well-being of mankind. These principles will be referred to frequently in this text and hopefully, as depth in their understanding increases, their usefulness will also.

But first, what is a principle? How are principles different from procedures and policies?

PRINCIPLES, PROCEDURES, AND POLICIES

There is a difference of opinion as to the meaning of the word "principle" and also as to what is credited with being a principle. This text defines a *principle* as a truth developed after careful and controlled investigation of a particular phenomenon. A principle will stand up to scientific testing. This characteristic separates a popular belief or so-called common sense approach from a principle. A popular belief will not necessarily survive scientific inquiry. It has been estimated that popular beliefs or common sense statements will have a fifty-fifty chance of being correct when scrutinized carefully. This represents considerable risk, especially when the safety of a patient is at stake.

Principles serve as guides to action; they do not specify what must be done. However, depending on desired results, they help in decision-making to determine the action that is necessary. Principles assist one to predict what will happen in a new situation. They are indispensable for the nurse in making judgments and in reaching decisions concerning the selection of nursing care a particular patient needs.

Following are a few examples of principles. Examples show how they act to guide action and how they can be used to predict what will happen in new situations.

From the science of microbiology, we learn that microorganisms in the nose and throat can be transmitted by coughing, sneezing, or talking, or by direct contact. This fact serves as a principle that guides much common action. We cover our nose and mouth when sneezing or coughing; the surgeon and his assistants wear face masks when operating, to prevent droplets from spreading to the working area; a patient with an uncontrollable cough will be separated from others; persons with a cold are advised to stay away from others and treat respiratory secretions as infectious; and so on. The predictive value of this principle is illustrated when it can be anticipated, for example, that one child in a crowded classroom can spread his cold to others by coughing and sneezing. Also, when someone is found to have pulmonary tuberculosis with positive sputum, his associates and family are examined since it can be anticipated that some of them could have contracted the disease from the patient by respiratory droplets.

A *law* of science is defined as a rule, stating that a particular phenomenon always occurs when certain conditions are present. For example, Pascal's law from the science of physics states that an increase in pressure on an enclosed liquid will be distributed uniformly and undiminished to all parts of the liquid. Using this law as a principle guides action in a variety of situations. For example, a water-filled mattress distributes pressure evenly over the body surface in contact with it. This decreases the tendency for patients to develop pressure sores. One can predict blindness when persons with glaucoma, an eye disease characterized by increased pressure within the eye, do not receive treatment since the pressure distributed throughout the eye will eventually and permanently damage vital eye structure. Hydraulic brakes and lifts operate on the principal of Pascal's law. Note Figure 3-1 which illustrates how Archimedes' law functions in two different situations.

A *theory*, unlike a law, lacks absolute or direct proof. A theory begins with an educated guess but when sufficient research supports that guess, eventually it becomes a theory. When data are uncovered that dispute a theory, revising or discarding the theory becomes necessary. For example, certain theories concerning the geology of the moon had to be revised when the moon-visiting astronauts collected data that could not support the original theories.

One example of a theory used as a principle is

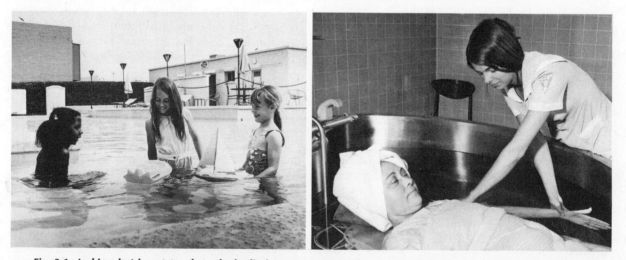

Fig. 3-1. Archimedes' law states that a body displaces an amount of water equal to its own volume. This law explains why the children's boats remain afloat in the pool. The same law is in effect when patients are placed in water in order that their extremities may be manipulated more easily since the loss in weight of a submerged body is equal to the weight of water displaced. (Photos by Ted Hill, Arizona)

the relationship of smoking to cancer of the lungs. There is evidence that heavy smoking often is present in the history of patients who develop lung cancer. However, there are some heavy smokers who do not develop lung cancer. To date, there is no absolute or direct proof that smoking causes cancer of the lungs. However, until more evidence of cause and effect are brought forth, it seems best to adhere to the theory that reduction of the irritation to lungs caused by smoking will reduce the chances of lung cancer.

A *moral doctrine* is concerned with the teaching or advocation of behavior which is considered right or good. As members of society, we arrive at standards of conduct from a variety of sources, such as our family, religion, education, and social and cultural groups, and we use these as principles in our daily living. An example of a moral doctrine accepted by our society is that every effort is made to save the life of another person. A lay person at the scene of an accident gives whatever aid he can until professional help arrives. Health practitioners continue to care for a patient until death occurs. The heroic efforts of people who save the lives of others in times of crisis are described regularly in our news media.

A moral doctrine may have to be suspended under certain extraordinary circumstances. The civil defense plan that would be put into action if this country suffers nuclear attack provides an example. Those with medical authority would separate persons who are injured beyond hope of recovery from those who have a chance of surviving and give preference to the latter. The logic of this system of priorities in civil defense programs is understood. Nevertheless, it is likely to create mental conflict and anguish for those having to make the decision because it is inimical to a fundamental moral doctrine to ignore a person who is likely to die.

A *procedure* is a mode of conducting a particular process. This text will not attempt to describe procedures typically written by health agencies for employee use. Agencies have procedure manuals so that there is as much uniformity in practice as is feasible. It would be economically unsound to allow for many varieties in personal preferences, for example, in the selection of equipment. Also having each nurse use a different method may not add to the patient's feelings of security.

Policies usually refer to directives enforced by a particular health agency. They spell out a definite course of action. Ordinarily, they cannot be varied except by administrative authority. They often act as a safety measure for the agency and the patient.

Policies in relation to a patient's valuables, for instance, are designed to protect both the health agency and the patient. Another example of a policy concerns visiting hours: which hours visitors may see a patient, how many may visit at one time or in one day, who visitors may be, and so forth. They are adopted as being expedient under the circumstances and agency employees, including students, are expected to observe them.

Consider an example that illustrates principles, procedures, and policies operating together in a particular situation. A nurse working in a hospital has two patients who are to have their baths given to them in bed. One is not permitted to bathe herself because of the possibility of heart strain. She is able to move about easily and is not receiving any treatments at this time. The other patient, who is elderly, has severe limitations to the extent that she cannot move and in addition requires several treatments. The nurse would observe hospital procedure concerning equipment, use of linen, and so on. However, guided by principles, the nurse would make variations in the way she bathes these two patients. For the patient who has heart impairment, the nurse would give the bath and make the bed so that as few movements as possible, such as turning or sitting upright, are required of the patient. (Increased effort increases heart action.) For the helpless patient it would be beneficial to be turned more than the other patient. (Decreased activity causes stasis, pressure on areas, decreased respirations, and so on.) Also, for the second patient the nurse would want to do the treatments which could soil the bed linen, such as irrigating the catheter and changing the dressing before the bath rather than at the completion of it and making the bed.

In this same hospital there is a policy which states that all patients over 65 years of age must have bed siderails up at all times. The nurse must comply even though her elderly patient is incapable of turning or moving herself. Her other patient is not 65 years of age but must remain in the sitting position at all times and receives medications that make her feel drowsy. The nurse decided to keep this patient's bed siderails up also. The nurse identified a problem and took action.

What are some of the principles underlying the action of the nurse in placing siderails up for the patient who is not 65 years of age? First, a person is incapable of maintaining a position which requires conscious effort when dozing or sleeping. Secondly, the body will move in the direction of greatest gravitational pull. If this pull should be toward the edge of

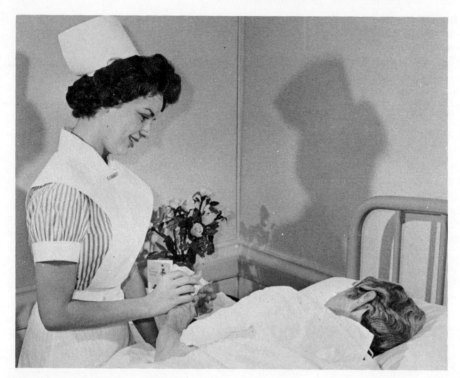

Fig. 3-2. Nursing is caring. It is showing concern and interest for the patient. After turning this patient, the nurse takes the patient's outstretched hand and smiles; both gestures illustrate caring.

the bed, the patient could fall out of bed if the line of gravity goes out of her base of support. Thirdly, with the bed as high as it is, a fall from that distance to a hard surface could result in injury.

Neither clearly written procedures or policies are sufficient to sustain a lack of awareness of principles as this example illustrates.

The remainder of this chapter discusses the three basic principles referred to in the introduction of this chapter.

MAN AS A UNIQUE HUMAN BEING

Every individual is unique and therefore has inalienable rights as a human being.

While it is true that there are many common characteristics of humans, no two individuals are alike. A large variety of factors make up the unique composite of each individual which results in there being no one else quite like him anywhere in the world. Uniqueness is a highly valued and a precious characteristic of every human being. It is largely responsible for our placing such a high worth on man's individuality and his inalienable rights as a human being.

A distinctly human characteristic is the ability to change. Man possesses tremendous energies to grow, to adapt, to adjust, to move forward, to retreat, to

feel "up" or to feel "down", *ad infinitum*. Moreover, just as each individual is unique, he changes in his own unique manner also.

One of the basic premises of a democratic form of government is respect for the individual. This tenet awards dignity and value to each human regardless of race, age, sex, creed, or social or economic status. While respect for man's rights has general and wide acceptance in society, it is often selective in practice. Leaders working for racial justice, for solutions to problems of poverty, for women's liberation, for greater participation of senior citizens in our society, and for many other causes as well, remind us in newspaper articles almost daily how far removed this country is in implementing equality.

Within recent times, it has become increasingly accepted that one right of man is his right to health. The World Health Organization, one of the special agencies of the United Nations, states in the preamble of its constitution that health is "... one of the fundamental rights of every human being without distinction of race, religion, political belief, economic or social condition."

In recent years man has become increasingly involved in his own health care. The consumer's heightened sophistication and assertiveness have changed the focus of health care from "doing for" to "doing with." The citizens of this country are taking much more active roles in identifying their health needs and in participating in meeting them as Chapter 2 describes.

High quality nursing practice reflects constant respect for man's dignity and value regardless of race, age, sex, creed, or social or economic status. Such practice also is guided by knowledge of the abilities of man to contribute and to change, and nurses will find many opportunities to utilize these capacities when promoting an individual's well-being.

This first principle can also be expressed well for nurses by the phrase, *nursing is caring*. Nursing is much more than keeping patients clean, clothed, fed, and protected. It is more than interest in caring for the physically and mentally handicapped. It is more than giving a bath, administering a medication, or rubbing a back. Nursing includes these things but it is also accepting of others as human beings. It includes listening, touching, bolstering self-esteem, and helping others in a time of crisis. Nursing has been called a beautiful adventure when it takes interest in the welfare, value, and dignity of each human being. If one *cares* for a person, than one has respect for him, regardless of the situation that exists. Nursing is not really nursing unless it is *caring*.

MAN AS AN ORGANISM

Well-being is attained when the body's physiologic and psychologic needs are being met satisfactorily.

A *need* is a necessity or a requirement. Most people have at least some understanding of human needs through education and experience. They come to realize, for instance, that the loss of sleep produces fatigue; excessive perspiration produces thirst; cutting off oxygen supply can quickly produce suffocation; the loss of loved ones causes feelings of grief

and loneliness; fear and anxiety mount when threatening situations exist; self-esteem may be shattered when a person feels disliked or ridiculed; and so on.

Although this second principle speaks of the physiologic and the psychologic needs of the human organism, they cannot be viewed as separate entities. They are related and constantly interrelating which adds to the complexities of understanding the workings of the human organism. Persons in the various health services soon become aware that it is almost impossible to observe a physical need without being aware of its psychologic implications; and vice versa.

Students of the human organism realize that much of the body's functioning is still not understood despite constant research and an already overwhelming body of knowledge. Some physiologic and psychologic processes for which there is considerable knowledge include the necessity of making oxygen available to body cells; eliminating wastes through the gastrointestinal, urinary, respiratory, and integumentary systems; providing opportunities for self-expression and enjoying satisfying personal relationships with others; and so on. However, questions to which answers remain elusive are still innumerable. For example, what causes the unruly growth of certain cells? What is responsible for the process of aging? Is there a biological cause for some mental illness? Why do persons exposed to very similar environments often develop such varied personalities?

It is known that the body has the ability to function in a systematic and life-sustaining manner within some rather broad limits. The body is capable of enhancing one function to compensate for another when necessity arises. This compensation is known as *adaptation*. Here are a few examples of adaptation. The kidney tubules reabsorb increased amounts of fluid when liquid intake is low or liquid loss is high in order to aid in preserving the body's fluid balance.

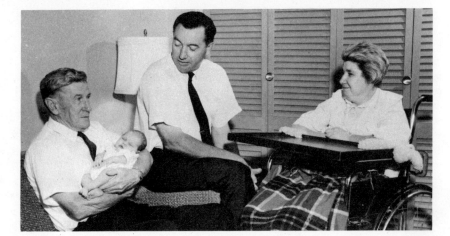

Fig. 3-3. A patient is not an isolated individual; he is part of a family, a neighborhood, a community. A community health nurse supervises the care of this chronically ill patient. As a result, the patient can remain in her home and be with her family and friends. In this way, many of her psychosocial needs are met more easily and pleasantly than if she were hospitalized.

Constriction of peripheral blood vessels when entering a cold environment is the process by which the body attempts to conserve its heat. When blood vessel resistance increases, the myocardial wall of the left ventricle ultimately becomes thicker in order to increase the force with which the blood is pushed out of the heart; this assists in keeping peripheral circulation adequate for cell survival. A person in need of and seeking personal recognition may exhibit exaggerated behavior in order to gain the attention he needs. The body triggers mechanisms that enable a person to be ready and able to avoid or withdraw from a threatening situation.

Adaptation varies from one person to another and even with the same person at different times. The developmental stage of the person, his general health status, and the presence or absence of supportive factors are examples of circumstances which influence man's adaptive ability. For instance, a child more frequently contracts communicable diseases than adults do because his body has not yet adequately developed his defense system of antibodies to provide protection. The elderly person may need more frequent rest periods as his energy reserves decrease. A person with a chronic disease or in a poor nutritional state will generally have less adaptive ability to heal a fractured bone. Persons who have family or friends whom they can trust and confide in usually experience more adaptive ability than persons without these supportive elements in their environment.

While the body's capacity to adapt is normally quite extensive, there are times when it needs assistance to maintain well-being. For example, when the body is unable to handle an infection, drugs may be given to provide an assist. Increased body temperature is a normal adaptive defense and desirable in many instances, but if it reaches extremes that could result in tissue damage, steps are taken to halt the body's adaptive process before it reaches a dangerous level. When an individual is no longer able to adapt to stresses in his life, he may seek the assistance of those who can help him to cope.

Does the presence or absence of sufficient ability to adapt determine the difference between illness and health? In this text, health and illness are considered to be on a continuum, as was described in Chapter 2. Or, stated in another way, people are neither totally healthy nor totally ill. Health and illness are dynamic and ever-changing states, and people find themselves at various points on the continuum at different times. Adaptation enables people to move toward the health end of the continuum and hence, the capacity to adapt may be considered a part of health.

This second principle indicates that health prac-titioners, including nurses, need to have a sound knowledge of human needs to provide society with high quality services. In later chapters in this text, basic human needs are discussed. Also, learning what to expect when needs are not met will be an important part of this text and of the entire educational program in nursing.

MAN AND HIS ENVIRONMENT

The environment influences an organism's well-being.

Man and his environment are constantly interacting. The environment influences man and man influences his environment at all times. The relationship between man and his environment is never static, always changing.

Our *environment* may be defined as the aggregate of people, things, conditions, or influences surrounding us. The *biological environment* considers all living things other than man. The *social environment* is unique to man and it is created by him. *Sociology* is concerned with the relationships between humans in their environment. The *physical environment* consists of nonliving portions of the environment such as air, water, and land. The science that concerns itself with relationships between all living organisms including man and their surroundings is called *ecology*.

The above principle concerning man and his environment implies than any environmental condition that interferes with well-being is a threat to the human organism when he is no longer able to cope with it sufficiently well. Some people tolerate their environment better than others. Also, each individual may experience variations in ability to tolerate certain conditions, depending on other factors in the situation at hand. "The last straw" often describes a factor which under other circumstances, would have been tolerable to the individual, but in a certain instance precipitates a crisis.

While sociology and biology have been well-known disciplines for some time, ecology has become a household word only recently. Concern for the physical as well as the sociological environment is global in nature. In a report to Congress on U. S. Foreign Policy for the 1970s, President Nixon said, "... What is new is the fact that we now face an increasing range of problems which are central to our national well-being, but which are, by definition, global problems ... Of greater import, however, is our shared and transcendent interest in the livability of our common home, the earth. To these problems, and the opportunities they present, that interest must be our guide and guide of others. The nurturing of that interest has now become a prime task of American leadership."

The United Nations' first Conference on the Human Environment was held in Stockholm in the spring of 1972. Approximately 1,200 diplomats representing 112 nations, several thousand scientific experts from about 550 non-governmental organizations, and innumerable environmental enthusiasts of every variety attended. Because of many conflicting philosophies among attendants, approval of resolutions was difficult. However, the conference did highlight the ever increasing concern of mankind in working for an environment that promotes well-being and demonstrated that a start could be made on problems generally considered too long ignored.

A few examples will show some of the implications of this principle which concerns itself with man and his environment.

The human organism enjoys optimum functioning when the air he breathes is sufficiently free of physical and chemical pollutants so that irritation to tissue is absent or at least negligible. In some metropolitan areas with high levels of air pollution (examples: Los Angeles, Tokyo) some people find it difficult to be outdoors because of irritation to eye and respiratory tissue. Uncontaminated water is essential to health. Water ladened with disease-producing organisms or chemical poisons will often lead to illness. Although the human organism is able normally to tolerate noise safely within a rather wide decibel range, it has been shown that exposure for long periods of time to loud noise may produce tension as well as damage to the ear. For example, teenagers enjoying the loudness of rock music have suffered damage to the inner ear after prolonged exposure. Their parents, on the other hand, usually cannot tolerate the loudness of the music either physically or psychologically. Variations within one individual in his ability to cope with environmental factors are shown by the commuter who tolerates heavy traffic patiently to and from work every day of the working week but becomes irritated and aggressive when he encounters similar traffic while traveling on a holiday. Human beings can adjust to change in their social environment until these changes occur too rapidly, at which point psychological tensions may become evident. The burden of adaptation placed on a person reared in a slow-paced rural environment may become intolerable when he moves to the faster-paced living characteristic of many metropolitan areas.

Within recent years, the world population growth and migration of many people to large urban areas

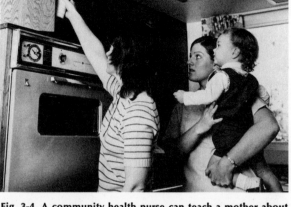

Fig. 3-4. A community health nurse can teach a mother about dangerous household items and the importance of keeping them from the reach of a toddler's natural curiosity. (Photo by Ted Hill)

have become common phenomena of concern. Research has attempted to answer questions such as these: How much space does man need to experience well-being? Is well-being in jeopardy when man is denied access to the beauties of nature? Is being able to "get-away-from-it-all" important for health? Are recreational activities and the time to enjoy them essential for well-being?

The nurse will concern herself with many additional environmental factors as she takes action to promote a healthful environment for her patients. An example is the practice of washing her hands thoroughly whenever indicated in order to help control the spread of infection. Also, the nurse knows that oxygen supports combustion and takes appropriate measures to decrease the likelihood of fire in the room of someone receiving oxygen therapy. As another example, she teaches parents that normal curiosity can result in tragedy when frayed electrical cords, medications, or household cleaning solutions are within easy reach of children.

Because of their concern for health, nurses cannot lose sight of the importance of a healthful environment. As citizens, their role can well be one of leadership in working for the kind of environment that promotes well-being.

CONCLUSION

As each nursing care activity is encountered, it will be helpful for the nurse to question how each of the three principles functions. In this way, it becomes possible to recognize rather quickly that while all are involved, they are not necessarily involved to an equal extent in every situation. Each one will guide actions according to the needs of the specific situation.

The complexities of the human being and the continuing search for increased understanding of how he functions point up that nurses, as well as other personnel offering health services, must study the human organism on a continuing basis. A course in anatomy and physiology or in psychology and anthropology cannot sustain the nurse in her practice for life. She must constantly be on the alert to keep abreast of new knowledge. The three basic principles presented in this chapter will serve as a sound base as the nurse strives to increase her knowledge and to offer the highest possible level of service to the people she serves.

Study Situations

1. Nurses are involved in various ways to help solve problems related to environmental pollution. The following references describe the measures some nurses are taking.

   Nurses play a major role in air pollution study. **Am. J. Nurs.,** 71:871; 872; 1000, May, 1971.

   Why does Dr. Calafiore feel that nurses are especially valuable in assisting with a study of community environmental pollution, such as the study on which she is working?

   Effects of pollution on pre-schoolers under investigation. **Am. J. Nurs.,** 71:872, May, 1971.

   Why did the investigation of pollution, described in the preceding reference, choose to work with the preschool age group?

   Letters: fighting pollution. **Am. J. Nurs.,** 71:254; 256, Feb., 1971.

   What are nurses described in this letter doing to help control environmental pollution?

2. The following quote is taken from a letter to the editor, written by Dorothy Welty, in the **Am. J. Nurs.,** 71:904, May, 1971:

   "Death does not always come with the last breath, the final heartbeat. Death can and does come sometimes long before that moment. You've stopped living—or you have never really started—when you can't look past the ugliness, or oldness, or fatness, or color and see a soul. Death is there if you build a pride so big it keeps you from saying, 'I'm sorry,' or 'I love you,' or just a simple 'thanks.' . . . You have never really been alive if you aren't aware of all the really nice people in this old world . . ."

   How does the philosophy expressed in this message support the principle described in this chapter that deals with man as a unique human being?

   Discuss how this same first principle was used in the care of Mr. C., as described in the following article:

   Lenarz, D. M.: Caring is the essence of practice. **Am. J. Nurs.,** 71:704–707, Apr., 1971.

3. The following book had a wide readership but also provoked certain controversies concerning man's survival and his ability to adapt:

   Toffler, A.: Future Shock. 562 p. New York, Bantam Books, 1970. (A condensation of the major ideas of this book appeared in this publication: Toffler, A.: Coping with future shock. **Reader's Digest,** 99:81–86, Aug., 1971.)

   What implications for nursing do you find in the author's description of dangers of future shock? What are the author's strategies for survival?

   Lothair, a German king in the ninth century is credited with having said, "All things change, and we must change with them." Do you believe previous generations were as concerned with man's well-being and his survival on earth as the present one is?

4. Describe how the three basic principles discussed in this chapter guided action in promoting total patient well-being, as reported in the following article:

   Murray, R. L. E.: Caring. **Am. J. Nurs.,** 72:1286–1287, July, 1972.

References

1. Bircher, A. U.: Mankind in crisis: an application of clinical process to population-environmental issues. **Nurs. Forum,** 11:10–33, No. 1, 1972.

2. Blowers, J. H.: The United States' position on environment. **Am. J. Public Health,** 62:634–638, May, 1972.

3. Dennis, R. J.: Ways of caring. **Am. J. Nurs.,** 64:107–108, Feb, 1964.

4. Eipper, A. W.: Pollution problems, resource policy, and the scientist. **Science,** 169:11–15, July 3, 1970.

5. Gress, L.: The aged—a nursing gap? **Nursing '72,** 2:4, May, 1972.

6. Jamann, J. S.: Health is a function of ecology. **Am. J. Nurs.,** 71:970–973, May, 1971.

7. Lave, L. B., and Seskin, E. P.: Air pollution and human health. **Science,** 169:723–733, Aug. 21, 1970.

8. Levine, M. E.: Holistic nursing. In **The Nursing Clinics of North America.** Philadelphia, W. B. Saunders, 6:253–264, June, 1971.

9. Long, K. R.: Pesticides—as occupational hazard on farms. **Am. J. Nurs.,** 71:740–743, Apr., 1971.

10. Pastiche. **Am. J. Nurs.,** 70:501, Mar., 1970.

11. Sargent, F., II: Man-environment-problems for public health. **Am. J. Public Health,** 62:628–633, May, 1972.

12. Schorr, T. M.: Ages of usefulness (Editorial). **Am. J. Nurs.,** 71:1129, June, 1971.

13. ———: Issues of conscience (Editorial). **Am. J. Nurs.,** 72:61, Jan., 1972.

14. Sullivan, C., et al.: Nursing in a society in crisis. **Am. J. Nurs.,** 72:302–304, Feb., 1972.

CHAPTER 4

Legal and Ethical Components of Nursing

GLOSSARY · INTRODUCTION · DEFINITION OF LAW · SOURCES OF
LAWS · TORTS AND CRIMES · NEGLIGENCE AND MALPRACTICE ·
SLANDER AND LIBEL; FALSE IMPRISONMENT; INVASION OF PRIVACY;
ASSAULT AND BATTERY; FRAUD · CRIMINAL ACTS · ADDITIONAL
LAWS OF INTEREST TO NURSES: THE NURSING STUDENT'S LEGAL
STATUS; GOOD SAMARITAN LAWS; NARCOTIC LAWS; FEDERAL FOOD,
DRUG AND COSMETIC ACT; WILLS · DEFENSE OF THE ACCUSED ·
NURSE PRACTICE ACTS · ETHICS AND THE CODE OF ETHICS FOR
NURSES · CONCLUSION · STUDY SITUATIONS · REFERENCES

GLOSSARY

Administrative Law: Law made by administrative or executive agencies of the government.

Assault: A threat, or an attempt, to make bodily contact with another person without that person's consent.

Battery: An assault that is carried out.

Civil Law: See **Private Law**.

Common Law: Law that results from court decisions that are then followed when other cases involving similar circumstances and facts arise. Common law is as binding as civil law.

Constitutional Law: Law stated in the federal and state constitutions.

Crime: An offense against persons or property. The act is considered to be against the government, referred to in a lawsuit as "The People," and the accused is prosecuted by the state.

Defamation: Wrongs of slander and libel.

Defendant: Person being accused of a tort or crime.

Ethics: A discipline that concerns itself with human actions in respect to their being right or wrong.

Expert Witness: A person having special training or experience who assists a judge and jury to formulate standards of care.

False Imprisonment: Unjustifiable retention or prevention of the movement of another person without proper consent.

Felony: A crime punishable by imprisonment in a state or federal penitentiary for more than one year. Felony is also described as a crime of deeper offense than a misdemeanor.

Fraud: Willful and purposeful misrepresentation that could or has caused loss or harm to persons or property.

Good Samaritan Law: Law that holds physicians and nurses harmless when undertaking to aid a person in emergency situations.

Invasion of Privacy: A wrong that invades the right of a person to be let alone.

Jurisprudence: The philosophy or science of law.

Law: Rules of conduct established and enforced by the government of a society.

Lawsuit: A legal action in a court of law.

Libel: An untruthful written statement about a person that subjects him to ridicule or contempt.

Litigation: The process of a lawsuit.

Malpractice: An act of negligence as applied to a professional person, such as a physician, nurse, and dentist.

Mandatory Nurse Practice Act: A law that requires that a nurse be licensed in order to practice nursing.

Manslaughter: Second degree murder.

Misdemeanor: A crime, of lesser offense than a felony, punishable with fines, or imprisonment, or both usually for less than one year.

Murder: Illegally killing another person.

(First degree murder: Murder with malice aforethought.)

(Second degree murder: Murder without previous deliberation, sometimes called manslaughter.)

Negligence: Performing an act that a reasonably prudent person under similar circumstances would not do, or failing to perform an act that a reasonably prudent person under similar circumstances would do.

Permissive Nurse Practice Act: A law that allows the licensed nurse to refer to herself as a **registered nurse** but does not require that the nurse be licensed to practice.

Plaintiff: Person or government bringing a lawsuit against another.

Precedent: The first case that sets down a common law.

Private Law: Rules that regulate relationships among people. Also called civil law.

Privileged Communication: Information that need not be revealed in court by the person receiving it.

Public Law: Rules that regulate relationships between individuals and their government.

Respondeat Superior: The master-servant rule that states that an employer is legally liable for his employee's acts.

Slander: An untruthful oral statement about a person that subjects him to ridicule or contempt.

Standard of Care: A description of conduct that illustrates what a reasonably prudent person would have done, or would not have done, under similar circumstances.

Stare Decisis: A Latin phrase meaning "Let the decision stand." **Stare decisis** is the basis for common law.

Statutory Law: A law enacted by a legislative body.

Testator: One who makes a will.

Tort: A wrong committed by a person against another person or his property.

INTRODUCTION

Accountability for practice has become a generally accepted principle in nursing, as indicated in Chapter 1. In the past, physicians and hospitals assumed much more responsibility for a nurse's action than is true today. However, as the nurse's role expanded, and as it continues to do so, the responsiblity of being accountable for her action increases for the nurse and takes on increased legal implications.

There is a public trust involved for health practitioners in administering health care services. Society rightfully expects that practitioners assume responsibility to give services that are skillfully done and executed with sound judgment. To offer less than that violates that public trust in which case the health practitioner is expected to be held accountable and liable.

A detailed discussion of the legal and ethical aspects of nursing generally is included in curricula of schools of nursing near the time when students are to graduate. Hence, the discussion here will be brief. However, because certain aspects of the law involve nurses from the time they begin their education in nursing, it seems appropriate to include an early overview. For example, in later chapters this text will discuss making entries on patients' records, caring for patients' clothing and valuables, obtaining consents, and reporting errors and injuries, all of which have legal implications.

DEFINITION OF LAW

A *law* is a rule of conduct established and enforced by the government of a society. (Note how this legal definition differs from the definition of a law, as used in science and as described in Chapter 3.) Laws are applicable to the people living in a governmental jurisdiction, such as the city, county, state, and country, over which authority is exercised by that government. Laws are intended primarily to protect the rights of the public. For example, nurse practice acts are intended primarily to protect the public and secondarily, to provide the nurse with protection. Of particular importance is that laws are not only promulgated by governmental processes but are also enforceable by authority of that government.

Laws may be referred to as standards of conduct. They make it possible for men to live together peacefully. The philosophy or science of law is called *jurisprudence.*

Public law is law in which the government is directly involved. It regulates the relationships between individuals and the government. Also, an important body of public law describes the powers of the government in authority. *Private law*, also called *civil law*, regulates the relationships among people. Examples of civil law include laws relating to contracts, ownership of property, the practice of nursing, medicine, pharmacy, dentistry, and so on.

SOURCES OF LAWS

There are four main sources of laws or rules of conduct in our country. These sources are the constitutions, the legislatures, the judiciary system, and administrative regulations.

Constitutions

In any society there must be an authoritative body if chaos is to be prevented. Although authority comes from the people, each individual relinquishes certain rights in order that a form of government can be established and given the authority to govern. The government is charged with the responsibility of maintaining order and protecting the general welfare of its people.

The constitution of the federal government and of each state indicates how its government is created and given authority. These constitutions state the principles and provisions for establishment of specific laws. Although they themselves contain relatively few laws (called *constitutional laws*), they are constant guides to legislative bodies. In our country each state constitution directs the governing of a specific geographic area, but it can in no way violate principles set down in the federal constitution.

Although individuals relinquish certain rights in order that a government can be created, the constitutions are not without their limits. For example, the first ten amendments of the federal constitution are referred to as the Bill of Rights. These amendments restrict the passage of laws that infringe on certain basic liberties; for example, freedom of worship, freedom of speech, freedom from unwarranted search and seizure of our homes and persons, and the like. Each state constitution sets similar limitations.

The Legislatures

Our government under the Constitution has created legislative bodies that are responsible for enacting laws. These bodies are called the Congress at the federal level and legislatures at the state level. Certain legislative bodies at the local level (county, municipalities, and the like) may be established also. A law enacted by a legislative body is referred to as *statutory law*. These laws must be in keeping with the federal constitution and, within each state, with that state's constitution as well. The Nurse Practice Acts are statutory laws.

The Judiciary System

Our government provides for a judiciary system which is responsible for reconciling controversies and conflicts. It interprets legislation as it has been applied in specific instances and makes decisions in relation to law enforcement. Over the years, a body of law known as *common law* has grown out of these accumulated judiciary decisions.

Common law is based on the principle known as *stare decisis*, or "Let the decision stand." In other words, once a decision has been made in a court of law, that decision becomes the rule to follow when other cases involving similar circumstances and facts arise. The case that first sets down the rule by decision is called a *precedent*. Court decisions can be changed but only when strong justification exists. Common law helps prevent one set of rules being used to judge one person, and another set being used to judge another person in similar circumstances.

Common law directly concerned with nursing exists. Under common law, for example, students in hospital-controlled schools of nursing have been considered employees of the hospital.

Administrative Regulations

One responsibility of the executive branch of our government is to execute the law of the land. Executive power resides in the president of the United States, the governors of the states, and the mayors, or their equivalents, at the municipal level. These chief executive officers administer various agencies that, among other things, are responsible for law enforcement. These agencies have power to make administrative rules and regulations in conformity with enacted law. The rules and regulations act as laws themselves and are enforceable just as any law in the country. They are referred to as *administrative laws*.

Examples of federal administrative agencies include the Federal Trade Commission, the Federal Communications Commission, and the Interstate Commerce Commission. The boards of nursing are examples of administrative agencies at the state level. An example of a municipal administrative agency is a city's board of health.

TORTS AND CRIMES

A *tort* is a wrong committed by a person against another person or his property. In most instances, the court in a civil case (that is, a case involving a tort) will settle damages in terms of money but rarely in terms of imprisonment. Torts may be intentional or unintentional acts of wrongdoing.

A *crime* is also a wrong against a person or his property but the act is considered to be also against the public. In a criminal case, the government (referred to as "The People") prosecutes the offender. When a crime is committed, the factor of intent to commit wrong is present. A crime is punished either by fines or imprisonment or both.

An act generally considered a tort may, because of its severity, be classed as a crime. For example, negligence of a gross nature that demonstrates the offender as guilty of complete disregard for another's life may be tried as both civil and criminal action. It is then prosecuted under criminal as well as civil law. By its very nature, a wrong tried as a crime implies a more serious offense with more legal implications than a tort.

There are some specific laws that define action of violators of such laws as crimes. For example, failure to observe the Federal Food, Drug and Cosmetic Act may constitute a crime, whether there was intent or not.

NEGLIGENCE AND MALPRACTICE

In the eyes of the law, negligence is carelessness. *Negligence* is defined as performing an act that a reasonably prudent person under similar circumstances would not do, or stated conversely, failing to perform an act that a reasonably prudent person under similar circumstances would do. As the definition implies, an act of negligence may be an act of omission or commission.

In order to determine negligence, a *standard of care* is determined by deciding first what a reasonably prudent person would have done, or would not have done, under similar circumstances. In order to assist juries and judges, standards of care are given by an *expert witness*. An expert witness is a person having special training or experience that assists a judge and jury to formulate standards of care. In instances involving nursing practice, a nurse may be requested to act as an expert to describe what standards of care could be expected under similar circumstances. The expert witness is not called upon to testify either for or against the person charged with negligence. He merely describes standards of care to assist the court in arriving at its decision.

Two important additional items are involved in determining negligence: knowing that failure to observe the standard of care could cause harm and demonstrating that harm resulted because of improper care.

Table 4-1 aids in the understanding of negligence. Examples of negligent acts for which nurses have been held liable include injuries to patients resulting from burns, falls, overlooked sponges in surgical procedures, medication errors, and failure to communicate.

The following is an example of a nursing act that could result in a lawsuit. A nurse is about to administer penicillin to a patient. As the nurse approaches the patient with the medication, the patient says, "I hope that isn't penicillin because I am allergic to it." If the nurse gives the medication anyway and if the patient has an allergic reaction, that nurse's act could be considered one of negligence. A reasonably prudent nurse would be expected to know that postpenicillin reactions can be very dangerous and the nurse could be expected to foresee potential harm if penicillin is administered to a person allergic to it.

TABLE 4-1: Guidelines on negligence* †		
Elements of liability	*Explanation*	*Example— Giving medications*
Duty to use due care (defined by the standard of care)	The care which should be given under the circumstances (what the reasonably prudent nurse would have done)	A nurse should give medications: accurately and completely and on time
Failure to meet standard of care (breach of duty)	Not giving the care which should be given under the circumstances	A nurse fails to give medications: accurately or completely or on time
Foreseeability of harm	Knowledge that not meeting the standard of care will cause harm to the patient	Giving the wrong medication or the wrong dosage or not on schedule will probably cause harm to the patient
Failure to meet standard of care (breach) *causes* injury	Patient is harmed because proper care is not given	Wrong medication causes patient to have a convulsion
Injury	Actual harm results to patient	Convulsion or other serious complication

* Adapted from Springer, E. W., ed.: Nursing and the Law. p. 4. Pittsburgh, Aspen Systems Corporation, 1970.
† Professional negligence is malpractice.

Malpractice is the term generally used to describe negligence of professional personnel. As one authority wrote, "Malpractice is only a term of limited nomenclature. Negligence is all-inclusive. In other words, malpractice and negligence are not two separate torts, but one and the same. What is necessary to constitute an act of negligence is essential to constitute an act of malpractice." (8:235)

SLANDER AND LIBEL; FALSE IMPRISONMENT; INVASION OF PRIVACY; ASSAULT AND BATTERY; FRAUD

A person committing an intentional tort is considered to have knowledge of the permitted legal limits of his words or acts. Violating these limits is grounds for prosecution.

Slander and Libel

Slander and libel are sometimes called the wrongs of *defamation*. Slander is an untruthful oral statement about a person that subjects him to ridicule or contempt. Libel is the same, except that the statement is in writing, signs, pictures, or the like. For example, false statements that indicate someone is unfit for the practice of his profession can be held as slander or libel. Falsely accusing someone of committing a crime constitutes slander or libel. Nurses who make false statements about their patient or their co-workers, for example, run the risk of being sued for slander or libel.

A person charged with slander or libel is not liable if he can prove that his oral or written statement is true. Also, *privileged communication* is legally acceptable defense for defamation. Privileged communication protects information exchanged between certain people, and the information need not be disclosed in a court of law. Communication between an attorney and his client has long been recognized as privileged. Many states have statutes that recognize privilege in a physician-patient or a priest-communicant communication. Three states (New York, New Mexico, and Arkansas) mention nurses in privileged communication laws as late as 1970. Privilege is based on the supposition that professional persons cannot give adequate care without the person's complete disclosure of facts in relation to his problems. Privileged communication is a complex subject, but the nurse should at least be aware of the existence of laws in relation to confidential information coming to her knowledge when attending patients.

False Imprisonment

Unjustifiable retention or preventing the movement of another person without proper consent can constitute *false imprisonment*. The indiscriminate and thoughtless use of restraints is an example of an act that can constitute false imprisonment. The amount of restraint can be only reasonable under the circumstances that warrant restraint. Occasionally a delicate balance of judgment is required in the use of restraints.

A person cannot be held legally against his will for his failure to pay for services rendered. Nor can he be legally forced to remain in a health agency (such as a hospital) if he is sound of mind, even when health practitioners believe the person should remain for additional care. Health agencies have special forms to use in such cases which the person signs indicating he will not hold the agency responsible for any harm that may result from his leaving. A

mentally ill patient or a person with certain communicable diseases can legally be kept in an agency if he presents a danger to society.

Invasion of Privacy

The U. S. Supreme Court has interpeted the right against invasion of privacy as inherent in the Constitution. The First Amendment, it held, was an effort to protect citizens by giving them the right of privacy and the right to be let alone.

Necessary exposure for caring for a patient by procedures essential to his care does not constitute grounds for invasion of privacy. If a patient is exposed to the public, either personally or through pictures, the person responsible for the exposure can be held liable. This does not hold if the patient has given consent for the exposure. Unauthorized exposure even after death may constitute invasion of privacy.

Health practitioners should recognize that unnecessary exposure of patients, while moving them through corridors or while caring for them in shared rooms, can constitute invasion of privacy. Personnel who gossip or discuss information concerning patients with persons not entitled to the information may be charged with invasion of privacy. Information on patients' charts is considered confidential and should not be discussed with unauthorized persons. Special care to protect a patient's privacy is recommended in the use of tape recorders, Dictaphones, computer banks, and so on. Nurses who prepare class assignments (written or oral) are advised to conceal the real identity of patients in order to prevent invasion of privacy.

Assault and Battery

Assault is a threat, or an attempt, to make bodily contact with another person without that person's consent. *Battery* is an assault that is carried out. Every person is granted freedom from bodily contact by another unless consent has been granted. In the field of health, a person operated on without his consent can sue the surgeon, or the health agency involved, or both. Hospital personnel cannot force patients to do things, or submit to things, against their will, unless consent has been granted, without fear of legal suit.

Every individual has the right to be free from invasion of his person. For health practitioners, an awareness of this principle and of requirement for consent is extremely important. Consent will be mentioned in this text as it applies to the subject under discussion. Table 4-2 offers guidelines on consent.

TABLE 4-2:   Guidelines on consent*

What is it	Permission to touch	
When it is needed or not needed	Needed: Routine hospital services, diagnostic procedures and medical treatment Any nonroutine medical or surgical treatment	Not needed: Emergency *if:* immediate threat to life or health experts agree that it's an emergency patient unable to consent and legally authorized person can't be reached Action in response to a complication during an operation if legally authorized person can't be reached When patient voluntarily submits
Consequences of not having consent	Nurse and doctor may be liable for battery Hospital is liable for battery because it has a duty to protect patients or it's responsible for its employees' actions	
Criteria for valid consent	Written (oral, if can be proved in court) Signed by patient or person legally responsible for him Patient (or signer) understands the nature of the procedure, the risks involved and probable consequences Procedure performed was one consented to	
Who signs	Patient signs when able Others sign When patient is physically unable, legally incompetent, a minor, unless married or self-supporting When patient's reproductive capability will be ended, spouse should sign	
Failure to sign	A patient has the right to refuse, but should sign a release form as proof of his refusal A hospital may request a court order to act when a patient's refusal endangers his life	

* Adapted from Springer, E. W., ed.: Nursing and the Law. p. 29. Pittsburgh, Aspen Systems Corporation, 1970.

Fraud

Fraud is willful and purposeful misrepresentation that could or has caused loss or harm to persons or property. Misrepresentation of a product is a common fraudulent act. In nursing, persons fraudulently misrepresenting themselves in order to obtain a license to practice may be prosecuted under nurse practice acts. Also, misrepresenting the outcome of a procedure or treatment may constitute fraud.

Table 4-3 aids in understanding intentional torts.

CRIMINAL ACTS

A *crime* is an offense against persons or property. It is a more serious offense than a tort and is considered to be against the government representing the people. Hence, in a lawsuit, the plaintiff (that is, the one bringing suit) is referred to as "The People" and the accused is prosecuted by the state.

In most states, criminal law is statutory law and only infrequently, common law. Crimes are classified as *felonies* or *misdemeanors*. Misdemeanors are crimes of a less serious nature than are felonies. Felonies are punishable by imprisonment in a state or federal penitentiary for more than one year. Misdemeanors commonly are punishable with fines or imprisonment, or both for less than one year.

TABLE 4-3:   Intentional torts important to the nurse*

Legal term	Definition	Example
Assault†	Placing a person in fear of being touched without his consent	Threatening to hit someone
Battery†	Actually touching someone without his consent	Hitting someone
False imprisonment	The unlawful detention of a person against his wishes	Keeping a patient hospitalized until he has paid his bill
Invasion of privacy	Violation of a person's right to be left alone and to have certain personal matters kept out of the public view	Taking pictures of a malformed child without parental permission
Defamation	Injuring the good name of another person by telling falsehoods about him to a third person	
Libel	Oral defamation	Saying someone is a thief
Slander	Written defamation	Writing that someone is a thief

* Adapted from Springer, E. W., ed.: Nursing and the Law. p. 52. Pittsburgh, Aspen Systems Corporation, 1970.

† They usually occur together, so the popular term for such a wrong is "Assault and Battery." But either act may occur separately: threatening to strike somebody, an assault; touching someone without consent or warning, a battery without assault.

First degree murder is illegally killing another person with malice aforethought. *Second degree murder* is killing another person but without previous deliberation. In some states, second degree murder is referred to as *manslaughter*. First and second degree murders are felonies.

A person practicing nursing (or medicine) unlawfully and whose patient dies as a result of the illegal practice can be tried for the felony of manslaughter. Additional examples of crimes include rape, mayhem, robbery, accessories to crime, extortion, and blackmail.

ADDITIONAL LAWS OF INTEREST TO NURSES: THE NURSING STUDENT'S LEGAL STATUS; GOOD SAMARITAN LAWS; NARCOTIC LAWS; FEDERAL FOOD, DRUG AND COSMETIC ACT; WILLS

The Nursing Student's Legal Status

In hospital-controlled programs, the nursing student has been considered an employee of the agency. The student is responsible for her own act of negligence if injury to a patient results. The hospital can also be held liable under the principle of *respondeat superior*, which states that an employer is responsible for his employee's acts. The status of students enrolled in college and university programs is not clear since there appears to be no evidence of the status having been defined in a court of law.

Patients harmed by student acts may bring suit for damages against an instructor-supervisor also. An instructor-supervisor can be held responsible for reasonable and prudent supervision of students. Through student assignments, she is vouching for fitness and competency. If standards of supervision are violated, negligence may be charged. If students feel their assignments are beyond their competency, it is recommended that they call attention to this to the instructor-supervisor responsible for the assignment.

This is the way one author on the subject discussed student negligence: "Although it may seem a harsh rule at first, a student nurse is held to the standard of a competent professional nurse in the performance of nursing duties. In several judicial decisions, the courts have indicated that anyone who acts as a nurse by performing duties customarily performed by professional nurses is held to the standards of a professional nurse. . . From the patient's point of view, it would be unfair to deprive him of the opportunity to recover from the injury because the hospital uses students to provide nursing care to him." (12:8)

A student nurse cannot safely assume that an employer (health agency or another health practitioner) has malpractice insurance to cover her in a manner satisfactory to her. Investigation of the policy is urged. After examination, the student may feel more secure if she has her own insurance also. Since there are records of students being sued, it may be desirable to consider malpractice insurance. Malpractice insurance is available from many commercial insurance companies. It is also available for students through the National Nursing Students' Association, and for graduate nurses through the American Nurses' Association.

Good Samaritan Laws

Good samaritan laws are laws designed to hold physicians and nurses harmless when they undertake to give aid to persons in emergency situations. For example, if a physician happens onto the scene of an auto accident, he may give emergency care as he deems necessary without fear of legal suit, unless he performs in a grossly negligent fashion.

Most states have a good samaritan law although they vary considerably. Nurses are covered in some states, while in others, they are not. So far, there appears to be no common law resulting from decisions based on these statutes. As a result, the manner in which these laws would be interpreted in a court case remains speculative. Many laws give certain persons immunity, and some provide standards of care in emergency situations with phrases such as actions in "good faith" or actions "without gross negligence." These descriptions of standards and the immunities would appear to decrease likelihood of liability and hence, tend to encourage health practitioners to render assistance at the scene of an emergency.

There remains considerable dilemma in emergency situations involving not only legal implications but moral and ethical considerations as well. No person has a legal obligation to help another and a health practitioner, as any other person, may choose to help or to leave the scene of an emergency. However, in many situations, there would seem to be a moral or ethical responsibility to assist. When health practitioners do assist and consent is not possible prior to giving care, they are expected to use good judgment in determining whether an emergency exists and to give care that a reasonably prudent person with a similar background and in a similar circumstance would give.

Narcotic Laws

The Harrison Narcotic Act is a federal law having as its primary purpose to control and suppress the illegal use and distribution of narcotics. In turn, states have their own Uniform Narcotic Drug Act to further regulate narcotics. Violators of these acts are prosecuted either under federal or state law as indicated. Wrong acts are considered as acts of crime.

Narcotic laws provide for the registration of those who may prescribe narcotics, such as physicians, dentists, and veterinarians. Nurses ordinarily act under the supervision of a registered person in the eyes of the laws and hence, are not required to be registered to administer prescribed narcotics. Narcotic laws are specific and violations are serious offenses.

Federal Food, Drug, and Cosmetic Act

Among other things, this act is concerned with non-narcotics, such as hypnotic and barbiturate drugs, and with certain other "dangerous" drugs. Only qualified persons, such as physicians and dentists, may prescribe drugs described in this law. The nurse's role relates to the administration of these drugs.

Wills

State laws regulate requirements for a will. Nurses sometimes are asked to witness a will. By so doing, the nurse, as a witness, indicates that the will was signed by the *testator*, the person who made the will in which he describes intentions which he wishes to be carried out upon his death. Also, the witness to a will indicates that to the best of his knowledge, the testator was of sound mind and that he acted voluntarily.

Wills occasionally specify intention in relation to autopsies and organ donations. Consent necessary when wills do not specify wishes will be discussed in Chapter 31.

DEFENSE OF THE ACCUSED

A *lawsuit* is a legal action in a court. *Litigation* is the process of a lawsuit. The person or government bringing suit against another is called the *plaintiff*. The one being accused of a tort or crime is called the *defendant*. The defendant has every opportunity in our courts of law to defend himself and certain specific defenses for torts and crimes have already

been mentioned. Philosophically, a defendant is presumed innocent unless proven guilty. Recent U. S. Supreme Court decisions, some of which gained considerable publicity, were predicated on the tenet that in our country every effort shall be directed toward justice for the accused. Hence, being accused of a tort or a crime does not imply guilt.

NURSE PRACTICE ACTS

It has been pointed out that the federal and state constitutions provide for governments that we as individuals charge with the responsibility of securing the public welfare. Legislative bodies have used this principle to enact laws that control certain occupational and professional groups. In other words, to secure public welfare, laws governing these groups are designed to prevent incompetent persons from practicing by establishing minimum standards which qualified practitioners must meet. In general the goal of these laws is accomplished through two channels: schools preparing practitioners must maintain certain minimum standards of education; and graduates of the educational programs may be licensed only after satisfactory completion of an examination. In addition, these laws include certain other requirements, such as citizenship.

Nursing is one group operating under state statutory laws that were designed in keeping with federal and state constitutional principles to promote the general welfare. The first law in the United States dealing with the practice of nursing was enacted in 1903 in North Carolina. At the present time there are nurse practice acts in the 50 states, the District of Columbia, Puerto Rico, and the Virgin Islands.

The laws vary considerably from state to state. Some laws define nursing, while others describe what a nurse may or may not do in the practice of nursing. In some states the law requires that a nurse be licensed in order to practice; such a law usually is referred to as a *mandatory nurse practice act*. In other states, the law merely allows the licensed nurse to refer to herself as a registered nurse or an R.N.; such a law usually is referred to as a *permissive nurse practice act*, since a license is not required in order to practice.

The administrative agency in each state that has power to make regulations in relation to nurse practice acts is the state board of nursing. The regulations made by these boards become laws in themselves, as previously described. Some typical responsibilities of these state boards include determining minimum standards for education for nursing, setting requirements for licensure, and deciding when a nurse's license may be suspended or revoked.

Nurses who actively supported and worked hard for enactment of nurse practice acts are worthy of much credit. But modifications in earlier laws continue. For example, a change, actively being sought in many states, would broaden the legal definition of nursing in order that nurses may assume greater responsibilities legally as their roles expand. In some states, this has already been accomplished, as a study situation at the end of this chapter illustrates.

Nurses also have a responsibility to work toward the defeat of proposed legislation which would appear to be against nursing and the public welfare. A study situation refers to legislation under consideration in certain areas which many nurses feel is regressive in nature.

ETHICS AND THE CODE OF ETHICS FOR NURSES

The word ethics has its origin in the Greek word *ethos*, meaning customs or habitual modes of conduct. *Ethics* is now referred to as a discipline that concerns itself with human actions in respect to their being right or wrong.

The ethics of various professions are described in codes. Through its code, each professional group sets standards of practice for its members. The purpose of a code is to promote high standards of competence among its members. An ethical code derives from the dignity and the rights of the patient as a person. It indicates acceptance of the trust and of the responsibility the patient places in the profession.

Ethical codes cannot be enforced by committees and panels. Rather, each practitioner is expected to assume the obligation to uphold and adhere to the code of her professional society. Enforcement depends on one's conscience and heart rather than on a law-enforcement officer.

The code of ethics for nurses, adopted by the American Nurses' Association in 1950 and revised in 1960 and 1968, consists of 10 statements, as follows:

1. The nurse provides services with respect for the dignity of man, unrestricted by considerations of nationality, race, creed, color, or status.

2. The nurse safeguards the individual's right to privacy by judiciously protecting information of a confidential nature, sharing only that information relevant to his care.

3. The nurse maintains individual competence in nursing practice, recognizing and accepting responsibility for individual actions and judgments.

4. The nurse acts to safeguard the patient when his care and safety are affected by incompetent, unethical, or illegal conduct of any person.

5. The nurse uses individual competence as a criterion in accepting delegated responsibilities and assigning nursing activities to others.

6. The nurse participates in research activities when assured that the rights of individual subjects are protected.

7. The nurse participates in the efforts of the profession to define and upgrade standards of nursing practice and education.

8. The nurse, acting through the professional organization, participates in establishing and maintaining conditions of employment conducive to high-quality nursing care.

9. The nurse works with members of health professions and other citizens in promoting efforts to meet health needs of the public.

10. The nurse refuses to give or imply endorsement to advertising, promotion, or sales for commercial products, services, or enterprises.

A copy of the code and an interpretation of each of the 10 statements may be obtained from the American Nurses' Association or from your state nurses' association. The code and an interpretation can be found in the appendix of the book, *The Nurse and The Law*, by Harvey Sarner; additional information concerning this book appears in Reference entry 11 at the end of this chapter. In addition, the same material appeared in the *American Journal of Nursing* in December 1968; additional information for this article appears in Reference entry 1 at the end of this chapter.

CONCLUSION

Chapter 3 described three principles serving as guides to practitioners offering society health care services. These three principles are directly related to legislation concerning nursing practice also. For instance, the first principle—each person is a unique human being—serves as a guide to legislators when laws are enacted to protect man's uniqueness and his rights as a human being. Laws prohibiting such wrongs as invasion of privacy and false imprisonment are examples.

Consider the second and third principles relating to man as an organism and man and his environment. Nurse practice acts provide that licensed nurses have met certain minimum requirements, including a knowledge of the functioning of the human body,

FUNDAMENTALS OF NURSING

and can be expected to give prudent care. Nurses are also expected to know what environmental factors may interfere with well-being and give care safe from environmental injury and harm to the extent possible under given circumstances. Note that the law protects society by holding the nurse responsible if care fails to meet reasonable standards.

Graduate and student nurses, as individuals and as members of their profession, are legally and ethically responsible for their acts and are committed to the promotion of the public welfare. While discussion on the legal and ethical aspects of nursing is necessarily brief in this text, the reader is urged to study references and news media reports, especially reports appearing in nursing periodicals, to keep informed and up to date on the legal and ethical components of nursing.

Study Situations

1. The following editorial refers to institutional licensure, that is, the licensing of practitioners by employing agencies (such as a hospital) which would judge the practitioner's competency to practice:

Schorr, T. M.: Back to the dark ages? (Editorial). **Am. J. of Nurs.,** 72:1071, June, 1972.

Ms. Schorr ends the editorial by stating that "Abdicating accountability to the employing institution is a regressive act and one that professionals should not agree to." Do you agree with the statement? Why?

2. "The law does not require that a person be provided absolute protection from injury." This quote is taken from the following article:

Hershey, N.: Safety of the difficult patient. **Am. J. Nurs.,** 71:1766–1767, Sept., 1971.

How does the author explain the statement given above? Note in the case cited, the court concluded that an emergency was created by the patient and not by negligence of personnel.

3. The **American Journal of Nursing** has a section entitled "NEWS." Refer to this section in 6 or 8 recent issues of the magazine and review reports concerned with legislation with implications for nursing. Here are a few examples to begin your review:

• ANA calls for moratorium on licensure of new types of health workers. 71:1487, Aug., 1971.
• Governor vetoes New York nursing bill, NYSNA responds: "shocking rejection." 71:1485, Aug., 1971.
• Rockefeller signs NYSNA nursing bill vetoed last year. 72:615, Apr., 1972.
• Amendment to Arizona nursing practice law broadens definition of professional nursing. 72:1203, July, 1972.

After reading several reports similar to those cited

above, how effectual do you believe nursing is in influencing legislation in relation to the practice of nursing? How did nurses in New York and Arizona believe modifications in their nurse practice acts benefited society and nursing?

4. A legal authority was quoted on page 44, concerning negligence and the student nurse. The following article describes cases in which nursing students were alleged to have fallen short of competent nursing standards:

Hershey, N.: Routine procedures and the standard of practice. **Am. J. Nurs.,** 70:529–30, Mar., 1970.

5. In the following article, the author proposes consumer input in the setting and securing of ethical standards for nursing:

Levin, L. S.: Time to hear a different drum. **Am. J. Nurs.,** 72:2007–2010, Nov., 1972.

Describe how you react to what the author calls a precedent-setting opportunity for nurses and consumers to join forces in dealing with matters related to quality of nursing performance.

References

1. Code for nurses. **Am. J. Nurs.,** 68:2581–2585, Dec., 1968.
2. Creighton, H.: Law Every Nurse Should Know. ed. 2. Philadelphia, W. B. Saunders, 1970.
3. Donahue, J. C., guest ed.: Symposium on the nurse and the law. In **The Nursing Clinics of North America.** Philadelphia, W. B. Saunders, 2:115–197, Mar., 1967.
4. Gibbs, G. E.: Will continuing education be required for license renewal? **Am. J. Nurs.,** 71:2175–2179, Nov., 1971.
5. Hershey, N.: Prudence and the coffee break. **Am. J. Nurs.,** 70:2389–2390, Nov., 1970.
6. ———: When is a communication privileged? **Am. J. Nurs.,** 70:112–113, Jan., 1970.
7. ———: Who and what next in licensure? **Am. J. Nurs.,** 71:105–107, Jan., 1971.
8. Lesnik, M. J., and Anderson, B. E.: Nursing Practice and The Law. ed. 2. Philadelphia, J. B. Lippincott, 1962.
9. McGriff, E. P.: A case for mandatory continuing education in nursing. **Nurs. Outlook,** 20:712–713, Nov., 1972.
10. Miller, C.: Nurses and the Law. Danville, Ill., Interstate Printers and Publishers, 1970.
11. Sarner, H.: The Nurse and the Law. Philadelphia, W. B. Saunders, 1968.
12. Springer, E. W., ed.: Nursing and the Law. Pittsburgh, Aspen Systems Corporation, Health Law Center, 1970.
13. Willig, S.: Nursing and the law. In Orem, D. E.: Nursing: Concepts of Practice. pp. 175–220. New York, McGraw-Hill, 1971.
14. ———: The Nurse's Guide To The Law. New York, McGraw-Hill, 1970.

UNIT 2

The Nursing Process System

CHAPTER 5

Description of the Nursing Process System

GLOSSARY · INTRODUCTION · GENERAL SYSTEMS THEORY · THE
NURSING PROCESS SYSTEM · ENVIRONMENTAL INFLUENCES ON
THE NURSING PROCESS SYSTEM · VALUES OF USING THE NURSING
PROCESS SYSTEM · CONCLUSION · STUDY SITUATIONS ·
REFERENCES

GLOSSARY

Closed System: A system that does not exchange stimuli with its environment.

Constraint: A limitation in resources available to a system.

Criterion: A standard of measurement.

Evaluation: The measurement of success or failure.

Feedback: The procedure of placing certain information back into a system. Information is obtained by comparing the output of a system or subsystem with performance criteria.

Input: Information that enters a system or subsystem.

Nursing Process: Sum total of nursing care activities performed to aid in promoting the patient's well-being.

Nursing Process System: A set of actions used to determine, plan, and implement nursing care.

Open System: A system that is exchanging stimuli with its environment.

Output: The end product of a system or subsystem.

Performance Criteria: Standards of measurement.

Process: A set of actions leading to a particular result.

Stimulus: An incentive or spur to action.

Subsystem: A lesser system which is part of a whole system.

System: A set of interrelated or interacting thing or parts, forming a unified whole.

Trade-off: An alternative method of accomplishing a system's purpose.

INTRODUCTION

A study of nursing demonstrates that it is no longer sufficient for the nurse to be skillful in carrying out such actions as giving an injection and cooling a fevered brow. In her present role, the task of promoting high-level wellness for the patient she serves is almost always a complex and intricate process. As Chapter 3 indicates, each human being is unique, multifaceted in structure and function, and constantly relating and interrelating to an ever-changing environment. The nurse must be able to analyze, critically, factors within each situation and make sound, creative decisions relative to dealing with the many variables involved.

Nurses have worked and continue to work in developing approaches to providing nursing care that is high in quality and geared to the needs of each patient. Various approaches have been researched and tried. Within the last decade or so, the nursing process system has been analyzed in greater detail as one means of providing high quality nursing care.

This text uses the phrase *nursing process* to refer to the sum total of nursing care activities performed to attain and maintain high-level wellness for the patient. The nursing process system, defined and described later in this chapter, has been developed from general systems theory. A brief orientation to systems theory is helpful to an understanding of the nursing process system.

GENERAL SYSTEMS THEORY

A *system* is a set of interrelated or interacting things or parts forming a unified whole. For example, a railroad system has parts such as trains, tracks, stations, and signals. Each part has its own purpose; each part is related to all other parts, and all of the parts together form the unified whole, namely the railroad system. Most systems are composed of lesser systems commonly referred to as *subsystems*. In the railroad system, the train may be thought of as one subsystem. It has parts: the engine, caboose, freight cars, passenger cars, and so on. Each part of the train is related to all other parts of the train. The sum of these parts is equal to the whole, namely the train. Each subsystem has its purpose. For example, the purpose of the train is to carry freight and passengers; the purpose of the tracks is to carry the train, and so on. The purpose of the railroad system, transportation of passengers and freight, has been achieved when the purpose of each subsystem has been achieved.

Input is the material or information which enters a system. It is used in whatever manner is appropriate to achieve the purpose of the system. Assume you wish to select a dessert for a dinner party you are giving. You would need certain information, such as the number of people attending your party, the amount of time you have to prepare a dessert, the amount of money you can afford to spend, and preferences of your guests. All the information just cited would be important to consider when you select the dessert. That information is the input for your system.

Output is the end product of a system. In the example given above, the output of the system is the selection of dessert that you will prepare and which you will then serve to your guests.

Evaluation is the measurement of success or failure. General systems theory uses continuous evaluation; that is, there is not a separate subsystem devoted to evaluation. The nursing process system, developed from general systems theory, does not consider evaluation separately but treats it as a part which is constantly functioning in the entire system, as well as in each subsystem.

How does one evaluate in order to determine success or failure? A *criterion* (plural: *criteria*) is a standard of measurement. Standards of measurement are specific descriptions of the expectations of the system's output. Usually, the phrase *performance criteria* is used in general systems theory and will be used in the nursing process system as well, to describe standards of measurement.

Remember the county fairs when favorite baked goods were entered and prizes were awarded for the best goods? The judges of the pies, for example, decided that pies would be judged on the basis of appearance, texture of the crust, texture of the filling, and taste. These standards on which the pies were judged served as performance criteria.

In systems theory, how does one use the information one obtains after comparing the output of a system or one of its subsystems with performance criteria? Stated in another way, how does one use the results of evaluation in systems theory? It is used in the procedure called *feedback*. If the output of the system does not meet performance criteria, that information is fed back into the system and appropriate adjustments or modifications are made. If evaluation demonstrates that the purpose of the system is being achieved, that information is fed back into the system to tell the operator to continue with the action until the purpose of the system is met. This latter feedback tells the operator that he is on the right track. If evaluation demonstrates that the purpose of the system has been achieved, the system process can be terminated by the operator.

Recall the example when systems theory was used to select a dessert. When you compared your selection with your performance criteria, assume you became aware that the dessert selected was inappropriate since you did not have time to prepare that particular dish. That information—lack of sufficient time to prepare it—is fed back into your system. The selection process and feedback will continue until you find a dessert that meets all of the performance criteria you have set. If feedback tells you that you are on the right track, you continue your search in the manner you have been using. When the dessert that meets performance criteria is selected, the systems process is discontinued since you have then achieved your purpose.

As this unit illustrates, feedback is an important part in the selection and carrying out of nursing care activities that are appropriate to meet a particular patient's needs.

A *stimulus* (plural: *stimuli*) is an incentive or spur to action. A system is considered to be *open* when it is exchanging stimuli with its environment. Because of the mutual, continuing interaction between man and his environment, any system which involves human beings has to be an open system. Nursing involves humans and therefore, the nursing process system is an open system. A *closed* system is one that is not influenced by its environment. Combining chemical constituents in a controlled laboratory experiment is an example of a system which does not exchange stimuli with its environment and therefore, is closed.

Figure 5-1 illustrates a general system.

There are occasions when a solution to a problem may be identified but is unsuitable for one reason or another. For example, a youngster requiring hospitalization is crying because she is lonesome for her parents who left after visiting hours had ended. Calling the parents to return is considered an unsuitable solution since it is not consistent with

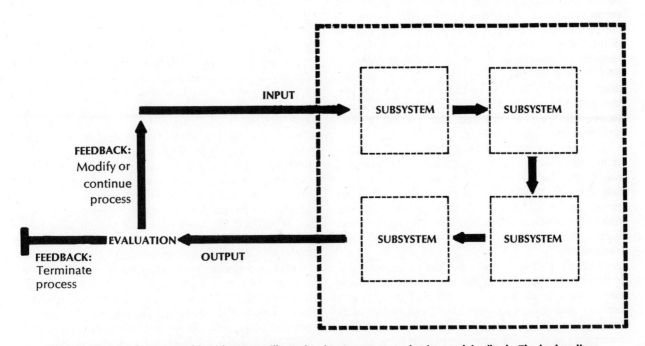

Fig. 5-1. A general system and its subsystems, illustrating input, output, evaluation, and feedback. The broken lines in the diagram are used to indicate that the system is open and hence, environmental influences are constantly affecting the system.

hospital policy. A limitation in resources available to a system, as in this example, is referred to as a *constraint*.

Possibly an alternative solution can be found to comfort the child. Will staying with the child and reading to her be a solution? An alternative method that circumvents the constraint but still accomplishes the system's purpose is referred to as a *trade-off*. Nurses often find that realistic limitations exist in patient situations and in health care settings. Hence, alternative methods frequently must be chosen.

Applications of general systems theory exist all around us. It is used in biology, physics, mathematics, psychology, sociology, engineering, business, and countless other areas. Systems are used to reserve a hotel room or an airplane ticket from any point in the world. They play an important role in the design of next year's models of automobiles and have been of dramatic significance in making space travel an accomplished fact. They have been used to explain and predict man's ability to maintain a constant body temperature in environmental conditions with thermometer readings above and below his temperature. In short, general systems theory has universal applications.

THE NURSING PROCESS SYSTEM

A *process* is defined as a set of actions leading to a particular result. For example, the process of sewing a dress consists of all necessary actions from threading a needle to tying the last knot in the thread used in the hem. The *nursing process system* is a set of actions used to determine, plan, and implement nursing care. The actions are dynamic; that is, they change, influence each other, and constantly interrelate with one another. The purpose of the nursing process system, as we said, is to give that care which will aid the patient to attain and maintain high-level wellness. The input (that is, the information that enters the nursing process system) is data about the patient and his environment. The output of the nursing process system describes the patient's health status. The performance criterion is evidence that the patient's state of wellness has been improved or maintained.

When the patient's health state is compared with performance criteria, the nurse then has information for feedback. She will make decisions during the procedure of feedback as follows. The nurse decides that the purpose of the system has been met, and then the nursing process system ends since the patient no longer requires the care the nurse has been giving. Or, the nurse decides the patient is progressing toward the goal of the nursing process system in a satisfactory manner, and the process is continued until the goal is reached. Or, she decides that the goals of the system are not being met, and so she retraces her steps in the nursing process system and revises and modifies as necessary. An example will help to illustrate the nursing process system as just described.

A nurse is to care for an acutely ill patient. One of her observations is that the patient's mouth and gum tissues appear dry and very red. Dried mucus is lodged on his teeth. The patient indicates that his mouth feels sticky and dry. The nurse's observations and the patient's comments are part of the data that is fed into the nursing process system; it is the system's input.

From her study of anatomy and physiology and from her own experience, the nurse is familiar with the appearance of normal mouth and gum tissues and of the teeth when good oral hygiene has been observed and when acute illness is not present. Her conclusion is that this patient's mouth is in an unhealthy state. She decides he needs nursing services that include special mouth care. The goal of giving the mouth care is to attain and maintain good oral health. The nurse then designs a plan of care with the patient to achieve that goal and puts her plan of care into action.

After giving mouth care for several days, the nurse observes that the teeth are clean of mucus and the tissues do not appear dry nor are they as red as they were before mouth care was started. Also, the patient states his mouth now feels clean and comfortable. These are examples of responses to the special mouth care the nurse gave and are part of the output of the nursing process system for this patient.

The nurse is now ready to compare these responses with the performance criterion. She notes that the patient's level of wellness has been increased. The performance criterion has been met. This information is now used in the procedure of feedback. The nurse will continue with the care she is giving in order to maintain clean and healthy mouth tissues and teeth if factors in the patient's total situation indicates that without such care, the health of the patient's mouth is likely to deteriorate again. This could occur, for example, if the patient continues to be acutely ill. Or, the nurse will discontinue the special mouth care since the purpose for giving it has been met and in her opinion, the patient no longer requires the care.

As we have learned, a patient's optimum level of wellness is based on knowledge of realistic limitations he may have. The nurse learns that, for some patients, maintaining the same level of wellness is an achievement when that level would decrease without nursing assistance. For example, when caring for a patient whose life is ebbing, high-level wellness may be maintained when the patient feels comfortable and has reached the point of accepting his condition. This is true also at times for patients with chronic diseases. For example, the patient who has permanent physical handicaps because of an arthritic condition is often maintaining his highest level of wellness when handicaps do not further limit his ability to care for his own daily hygienic needs.

There will be times when the patient feels that his progress toward high-level wellness is too slow. Possibly the goals were unrealistic to begin with, or he did not understand the anticipated amount of time it would take to note progress. Perhaps no one had predicted the time required because other problems arose in the situation that delayed progress. In such instances, the nurse will wish to retrace her steps and redefine goals of care with the patient that are more realistic and less frustrating in terms of time for noting progress and for accomplishing the goal.

The nursing process system is composed of four subsystems: *data gathering, assessment, planning nursing care,* and *nursing intervention.* These subsystems are described in the next four chapters of this unit. After reading those chapters, it is recommended that you return to the example given earlier concerning the patient who required and was given special mouth care. You will note that although they were not specified and defined in the example, the four subsystems can be readily identified.

A diagram of the nursing process system appears in Figure 5-2.

ENVIRONMENTAL INFLUENCES ON THE NURSING PROCESS SYSTEM

Human beings are constantly being influenced by their environment; therefore, environmental influences may affect the nursing process system at any point and necessitate changes, since the system is an open system. For example, a nurse who has been supervising a woman's prenatal care will need to make adjustments when the patient reports that her husband has just learned that he has pulmonary tuberculosis. A nurse may need to make certain modifications in her care of a family when she learns

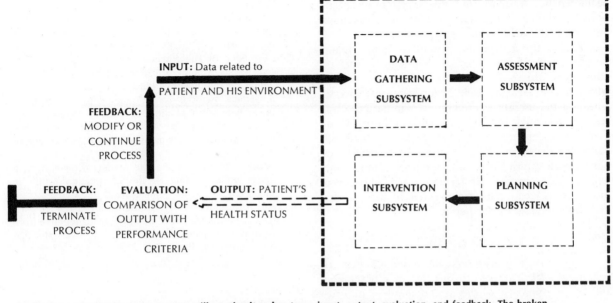

Fig. 5-2. The nursing process system, illustrating its subsystems, input, output, evaluation, and feedback. The broken lines in the diagram are used to indicate that the system is open and hence, environmental influences are constantly affecting the system.

that one of the teen-age members of the family is using illicit drugs. A community health program will be influenced by the effects of a flood in the community. A hospitalized patient learns that his father is seriously ill, and his nursing care requirements change when the patient demonstrates anxiety and concern. A spell of dry, windy weather may influence the care of a patient who has hay fever. Any number of additional examples could be cited.

In the succeeding chapters that describe the subsystems of the nursing process system, in order to avoid unnecessary duplications, environmental influences are not described in separate sections. However, it must be emphasized that the influences are constantly there. Hence, the nurse will have to remain alert to them, treat them as new data entering the subsystem, and modify nursing care accordingly.

VALUES OF USING THE NURSING PROCESS SYSTEM

While on first reading, the nursing process system may seem complicated, with practice the use of the system can become an invaluable tool for the nurse. One of its greatest values is that it can be used in any situation in which a nurse gives care. It is adaptable to every patient even though no two individuals are alike. The great practicality and adapt-

ability of the nursing process system not only saves time but contributes to high quality and individualized care.

Another value in using the nursing process system is that it provides for constant evaluation which in turn serves as a basis for improving care at all stages. Traditionally, the basis for evaluating much of the nursing care being given was the nurse's efficiency. Currently, emphasis is placed on the patient's level of wellness. The nursing process system's built-in evaluation focuses on each phase of the process and on the *patient* and his health status.

The nursing process system is responsive to changes within the person and to environmental influences. There is allowance for constant new input since it is an open system. It makes allowances for constraints or limitations, as well as for possible trade-offs or options, two particularly significant features that help to individualize the care of each person.

It has often been said that the difference between mediocre nursing care and high quality care is dependent on the quality of decisions the nurse makes. The nursing process system is a logical, organized way of approaching a nursing care problem and allows for great creativity, limited only by the potential of the nurse giving care. It is oriented toward attaining objectives. It demands critical thinking and objective evaluation. Helping a human being with a health problem is a complicated matter. The characteristics of the nursing process system just mentioned will help the nurse to make wise decisions and give high quality care.

This is the age of the computer. While many people are fearful of the dehumanizing effects of computers, this will occur only if man allows it. Many health facilities have begun extensive investigation of the usefulness of computers in patient care, and progress holds much promise for the future. General systems theory has been used as the basis for computer development. The nurse who familiarizes herself with the theory and its application to nursing will be preparing herself for that time when even more use will be made of computers in the delivery of health services to the public.

CONCLUSION

The nursing process system, based on general systems theory, is offered in this text as a systematic and sound approach to the development of individualized nursing care. It provides a framework of functioning for the novice in nursing and for the experienced practitioner. Expertise in its use will come with practice and with the acquisition of new knowledge and skill in the nurse's daily nursing practice.

Study Situations

1. The following programmed book gives a "fun" approach to explaining systems analysis and design as applied to engineering:
   Corrigan, R. E., and Kaufman, R. A.: Why System Engineering. 71 p. Palo Alto, Calif., Fearon Publishers, 1966.
   Read it and see if you can select the right answers. After you have finished, think about its application to the nursing process system.

2. "To be therapeutic the nurse must contribute to the wholeness of man, to the person's here-and-now as well as to his future, to the health of all the parts so that the person may attain and maintain his highest potential."
   This quote was taken from the following article:
   Lewis, L.: This I believe . . . about the nursing process—key to care. **Nurs. Outlook,** 16:26–29, May, 1968.
   How does the nursing process system aid in meeting this author's objective of nursing care, as stated in the quote? Describe the author's definition of the nursing process and compare it with the definition given in Chapter 5?

3. The author of the article given below wrote that nursing is a system in which there are at least two components: the patient and the nurse. She also refers to a family system, political systems, health care systems, economic systems, cultural systems, and so on.

After reading the article, identify some of the subsystems that you believe exist in these systems.
   Hazzard, M. E.: An overview of systems theory. *In* **The Nursing Clinics of North America.** Philadelphia, W. B. Saunders, 6:385–393, Sept., 1971.

4. In the issue of **The Nursing Clinics of North America** referred to in Study Situation 3, there are articles in which various health problems are approached with a systems method. Even though you may be unfamiliar with some of the diagnoses of patients in the articles, look for the systems methods used. Note the diagrams and compare them with the figures used in Chapter 5.

5. A study technique to aid the reader in developing a better understanding of the information found in this chapter is recommended. Read this chapter again and in instances where examples are given to illustrate a particular point, describe an experience from your own nursing practice that will illustrate that point equally well.

References

1. Banathy, B. H.: Instructional Systems. Palo Alto, Calif., Fearon Publishers, 1968.
2. Byrne, M. L., and Thompson, L. F.: Key Concepts for the Study and Practice of Nursing. St. Louis, C. V. Mosby, 1972.
3. Carlson, S.: A practical approach to the nursing process. **Am. J. Nurs.,** 72:1589–1591, Sept. 1972.
4. Carrieri, V. K., and Sitzman, J.: Components of the nursing process. *In* **Nursing Clinics of North America.** Philadelphia, W. B. Saunders, 6:115–124, Mar., 1971.
5. Cornell, S. A., and Brush, F.: Systems approach to nursing care plans. **Am. J. Nurs.,** 71:1376–1378, July, 1971.
6. Finch, J.: Systems analysis: a logical approach to professional nursing care. **Nurs. Forum,** 8:176–190, No. 2, 1969.
7. Goshen, C. E.: Your automated future. **Am. J. Nurs.,** 72:62–67, Jan., 1972.
8. Interdisciplinary sessions consider systems approach. **Am. J. Nurs.,** 71:880, May, 1971.
9. Lewis, L.: This I believe . . . about the nursing process—key to care. **Nurs. Outlook,** 16:26–29, May, 1968.
10. McKay, R.: Theories, models, and systems for nursing. **Nurs. Research,** 18:393–399, Sept.–Oct., 1969.
11. Mauksch, I. G., and David, M. L.: Prescription for survival. **Am. J. Nurs.,** 72:2189–2193, Dec., 1972.
12. Mayr, O.: The origins of feedback control. **Sci. Am.,** 223:110–118, Oct., 1970.
13. Pierce, L. M.: Usefulness of a systems approach for problem conceptualization and investigation. **Nurs. Research,** 21:509–513, Nov.–Dec., 1972.
14. von Bertalanffy, L.: General System Theory: Foundations, Development, Application. New York, George Braziller, 1968.
15. Zimmerman, D. S., and Gohrke, C.: The goal-directed nursing approach: it does work. **Am. J. Nurs.,** 70:306–310, Feb., 1970.

CHAPTER 6

Data Gathering

GLOSSARY · INTRODUCTION · THE PROCESS OF DATA GATHERING ·
FEEDBACK · CONCLUSION · STUDY SITUATIONS · REFERENCES

GLOSSARY

Health State Profile: Outline or diagram of a patient's illness-wellness status.

Inspect: To examine systematically for a purpose. *Prob.-Solv. Approach*

Interview: To talk over something with a person or persons, usually in a face-to-face meeting. *assessment*

Observe: To watch carefully for facts that may be significant.

Relevant: Having a bearing upon, having influence, or being connected in some way with the situation under consideration.

Validate: To confirm or to verify.

INTRODUCTION

Data gathering is the first subsystem in the nursing process system. It is totally vital. Without accurate and appropriate data, the system cannot function properly to provide nursing care that will meet the patient's needs. It is the means to put the nursing process system into action. There is no one point at which data gathering stops. New information continues to be collected and added as it becomes evident and necessary to assist in meeting patient needs. If the total of patient care needs is viewed as a mosaic, the data are pieces playing a critical role in completing the picture.

The *purpose* of data gathering is to collect and organize information related to the patient's state of health. The *input* of data gathering is that information. A *profile* is an outline or diagram of collected data. The *output* of data gathering is the *health state profile*, that is, an outline or diagram of a patient's illness-wellness status. The *performance criteria*, or the standards used to judge the profile, are appropriateness and accuracy of data. Figure 6-1 illustrates data gathering input, process, output, performance criteria, and feedback.

THE PROCESS OF DATA GATHERING

The process of data gathering is described in six phases: selecting appropriate data; organizing the data; selecting methods to gather data; the gathering of data; validating data; and evaluating data by comparing them with performance criteria. Figure 6-2 is a flow chart illustrating the data-gathering process.

Selecting Appropriate Data

Analyzing a situation that involves humans can be a complicated and difficult procedure because of man's very complex nature. Data gathering concerning a patient would be endless if one wished to amass every piece of information that could be found. Before starting, the nurse needs to make a decision by asking the question, What data are appropriate in *this* patient's situation?

Appropriate data are *relevant* data, that is, having a bearing upon, an influence on, or some connection with the situation under consideration. Here are some questions, the answers to which will aid in the selection of relevant data. Who is the patient? For what reason is he being considered for receiving nursing care? What factors in this patient's life are playing a part in his present situation?

As mentioned earlier in this text, the patient may be an individual, a family, a neighborhood, a community, or others. A single patient may be encountered in a variety of settings, as for example, in a hospital, a community health center, a clinic, a physician's office, or at home. When a community is the nurse's responsibility, she might be concerned with all persons living in a housing development, a neighborhood, or a government-determined area such as a county, city, or state.

To illustrate, if the nurse is responsible for health care in a rural county, she would probably focus her attention on environmental factors related to the

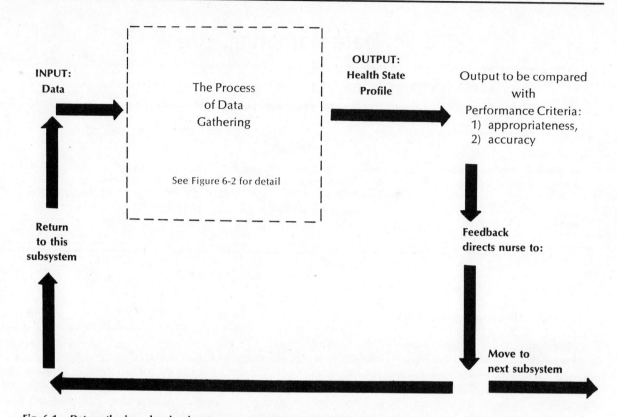

Fig. 6-1. Data gathering, showing input, process, output, performance criteria, and feedback. Broken line indicates environmental influences may affect process at any time, as described in Chapter 5.

health of its citizens. For example, she may collect data on the incidence of injuries occurring while using farm machinery or on the purity of common water supplies. If she is caring for a family, relationships among family members may need study when, for instance, there are young children in the home and the mother has a degenerative disease. As these examples illustrate, knowing who the patient is will aid in the selection of data relevant to the situation.

The reason for which the patient is to receive care helps determine a framework for data gathering. Providing care for the patient who has come to the industrial nurse's office after he has had an on-the-job injury requires information different from that needed when giving immunizations to children being cared for by the school nurse. The nurse caring for a patient who has premature labor contractions in the maternity unit of a hospital requires a particular kind of data. Still different information is needed by

the community health nurse serving a neighborhood with a high population of women in childbearing years when it is learned that there is a threat of an increase in the incidence of rubella (German measles). The nurse caring for a patient with severe head injuries following an automobile accident would need still different data from that required in any of the foregoing examples.

The nurse's general knowledge helps her to select appropriate data. For example, she learns that cow's milk contains no iron and that babies who do not have iron-containing food added to their diets after their maternal supply is depleted will generally develop anemia. This knowledge helps the nurse to determine what information is pertinent to gather in relation to a one-year-old child's diet. As another example, the nurse who knows what complications commonly are associated with diabetes mellitus, and how they can be prevented, will gather data about a

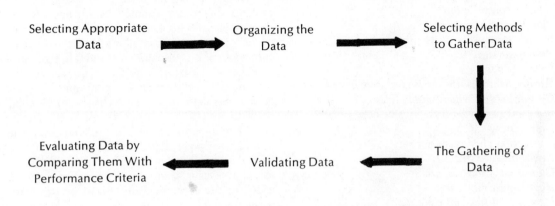

Fig. 6-2.   Flow chart illustrating data gathering process.

patient's understanding of his therapeutic regimen.

Because people interpret new situations by drawing upon past experiences, the nurse will attempt to gather data from the patient's past experiences that may have an influence on his present situation. For example, the manner in which a person coped with an emergency appendectomy three years ago may influence his response to surgery today. The manner in which a community organized itself to promote polio immunizations would undoubtedly be significant information when plans are being made to implement a veneral disease education program for the same community.

The nurse's own past experiences also influence her observations, and she should be careful not to jump to conclusions. For example, a nurse had an experience with an elderly lady, with disheveled hair, who said she had no interest in her personal appearance. When the nurse next cared for an elderly patient with uncombed hair, she concluded that the patient was uninterested in her personal appearance. Had she investigated further, she would have learned that the second patient could not comb her hair because of arthritis in her shoulders. Not all patients are alike; things are not always what they appear to be. The nurse should recognize her own biases and attempt to make objective conclusions based on accurate data presented by each patient.

The three basic principles described in Chapter 3 of this text will serve as aids in the collection of appropriate data. Recognizing that a patient is a unique individual, that he has psychosocial and physiologic needs, and that he comes from a distinct type of environmental setting is important in data gathering. There may be times when all three principles will guide decision-making with equal weight.

At other times, one or two of the principles will influence decision-making to a greater extent. For example, all three principles may require equal weight in making decisions in the care of a man with injuries necessitating a long convalescence. The nurse will need to consider such factors as the injury itself and the physiologic effects it may have on the patient's normal functioning. However, of equal importance will be the effects of long convalescence on his psychological needs and his personality, and how well he is able to adapt to a setting in which his independence is limited. On the other hand, a nurse seeing another patient at the time of his annual physical examination may focus almost entirely on his physical health status.

Various authorities have developed outlines of types of information to help the nurse in the data-gathering process. The following examples serve as illustrations:

DATA AREAS PERTAINING TO THE INDIVIDUAL PATIENT[1]
Personal data: age, religion, marital status
Socio-economic and cultural influences
Concept or perception of self
Physiologic status
Adaptation to illness
　　Current illness and life pattern of illness
　　Hospital setting or health team
Understanding of treatments and procedures
　　during hospitalization
Specific fears, i.e., fear of death, procedures

[1] Carrieri, V. K., and Sitzman, J.: Components of the nursing process. *In* The Nursing Clinics of North America. Philadelphia, W. B. Saunders, 6:116, Mar., 1971.

DATA AREAS PERTAINING TO THE FAMILY[2]

Family constellation
Family health history
Health status of each family member
Economic situation
Living conditions
Family relationships, attitudes, and interaction
Community in which family lives

DATA AREAS PERTAINING TO THE COMMUNITY[3]

Community
Population characteristics
Environmental factors
Communication resources
Health information
Health facilities and resources
Community health nursing services

Organizing the Data

Once the nurse has made a decision concerning the kinds of data to gather, tentative categories are developed so that data can be organized as it is gathered. The nurse may wish to make modifications of the categories later, but the approach of tentatively preparing categories provides a system to follow and tends to prevent omission of necessary facts.

Generally, data are organized in groups with related items or topics placed together. For example, information on an individual's daily living habits might be one category; it will include the patient's eating, sleeping, exercising, and elimination habits. Items referring to a patient's understanding of his health state and related health practices could be another category and include data describing the patient's knowledge of his diagnosis, dietary restrictions, prescribed medications, and so on. Current clinical findings, including laboratory test results, body temperature, blood pressure, and overt signs, might be still another category.

If the nurse is caring for a family, one category might be family relationships. Characteristically, family members assume certain roles, the primary decision-maker being an example of one. Another category might be the family's attitudes toward health practices such as periodic health examinations and immunizations. The family's religious beliefs that may affect certain attitudes toward health practices could be included in this category.

[2] Sobol, E. G., and Robischon, P.: Family Nursing: A Study Guide. pp. 6–9. St. Louis, C. V. Mosby, 1970.
[3] Tinkham, C. W., and Voorhies, E. F.: Community Health Nursing: Evolution and Process. pp. 287–305. New York, Appleton-Century-Crofts, 1972.

Data relating to a neighborhood might have a category describing common health hazards, such as the amount and kind of air pollution and the number of active cases of tuberculosis in the neighborhood. Information on the number and kind of hospitals and clinics located within reasonable distances, public recreational facilities, active community service organizations with an interest in health promotion, and so forth, might be placed in still another category.

Many types of guides are available that are useful as aids in organizing and recording data. Most health agencies adopt specific guides for their own use. These usually are developed by persons experienced in the common care offered by the particular agency and hence, while appropriate for one setting, may not be useful elsewhere without modification. These guides are often referred to as nursing histories, community survey guides, family health histories, and so on. The guide may be a brief topical outline. Some require the nurse to write an answer to questions; other types may ask the nurse to check a response that most nearly describes the situation, and so on. References which include examples of guides and suggestions for organizing types of data are given at the end of this chapter.

The nurse should remember that suggested guides serve as aids only. The question remains: what kind of data are appropriate for *this* patient and how shall they be organized? She will want to determine also what suggested categories on a guide are appropriate for a particular patient and which are not. In addition, she will want to identify data which are pertinent for this patient but which are not asked for on the guide and then add them to her organizational scheme. Regardless of the type of guide, the final responsibility and accountability for determining the collection and organization of appropriate data belong to the nurse. The pattern for organizing data should always provide an objective and workable base for the nurse to draw relationships among the data and to make sound judgments from them.

Selecting Methods to Gather Data

Accuracy and economy of time and effort are factors to consider when deciding on methods of gathering data. Determination of the method of gathering data also is based, to a large extent, on the type of data desired.

Data-gathering methods most commonly used in nursing are observation, interviewing, and physical inspection. One or more of these methods may be used in any situation since there is usually overlap-

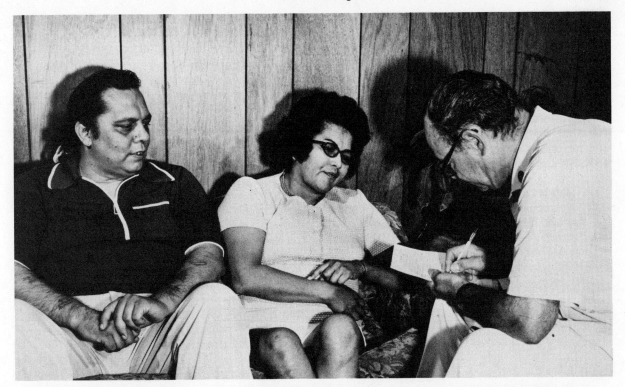

Fig. 6-3. The community health nurse is interviewing this couple to gather data he will use for assessing the family's needs and for planning nursing care. Note that the nurse has a form on which he is recording information during the interview. (Photo by Ted Hill, Arizona)

ping among them. For example, the interview and physical inspection both contain the element of observation.

To *observe* means to watch carefully for facts that may be significant. The nurse is observing when she sees a patient cry or when she sees homes in an urban ghetto in a state of disrepair. The nurse may also be observing when she listens to a person's cough or is aware of the particular odor from the discharge of a wound.

To *interview* is to talk over something with a person or persons, usually in a face-to-face meeting. When nurses interview patients, the goal is to obtain data that will be used for planning nursing care. A patient with a chronic muscle disease may be interviewed by a nurse, for example, to determine how he manages his motion with a minimum of problems. Observation and interviewing are discussed further in Chapter 13.

To *inspect* is to examine systematically, for a purpose. Physical inspection is the examination of a person. A mother uses the method when she feels a baby's forehead to detect skin temperature. The

nurse makes a systematic examination when she touches the toes of a leg in a cast to compare their temperature with that of the toes on the other extremity. As another example, the nurse is inspecting when she removes a dressing from a wound to determine whether drainage is present.

There are many tools or instruments available that help to gather data in relation to physiological functioning of the body. They vary in sophistication from the simple glass thermometer or the stethoscope to complex monitoring devices. Techniques for the use of some of these instruments are discussed in later chapters in this text.

The Gathering of Data

After completing the first three phases in the data-gathering process the nurse is ready to start the actual collection of information. To which sources should she turn for gathering data?

In most cases, the nurse will go to the patient, especially for some of the initial information she seeks. The patient's descriptions of his situation and of his state of health as he sees it, are important in understanding him as an individual.

Current records prepared by health practitioners and those kept by health agencies the patient has visited in the past are additional important sources of data. It is suggested that the nurse review available information early when gathering data and in some instances before her first contact with the patient. Then, she will wish to go on to confirm and amplify data obtained from other sources and return to the patient as necessary. Using available data helps to prevent the gathering of duplicate information. Patients who are asked the same questions again and again become understandably annoyed and fatigued. It is a waste of everyone's time, and the patient may feel distrustful of the health practitioner's interest in and ability to care for him.

Other persons who know the patient often are helpful. Family members and close friends often can make meaningful and useful contributions. Care must be taken, however, to determine that the patient does not object to information being gathered from these sources and that these other persons wish to participate. A clear understanding by the patient, his family, and friends concerning the confidential nature of the data is also important.

Other health practitioners frequently secure data that are useful to the nurse's purpose. Physicians, social workers, physical therapists, nursing personnel, and others often have information which is mutually helpful when shared. Conferences are important in the process of sharing and exchanging data.

While gathering data, the nurse should record her findings. The guides most agencies have, as mentioned earlier, usually provide space for the recording of the data. Some health agencies provide dictating facilities; that is, material is dictated and then transcribed by a secretary on an appropriate form for health practitioner use. Recording equipment may be used in some situations and is especially helpful when the nurse wishes a verbatim record of conversations she has with the patient. The nurse should inform the patient when she is taping conversations and explain their confidential nature so that she has his cooperation and permission to do so. Computers are now being used for the storage of much recorded data.

Recording data properly and accurately enhances the degree of its accuracy and completeness. Also, proper records provide a good means of communication among various health practitioners. One has only to recall how much information one tends to forget when it is not recorded to recognize the importance of record keeping in relation to patient care.

Validating the Data

Validation is the act of confirming or verifying. The purpose of validating the data is to keep the data as free from error, bias, and misinterpretation as possible. When validation suggests that certain data are inaccurate, the nurse should take steps to correct errors.

Validation of all data is neither possible nor necessary. It would be repetitious and wasteful of time and energy to attempt to do so, both for the nurse and for the patient. Consequently, the nurse should decide which items need verifying. There are several guides the nurse can use in helping her to decide which data to validate.

Validation is necessary when the nurse notes that certain data contain discrepancies. For example, a patient tells the nurse that he is fine and has no concerns, but the nurse notes that he demonstrates tense body musculature and seems curt in his responses to her comments. There is a discrepancy between what the patient is saying and what the nurse is observing and validation is indicated to determine accuracy.

It is best to validate data that has been used to make judgments or draw inferences. For example, a nurse suspects that the patient hears from one ear but does not hear well from the other. She should validate her judgment and determine whether the patient does actually have a hearing problem, and if so, what the problem is.

When there is any doubt of the accuracy of the data or when there appears to be a lack of clarity, validation is necessary. For example, a mother states that her child "hasn't eaten for a month." However, the child does not appear to be ill or undernourished, and so validation is indicated.

Very often, the patient is the best source for validating data. For example, the nurse can ask the patient if her perception of the situation is accurate. When the patient is unable to validate information, a family member or others who know the patient may be able to do so. Other health practitioners and the patient's records are also important validation sources. Certain instruments are useful for confirming data; for example, a scale can validate the patient's weight and so on. When information seems vague or indefinite, observations of the patient, his behavior, his symptoms, and his reactions and responses to nursing care may serve to validate.

The nurse may want to validate some data as she collects them, or, she may want to do so at the end of the procedure, summarizing with the patient. Certain data might be validated at a later time, rather than when gathered, as the nurse's judgment may dictate. This step in the data-gathering process often takes little time, but it is an extremely important one because it detects inaccuracies that can lead to inadequate nursing care planning.

Evaluating Data by Comparing Them with Performance Criteria

It will be recalled that the output of data gathering is a health state profile. In this last phase in the data-gathering process, the nurse should compare the profile she has prepared with the performance criteria to determine whether it is appropriate and whether it is accurate.

Determining appropriateness and accuracy requires that the nurse review all data collected for organization and omissions. Then, she should answer several questions. Does the health state profile accurately reflect the patient's present state of health? Are all relevant factors in the patient's situation being considered in the profile? Are the relationships between various factors in the patient's situation appropriate and accurate? Answers to these questions require that the nurse be honest and objective. Her skill in making judgments will increase with practice. However, failure to stop at this point in the nursing process system for an honest appraisal of the patient's health state profile can result in care that may be inappropriate.

If in the nurse's judgment, the health state profile does not meet the criteria of appropriateness and accuracy, she then becomes responsible for modifications. More data may be needed. Possibly some data appear in conflict and additional validation is necessary. The profile may not accurately reflect a particular problem area sufficiently well and needs restating or additional data. Irrelevant data may be distorting the picture. Just as an artist stands back from his painting to view his work in toto, the nurse stands back and appraises the patient's health state profile. If a change is necessary, this is made before she proceeds to the next part in the nursing process system, that of assessment which will be discussed in the next chapter.

FEEDBACK

When an evaluation of the health state profile by comparing it with the performance criteria indicates that the profile is inaccurate or inappropriate, the nurse retraces her steps. She goes back to the beginning of this subsystem.

When evaluation indicates a satisfactory health state profile, the nurse goes on to the next subsystem which, in this case, is the assessment subsystem.

Look again at Figure 6-1 on page 56. Note that the courses of action the nurse has at her disposal in the feedback procedure are diagramed at the right-hand side of the figure where one line divides into two: the nurse returns to the beginning of this subsystem; or she goes on to the next subsystem.

CONCLUSION

To acquire skill in gathering appropriate and accurate data, the nurse must train herself to respond to clues, to be objective, and to be accurate. Behavioral scientists tell us that our senses are constantly bombarded with stimuli, but that only those stimuli to which we are sensitive are actually transmitted to a level of consciousness. In order to use her senses as better detection devices, the nurse must practice cultivating sensitivity to those stimuli that are appropriate to the situation.

The skill of drawing relationships plays an important part throughout the nursing process system. When gathering data, it is especially important in organizing the information so that it has relevancy and meaning. For example, determination of the desirable weight gain of an infant is based upon his birth weight. A 6-weeks-old infant and a 12-weeks-old infant could weigh approximately the same, and both could be progressing normally. However, if the nurse failed to secure birth weights, she may have an inadequate basis for drawing a conclusion concerning the significance of the weight of either baby.

Communication skills are important when interviewing patients and when attempting to discern unspoken feelings and thoughts. Communication is further discussed in Chapter 13.

The nurse needs to demonstrate a sufficiently strong belief in the purpose of data gathering so that the patient will be confident that it will be used intelligently and to his advantage. Because data gathering generally starts very early in the nurse-patient relationship, the nurse can set the climate for a meaningful relationship as well as demonstrate to the patient that he can play a role in determining the care he needs.

Study Situations

1. As this chapter pointed out, the nurse uses her knowledge of health and illness as a guide in selecting the data she will gather. Read the following articles and identify the data the authors considered important to gather in order to provide effective nursing care.

    Blake, F. G.: Immobilized youth: a rationale for supportive nursing intervention. **Am. J. Nurs.,** 69:2364–2369, Nov., 1969.

    Craven, R. F., and Sharp, B. H.: The effects of illness on family functions. **Nurs. Forum,** 11:186–193, No. 2, 1972.

    Pranulis, M. F.: Loss: a factor affecting the welfare of the coronary patient. In **The Nursing Clinics of North America.** Philadelphia, W. B. Saunders, 7:445–455, Sept., 1972.

2. The nurse may use data-gathering guides developed by other nurses, or she can develop her own. These sources contain examples of guides as well as information concerning the process of designing your own guide:

    Little, D. E., and Carnevali, D. L.: Nursing Care Planning. 245 p. Philadelphia, J. B. Lippincott, 1969.

    Mayers, M. G.: A Systematic Approach to the Nursing Care Plan. 304 p. New York, Appleton-Century-Crofts, 1972.

3. Compare and contrast the work of these two authors who illustrate still other types of data-gathering guides:

    Beland, I. L.: Clinical Nursing: Pathophysiological and Psychosocial Approaches. pp. 18–23. New York, MacMillan, 1970 (2nd ed.).

    McPhetridge, L. M.: Nursing history: one means to personalize care. **Am. J. Nurs.,** 68:68–75, Jan., 1968.

4. The author of the book referred to below talks of the difficulty beginning students have in learning to observe a patient, because of the many new challenges and adjustments that have to be made simultaneously. Read her book for further suggestions concerning data gathering and then practice increasing your perception skills as you give nursing care.

    Byers, V. B.: Nursing Observations. 106 p. Dubuque, Iowa, William C. Brown, 1973 (2nd ed.).

5. After reading the following article, describe how the nurse validated her perceptions of a patient:

    Schmidt, J.: Availability: a concept of nursing practice. **Am. J. Nurs.,** 72:1085–1089, June, 1972.

6. After reading the following article, describe how the patient information categorized in Table 1 is significant in carrying out the plan of care in Table 2:

    Griffith, E. W.: Nursing process: a patient with respiratory dysfunction. In **The Nursing Clinics of North America.** Philadelphia, W. B. Saunders, 6:145–154, Mar., 1971.

7. As for Chapter 5, a study technique to help the reader to develop a better understanding of the information presented in this chapter is recommended. Read this chapter again, and in instances where examples are given to illustrate a particular point, describe an experience from your own nursing practice that will illustrate that point equally well.

References

1. Attneave, F.: Multistability in perception. **Sci. Am.,** 225:63–71, Dec., 1971.
2. Bower, F. L.: The Process of Planning Nursing Care: A Theoretical Model. St. Louis, C. V. Mosby, 1972.
3. Brinton, D. M.: Value differences between nurses and low-income families. **Nurs. Research,** 21:46–52, Jan.-Feb., 1972.
4. Brown, E. L.: Newer Dimensions of Patient Care: Part 3: Patients as People. New York, Russell Sage Foundation, 1964.
5. Eckelberry, G. K.: Administration of Comprehensive Nursing Care: The Nature of Professional Practice. New York, Appleton-Century-Crofts, 1971.
6. Garant, C.: A basis for care. **Am. J. Nurs.,** 72:699–701, Apr., 1972.
7. Gomrich, E. H.: The visual image. **Sci. Am.,** 227:82–96, Sept., 1972.
8. Harpine, F. H.: Assessing the needs of the patient. pp. 21–43. In Yura, H., and Walsh, M. B., eds.: The Nursing Process: Assessing, Planning, Implementing, Evaluating. Washington, D. C., Catholic University of America Press, 1967.
9. Henderson, V.: Basic Principles of Nursing Care. London, International Council of Nurses, 1960.
10. Keegan, L. G.: A climate of creativity brought . . . change in action. **Nurs. Outlook,** 18:42–43, Dec., 1970.
11. King, J. M.: The initial interview: basis for assessment in crisis intervention. **Perspect. Psychiat. Care,** 9:247–256, No. 6, 1971.
12. LaFargue, J. P.: Role of prejudice in rejection of health care. **Nurs. Research,** 21:53–58, Jan.-Feb., 1972.
13. Little, D., and Carnevali, D.: The nursing care planning system. **Nurs. Outlook,** 19:164–167, Mar., 1971.
14. McCain, R. F.: Nursing by assessment—not intuition. **Am. J. Nurs.,** 65:82–84, Apr., 1965.
15. Noton, D., and Stark, L.: Eye movements and visual perception. **Sci. Am.,** 224:34–43, June, 1971.
16. Orlando, I. J.: The Dynamic Nurse-Patient Relationship. New York, G. P. Putnam's Sons, 1961.
17. Shumway, S. M., and Wisehart, D. E.: How to know a community. **Nurs. Outlook,** 17:63–64, Sept., 1969.
18. Sobol, E. G., and Robischon, P.: Family Nursing; A Study Guide. St. Louis, C. V. Mosby, 1970.
19. Tinkham, C. W.: The plant as the patient of the occupational health nurse: a survey guide. In **The Nursing Clinics of North America.** Philadelphia, W. B. Saunders, 7:99–107, Mar., 1972.
20. Tinkham, C. W., and Voorhies, E. F.: Community Health Nursing: Evolution and Process. pp. 130–145; 205–219; 279–305. New York, Appleton-Century-Crofts, 1972.

CHAPTER 7

Assessment

GLOSSARY

Assessment: Process by which an estimate of the value or merit of something is made, relative to a standard.

Norm: Synonym for standard.

Nursing Assessment: Sum total of conclusions reached by the nurse after estimating the merit or value of something, relative to a standard, concerning a patient's health-illness status.

Nursing Diagnosis: Synonym for nursing assessment.

Standard: A generally accepted rule, measure, pattern, or model that can be used as a basis for comparing things in the same class or category.

INTRODUCTION

Assessment is the second subsystem in the nursing process system. Like data gathering, assessment involves a process that requires the nurse to make judgments in relation to a specific patient. When assessment is skillfully executed, the nurse has a sound basis on which to develop a nursing care plan.

Assessment is the process by which a judgment is made concerning the value or merit of something when it is compared with a standard.

The *purpose* of assessment is to judge the items on the health state profile in relation to the patient's health-illness status. The *input* for assessment is the health state profile which was the output for the data-gathering process. The nurse judges the health state of a patient when she compares his health state profile with certain standards. Standards are described later in this chapter. When the patient appears to meet a standard, the nurse concludes that the patient has a strength in a particular area, and this strength contributes to his level of wellness. When the patient appears not to meet certain standards, the nurse concludes that the patient most probably has a limitation in this aspect of his level of wellness and needs professional services. She then uses the patient's strengths in assisting him to meet needs in areas where problems may exist. As an example, assume a patient is hard of hearing. This information will be important to consider in planning his nursing care. Assume this same patient's profile indicates that his eyesight is excellent. The nurse can then consider this as a strength and build upon it when helping the patient to solve at least some problems he may have because of his hearing limitation.

The *output* of the assessment process is called the *nursing assessment*.[1] It consists of the conclusions the nurse reaches after she has estimated the merit of something, relative to a certain standard, concerning the patient's health status. The nursing assessment in the example given above would be that the patient is likely to have problems because he is hard of hearing but that he has a strength because his eye sight is excellent. The *performance criteria* used to evaluate the nursing assessment are appropriateness and accuracy of the assessment. Figure 7-1 illustrates assessment input, process, output, performance criteria, and feedback.

THE PROCESS OF ASSESSMENT

The process of assessment will be described in five phases: selecting a standard; comparing the health state profile with standards; stating the nursing assessment; validating the nursing assessment; and evalu-

[1] Some authors refer to the output of the assessment process as the *nursing diagnosis*. "Diagnosis" is most commonly employed in the medical context. To obviate misunderstanding the authors prefer the form "nursing assessment." Also, assessment includes identifying strengths of the patient as well as his inadequacies or needs.

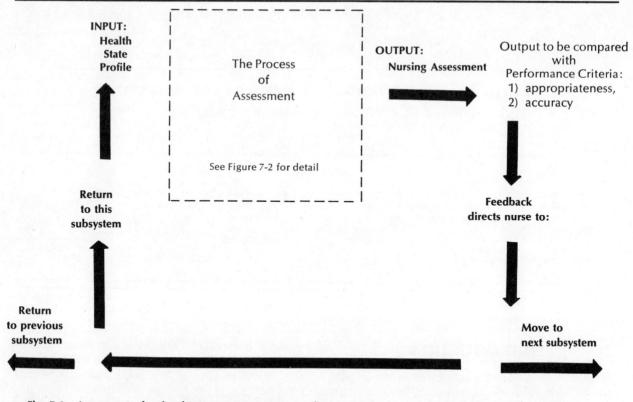

Fig. 7-1. Assessment, showing input, process, output, performance criteria, and feedback. Broken line indicates environmental influences may affect process at any time, as described in Chapter 5.

ating nursing assessment by comparing it with performance criteria. A flow chart illustrating the assessment process appears in Figure 7-2.

Selecting a Standard

A *standard* is defined as a generally accepted rule, measure, pattern, or model which can be used as a basis for comparing things in the same class or category. The word *norm* is a synonym for the word standard. During the assessment process, standards are selected that are relevant and appropriate to a particular situation. A few examples will illustrate.

One often hears that one cannot compare apples with oranges; that is, an orange is not a relevant standard when one wants to judge an apple. The same principle applies when comparing items from the health state profile with a particular standard. For example, comparing the annual number of deaths from respiratory diseases in an urban area with a norm established for a rural area would lead to inaccurate conclusions. In this case, a relevant norm would be death rates from respiratory diseases estab-

lished for urban areas. Comparing a child's daily dietary intake with a dietary norm established for adults illustrates the use of an irrelevant norm. A relevant norm in this instance would be one established for healthy children.

When the patient's health state profile describes a general or broad item, a relevant norm is one that is also general or broad in nature. For example, the patient's health state profile indicates that the patient is completely immobile in bed. A relevant and appropriate standard would be the fact that immobility has been observed to contribute to cardiovascular, respiratory, gastrointestinal, motor, urinary, metabolic, and psychosocial dysfunctioning.

A more specific item requires a more specific standard for comparison. For example, a diagnostic test indicates that a six-year-old child's white blood cell count is 22,000 per cu. mm. of blood. An appropriate and specific standard for comparison purposes would be a norm that describes the average number of white blood cells per cu. mm. of blood normally found in healthy children of that age.

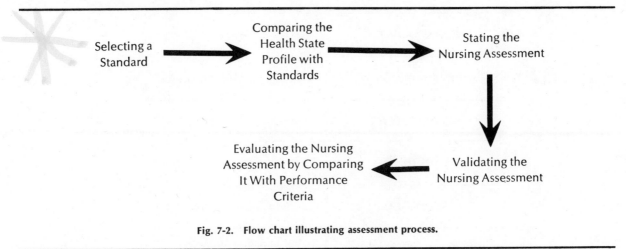

Fig. 7-2. Flow chart illustrating assessment process.

There are many types of standards from which the nurse can choose. Here are some examples when theories, principles, and averages are used as standards.

A *theory*, as defined and described in Chapter 3, can serve as a standard with which one may compare certain items on a patient's health state profile. For example, Abraham Maslow has developed a theory of human motivation that can be used as a standard. Dr. Maslow theorizes that every human being has common needs that motivate his behavior. These needs, he observes, fall into a characteristic order or hierarchy, and are described as physiologic needs, safety needs, belongingness and love needs, esteem needs, and self-actualization needs. When an individual experiences at least some satisfaction at one level, he generally then moves on to the next level where he again seeks satisfaction.

A community health nurse visited a home to discuss the role of discipline in a child's development with the mother. However, the mother was concerned and preoccupied because she knew the family's diet was inadequate due to insufficient money to buy food. If the nurse had used Maslow's theory of motivation as an assessment standard, she might have made a more appropriate decision, that is, to focus on aiding the family to meet basic physiologic needs before proceeding to consider safety and security needs. Dr. Maslow's book, describing his theory in detail, is included in the references at the end of this chapter.

Erik Erikson has developed a theory of human psychosocial development. In each of eight ages, man attempts to resolve certain conflicts, according to

Dr. Erikson. Figure 7-3 illustrates each age with its conflict and resolution.

According to Erikson's theory for example, a toddler works to develop feelings of autonomy (synonym: independence). The child can develop feelings of independence from learning that he has a way of expressing and controlling himself apart from the mother's control. As he acquires autonomy, he resolves feelings of shame and doubt when the uncertainty of not being a part of his mother occurs.

A conflict at a particular age may be resolved with relative ease and satisfaction. The person then moves on to the next age where a new conflict is to be resolved. Or a person may not resolve a conflict in a suitable manner while still moving on to the next chronological age. The outcome of previous conflict resolutions in each age of man will influence the manner in which the person copes with the developmental tasks and conflicts of his current life stage. For example, the adolescent who does not resolve role confusion during his teens will go on to young adulthood while struggling with the conflict of an earlier age. As another example, resolving shame and doubt satisfactorily and developing autonomy during the toddler age helps to develop initiative at the next developmental age. Erikson's theory can serve as a standard for the nurse to assess a patient's developmental age and primary conflicts to be resolved at each age. It can also assist her in determining how the person's health state may contribute to or inhibit resolution of developmental conflicts.

The theories of Maslow and Erikson attempt to describe psychosocial development in man but from somewhat different views. For example, Maslow

ELDERLY ADULT:	*Ego Integrity vs. Despair*
MIDDLE AGE ADULT:	↑ *Generativity vs. Stagnation*
YOUNG ADULT:	↑ *Intimacy vs. Isolation*
YOUTH:	↑ *Identity vs. Role Confusion*
SCHOOL AGE:	↑ *Industry vs. Inferiority*
YOUNG CHILD: (PRESCHOOL)	↑ *Initiative vs. Guilt*
TODDLER:	↑ *Autonomy vs. Shame and Doubt*
BABYHOOD:	↑ *Basic Trust vs. Basic Mistrust*

Fig. 7-3. Erikson's ages of man (Adapted from Erikson, E. H. Childhood and Society, pp. 247–274. New York, W. W. Norton, 1963.)

speaks of needs while Erikson speaks of tasks. Both theories describe man's attempt to adapt and when man does so satisfactorily, he is in a position to utilize his resources to their fullest and experience well-being while doing so.

Many norms used in nursing come from *principles* gained in the study of the psychosocial and physiologic sciences. Consider this principle from psychology: intense emotion influences the decision-making ability of an individual. This principle could be used as an appropriate standard in the following example. A patient's health state profile, developed in the physician's office, revealed that the patient was fearful of losing his job and was very worried about inadequate financial resources to support his family. His emotional state could well influence his decision-making ability when hospitalization for extensive diagnostic examinations was advised.

A principle from the field of physiology is that normal cellular functioning requires an environment having a pH value of approximately 7.4 (pH refers to the hydrogen ion concentration within a substance). This principle may be an appropriate standard when assessing a patient whose blood serum has a pH of 7.2.

Probably among the most common types of

standards are *averages* compiled from data gathered from large numbers of examined subjects. Very often, an average is reported within a range; that is, most examined subjects fall within a range of the item being studied. Here are some examples of averages and of average ranges. The average normal body temperature of adults, when measured orally, is 98.6°F. (37°C.). The average intelligence quotient of Americans, measured by using an examination such as the Stanford-Binet intelligence test, is 90 to 110. The average amount of urine an adult produces in 24 hours is 1,000 to 1,500 c.c. Normal bleeding time is approximately one to three minutes. The nurse selects the standard most directly related to the data she is assessing.

In some instances, tools have been developed from commonly used standards to make the assessment process faster, more consistent, and accurate. The tools usually provide space to record the patient's data and some type of a calculation reflecting variations from the standard. More than one standard can be included in the same tool. Several examples follow.

Most hospitals use graphs on which the patient's temperature, pulse rate, and respiratory rate may be plotted. Some of these graphs also indicate normal

FAMILY COPING ESTIMATE

Family_____ Nurse_____ Date_____

Initial_____ Periodic_____ Discharge_____

COPING AREA	RATING x-status 0-est. change Poor ....Exc.					JUSTIFICATION
Physical Independence	1	2	3	4	5	
	Not Applicable ☐					
Therapeutic Independence	1	2	3	4	5	
	Not Applicable ☐					
Knowledge of Condition	1	2	3	4	5	
	Not Applicable ☐					
Application of Principles of Personal Hygiene	1	2	3	4	5	
	Not Applicable ☐					
Attitude Toward Health Care	1	2	3	4	5	
	Not Applicable ☐					
Emotional Competence	1	2	3	4	5	
	Not Applicable ☐					
Family Living Patterns	1	2	3	4	5	
	Not Applicable ☐					
Physical Environment	1	2	3	4	5	
	Not Applicable ☐					
Use of Community Resources	1	2	3	4	5	
	Not Applicable ☐					
Comments						

Fig. 7-4. Family Coping Estimate. (Freeman, R. B. Community Health Nursing Practice. Philadelphia, p. 60. W. B. Saunders, 1970. Developed jointly by the Richmond IVNA City Nursing Service and the Johns Hopkins School of Hygiene and Public Health, 1964.)

ranges for these data. Some laboratories report test results on graphs similar to the one just described. For example, a patient's red and white blood cell count will be reported by the laboratory on a graph that also indicates normal average ranges for red and white blood cell counts. As another example, schools usually report a student's scores on aptitude tests on a graph that simultaneously illustrates how the stu-

dent's results compared with national norms.

The Family Coping Estimate, shown in Figure 7-4, is an example of an aid that helps the nurse both to gather and assess certain data. This form is based on the premise that knowledge of the family's ability to cope with its health problems is the key to determining its health status. The family's ability to deal successfully with each of the nine categories is judged

Sign	0	1	2
HEART RATE	ABSENT	SLOW (LESS THAN 100)	OVER 100
RESPIRATORY EFFORT	ABSENT	SLOW, IRREGULAR	GOOD CRYING
MUSCLE TONE	FLACCID	SOME FLEXION OF EXTREMITIES	ACTIVE MOTION
REFLEX IRRITABILITY	NO RESPONSE	CRY	VIGOROUS CRY
COLOR	BLUE, PALE	BODY PINK, EXTREMITIES BLUE	COMPLETELY PINK

Figure 7-5. Apgar Scoring Chart. (Fitzpatrick, Elise, et al, Maternity Nursing, J. B. Lippincott Company, Philadelphia, 1971, p. 275.)

by the nurse on a range from 1 to 5, that is, poor to excellent. She determines the family's current status of coping and then estimates changes in coping with nursing care. Comments in the justification column are specific, supportive statements relating to placement on the scale. The completed Estimate is a profile of the family's abilities to manage its health problems.

The Apgar Scoring Chart, illustrated in Figure 7-5, is an example of a tool for assessing a newborn infant's physiologic status. When using it, the nurse observes each of the five signs one minute after delivery. A similar observation is made five minutes later. The infant is scored on each sign following each observation. After each observation, the scores are totaled and then assessed by comparing them with a scale that accompanies the chart. The maximum score is 10. A score of 7 to 10 indicates the infant's condition is good and no special action needs to be taken. A score of 4 to 6 means the baby is in fair condition and certain recommended procedures should be followed. A score of 3 or less means the baby is in serious condition and emergency measures are needed.

The sources of standards are about as numerous as the standards themselves. Legitimate and reliable authorities can be sources of standards. Books, periodicals, and other published material are often good sources. The expertise of experienced health practitioners can be used as sources for standards. The Bureau of the Census, U. S. Department of Commerce, publishes many statistics that have implications for health care, as Chapter 2 illustrates. As the nurse becomes more knowledgeable and experienced, her own background may provide her with some standards. Because of the importance of objectivity and accuracy, reasonable safeguards should be observed to make certain the sources of standards are reliable.

While many standards are available, more are always in the process of being developed as knowledge grows. For this reason, the nurse will wish to update and add to her knowledge regularly in order to have objective and meaningful norms to use in the assessment process.

Comparing the Health State Profile with Standards

After a standard is selected, the nurse is ready to compare the health state profile with that standard. The process of comparing involves bringing items together so that they can be examined. The purpose is to draw conclusions about the items being compared with the norm.

The nature of the conclusion will depend on the type of items and the standard with which it is being compared. The conclusions generally are of two types. One type of conclusion indicates the similarities or differences between the profile item and the norm. For example, a patient's body temperature, pulse rate, and respiratory rate are compared with norms. The patient's signs may fall either within the normal range, or outside it. A community's population characteristics may be similar to a national norm, or they may be very different from that norm.

A second type of conclusion has predictive value;

that is, the nurse anticipates that something may occur. For example, a patient displays signs of a wound infection but laboratory results show that his white blood cell count has not increased as is usual when an infection of this nature is present. The nurse concludes that the body is apparently not building up normal defenses to combat the infection. She then predicts certain problems, such as a longer wound healing period than would normally be expected. This has many implications for nursing care, for example, in relation to the patient's diet, fluid intake, urinary output, mobility, and so on.

As another example of a conclusion having predictive value, assume a well child's health state profile completed in a pediatrician's office is compared with certain developmental norms. The nurse concludes that the child is developing normally. She can then predict that barring unusual illness or injury, this child will most likely continue to develop normally.

Stating the Nursing Assessment

The nursing assessment is the sum total of conclusions the nurse reaches about the significance of various aspects of the patient's health state profile in relation to high-level wellness. The nursing assessment should be objective and accurate and should identify the patient's strengths as well as his limitations. The conclusions may be general or quite specific, depending on the data collected. They should be stated as briefly and precisely as possible.

The following statements are possible conclusions that the nurse could have drawn from the examples of standards used in this chapter. Then, each statement could be part of a nursing assessment.

• The community death rate from respiratory causes during the past year is lower than the national rate.

• The child's average dietary intake is not adequate to meet the normal growth requirements for his age.

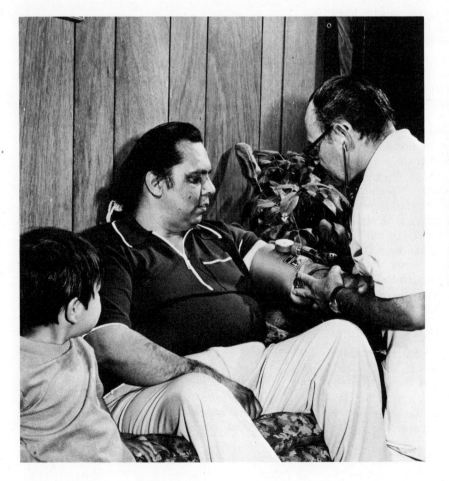

Fig. 7-6. This photo illustrates a community health nurse in the process of assessing. After the patient's blood pressure is determined, the nurse compares his findings with a standard that describes normal, average adult blood pressure readings. Then the nurse judges whether the patient's blood pressure presents a problem and a need for planning nursing intervention. The nurse's judgment also may include communicating with other members of the health team. (Photo by Ted Hill, Arizona)

• The immobilized patient is likely to develop cardiovascular, respiratory, gastrointestinal, motor, urinary, metabolic, and psychosocial disabilities.

• The mother will probably be unable to focus effectively on child discipline until food needs of the family are met.

• The man will probably have difficulty making a decision regarding hospitalization because of his job-related worries.

• The patient's red blood cell count is within the normal range at this time.

• The family's ability to cope with their health problems related to living patterns and use of community resources would probably be improved with nursing care.

• The newborn infant's condition is good and does not require special care at this time.

Validating the Nursing Assessment

The purpose of validation is to minimize the occurrence of errors, biases, and misinterpretations. Usually it is not practical or possible to validate all of the items making up the nursing assessment; however, the more that are validated, the more effective nursing care planning is likely to be. Because of the potential for human error in each step of the assessment process, a high percentage of validations is recommended, especially for beginners. With more experience, the nurse may become more selective when she validates.

As in the data-gathering process, the patient is a good source for validating some of the nursing assessment statements. If the patient is unable to confirm the statements because of age or degree of illness, family members can sometimes do so. Some statements cannot be validated by the patient or family because of lack of knowledge. Patients' records can sometimes also be used for validation. Some statements can be validated by other nurses or by the physician, dietitian, and others. Views of authorities on a particular subject may be useful validators. If the nurse takes care to be objective, her own past experiences can sometimes be used for validation purposes.

In the previous example describing a mother who was concerned about food in contrast to child discipline, the nurse's conclusion could be validated by the mother. The nurse who drew the conclusion about the family's coping ability may want to validate her judgment with another nurse. Reference books could be used as validation sources for the

conclusions concerning the child's dietary needs and the patient's red blood cell count.

While the primary purpose of validation is to insure the accuracy of judgments upon which a patient's care will be planned and provided, it has an additional benefit for the nurse. Validation can provide immediate, positive or negative evidence of her judgment skills. Either result can be helpful in her continued efforts to perfect her nursing skills.

Evaluating Nursing Assessment by Comparing It with Performance Criteria

The output of the assessment process is the nursing assessment. In this phase in the nursing process, the nurse should compare the nursing assessment she has prepared with the performance criteria to determine whether it is appropriate and whether it is accurate.

The procedure of evaluating the nursing assessment is similar to that described in Chapter 6 when evaluating the health state profile. The nurse will wish to answer several questions such as the following. Does the nursing assessment reflect the patient's present health-illness status? Are all relevant factors in the patient's situation considered in the assessment? Are strengths stated as well as the patient's limitations?

If in the nurse's judgment, the nursing assessment does not meet the criteria of appropriateness and accuracy, she then becomes responsible for making modifications.

FEEDBACK

In this subsystem, the procedure of feedback provides the nurse with three options. If the nursing assessment satisfies the performance criteria, the nurse proceeds to the next subsystem which is planning nursing care. If the nursing assessment does not satisfy the performance criteria, the nurse has two options. She returns either to the beginning of the assessment subsystem, or to the data-gathering subsystem. Her decision is made on the basis of the evaluation she has made. For example, if her evaluation tells her she has used an inappropriate standard when she studied the patient's health state profile, she returns to the process of selecting an appropriate standard. If, on the other hand, evaluation illustrates that her data appear inaccurate or incomplete, she returns to data gathering to correct the error.

Look again at Figure 7-1 on page 64. The courses of action the nurse has at her disposal in the feedback procedure are diagrammed at the lower part of the figure that illustrates feedback leading to three alternative routes.

CONCLUSION

Developing a nursing assessment using the process described in this chapter may seem complex, especially to the beginner in nursing. The process requires deliberate effort and attention in all of its phases. However, once the nurse has developed skill in drawing up a nursing assessment, she learns that it is an essential aid in taking the next step in the nursing process system—that of developing a plan of nursing care which is described in the next chapter.

Study Situations

1. The following reference describes a variety of patient situations; however, the assessment process was applied in different ways. Read several of the articles and see if you can identify the phases of the assessment process, as described in this chapter, even though the phases may be referred to by different names.
   Giblin, E. C., guest ed.: Symposium on assessment as part of the nursing process. *In* **The Nursing Clinics of North America.** Philadelphia, W. B. Saunders, 6: 113–209, Mar., 1971.
2. The author of the article given below uses the terms, evaluation and diagnosis, to describe the assessment process and shows how essential they are to effective nursing care. Read the article and compare the ideas with those expressed in this chapter.
   Rothberg, J. S.: Why nursing diagnosis? **Am. J. Nurs.,** 67:1040–1042, May, 1967.
3. The natural and social science principles included in the book referred to below can serve as standards for the assessment process.
   Nordmark, M. T., and Rohweder, A. W.: Scientific Foundations of Nursing. 388 p. Philadelphia, J. B. Lippincott, 1967 (2nd ed.).
   Practice identifying standards by selecting those which are pertinent to a patient for whom you have recently cared.
4. When statistics are used as standards, at times they may seem confusing. The following article offers some cautionary measures and guidelines when using statistics:
   Means, R. K.: Interpreting statistics: an art. **Nurs. Outlook,** 13:34–37, May, 1965.
5. Chapters 7 and 12 of the following book discuss ways

of determining a family's and a community's nursing requirements:
Tinkham, C. W., and Voorhies, E. F., Community Health Nursing: Evolution and Process. 320 p. New York, Appleton-Century-Crofts, 1972.
Read the chapters and identify the similarities and differences when implementing the assessment process for the individual, the family, and the community.
6. As was recommended for the previous chapters in this unit, read this chapter again, and in instances where examples are given to illustrate a particular point, describe an experience from your own nursing practice that will illustrate that point equally well.

References

1. Aguilera, D. C.: Sociocultural factors: barriers to therapeutic intervention. **J. Psychiat. Nurs. and Mental Health,** 8:14–18, Sept.–Oct., 1970.
2. Bower, F. L.: The Process of Planning Nursing Care: A Theoretical Model. St. Louis, C. V. Mosby, 1972.
3. Burtt, E. A.: Employee assessment of the young and the older worker. *In* **The Nursing Clinics of North America.** Philadelphia, W. B. Saunders, 7:109–119, Mar., 1972.
4. Carlson, C. E., coordinator: Behavioral Concepts and Nursing Intervention. Philadelphia, J. B. Lippincott, 1970.
5. Erikson, E. H.: Childhood and Society. ed. 2, revised, pp. 247–274. New York, W. W. Norton, 1963.
6. Fitzpatrick, E., et al.: Maternity Nursing. ed. 12, pp. 274–275. Philadelphia, J. B. Lippincott, 1971.
7. Freeman, R. B.: Community Health Nursing Practice. Philadelphia, W. B. Saunders, 1970.
8. Freeman, R. B., and Lowe, M.: A method for appraising family public health nursing needs. **Am. J. Public Health,** 53:47–52, Jan., 1963.
9. Gardner, M. A. M.: Responsiveness as a measure of consciousness. **Am. J. Nurs.,** 68:1035–1038, May, 1968.
10. Helvie, C. O., et al.: The setting and nursing practice. **Nurs. Outlook,** 16:35–38, Sept., 1968.
11. Knowles, L. N., guest ed.: Symposium on putting geriatric nursing standards into practice. *In* **The Nursing Clinics of North America.** Philadelphia, W. B. Saunders, 7:201–309, June, 1972.
12. Kraegel, J. M., et al.: A system of patient care based on patient needs. **Nurs. Outlook,** 20:257–266, Apr., 1972.
13. Levine, M. E.: Introduction to Clinical Nursing. ed 2. Philadelphia, F. A. Davis, 1973. (Content at end of each chapter, in section entitled "Essential Science Concepts," could be used as standards in assessment process.)
14. Lewis, L.: Planning Patient Care. Dubuque, Ia., William C. Brown, 1970.
15. Lewis, L.: This I believe . . . about the nursing

process—key to care. **Nurs. Outlook,** 16:26–29, May, 1968.

16. McCabe, G. S.: Cultural influences on patient behavior. **Am. J. Nurs.,** 60:1101–1104, Aug., 1960.

17. McCain, R. F.: Nursing by assessment—not intuition. **Am. J. Nurs.,** 65:82–84, Apr., 1965.

18. Maslow, A. H.: A theory of human motivation. **Psychol. Rev.,** 50:370–396, July, 1943.

19. ———: Motivation and Personality. ed. 2, pp. 35–58. New York, Harper and Row, 1970.

20. Mayers, M. G.: A search for assessment criteria. **Nurs. Outlook,** 20:323–326, May, 1972.

21. Poland, M., *et al.*: PETO: a system for assessing and meeting patient care needs. **Am. J. Nurs.,** 70:1479–1482, July, 1970.

22. Robischon, P., and Scott, D.: Role theory and its application in family nursing. **Nurs. Outlook,** 17:52–54, July, 1969.

23. Roy, Sr. C.: Adaptation: a basis for nursing practice. **Nurs. Outlook,** 19:254–257, Apr., 1971.

24. Standards for geriatric nursing practice. **Am. J. Nurs.,** 70:1894–1897, Sept., 1970.

25. Tapia, J. A.: The nursing process in family health. **Nurs. Outlook,** 20:267–270, Apr., 1972.

26. Tinkham, C. W., and Voorhies, E. F.: Community Health Nursing: Evolution and Process. pp. 146–158; 220–235. New York, Appleton-Century-Crofts, 1972.

27. Wagner, M. M.: Assessment of patients with multiple injuries. **Am. J. Nurs.,** 72:1822–1827, Oct., 1972.

28. Yura, H., and Walsh, Mary B.: The Nursing Process: Assessing, Planning, Implementing, and Evaluating. ed 2. New York, Appleton-Century-Crofts, 1973.

29. Zimmerman, D. S., and Gohrke, C.: The goal-directed nursing approach: it does work. **Am. J. Nurs.,** 70:306–310, Feb., 1970.

CHAPTER 8

Planning Nursing Care

GLOSSARY • INTRODUCTION • THE PROCESS OF PLANNING •
NURSING CARE • FEEDBACK • CONCLUSION •
STUDY SITUATIONS • REFERENCES

GLOSSARY

Alternative: A choice between things.

Goal: Synonym for objective.

Nursing Care Plan: A scheme or guide for nursing care actions.

Nursing Order: A description of what specific nursing care is to be given.

Objective: An aim or an end.

Plan: A scheme or guide for action.

INTRODUCTION

Planning the patient's nursing care is the third subsystem in the nursing process system. As in the previous subsystems, described in Chapters 6 and 7, planning involves a process and requires the nurse to make judgments in relation to a specific patient. The plan for nursing care becomes the guide for nursing intervention, the actual giving of nursing care.

As this text emphasizes, planning nursing care in collaboration with the patient is an essential part of high quality nursing. Unless planning involves the patient, the nurse runs the risk of devising a plan that may be unacceptable or inappropriate for the patient. Also, involving the patient usually carries the added advantage of encouraging him to assume more responsibility for his own health and for gaining more independence in attaining and maintaining the goal of high-level wellness.

A *plan* is a scheme or guide for action. This chapter will describe the process of developing a scheme or guide for the provision of nursing care.

The *purpose* of planning nursing care is to develop a rational scheme or guide designed to help the patient to attain and maintain high-level wellness. The *input* for planning nursing care is the nursing assessment, the output of the assessment process as described in the last chapter. The *output* of the process of planning nursing care is the nursing care plan.

There are two *performance criteria* for planning nursing care. The first criterion is that there should be evidence of a direct relationship between the nursing assessment and the nursing care plan. The second is that the nursing care plan should be acceptable to the patient. Figure 8-1 illustrates the input, process, output, performance criteria, and feedback of planning nursing care.

THE PROCESS OF PLANNING NURSING CARE

The process of planning nursing care is described in six phases: determining areas where the patient requires nursing care and establishing their priorities; determining objectives of nursing care; identifying alternatives of nursing care and selecting from alternatives that care which will best aid in meeting objectives; writing nursing orders; developing a nursing care plan; and evaluating nursing care plan by comparing it with performance criteria.

Determining Areas Where the Patient Requires Nursing Care and Establishing Their Priorities

The nursing assessment contains conclusions that point out the strengths and the weaknesses or disabilities in relation to the patient's health-illness

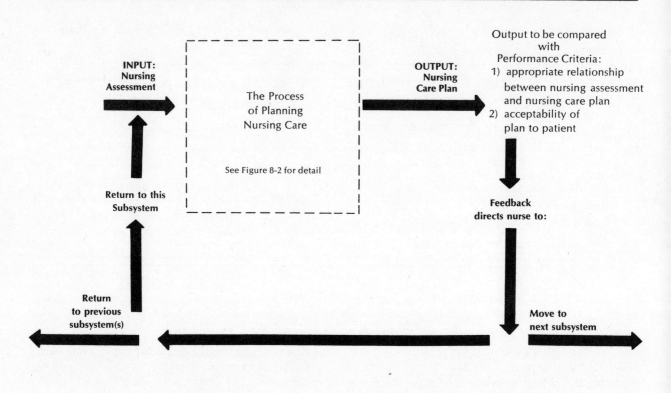

Fig. 8-1. Planning nursing care, showing input, process, output, performance criteria, and feedback. Broken line indicates environmental influences may affect process at any time, as described in Chapter 5.

status. From these conclusions, the nurse next defines areas in which the patient requires services of the nurse and establishes priorities among these areas in a hierarchy ranging from those considered most urgent to those of least importance.

As the nurse identifies areas requiring nursing services, she will note that in general these areas fall into several common categories. One contains areas that define the patient's inability to meet his own physical and psychosocial needs. The patient may lack physical, intellectual, emotional, or material resources. The patient may be too ill, physically or mentally, to be able to eat by himself or keep himself clean without assistance. Another patient may lack dexterity of his fingers and hence, cannot apply a bandage to his leg. A patient may lack the intellectual capacity to determine whether or not he is taking the proper dosage of a prescribed medication.

Another may lack the finances to purchase the solution and equipment necessary to irrigate his wound.

A second category where services often are necessary includes areas that define the patient's unawareness of a need. For example, many persons are often unaware of the implications of a particular symptom. Consider the mother who does not know the normal developmental progression in children and therefore, does not realize the implications when there is a delay in her child's learning to hold his head, sit, stand, or walk. Another mother may not know that a child's sore throat caused by the streptococcus organism can be predisposing to rheumatic fever and heart damage. Young couples who are planning for children are frequently unaware of genetically caused conditions such as sickle cell anemia, Tay-Sachs disease, or phenylketonuria. Or these couples may be unaware of detection methods that

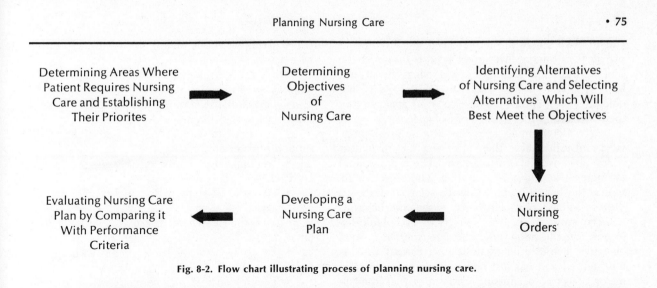

Fig. 8-2. Flow chart illustrating process of planning nursing care.

will help to establish whether they are carriers of hereditary diseases. As still another example, a neighborhood or a community may be unaware of the long-range implications of extreme noise pollution on hearing.

Another category where services are necessary includes those health-illness situations that are being handled in a manner that is not conducive to high-level wellness. For instance, the person who follows a poorly balanced diet to lose weight may cause kidney damage. A person who habitually takes laxatives may depress his own intestinal activity to a serious degree. The patient who frequently uses bicarbonate of soda from the kitchen to relieve his indigestion may cause a disturbance in his blood chemistry.

After a requirement for nursing care has been defined, identifying the reason for the problem will usually suggest the selection of appropriate nursing care. For example, following major abdominal surgery, three patients may remain in bed and demonstrate reluctance toward physical activity. These patients all require nursing care that will promote activity. One has rheumatoid arthritis and is reluctant to move because she says she feels too stiff to move. Another says that she is too tired to move and wants to use this period of hospitalization as a time to get a complete rest. The third patient is fearful that physical activity may damage her wound since "father's stitches broke when he turned on his side after an operation 30 years ago." Although these three patients need to increase their activity, specific nursing measures needed to bring this about will undoubtedly be quite different.

Ranking the needs for nursing services in order of their priorities will take into account both the patient's and the nurse's opinions. Little can be accomplished if the nurse chooses to ignore what the patient feels is important. She will generally find that whenever possible, if she defers to the patient's ranking, she will have a much more secure and satisfied patient. At times she will not be able to do so and will have to attempt to help the patient understand the reasoning behind her judgment. In such instances, possibly a compromise can be worked out that is both suitable and acceptable to the patient and the nurse.

The patient brings his past experiences and values to the job of establishing priorities. For example, a patient, who has in the past experienced pain so severe that he became nauseated and vomited, may place the relief of pain high on his list of priorities. A person who is modest and too embarrassed to discuss intestinal elimination would place a high priority on measures to prevent constipation in order to avoid the need for a cleansing enema.

While still considering the patient's feelings about priorities, the nurse determines them largely on the basis of her knowledge of the needs and functions of human beings and on past nursing experience. Nursing assessment of very low priority may not be dealt with. The urgency of meeting basic physiological needs over others is paramount.

Determining Objective of Nursing Care

An *objective* is an aim or an end; it expresses an unmet need. Effort is exerted to attain the aim or end so as to satisfy the unmet need. For example, a person feels hungry; his unmet need is the satisfying and comfortable feeling he has when he is not hungry; therefore, he directs his efforts toward the objective of obtaining food. The word *goal* is often used as a synonym for the word objective.

After determining areas that require nursing services and establishing their priorities, the nurse next states objectives of nursing care. There are several characteristics of a good objective. The objective describes the behavior one wishes to occur; it describes the conditions under which one wishes the behavior to occur; and it describes criteria of acceptable behavior. To illustrate these characteristics of a good objective, consider an example of a patient who is hospitalized and has just had a leg amputation. The major objective of nursing care states that the patient will be employed and that employment will be satisfactory to both the employer and employee. When the objective is attained, the patient's behavior will demonstrate that he is fully employable; this is the behavior one wishes to occur. The person will be not only employable but also employed; this is the condition under which one wishes the behavior to occur. The person's behavior on the job will be satisfactory to the person and to the employer; this states criteria of acceptable behavior.

Objectives may be short-term or long-term in nature. Usually long-term objectives tend to cover a larger area than short-term objectives. The objective of care stated above for the patient with the leg amputation is an example of a long-term objective.

While long-term objectives are necessary and useful when planning patient care, the more precise short-term objectives which lead the way to the long-term objectives are especially important. Short-term objectives will illustrate exactly what should be accomplished along the way and will show even small increments of progress. Since they are usually quicker to attain, the patient as well as the nurse can enjoy the satisfactions of observing progress enroute. In addition, there is less likelihood of the patient being off track and reinforcing poor habits on the way to the long-term goal. An additional advantage of stating short-term goals is that they are much easier to adjust in order to plan care that will meet an individual's needs as they change from day to day or week to week. Whether the objectives are short- or long-term, the characteristics of a good objective, as described previously, apply.

In the case of the amputee cited above, these short-term goals will aid in directing the course toward the desired end more accurately and precisely.

• To move from sitting to standing position with assistance of nurse.
• To move from sitting to standing position without assistance.
• To stand for 5 minutes at side of bed with support of nurse.
• To stand for 5 minutes at side of bed with support of chair or table.
• To stand for 10 minutes with the aid of crutches.
• To walk 10 steps with crutches with nurse's assistance.
• To walk 10 steps with crutches without assistance.
• To apply artificial leg correctly with nurse's assistance.
• To apply artificial leg correctly within 10 minutes without assistance.
• To stand alone on artificial leg for 5 minutes.
• To walk 10 steps alone with artificial leg. And so on.

These examples illustrate objectives expressed in terms of activities the patient will be able to do in relatively short periods of time, unless complications occur. They are clear and concise. It will be relatively simple to evaluate the progress the patient makes at each step and to recognize when additional time is necessary before the patient can proceed to the next. Short-term objectives have the advantage of being able to spot troubles almost as soon as they begin so that the patient does not reinforce poor learning or become frustrated while exerting efforts to reach his long-term goals.

Objectives stated clearly and concisely and in terms of specific, expected behavior are important for communicating a plan of action to other members of the nursing team. Reconsider the example of the patient with the leg amputation. Think about this objective: the patient will be able to stand. Stand where and how? Stand with or without assistance? For how long? It can be seen that the objective just stated hampers communication among health practitioners concerning the patient's progress. Without clear communication, health team members cannot reinforce each other's efforts.

Objectives and evaluation are discussed also in Chapter 16 which describes the role of the nurse as a health teacher. References and study situations at the end of this chapter will be of special help in aiding the nurse to prepare objectives. Although much literature on objectives is designed for the field of education, the same principles can be applied to nursing situations.

Identifying Alternatives of Nursing Care and Selecting from Alternatives the Type of Care Which Will Best Meet Objectives

An *alternative* offers a choice of things. In this phase of the process of planning nursing care, the nurse will identify various kinds of care that could be used to meet the objectives and then will select from those alternatives the care which she believes will best serve to meet the objectives. Some alternatives may be unrealistic and therefore will not be considered. A person has many options, for example, when traveling from New York to San Francisco; he may travel by boat, plane, bicycle, on foot, automobile, and so on. However, if a man wishes to make the trip when he has business one day in New York and business in San Francisco two days later, any choice other than using a plane is unrealistic.

In Chapter 5, constraints were described. Unrealistic options to reach an objective are constraints and in nursing, for example, may include such constraints as lack of available time, skilled personnel, or financial resources. In some instances, an agency's policies may act as a constraint. For example, a nurse may feel that a relative might well be of great assistance if allowed to stay overnight with a hospitalized patient. If the agency's policies forbid the practice, the nurse will seek a *trade-off* or alternative method to accomplish the goal. A patient unable to get in and out of a tub may use a shower bath as a trade-off. If a patient is on a low cholesterol diet and does not care for fish, one trade-off is to use cheese as a substitute.

At times a nurse may realize that she does not have sufficient knowledge to handle a particular problem. She may then consult with other personnel who may be more experienced than she for assistance in finding a suitable trade-off. The nurse may also confront legal constraints in her practice which provide for no trade-offs. For instance, certain diseases (pulmonary tuberculosis being one common example) must be reported to an official health department, according to law. For this type of constraint no alternatives are possible.

In considering the various nursing care alternatives to accomplish an objective, the nursing assessment with its conclusions describing the patient's strengths is often very helpful in making a final choice. For example, a patient who is demonstrating difficulty in adjusting to blindness may have family members who are willing to assist the patient to gain as much independence as possible. The nurse will wish to use this information in assisting the patient. A nurse can build on a patient's manual dexterity when he is now required to administer his own injections. Or, the nurse can make the most of a patient's good respiratory functioning after a laryngectomy (removal of the voice box) in assisting the patient in learning to speak again.

Involving the patient when choices are made is essential when selecting appropriate care for achieving a particular objective. Many times a patient will have his own ideas on how best to achieve an objective. For example, an arthritic patient may tell the nurse that he can feed himself and carry out his prescribed exercises more effectively if he can soak in a tub of warm water first. As another example, community leaders in a neighborhood may have had a previous, successful experience with publicizing a mobile chest x-ray visit to the area by distributing information through school children and through signs in the grocery stores. The nurse who fails to consider this experience may find her alternative of using other publicity media unsuccessful in achieving the goal.

Involving other nursing and health team members is also recommended when selecting care for a particular patient. This practice often serves to reinforce each other's efforts. Also, an alternative one person may propose may generate still more ideas from others. A proposal for care that has not been successful when used by one nurse may enable another to make a choice.

Knowledge of the patient's cultural and religious backgrounds is useful in selecting care, such as dietary customs observed by practicing Orthodox Jews. As another example, certain cultures stress close physical contact between mother and child in their child-rearing customs; others practice a good deal of physical restraint. These examples may remind the nurse that her own cultural and religious customs may be inappropriate as norms when selecting care for patients holding different beliefs from her own. Chapters 14 and 15 discuss cultural and religious considerations when planning nursing care.

The nurse together with the patient then makes a final decision on the best way to meet an objective by selecting the care that has the greatest probability of resulting in desirable effects. Statistical consideration for the probability of success sometimes is used. For example, if from statistical studies a particular action is considered highly likely to succeed, it can be predicted that success will occur in about seven of ten cases. If it is considered moderately likely to succeed, it can be predicted that success will occur in about four of seven cases. Low probability results in success in about one out of four cases. It is used

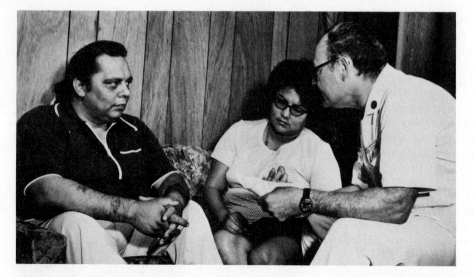

Fig. 8-3. The community health nurse in this photo has prepared a plan for nursing care for this man, his wife, and their family. He is discussing the plan with his patients so that they too will be knowledgeable about their needs for service and the recommended ways to obtain services that will be acceptable to them. (Photo by Ted Hill, Arizona)

often by the physician in predicting the prognosis or the outcome of certain illnesses. An example is that of a patient who received treatment very early, or very late, after he was diagnosed to have a malignant tumor. Predicting the probability of success with the use of certain drugs is also an example. There are nurses who are beginning to use probability of success in their practice, such as when considering approaches for relieving pain, for teaching patients, and for preventing decubiti (bedsores).

Identifying alternatives and then selecting best ways to meet an objective are stimulating and challenging experiences. Sometimes, the most effective way to give care is not the most obvious way. It requires creativity and ingenuity to look for alternate methods of care and avoid giving stereotyped care to everyone. However, the rewards of individualized service are well worth the efforts.

Writing Nursing Orders

Nursing orders are written on the basis of the nursing care selected for a particular patient. A *nursing order* tells what nursing care is to be done. It is particularly important that these orders be spelled out clearly and concisely. Carefully written nursing orders are essential to promote communications among team members in order that patient needs will be met as planned. A few examples will illustrate.

A hospitalized patient with an elevated body temperature needs a larger than usual fluid intake to prevent dehydration, a condition due to excess water loss from the body when fluid intake is insufficient to compensate for the loss. One nursing order states, "Force fluids." A better and much more precise order

would read, "Offer 200 c.c. of fluid every two hours while patient is awake to a total of 3,000 c.c. intake in each 24-hour period." Another patient had a nursing order that read, "Increase activity." A better statement of the order is, "Have patient walk length of hall three times daily."

A community health nurse wrote this nursing order for the children in a family, "Have children immunized." A better order would have stated the names of each child needing immunization, the exact type of immunization needed for each, and when the immunization was to be done.

Following a flood in a rural community, a nursing order read, "Check for drinking water contamination." A better way to write this order is, "Check safety of drinking water with city health department daily until water is reported to be free of contamination by department for 21 consecutive days."

A good nursing order is a written order. Depending on memory and on verbal communication of nursing orders is not safe. Oral orders may be forgotten, misunderstood, or incorrectly interpreted.

Developing a Nursing Care Plan

A *nursing care plan* is a guide or scheme for giving nursing care. Usually, health agencies have their own nursing care plan forms, which are helpful and the use of which is encouraged. Many suggestions for forms appear in the nursing literature and descriptions of various kinds of forms can be found in the references at the end of this chapter. The first study situation at the end of this chapter illustrates a nursing care plan and refers the reader to a publication that will be helpful in developing and evaluating nursing care plans. However, it must be remembered that the information called for on the form may not be appropriate or complete for every patient. Therefore, the nurse will use the form while making whatever adjustments are indicated for each patient.

These are basic pieces of information on a complete nursing care plan: the nursing care objectives; nursing orders; a statement of the patient's strengths on which to build and his limitations or disabilities that require nursing care; and the priorities of care. Some nursing care plans contain additional information, for example such as certain personal data concerning the patient, medical orders, agency routines, and the like.

Evaluating Nursing Care Plan by Comparing It with Performance Criteria

The final phase in the process of planning nursing care is to evaluate the plan by comparing it with the performance criteria. There are two performance criteria that will be used: appropriate relationship between nursing assessment and nursing care plan; and acceptability of the plan by the patient.

Assume, for example, that when the nurse gathers data, she learns that a patient has certain sensitivities (allergies). The nursing assessment states that the patient has a high degree of sensitivity to varied determined and undetermined substances. One objective of care is that the patient would not demonstrate sensitivity reactions during hospitalization. Then, nursing care would include actions to avoid common substances to which the patient may be sensitive. The nursing care plan includes one nursing order stating that a nondetergent soap be used when bathing the patient. A relationship can readily be seen between the nursing assessment statement and the nursing care plan.

During evaluation, the nurse will also wish to answer the question: Do the nursing orders utilize the strengths of this patient as these strengths are stated in the nursing assessment? If they do not, an appropriate relationship between assessment and planning may be questionable.

Evaluation to determine whether the plan is acceptable to the patient is usually a relatively easy step. The nurse will wish to consult with the patient as a starter. There will be times when the patient believes a plan is satisfactory but learns later that it is unacceptable. In such instances, a modification in the plan is made by using a trade-off. If the patient is unable to assist, a member of the family may be used.

A community health nurse developed a nursing care plan with a family. The man and his wife stated that the plan they and the nurse had devised was acceptable: one of the children was to be evaluated by a private psychiatrist. However, before the youngster saw the psychiatrist, the parents changed their minds and told the nurse that the plan was unacceptable. The trade-off in this case was to use a mental health clinic instead, a plan to which the parents concurred.

FEEDBACK

When evaluation of the nursing care plan by comparing it with the performance criteria indicates the nursing care plan is unsatisfactory, the nurse retraces her steps. She decides to return to the beginning of this subsystem, or she decides to return to any of the previous two subsystems. In the latter case, she may gather more data or may use different standards when making a nursing assessment.

If evaluation of the nursing care plan indicates that it is satisfactory, the nurse goes on to the next subsystem in the nursing process system, which is described in the next chapter.

Look again at Figure 8-1, on page 74. Note that the courses of action the nurse has at her disposal during feedback are diagrammed at the lower part of the figure. It illustrates three options: she returns to the beginning of this subsystem; she returns to any of the previous two subsystems; or she goes on to the next subsystem.

CONCLUSION

The development of a nursing care plan is a challenge that requires ingenuity and patience as well as the ability to make constant changes as nursing care needs change. The best plans are developed with the patient along with other members of the nursing and health teams. A nursing care plan is an essential bridge between knowing about a patient's nursing care needs and implementing the care the patient requires.

Study Situations

1. The following book discusses the planning of nursing care:

   Little, D. E., and Carnevali, D. L.: Nursing Care Planning. 245 p. Philadelphia, J. B. Lippincott, 1969.

   Chapters 6 (pages 105–160) and 8 (pages 169–186)

NURSING CARE PLAN

Objective (Patient Centered) _Satisfactory recovery from gall bladder removal surgery_

Assessment of Needs or Problems

Method of Approach

PRIORITY

#1. Comfort
Goal - Relief of pain and nausea with progressive ↓ of medications

1) Backrubs, repositioning q 2 hrs.; support wound with pillow, 5/15, 5/16
2) Observe for pain and nausea q 2 hrs., 5/15, 5/16 (pt. reluctant to complain.")
3) Ask pt. what comfort measures she prefers
4) Cue room dim when food trays served while nauseated
5) Keep window draperies closed, use soft lighting (upon light sensitive)

#2. Hydration
Goal - Oral fluid intake of 2000 cc./24 hrs. by 5/18

1) Oral fluid goals: 500 cc., 5/16; 1000 cc., 5/17; 2000 cc., 5/18 ⟶
2) Offer fluids between meals, preferns juices; no ice or milk
3) Offer bedpan or bathroom assistance q 2-3 hrs.
4) Teach pt. about importance of fluids and to keep own I and O record
5) Check intravenous infusion hourly (pt. fearful)

#3. Activity
Goal - Comfortable, progressive, of ambulation 3x daily by 5/20

1) Assist pt. to deep breathe and cough q 2 hrs. while awake, 5/15, 5/16
2) Isometric exercises of lower extremities for 5 mins. x 3, 5/15, 5/16
3) Encourage progressive self care starting 5/16
4) Dangle feet 5 mins., 5/15; Up in chair at bedside 5-10 mins. x 3, 5/16;
   to bathroom 20 mins. x 3, to bathroom, 5/17; Up for 60 mins. x 3, ambulate
   length of corridor, 5/18; increase ambulation, 5/19 ⟶
5) Stay with pt. during ambulation (fearful of fainting.)

#4. Understanding
Goal - Adequate knowledge and skill for safe, confident home self care

1) Demonstrate dressing technic; observe 3 satisfactory dressing changes
   by pt.; Assist with plans for home supplies
2) Call dietician to see pt. for diet instructions after 5/18
3) Plan home activity and rest schedule with pt.

Room # 415   Name SMITH, MRS. MARY   Doctor JOHN BROWN   Diagnosis cholelithiasis cholecystectomy 5/15

ALLERGIES
Adhesive tape

MEDS - (PLAN A)   PLAN B

Demerol 100 mgm. IM q 4 hr. PRN pain, 5/15-5/17
Compazine 10 mgm. IM q 4 hr. PRN nausea
Seconal gr. i/ss HS PRN for sleep

X-RAYS AND OTHER TESTS

5/13   Chest x-ray
5/13   Gall bladder series
5/14   CBC, UA
5/14   serum electrolytes
5/16   serum electrolytes

SPECIMENS

OPERATIONS
Cholecystectomy - 5/15

Acuity

Adm. # *48347*

Adm. Date *5/13*

RELIGION - *Protestant*

OCCUPATION - *Homemaker, secretary*

EDUCATION - *Business school graduate*

HOME TOWN - *Local*

EMERGENCY PHONE NUMBER
283-8094

FAMILY SOCIAL HISTORY -
Husband deceased
Son, age 23, daughter age 17, live at home, attend college and high school
Married daughter and 2 grandchildren out of state
"close" family relations

TREATMENTS
5/14   S.S. enema
5/14   skin prep.
5/15   2000 cc. 5% D/W   IV at 50 gtts./min.
5/16, 5/17   1000 cc. 5% D/W   IV at 60 gtts./min.
5/16   dressing change daily, use non-allergic tape

DIET *Clear liquid first named, Progress to low fat regular diet. Prefer juices, no ice or milk*

TPR - *q 4 hr; 5/15, 5/16* BP - *q 2 hr. until stable, then daily* *TID thereafter*

WT. - Yes (No)   *Admission 143#*

BATH. - *Pts. preference. Prefers own soap*

ACTIVITY - *Up 5/16, Increase according to pts. tolerance*

I & O - (Yes) No

REFERRALS *Dietician re low fat diet*

Rm # *415*   Name *SMITH, MRS. MARY*   Age *46*   Doctor *JOHN BROWN*   Diagnosis *Cholelithiasis*

GSH 00-0552

Fig. 8-4 Nursing Care Plan Cards.

discuss the written plan of care. After reading these chapters and again reviewing this chapter, evaluate the sample nursing care plan illustrated (Fig. 8–4) to determine if you feel it is satisfactory. Is all of the information needed for providing nursing care for Mrs. Smith included? Are the directives clear and specific? Is there other information you feel would be helpful in providing her care? Can the plan be used to evaluate the effectiveness of Mrs. Smith's care? What changes, if any, would you make in the plan?

2. The following two references discuss the planning process and give examples of patient situations. Both references have sections dealing with the selection of alternatives based on probability theory. After reading these sections, use this approach to select the nursing actions you will implement with your next patient care assignment.

   Bower, F. L.: The Process of Planning Nursing Care: A Theoretical Model. 139 p. St. Louis, C. V. Mosby, 1972.

   Lewis, L.: Planning Patient Care. 136 p. Dubuque, Iowa, William C. Brown, 1970.

3. What suggestions does the author of the following article make for dealing with common problems nurses encounter when preparing nursing care plans?

   Wagner, B. M.: Care plans—rights, reasonable, and reachable. **Am. J. Nurs.,** 69:986–990, May, 1969.

4. The author of the first article given below gives reasons why she believes nursing care plans are important. The author of the second article identifies some practical problems in the development of nursing care plans in a busy hospital.

   Harris, B. L.: Who needs written care plans anyway? **Am. J. Nurs.,** 70:2136–2138, Oct., 1970.

   Palisin, H. E.: Nursing care plans are a snare and a delusion. **Am. J. Nurs.,** 71:63–66, Jan., 1971.

   Read these authors' opposing views and think about your own experiences with patients to whom you have given care. What conclusions would you draw concerning nursing care plans?

5. The following three references are concerned with stating educational objectives:

   Mager, R. F.: Preparing Instructional Objectives. 60 p. Palo Alto, Calif., Fearon Publishers, 1962.

   Geitgey, D. A., and Crowley, D.: Preparing objectives. **Am. J. Nurs.,** 65:95–97, Jan., 1965.

   Gronlund, N. E.: Stating Behavioral Objectives for Classroom Instruction. 58 p. New York, Macmillan, **1970.**

After reading these references, practice writing objectives for the next patient for whom you will care, using the above authors' guidelines to assist you.

6. As was recommended for the previous chapters in this unit, read this chapter again and in instances where examples are given to illustrate a particular point, describe an experience from your own nursing practice that will illustrate that point equally well.

References

1. Ciuca, R. L.: Over the years with the nursing care plan. **Nurs. Outlook,** 20:706–711, Nov., 1972.

2. Cornell, S. A., and Brush, F.: Systems approach to nursing care plans. **Am. J. Nurs.,** 71:1376–1378, July, 1971.

3. Ellsworth, M. S.: Who was Molly? **Am. J. Nurs.,** 70:2406–2408, Nov., 1970.

4. Griffith, E. W.: Nursing process: a patient with respiratory dysfunction. *In* **The Nursing Clinics of North America.** Philadelphia, W. B. Saunders, 6:145–154, Mar., 1971.

5. Horvitz, I. A.: Unrecognized cues or the case of Mr. X. **Am. J. Nurs.,** 68:2133–2134, Oct., 1968.

6. Josten, L. V., *et al.:* Staff plan to minimize paper nursing. **Am. J. Nurs.,** 72:492–493, Mar., 1972.

7. Kelly, N. C.: Nursing care plans. **Nurs. Outlook,** 14:61–64, May, 1966.

8. Levine, M. E.: Introduction to Clinical Nursing. ed. 2. Philadelphia, F. A. Davis, 1973. (Outline entitled "Nursing Process" at end of each chapter gives examples of factors that could be used to guide planning of nursing care.)

9. Little, D. E., and Carnevali, D. L.: Nursing Care Planning. Philadelphia, J. B. Lippincott, 1969.

10. ———: The nursing care planning system. **Nurs. Outlook,** 19:164–167, Mar., 1971.

11. Mayers, M. G.: A Systematic Approach to the Nursing Care Plan. New York, Appleton-Century-Crofts, 1972.

12. Nordmark, M. T., and Rohweder, A. W.: Scientific Foundations of Nursing. ed. 2. Philadelphia J. B. Lippincott, 1967.

13. Smith, D. M.: Writing objectives as a nursing practice skill. **Am. J. Nurs.,** 71:319–320, Feb., 1971.

14. Tinkham, C. W., and Voorhies, E. F.: Community Health Nursing: Evolution and Process. pp. 159–175; 236–250. New York, Appleton-Century-Crofts, 1972.

15. White, M. B.: Importance of selected nursing activities. **Nurs. Research,** 21:4–14, Jan.–Feb., 1972.

CHAPTER 9

Nursing Intervention

GLOSSARY

Intervene: To come between.

Response: A reaction to a stimulus.

INTRODUCTION

Nursing intervention is the last subsystem in the nursing process system. To *intervene* means to come between. For example, a labor arbitrator intervenes to settle a strike. He comes between an employer and an employee. In nursing, a nurse intervenes to assist a patient with a health-illness problem. She comes between a problem and its solution by carrying out services to solve the problem.

Involvement of the patient to the greatest extent possible is important when giving nursing care. It has been demonstrated and described in nursing literature often that expressions of patient satisfaction are directly proportional to the patient's involvement in his care. Whether the nurse is caring for an individual, a family, or a community, there is a sense of accomplishment when the patient participates. Patient involvement takes more time; but in the long run, the expenditure of time is well worth it and generally helps the patient to become more independent in relation to meeting his own needs.

As was true for the earlier subsystems of the nursing process system, nursing intervention involves a process and requires the nurse to make judgments in relation to a specific patient. The *purpose* of intervention is to render appropriate patient care by putting the nursing care plan into action. The *input* of intervention is the nursing care plan which was the output of the planning process described in Chapter 8. The *output* is the patient's responses to the nursing care he has received. There are two *performance criteria* used in the nursing interven-

tion process: evidence that the patient is reaching objectives of nursing care or has reached them; and evidence of acceptability of the nursing care to the patient.

Figure 9-1 illustrates the input, process, output, performance criteria, and feedback of nursing intervention.

THE PROCESS OF NURSING INTERVENTION

The process of nursing intervention is described in three phases: putting nursing care plan into action; identifying patient responses to care; and evaluating responses to nursing care by comparing them with performance criteria. A flow chart illustrating the process of nursing intervention appears in Figure 9-2.

Putting Nursing Care Plan Into Action

The information contained in the nursing care plan becomes the basis for action. The specific action a nurse has planned to take will be guided by principles, as discussed in Chapter 3. For example, consider a patient who is receiving oxygen therapy. A physical principle states that oxygen supports combustion. Oxygen itself does not burn but any combustible material will burn in the presence of concentrated oxygen. This principle is used to guide the nurse in planning care for the patient in order to avoid accidents.

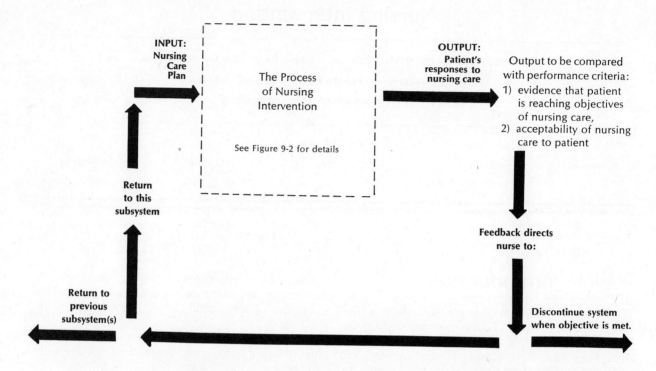

Fig. 9-1. Nursing intervention, showing input, process, output, performance criteria, and feedback. Broken line indicates environmental influences may affect process at any time, as described in Chapter 5.

The principle of maintaining the patient's individuality is considered during nursing intervention. There may be times when the nurse will make on-the-spot decisions in order to keep care individualized. For example, a nurse may be teaching a mother the essentials of a balanced diet for her family. She may find that it seems better to use a chart picturing the essentials of a balanced diet for this patient before presenting information in printed form. In another instance, a patient may appear to prefer reading something first before studying about it from a chart or discussing it during an interview. As another example, while continuing to observe microbiological and physics principles to apply a dressing to a wound, the nurse may adjust the exact placement of tapes holding the dressing in place to suit the patient's desires. A patient needs to exercise her arm following a mastectomy (removal of a breast).

She may prefer doing the exercise after lunch rather than before, and she is allowed to do so.

While patient involvement is important, care must be exercised so that inappropriate demands are not made on the patient. Some patients may be too frightened or fearful of involvement. Or, some may not have the emotional or physical resources to participate. Others may accept involvement only out of fear of being labeled "uncooperative." Refusal may cause the patient to fear that the nurse may retaliate. Sensitivity to the patient's feelings, with encouragement and support, are important as the nurse promotes patient involvement with his care.

Another precaution when involving patients with their care is to be sure that adjustments in care suggested by the patient will not interfere with objectives. For example, a patient may wish to postpone learning how to administer his own insulin

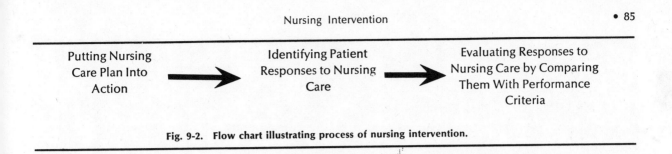

Fig. 9-2. Flow chart illustrating process of nursing intervention.

until after he has returned from a vacation. This arrangement may be unwise if postponement represents a threat to the control of his disease. To delay the teaching program in this example would defeat the overall objective of nursing care.

Identifying Patient Responses to Nursing Care

A *response* is a reaction to a stimulus. A person's reactions of joy (response) when he sees a long-time friend unexpectedly (stimulus) is an example.

Identifying responses to nursing care requires deliberate efforts to detect reactions in the patient as a result of care he received. Reviewing the objectives of care will aid the nurse to identify responses that indicate change has occurred. For example, an objective of care stated that the patient's intestinal elimination will occur on a daily basis within two weeks of beginning a bowel training program. The patient's responses to the training program are relatively easy to see: bowel elimination occurs or it does not in the manner stated in the objective. Other responses or changes in the patient may be more subtle and difficult to note. How a patient feels about adjustments he may need to make in his activities of daily living following a heart attack is difficult to gauge. The nurse will have to form her impressions out of a number of clues.

The methods used to identify patient responses to nursing care are those used when gathering data, as described in Chapter 6. The nurse needs to know what she is looking for in relation to patient responses; she must be alert to any clues, the subtle as well as the obvious; and she must be objective and honest in her appraisal of patient responses to care. The following examples will illustrate how nurses identified patient responses to care.

A nurse is caring for a patient who is nauseated and vomiting. He is unable to retain fluids or food. The objective of care is that there will be less nausea and vomiting and an increase in fluid intake to 2,000 c.c. within 24 hours. Once appropriate care has been given, the nurse will identify the responses of this patient to it in several ways. She may ask the patient to compare his current feelings about nausea with previous ones. If he states he feels no nausea and if there has been no vomiting, his responses to care have been demonstrated. The nurse will also observe the patient's appearance to detect changes in his skin coloring, his facial expressions, his mannerisms, and so on. For example, the pale appearance of his skin has disappeared; his facial muscles appear relaxed; he no longer wants an emesis basin at his side. In addition, the nurse notes that the patient's oral intake has reached 2,000 c.c. in the last 24-hour period; his urinary output has increased; his body temperature and his pulse and respiratory rates are within normal ranges; and laboratory reports indicate that his blood chemistry findings are within normal ranges. These examples illustrate responses to care.

Assume now that instead of the responses just described, the patient demonstrates the following signs: he states he still feels nauseated and he continues to vomit; he insists he needs an emesis basin at his side at all times; he appears pale and his facial muscles are tense. Also, the patient states he feels "bloated" and the nurse observes that his abdomen is distended (swollen); he is urinating much less than would be expected of an adult, and he is refusing fluids and food; his body temperature is elevated and his respiratory and pulse rates do not fall within normal ranges; laboratory reports indicate that his blood chemistry findings do not fall within normal ranges. These responses obviously indicate that care measures were unsuccessful.

Consider another situation. A community health nurse is planning expectant parent classes. Her data gathering illustrated that there has been an average of 202 babies born in a particular neighborhood annually for the last three years. In any one six-month period in the past two years, the average number of couples attending expectant parent classes was 31. From this information, the nurse concluded that many couples were not attending classes. She stated her objective as: to increase the number of expectant parents completing classes within the next

FUNDAMENTALS OF NURSING

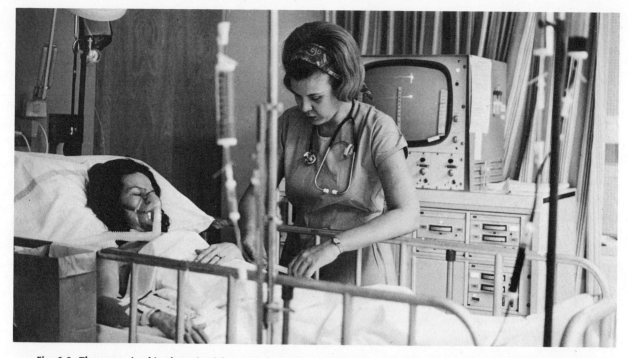

Fig. 9-3. The nurse in this photo is giving care that will aid in meeting the patient's needs. She also evaluates the care she is giving. Note the monitoring machine which aids the nurse in evaluating the patient's condition. Often, even the more subtle changes in the patient's condition may require the nurse to change and adapt care as she intervenes in order to help the patient overcome present problems and then take steps toward the ultimate goal of high-level wellness. (Good Samaritan Hospital, Phoenix, Arizona)

12 months by 50 percent. She developed and implemented a plan that included using a local newspaper and radio station to advertise that classes were being offered. After one year, the nurse identified certain responses to her plan. An average of 41 couples in the neighborhood had attended classes in each of the two six-month periods while the number of births had remained approximately the same as for the previous three-year period.

These examples illustrate that identifying responses to nursing care begins by looking at the nursing care objectives. Then the nurse searches for clues to tell her what her patient's responses have been.

Evaluating Responses to Nursing Care by Comparing Them with Performance Criteria

The final phase in the process of nursing intervention is to evaluate nursing care responses by comparing them with performance criteria. As stated earlier, the nurse must know what she is looking for and the objectives of care she has set.

The first performance criterion has been met when the nurse has evidence that the patient has reached or is reaching objectives of nursing care. Go back for a moment to the example of the patient who is having nausea and vomiting. The objectives of nursing care for this patient were met in the first instance. When, in the second instance, the patient's nausea and vomiting continued, his fluid intake failed to meet the objective, and he displayed additional signs that served as clues that his condition was becoming worse, the performance criteria had not been met.

In the example of the community health nurse preparing expectant parent classes, the nurse's objective was to increase attendance at the classes by 50 percent in a particular neighborhood within the succeeding 12-month period. The increase in attendance of approximately 32 percent falls short of the objective but suggests that the advertising appeared to help. Hence, the performance criterion was only partially met. The nurse concludes that the plan she implemented was only partially successful to date but she is making progress toward meeting her ultimate objective.

The preceding examples illustrate the importance of stating objectives of nursing care in precise and specific terms so that the nurse can clearly determine whether or not objectives were reached or the extent to which they have been reached. Had the nurse's objective in the example of expectant parent classes, for instance, not clearly stated what increase in attendance she planned for, the nurse would have been unable to estimate the extent to which the plan she used had succeeded.

The second performance criterion, acceptability of care to the patient, has been discussed in Chapter 5 since this criterion is used in evaluating the entire nursing process system.

FEEDBACK

Nursing intervention is the last subsystem in the nursing process system. When evaluation of patient responses to nursing care by comparison with the performance criteria indicates nursing care objectives are not being met, the nurse retraces her steps. She decides to return to the beginning of this subsystem. Or, she decides to return to any of the previous three subsystems. In the latter case, she may gather more data; use different standards when making a nursing assessment; or modify her nursing care plan.

Look again at Figure 9-1 on page 84. Because nursing intervention is the last subsystem in the nursing process system, there is no option to go on to a next subsystem. Rather, if evidence indicates that progress toward an objective of nursing care is progressing satisfactorily (that is, if an objective is partially achieved) the nurse continues until the objective is reached. Or, when an objective is reached, the requirement for the nursing care that has accomplished its goal is no longer necessary. The output becomes part of the total system output and when its objective is achieved, the system terminates.

CONCLUSION

Now that the four major subsystems in the nursing process system have been described, the nurse can observe how interrelated each subsystem is with every other one. Advantages of using the nursing process system, as discussed in Chapter 5, are now more obvious. For example, the nursing process system is responsive to changes within the patient and his situation; it is responsive to changes in the nurse's perceptions of needs for care; it can be used in any situation where a patient needs care. Also, it provides for constant evaluation; it is a logical and organized way of approaching nursing care problems while still allowing for great creativity on the part of the nurse.

Chapter 10, which completes this unit, will discuss communications among health practitioners, which are essential for the proper functioning of the nursing process system, as the previous discussions in this unit attempted to illustrate.

Unit 3 is concerned with the nurse-patient relationship. The information discussed in that unit is essential for the smooth functioning of the nursing process system. For example, unless the nurse has certain communication skills, as described in Chapter 13, she will be handicapped in every contact she has with patients. The nurse who is able to develop therapeutic relationships with patients, as described in Chapter 11, has invaluable and necessary tools for implementing the nursing process system. Being aware of the role of the patient (Chapter 12), observing principles from the social sciences (Chapter 14), respecting a patient's religious beliefs (Chapter 15) and preparing health teaching programs (Chapter 16) are all important in the use of the nursing process system. Units 4 and 5 will provide the nurse with much information essential to all phases in the nursing process system. The information in these units is more specifically related to descriptions of nursing care activities.

Immediately following this chapter, the reader is provided with an example of a patient's care, using the entire nursing process system.

The nursing process system is recommended in this text as the basis or the frame of reference that guides the nurse in her work in aiding patients to attain and maintain high-level wellness. With continued use and practice, the skills to use it effectively will result in nursing care that is individualized for each patient and that is high quality and professional in nature.

Study Situations
1. Articles in the following reference discuss factors the nurse must know in order to adapt care appropriately in relation to each patient's needs:
   Symposium on Current Surgical Nursing. In **The Nursing Clinics of North America.** Philadelphia, W. B. Saunders, 8:107–198, Mar., 1973.
   Recall several patients you have cared for recently and list factors you needed to consider in order to individualize patient care.

2. The authors of the following two articles give different points of view about the role of routines in nursing intervention:

Baziak, A. T.: Prospects for change in nursing. **Nurs. Forum,** 6:134–153, No. 2, 1967.

Ramphal, M. M.: Values of routines in nursing. **Nurs. Forum,** 6:335–340, No. 3, 1967.

After reading these two articles, think about routines with which you are familiar and consider their advantages and disadvantages in relation to patient care.

3. The author of the following book made some suggestions on how common factors in a hospital situation can be used by nurses to enhance patient care. The factors included the hospital environment, policies in relation to visitors, food service, and lounge facilities.

Brown, E. L.: Newer Dimensions of Patient Care; Part 1: The Use of the Physical and Social Environment of the General Hospital for Therapeutic Purposes. 159 p. New York, Russell Sage Foundation, 1961.

Describe a situation, with which you are familiar, when a nurse intervened to modify some aspect of a patient's hospital environment that resulted in an improvement in patient care.

4. The nurse who wrote the following article worked for her community by becoming a member of a community planning committee:

McNeil, H. J.: How to become involved in community planning. **Nurs. Outlook,** 17:44–47, Feb., 1969.

List ways in which you believe you may be able to intervene and help the community in which you live.

5. As recommended for the previous chapters in this unit, read this chapter again and in instances where examples are given to illustrate a particular point, describe an experience from your own nursing practice that will illustrate that point equally well.

References

1. Abdellah, F. G.: Criterion measures in nursing. **Nurs. Research,** 10:21–26, Winter, 1961.

2. Barnett, K.: A theoretical construct of the concepts of touch as they relate to nursing. **Nurs. Research,** 21:102–110, Mar.–Apr., 1972.

3. Durr, C. A.: Hands that help . . . but how? **Nurs. Forum,** 10:392–400, No. 4, 1971.

4. Levine, M. E.: Introduction to Clinical Nursing. ed. 2. Philadelphia, F. A. Davis, 1973. (Outline entitled "Nursing Process" at end of each chapter gives examples of factors that could be used to guide nursing intervention.)

5. Lewis, L.: Planning Patient Care. Dubuque, Ia., William C. Brown, 1970.

6. Mayers, M. G.: A Systematic Approach to the Nursing Care Plan. pp. 117–139. New York, Appleton-Century-Crofts, 1972.

7. Nordmark, M. T., and Rohweder, A. W.: Scientific Foundations of Nursing. ed. 2. Philadelphia, J. B Lippincott, 1967.

8. Pluckhan, M. L.: Space: the silent language. . . . **Nurs. Forum,** 7:386–397, No. 4, 1968.

9. Schmidt, J.: Availability: a concept of nursing practice. **Am. J. Nurs.,** 72:1086–1089, June, 1972.

10. Schwartz, D. R.: Toward more precise evaluation of patients' needs. **Nurs. Outlook,** 13:42–44, May, 1965.

11. Tinkham, C. W., and Voorhies, E. F.: Community Health Nursing: Evaluation and Process. pp. 176–192; 251–265. New York, Appleton-Century-Crofts, 1972.

EXAMPLE OF APPLICATION OF THE NURSING PROCESS SYSTEM

The following example is intended to illustrate one way in which the nursing process system can be implemented. There are many variations in its application. Information is given to demonstrate the characteristics of the system and its subsystems, but it is not intended to include all factors that could be involved with a patient's care.

Nursing Process System
    Purpose: To provide nursing care which will promote high-level wellness for the patient
    Input: Data about the patient and his environment
    Output: State of the patient's health
    Process Phases: Data gathering; assessment; planning; intervention
    Performance Criterion: Improvement or maintenance of the patient's state of wellness

SUBSYSTEM SUMMARY

DATA-GATHERING SUBSYSTEM

Purpose: To collect and organize data about the patient's health state
Input: Information items
Output: Health state profile
Process Phases: Selecting data; organizing data; selecting data gathering methods; gathering data; validating data; and comparing output with performance criteria
Performance Criteria: Appropriateness and accuracy

EXAMPLE OF APPLICATION

DATA ITEMS

Health Agency Record
    Name: Mr. B.
    Age: 74
    Grade school education
    Married for 43 years, no children
    Lived in same ground floor apartment with wife for past 21 years
    Physician's Report: ". . . one month post cerebrovascular accident (stroke) which resulted in right arm weakness and right homonymous hemianopsia (loss of vision in right half of both eyes)."
    Patient's Verbalization: ". . . can't see very well, nothing on the right side, . . . arm is so weak and hand shakes, never was any good at using my left hand, I'm such a burden, . . . wife is so good to me."
    Wife's Verbalization: ". . . feed and dress him at home because he's awkward and spills since he can't see well and his hand is so weak . . . do you think you can help him? Is there something else I can do?"
    Nurse's Observations: Patient dressed in pajamas and robe, wears glasses, turns upper part of body slightly when his attention is focused on something at his right. He moves left arm and hand with no difficulty; moves right hand and arm slowly and with trembling but appropriately upon request; raises right hand to shoulder height; unable to lift right arm over head. He talks slowly in a quiet voice with head down but responds readily and appropriately; tears well in his eyes as he talks about being ". . . a burden." Wife is small woman; appears younger than husband; glances at husband often as she talks; has tense facial muscles; answers questions and offers information readily.

VALIDATION

Direct question to patient: "You seem to be discouraged by not being able to see very well and not being able to feed yourself, is that right?"

HEALTH STATE PROFILE

Limited use of right hand and arm. No right field vision. Discouraged with poor self-image. Strong husband-wife relationship.

SUBSYSTEM SUMMARY	EXAMPLE OF APPLICATION

EXAMPLE OF APPLICATION

OUTPUT EVALUATION

Do any of the data areas receive too much emphasis in the profile? Are there any important data areas omitted in the profile? Are the profile statements correct?

Revise or continue subsystem process until performance criteria are met, or move on to the next subsystem.

ASSESSMENT SUBSYSTEM

Purpose: To judge the items of the health state profile in relation to the patient's health-illness status
Input: Health state profile
Output: Nursing assessment
Process Phases: Selecting standards; comparing profile with standards; stating nursing assessments; validating nursing assessments; and comparing output with performance criteria
Performance Criteria: Appropriateness and accuracy

STANDARDS

Head movements can increase the visual field.
Muscle weaknesses and loss of coordination of neurological origin can be temporary or permanent; muscle exercises and use can promote functional return and prevent further deterioration.
Independence is a fundamental human need and influences the self concept.
Older persons decrease their social contacts and develop increasing dependency on fewer significant persons; persons significant to an individual can influence his motivation.

NURSING ASSESSMENTS

Using adaptive head movements could compensate for Mr. B.'s vision disability.
Active use of Mr. B.'s right arm will reduce the likelihood of further impairment and may promote regaining its use.
Developing alternate behaviors which promote independence should enhance Mr. B.'s self concept.
The likelihood of Mr. B. learning new skills will be increased if Mrs. B. is involved in the effort.

VALIDATION

Ask another nurse, "Do you believe Mr. B. would be more likely to succeed in his therapy if we make certain Mrs. B. is involved?"

OUTPUT EVALUATION

Do the nursing assessments identify Mr. B.'s strengths and disabilities?
Are the nursing assessments correct as stated?

Revise or continue subsystem process until performance criteria are met or move on to the next subsystem.

PLANNING SUBSYSTEM

Purpose: To develop a scheme or guide for providing nursing care
Input: Nursing Assessment
Output: Nursing Care Plan
Process Phases: Determining nursing care requirements and their priorities; determining nursing care objectives; identifying alternative nursing actions and selecting ones to be implemented; writing nursing orders; developing nursing care plan; and comparing output to performance criteria
Performance Criteria: Illustrating relationship between nursing care assessment and nursing care plan; and illustrating plan is acceptable to patient

NURSING CARE REQUIREMENTS AND PRIORITIES

1. Activity of the right upper extremity.
2. Learning to feed himself.
3. Increasing self-esteem.

NURSING CARE OBJECTIVES

Patient will carry out prescribed right-arm and right-hand exercises within three days independently.
Patient will feed himself all meals unassisted with right arm within two weeks and express progressive feelings of self-satisfaction.

ALTERNATE NURSING ACTIONS CONSIDERED

(Starred items have been selected for implementation)
*Refer patient to physical therapist for arm and hand exercise regimen.
Teach wife to provide passive right arm movements, or,

SUBSYSTEM SUMMARY   **EXAMPLE OF APPLICATION**

*Teach patient to lift arm over head with left arm and en-
courage use of right arm.
*Observe patient for adequacy of hand and arm exercises.
*Encourage wife to be present during sessions with physical
therapist, *or,*
Discuss exercise plan and progress with wife after physical
therapy sessions.
*Provide for rest periods to prevent fatigue and discourage-
ment.
*Refer patient to occupational therapist for assistance with
eating.
*Arrange food in left visual field range.
*Pad handles of silverware.
*Prepare food in advance.
*Seat patient in comfortable, well-lighted area for eating.
*Encourage selection of easily handled foods; that is, avoid
food such as peas and jello.
Ask another recovering partially paralyzed patient to eat
with Mr. B., *or,*
Remain with patient and wife while he is eating, *or,*
*Encourage wife to be present at meals.

NURSING CARE PLAN

Patient's major strengths:
Alert; responsive; has supportive, interested wife; and has
normal use of three extremities.
Patient's major disabilities:
Impaired right-side vision, weak right arm, and feeling of
discouragement.
Objective No. 1:
Patient will carry out prescribed right-arm and right-hand
exercises within three days independently.
Nursing Orders:
Have patient ready for physical therapy at 10:30 A.M.
Wife to accompany him.
Encourage and give patient time to use right hand and
arm.
Observe and provide encouragement and any necessary
correction of exercises twice daily. (See prescribed
exercises in physical therapy report.)
Encourage patient to plan daily schedule of activities in-
cluding exercises and rest periods.
Objective No. 2:
Patient will feed himself all meals unassisted within two
weeks and express progressive satisfaction.
Nursing Orders:
Encourage selection of easily handled foods. Assist wife
to prepare and arrange food in left visual field.
Provide silverware with padded handles.
Seat patient in comfortable, well-lighted area.
Occupational therapist or nurse to spend short time with
patient during meals to provide encouragement or in-
struction.

OUTPUT EVALUATION

Is there a relationship between each of the nursing assessments and the nursing care plan?
Is the plan acceptable to Mr. B.?

SUBSYSTEM SUMMARY	EXAMPLE OF APPLICATION

Revise or continue subsystem process until performance criteria are met or move on to next subsystem.

NURSING INTERVENTION SUBSYSTEM

Purpose: To give care by putting nursing care plan into action.

Input: Nursing care plan

Output: Patient's responses to care

Process Phases: Putting plan into action; identifying patient responses; and comparing output with performance criteria.

Performance Criteria: Nursing care objectives reached or being reached; and care acceptable to patient

CLUES TO PATIENT RESPONSES

Objective No. 1:
Frequency of performed exercises.
Quality of performed exercises.
Degree of independence regarding exercise regimen.

Objective No. 2:
Amount of food ingested.
Adeptness of use of silverware with right hand.
Amount of food soiling of clothing.
Verbal and behavioral manifestations relating to eating.

OBSERVED PATIENT RESPONSES

Objective No. 1:
Performs morning exercises appropriately and on own initiative. Often needs to be reminded of afternoon and evening sessions and to complete the entire regimen. Does so with encouragement.
Performs exercises with greater interest when wife is present.
Able to touch top of head with right hand without pain.

Objective No. 2:
Selecting wider variety of foods and finishing all food on tray.
Beginning to manage simultaneous use of knife and fork.
Handles solid foods with few spills but still has difficulty raising cup to mouth with right hand with steadiness.
Smiles and converses with wife occasionally while eating.
States he "... doesn't feel so helpless anymore."

OUTPUT EVALUATION

Is Mr. B. carrying out the exercises independently within three days?
Is Mr. B. feeding himself unassisted within two weeks and expressing related progressive satisfaction?
Is Mr. B. satisfied with his nursing care?

Revise or continue subsystem process until performance criteria are met or determine if system purpose has been met.

System Output Evaluation
Has Mr. B.'s state of wellness been improved or maintained?
Continue system process until performance criterion is met, then terminate nursing care system.

CHAPTER 10

Communications Among Health Practitioners

GLOSSARY

Auditing: Using a record as an aid in evaluating the quality of patient care.
Baseline Information: Fundamental data on which care is built or developed.
Chart: Synonym for record.
Communication: An exchange of information.
Confer: To consult; to exchange ideas; to seek information, instruction or advice from another.
Consult: A synonym for confer.
Direct: To guide or order.
Problem-Oriented Records: Records that are prepared on the basis of a specific method of organizing data about a patient and that focus on a patient's specific problems.
Record: Sum total of forms that contain information about a patient.
Refer: To send or direct someone for action or help.
Referral: The process of directing or sending someone for action or help.
Report: To give an account of something that has been seen, heard, done, or considered.

INTRODUCTION

As the previous five chapters in this unit illustrated, communications among health practitioners are essential for determining, planning, and implementing the services required by patients. This chapter will describe common ways and means of communicating among health practitioners serving the patient.

The reader will note that Chapter 13 is also concerned with communications. Chapter 13 deals more specifically with the theory of communication and focuses on communications between the nurse and the patient.

PURPOSE OF COMMUNICATION AMONG HEALTH PRACTITIONERS

Communication is the exchange of information. The efforts of health practitioners are directed toward aiding the patient to attain and maintain high-level wellness. Effective communication among health practitioners helps in reaching that goal; for without

it, there would be utter chaos, with the patient being the loser.

The primary purpose of communication among health practitioners is to exchange information that will serve to promote coordination and continuity of patient care, resulting in a harmonious blending of whatever services the patient requires. Effective communication among health practitioners will enable personnel to supplement and complement each other's services and to avoid duplication, omissions, and unnecessary overlaps in care.

For example, consider a patient being cared for by a variety of health practitioners. A smooth transfer of responsibility and coordination of care is often important when the patient is hospitalized and acutely ill, from hour to hour and at change-of-shift time. When the patient receives services from various departments in the hospital, as for instance, the x-ray, operating room, laboratory, and physical therapy departments, good communication will coordinate the services of personnel in these various departments. Communications among health practitioners when the patient is discharged from the hospital remain

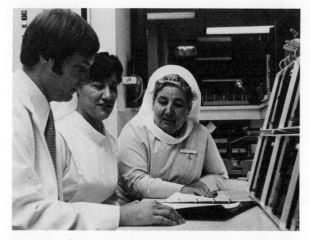

Fig. 10-1. The importance of health team colleagues exchanging information in relation to a patient has been discussed often in this text. Here, a social worker, a nurse, and a physician discuss the best way to coordinate their plans for a patient being cared for in the coronary care unit who will face problems when he is ready to return to his home and family. Even during the acute phase of the patient's illness, groundwork is being laid to provide for continuity of care. Mention has been made several times in this text of the increased use of sophisticated equipment that aids health practitioners in observing a patient's condition. The equipment on the right-hand side of the picture is a continuous coronary monitoring system. (St. Joseph's Hospital and Medical Center, Phoenix, Arizona)

important as the patient turns to various agencies in the community offering health services, as for example, a visiting nurse service, the health office at work or school, or an extended care facility. This same person, at home or while still hospitalized, may require services of a social worker; a physical, occupational, recreational, or speech therapist; a clergy-man; a person from a homemaker service; and others. As this example illustrates, continuity and coordination of care for the patient are important and require effective communications among all persons concerned.

METHODS OF COMMUNICATION COMMONLY USED BY HEALTH PRACTITIONERS

An exchange of information may occur in face-to-face meetings or indirectly through communication media. Communications of the latter type use the written word or certain mechanical devices such as the tape recorder.

Speaking directly to someone has several advantages. One can secure an immediate message, as well as its interpretation when indicated. Also, there is the added advantage of exchanging nonverbal messages that are often conveyed by tone, facial expressions, gestures, and the like. Nonverbal communications and their important role in information exchange are discussed in Chapter 13.

A face-to-face meeting for the purpose of exchanging information has disadvantages too. For example, the people communicating must be in the same place at the same time and have the time available for communicating then and there. Also, there generally is no permanent record of the information exchanged for use at a later date.

Telephone communication and messenger-relayed information, while direct, have limitations. Telephone communication cannot convey most forms

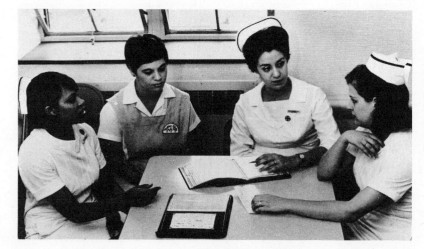

Fig. 10-2. Nursing team members often exchange information in conferences such as illustrated here. These team members are pooling information which they will then use to adjust care for each patient according to his needs. (Photo by Warren R. Vroom)

of nonverbal communication; only tone of voice, voice inflections, and the like, can be noted. A messenger also does not necessarily carry the original sender's nonverbal messages, and the information may become garbled in delivery. While using a messenger and a telephone have some of the advantages of face-to-face communication, they also have the disadvantages described in the preceding paragraph.

A common type of face-to-face communication occurs in groups, as for example, when team members confer, when health practitioners visit patients during rounds, or when a formal case presentation is made. Informal face-to-face meetings concerning patient care sometimes take place over a cup of coffee or during a meal.

Indirect communication, such as when using the written word or a tape recorder, has several advantages over face-to-face communication. The information can be exchanged at times convenient for the people involved and a record is available for later use. However, a disadvantage is that the sender of the message is not in a position to judge whether his message was interpreted as he intended it to be.

In general, communications among health personnel fall into four categories: reporting, directing, conferring, and referring.

To *report* is to give an account of something that has been seen, heard, done, or considered. Nurses report to other nurses who will assume patient care responsibilities at change-of-shift time, for instance. Another example is the progress record of a child's physical and mental development.

To *direct* is to guide or order. For instance, a nurse uses nursing orders to guide nursing care activities. The physician's order directs personnel concerning the care he wishes his patient to receive. An assignment sheet directs personnel to those activities for which they are responsible. When communication involves a directive, it is important to tell who does what and when. Often, directives are given verbally. However, there is greater safety when a directive is written in order to avoid errors and misunderstandings.

To *confer* is to consult with someone to exchange ideas or to seek information, advice, or instructions from another. For example, a nurse may consult with another nurse, as when a team leader consults with a clinical specialist about a particular patient's care. A school nurse may consult with a child's teacher or a psychologist about a behavior problem. A community health nurse and physician may confer about a patient's activity regimen. Health practitioners often confer in order to validate information concerning a patient. Validation was discussed in Chapters 6 and 7 of this unit.

To *refer* is to send or direct someone for action or help. The process of sending or guiding someone to another source for assistance is called a *referral*. A referral may be used among health agencies. For example, a patient may be referred by a hospital to a community health nursing service for assistance with home care. A school nurse may refer a student to a hospital emergency room. A community health nurse may refer a problem she encounters in a neighborhood to the department of health for action. A referral may be used within a particular agency also, as for example, a hospital outpatient clinic may refer a patient to the hospital's inservice facilities. A woman may be referred by a prenatal clinic to the agency's postpartum clinic after delivery.

The nurse's role as the patient's advocate was discussed in Chapter 1. Nurses often function in this capacity when they use referrals to seek assistance in meeting the patient's various needs. For example, the nurse may obtain services for a patient through a referral to an agency's dietary department or to a community social service agency. In such instances, the nurse will wish to discuss the referral with the patient so that he knows of the plan and gives his permission for the nurse to initiate action on his behalf.

Most health agencies have policies in relation to referrals. For example, the agency may have a special form that personnel are to use when making referrals. The policies usually indicate who may initiate a referral, how it is to be done, and so on.

It can be seen that referrals are especially important in providing continuity of care for patients needing a variety of services. It is essential, then, that health practitioners to whom a patient is referred be given information that is most useful to other practitioners and to do so with a minimum of break in its continuity. The key question is: What would I want to know about this patient if I were the person who had to continue his care at this point? The patient must of course know and approve of a referral to another agency or other health personnel for care.

Both direct and indirect communications may be used in any one or all of the four categories described above. Also, one communication experience may have parts that fall into each of these four categories. For example, a nurse and a physician may report, direct, confer, and/or refer in a face-to-face meeting or through a patient's record.

TYPES OF INFORMATION COMMONLY EXCHANGED AMONG HEALTH PRACTITIONERS

Information exchanged among health practitioners usually is of three types. Certain basic information, sometimes called *baseline information,* is one type. This is the fundamental data on which one builds patient care. Examples include the patient's name and address, age/birth date, marital status, name and address of next of kin, employer, religious preference, reason for seeking service, name of the physician, and data gathered in relation to the patient's present state of health. Examples of such data and the data-gathering process are described in Chapter 6.

A second type of information exchanged among health personnel describes the patient's needs and the plans for meeting them. Examples of this type of information and the processes to develop the information are described in Chapters 7 and 8.

A third type of information is in relation to the care given and the patient's responses to it. Examples and the process to develop the information are described in Chapter 9.

COMMON TOOLS OF COMMUNICATION USED BY HEALTH PRACTITIONERS

There is a wide variety of printed forms used by health agencies that are helpful in the promotion of effective communications among health practitioners. Health agencies usually place all forms used for one patient in a folder or binder and the sum total of the material is referred to as the patient's *record.* In hospitals, *chart* commonly refers to a patient's record. Each health agency has its own policies in relation to the patient's record or chart. For example, they will indicate which personnel are responsible for the recording on each form and may describe the order in which forms are to appear in the record. Additional examples include the frequency with which entries are to be made; whether routine nursing care is to be recorded; the manner in which health personnel identify themselves after making an entry; which types of abbreviations are acceptable; and the manner in which an error in recording is handled. The nurse should familiarize herself with the policies and observe them as described by the agency in which she is giving care.

Some of the forms in common usage have been described in earlier chapters in this unit, such as data-gathering guides and nursing care plans. Graphs and checklists have also been mentioned; they often are used to record information in relation to the patient's temperature, pulse and respiratory rates, blood pressure, physical development, vision and hearing test results, laboratory test results, administration of medications, and so on. Examples of other forms in common use include the physician's order sheet, medical and nursing history forms, referral forms, progress note forms, nurses' notes, consent for therapy forms, immunization records, and x-ray and physical therapy records.

As mentioned earlier, some agencies use mechanical devices to assist in communicating information, such as the Dictaphone which records information that is then transcribed onto the agency's appropriate form and entered into the patient's record. A patient's health history and progress notes are examples of material often dictated and transcribed. Dictaphones are used by nurses as well as by physicians. Tape recorders are used for preserving verbatim conversations between patients and health personnel. They also may be used for exchanging information among health personnel, as for example at change-of-shift time.

The various tools used to exchange information are indispensable in the delivery of health services. Their value will be enhanced when they are used appropriately and when information is accurate, relevant, concise, and clear.

THE LEGAL STATUS OF THE PATIENT'S RECORD

The patient's record may be viewed as a legal document, admissible in courts as evidence, hence, the importance of accuracy in recording information. Also, only appropriate and relevant information should be recorded and reported in order to protect the patient's privacy. Legal implications for invasion of privacy are discussed in Chapter 4.

Consent forms (that is, a form the patient signs authorizing the performance of certain therapy) are an important part of the patient's record. A patient may bring legal action if his consent has not been properly attained. The legal implications of care without consent are discussed in Chapter 4 in the section, "Assault and Battery."

There is a difference of opinion as to the legal status of nurses' notes. In some places, the nurses' notes are not kept after the patient is discharged from a health agency; in other places, the nurses' notes are preserved as a permanent part of the patient's record. The length of time records are retained depends primarily on state law. The nurse should familiarize herself with the laws in relation to the patient's record in the state where she works.

The use of verbal orders has legal implications. Local policy and law will guide the nurse in relation to the execution of verbal orders. In the past, problems have arisen primarily in relation to verbal orders given to nurses by physicians.

TRENDS IN THE USE OF VARIOUS COMMUNICATION TOOLS

Changes in Forms Being Used

Keeping records is time-consuming, involves many health practitioners, and is subject to human error. There is a trend toward using tools that will simplify record-keeping and insure greater objectivity and accuracy. For example, the lengthy descriptions commonly found in much of the patient's record are being replaced by the use of more graphic records, checklists, and so forth. This type of record-keeping not only saves time for the health practitioner but also tends to minimize heresay and subjective record-keeping.

It has been typical of most agencies to use a different form for each group of health personnel. For example, the nurses have one form, the physicians another, the physical therapists their own, and so on. A trend is toward a single form used by all team members. This method gives a record of events in the order in which they occur. A chronicle of this sort provides personnel with a more unified picture of the patient. The result is less fragmentation and better continuity in care when a single progress form is used.

Problem-Oriented Records

Credit is given to Dr. Lawrence L. Weed for developing the concept of problem-oriented records. Dr. Weed first used problem-oriented records in the field of medicine but they are presently being used by a variety of health disciplines, including nursing.

Dr. Weed's basic plan for organizing records contains four parts: a compilation of baseline information related to the patient; a description of the patient's problems or needs; a plan on how each problem is to be handled; and a record of the patient's responses to the care that was implemented. In Dr. Weed's plan, problems are specified and then classified according to a predetermined numbering system, and the patient's responses are also coded in a manner that reflects the initial problem and the care the patient received.

The nursing process system and problem-oriented recording complement each other. Note how each of the processes in the nursing process system can be used for problem-oriented records: the data-gathering process is used to collect baseline data; the assessment process is used to identify the patient's needs; the process of planning nursing care is used to develop a plan on how each of the patient's problems are to be handled; and the nursing intervention process includes the gathering of information and an evaluation of the patient's responses to the care he receives.

The component of feedback, as described in each of the previous chapters in this unit, can be of great assistance when problem-oriented records are kept. The results of feedback can be placed in the record and then used as a means to evaluate the quality of care that has been given and to improve on it as indicated.

Using records as an aid in determining the quality of care and as a guide to improving care is known as *auditing*. Both physicians and nurses use auditing in their practices for this purpose. Several entries in the references given at the end of this chapter describe auditing in more detail.

Computerization

The trend toward more computerization in the delivery of health care can be expected to continue. More and more, health agencies are finding the use of a computer for record-keeping a great time- and space-saver and a very convenient way to store information that can quickly and accurately be retrieved at any time health practitioners need it.

The development of problem-oriented records anticipated computerization. The technique Dr. Weed advocates takes a giant step from descriptive-type records to the use of a system that can be adapted with relative ease for computer storage. Evidence of the use of problem-solving records by nurses or the use of records kept in a similarly organized manner is evidence that nursing too is moving forward in this age of the computer.

CONCLUSION

Effective communication among all team members is essential for the use of the nursing process system and for the efficient functioning of the health and nursing teams. Communications alone cannot produce well coordinated and continuous care, but lack of good communications can very often result in inferior care.

Study Situations

1. The authors of the following articles discuss ways nurses can use referrals as a means of promoting continuity of care:

   Luc, M. M.: Working relationships between occupational health nursing and community agencies. *In* **The Nursing Clinics of North America.** Philadelphia, W. B. Saunders, 7:163–174, Mar., 1972.

   Johansson, M. S.: A migrant referral system for continuity of health care. *In* **The Nursing Clinics of North America.** Philadelphia, W. B. Saunders, 7:133–141, Mar., 1972.

   Describe patient care you have observed that, in your opinion, lacked continuity because of inadequate referrals.

2. The following article points up the need for good communications among health practitioners:

   Juntti, M. J.: Problem solving in arranging for comprehensive home care. **Nurs. Forum,** 8:103–109, No. 1, 1969.

   Note the number of people with whom the nurse communicated in order to promote a smooth transition from hospital to home for 2-year-old Stevie.

3. Problem-oriented records were discussed in this chapter. The following articles describe problem-oriented recording and give examples of its use in various settings:

   Bonkowsky, M. L.: Adapting the POMR to community child health care. **Nurs. Outlook,** 20:515–518, Aug., 1972.

   Bloom, J. T., et al.: Problem-oriented charting. **Am. J. Nurs.,** 71:2144–2148, Nov., 1971.

   Schell, P. L., and Campbell, A. T.: POMR—not just another way to chart. **Nurs. Outlook,** 20:510–514, Aug., 1972.

   After reading the articles, describe how this recording method and the nursing process system parallel each other.

4. The following report of a study describes communications that did and that did not contribute to patient care:

   Bates, B., and Kern, M. S.: Doctor-nurse teamwork: what helps? what hinders?. **Am. J. Nurs.,** 67:2066–2071, Oct., 1967.

   List suggestions the authors made that tended to promote good communications among health practitioners. Describe how you might use the suggestions in your practice.

References

1. Brown, E. L.: Newer Dimensions of Patient Care: Part 2: Improving Staff Motivation and Competence in the General Hospital. New York, Russell Sage Foundation, 1962.

2. Brown, V. B., et al.: A computerized health information service. **Nurs. Outlook,** 19:158–161, Mar., 1971.

3. Deakers, L. P.: Continuity of family-centered nursing care between the hospital and the home. *In* **The Nursing Clinics of North America.** Philadelphia, W. B. Saunders, 7:83–93, Mar., 1972.

4. Dunlap, L., and Matteoli, R.: A team function: developing a nursing care plan in a psychiatric setting. **J. Psychiat. Nurs. and Mental Health Services,** 8:19–23, Sept.–Oct., 1970.

5. Field, F. W.: Communication between community nurse and physician. **Nurs. Outlook,** 19:722–725, Nov., 1971.

6. Gallagher, J. J., and Gallagher, A. H.: A phantasy (with references). **Am. J. Nurs.,** 70:538–542, Mar., 1970.

7. Keller, N. S.: Care without coordination: a true story. **Nurs. Forum,** 6:280–323, No. 3, 1967.

8. Kelso, M. T., and Barton, D.: The nursing questionnaire as a facilitator of psychological care on medical and surgical wards. **Perspect. Psychiat. Care,** 10:123–127, No. 3, 1972.

9. Little, D. E., and Carnevali, D. L.: Nursing Care Planning. Philadelphia, J. B. Lippincott, 1969.

10. Lucido, P., et al.: Recording the home visit. **Nurs. Outlook,** 15:38–40, Feb., 1967.

11. Lynaugh, J. E., and Bates, B.: The two languages of nursing and medicine. **Am. J. Nurs.,** 73:66–69, Jan., 1973.

12. Melody, M., and Clark, G.: Walking-planning rounds. **Am. J. Nurs.,** 67:771–773, Apr., 1967.

13. Mershimer, R., and McNamara, K.: Automating the paperwork. **Am. J. Nurs.,** 71:1164–1167, June, 1971.

14. Mitchell, P. H.: A systematic nursing progress record: the problem-oriented approach. **Nurs. Forum,** 12:187–210, No. 2, 1973.

15. Phaneuf, M. C.: Nursing audit for evaluation of patient care. **Nurs. Outlook,** 14:51–54, June, 1966.

16. ——: The Nursing Audit: Profile for Excellence. New York, Appleton-Century-Crofts, 1972.

17. Radtke, M., and Wilson, A.: Team conferences that work. **Am. J. Nurs.,** 73:506–508, Mar., 1973.

18. Rubin, C. F., et al.: Nursing audit—nurses evaluating nursing. **Am. J. Nurs.,** 72:916–921, Mar., 1972.

19. Sharp, B. H., and Cross, E.: Rounds and rounds. **Nurs. Outlook,** 19:419–420, June, 1971.

20. Speed, E. L., and Young, N. A.: Scan: data processed printouts of a patient's basic care needs. **Am. J. Nurs.,** 69:108–110, Jan., 1969.

21. Stein, L. I.: The doctor-nurse game. **Am. J. Nurs.,** 68:101–105, Jan., 1968.

22. Unangst, C.: The clinician's use of nursing rounds. **Am. J. Nurs.,** 71:1566–1567, Aug., 1971.

23. Weed, L. L.: Medical Records, Medical Education, and Patient Care. Cleveland, Press of Case Western Reserve University, 1970.

24. Weil, T. P., and Weil, J. W.: The use of computer systems in patient care. **Nurs. Forum,** 6:206–217, No. 2, 1967.

25. Woody, M., and Mallison, M.: The problem-oriented system for patient-centered care. **Am. J. Nurs.,** 73:1168–1175, July, 1973.

UNIT 3

The Nurse-Patient Relationship

CHAPTER 11

Developing a Therapeutic Relationship

GLOSSARY

Covert: Concealed from view.

Expressive Factor: Behavior in social interaction that results in an influence on a group's emotional tone and indirectly moves the group toward its ultimate goal(s).

Functional Factor: Behavior in social interaction that directly moves the group toward its ultimate goal(s). Synonyms include utilitarian factor and instrumental factor.

Hierarchy: Process or system that places things or persons in graded order or rank.

Hierarchy of Needs: Process or system that places requirements or necessities in an order or rank.

Interaction: Action or behavior of one person that produces reaction or behavior in another.

Need: A necessity or requirement.

Need Gratification: Satisfying a necessity or requirement.

Nurse-Patient Relationship: Interaction between a nurse and a patient.

Overt: Open to view.

Psychosocial: Pertaining to a combination of psychological and social variables.

Relationship: An interaction of individuals with one another.

Social Interaction: A group of two or more people who interact with one another. (See definition of interaction.)

Therapeutic Relationship: Interaction that is considered beneficial by participants in moving them toward a common goal(s).

INTRODUCTION

As Chapter 3 points out, man cannot be separated into physical and psychological entities. Rather, the two entities function interdependently to form unity in each individual. While still recognizing the concept of the wholeness of man, this unit will be primarily concerned with the psychological and social, or *psychosocial*, needs of the patient.

Increasing emphasis is being placed on the relationships between patients and nurses. A *relationship* may be defined as an interaction of individuals with one another. A *therapeutic relationship* is an interaction that is considered beneficial by participants because it moves them toward a common goal(s). A

therapeutic relationship may be said to be one in which need gratification occurs, that is, it is satisfying to an individual's necessities or requirements. For example, the infant in need of love and affection experiences need gratification when his mother holds him securely and tenderly in her arms. The mother, in turn, experiences need gratification in her relationship with the infant as she feels needed and wanted in her motherly role. The relationship in this example may be said to be therapeutic in nature.

The goal or purpose of a therapeutic nurse-patient relationship is defined in terms of the patient's needs. Broadly speaking, examples of goals include increased independence for the patient, greater feelings of worth, and improved physical well-being. Depending on the goal, the nurse in turn selects nursing care activities that will move the patient toward the goal. As the patient's needs and goals change, so do the nursing care activities.

Satisfactory social interaction and psychosocial need gratification are interdependent and without a true beginning or end. Need gratification and social interaction, while discussed separately, are nonetheless completely intertwined.

NEED GRATIFICATION OF THE HUMAN ORGANISM

Maslow's theory of the human organism's hierarchy of needs is mentioned in Chapter 7. The concept is important to an understanding of the nurse-patient relationship since certain need gratifications have been observed when good relationships exist.

The word *hierarchy* is defined as a process or system that places things or persons in a graded order or rank. *Hierarchy of needs* may be defined as the placement of requirements or necessities in an increasing order of importance. Examples below will illustrate.

When a particular physiologic need that is high on the hierarchy of human needs is being met with a relative degree of satisfaction, other needs of lesser importance then take precedence. For example, when an individual is extremely thirsty, he activates every effort he can muster to satisfy the physiologic need for fluid which is high on the hierarchy of physiologic needs. Once his thirst has been satisfied, he then becomes occupied with some other need. The need may be physiologic, as for food, or if this has been satisfied, psychosocial in nature, as for love and affection.

As is true with physiologic needs, psychosocial needs may also wholly dominate behavior as an individual seeks to satisfy them. The person whose life is in danger will use every ounce of ingenuity and strength, for example, when confronted by a person wielding a gun in his face, by a blazing fire, or by a raging body of water. Until the immediate danger of survival and safety has subsided, physiologic needs or lesser ranking psychosocial needs will play little part in what he does.

Psychologists and sociologists have described the psychosocial needs of the human organism in much of their literature. While there are some differences of opinion among them, these are some common phrases used by Maslow to describe basic psychosocial needs: the need for security and survival; the need for belongingness, love, and affection; the need for self-respect and self-esteem; the need for self-fulfillment and self-actualization; the need to know and understand; and the need for aesthetics. When these needs are thwarted, humans tend to feel lonely, friendless, and rejected. They experience feelings of fear, weakness, and inferiority; they often feel dejected, anxious, and depressed.

The hierarchy of needs has been described in terms of the patient. The nurse's needs also are everpresent; however, if they take precedence over the patient's, nursing care is likely to deteriorate. For example, the nurse who seeks esteem and respect may describe a patient as uncooperative if his behavior does not indicate that such are forthcoming. As another example, the nurse seeking for a feeling of being wanted could use poor judgment in her nursing care of a youngster if she attempts to gain the child's love and affection for her gratification. The nurse who recognizes her needs and their order of importance gains much insight into her own behavior and better control over it. When the relationship between the nurse and the patient is a warm and comfortable one, when it demonstrates accepting the patient as he is, when it illustrates feelings of understanding, and when the nurse's needs are not dominating the relationship, then the nurse is helping the patient meet psychosocial needs as well as his physiologic needs.

SOCIAL INTERACTION IN THE NURSE-PATIENT RELATIONSHIP

Behavioral scientists have long shown interest in the nurse-patient relationship as a form of social interaction. *Social interaction* is concerned with a group of two or more people in which these people interact. *Interaction* is a reciprocal form of behavior. It is action by one that, in turn, produces action in another, and so on; that is, behavioral activity of one stimulates behavioral activity in another. The action or behavior may be *overt*, or open to view, such as the act of applauding or laughing. Or the action may be *covert*, that is, concealed from view. For instances, feelings of love, hate, and disgust are sometimes covert in nature.

Why should we be interested in the psychosocial aspects in the nurse-patient relationship? One social scientist stated it well: "The nurse's traditional patient care role includes motivating the patient to care for himself, and cooperating with those aiding him toward a cure. Motivation is psychological, and it is through social interaction with the patient that the nurse can affect the patient's motivation. Therefore, the social sciences are basic to nursing . . ." (18:3)

Study of social interaction is concerned with a variety of factors, two of which are of special concern to this discussion of the nurse-patient relationship: the functional factor (sometimes called the utilitarian or instrumental factor) and the expressive factor.

The *functional factor* in social interaction refers to action that is taken to move people toward a goal. A few examples will illustrate. A hospitalized patient tells a nurse that he is hungry, and the nurse serves him appropriate nourishment. Another explains to a school nurse that she cannot afford the dental care recommended for her child and the nurse prepares a referral to an appropriate social agency for financial assistance. A nurse observes on a home visit that a family's diet is lacking in essential nutrients and she confirms this observation during interviews with the mother. The nurse then proceeds with a teaching program to assist the family in better meal planning and food purchasing.

The *expressive factor* in social interaction refers to an emotional state. An emotional state may be described by many words—feelings, drives, attitudes, sentiments, and so on. The words "sentiments" and "feelings" will be used here. When sentiments and feelings of persons are unsatisfactory, their equilibrium may be upset, resulting in failure to reach common goals. When they are satisfactory, equilibrium is maintained. Satisfactory interaction preserves the integrity of individuals while promoting an atmosphere characterized by minimum fear, anxiety, distrust, and tension. Persons feel harmonious and contented with each other as they work cooperatively to reach common goals.

The functional and expressive aspects of social interaction must both be present. In successful relationships, they function harmoniously and interdependently as goals are attained. For example, the teaching program the nurse designs may be flawless in terms of organization, content, and teaching methods; that is, the functional element is satisfactory. However, unless the relationship is one in which the participants feel good and which is characterized with warmth, understanding, and acceptance of each other, teaching may be a failure for lack of concern for the expressive factor in the interaction.

Behavioral scientists have observed that when a relationship is satisfactory, social interactions of a similar nature tend to be repeated and continued. When a relationship is unsatisfactory, social interactions tend to be avoided. As an example, a patient began to break clinic appointments. He had not appeared to lack interest in his health when he began visiting the clinic. When a community health nurse called on the patient at home, he said, "The nurse at the clinic seems too busy; she just doesn't seem to care if I come or go. I don't like to go to that clinic." The lack of satisfactory interaction between the nurse and the patient discouraged the patient from continuing the relationships, even at the expense of his health. Had the nurse-patient relationship been satisfactory, breaking appointments probably would not have been a problem.

It has been observed that successful interaction is more likely to occur when there is a known and accepted division of labor among participants in the relationship and when there is leadership present. In the nurse-patient relationship, the roles of the nurse and the patient constitute a division of labor, and the nurse, by virtue of her role, generally takes the position of leadership. Consider an example when a misunderstanding concerning roles occurred due to poor cooperative planning between the patient and the nurse. A nurse who was otherwise competent failed to convey to the patient the importance of initiating self care. As a result, the patient felt that the nurse was refusing to assume her proper role of taking the leadership and administering his personal care without his assistance. He appeared dejected and commented: "The nurse doesn't like me and won't give me the care I need."

Leadership does not mean control in the restrictive or manipulative sense. The importance of including the patient in planning his care has been discussed several times in this text. When cooperative planning occurs with consideration of patient needs, then a labor division between nurse and patient is more likely to be mutually satisfactory. Leadership here implies taking the initiative in enlisting the patient's cooperation.

The emotional tone in interaction usually is heightened when a crisis occurs. Sentiments often become very intense between health practitioners and patients, for example, when patients are faced with urgent situations. When the interaction is positive in nature during crises, the resultant feelings can serve as great assists in the nurse-patient relationship after a crisis subsides. It is easy to forget the importance of the expressive factor in social interaction in a crisis when the functional factor may necessarily take precedence. But nonetheless, even in a crisis, the ex-

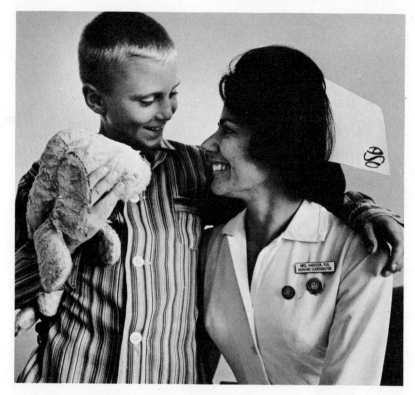

Fig. 11-1. To judge from the facial expression, this nurse appears to have established a warm and therapeutic relationship with her young patient. Note the child's favorite toy, which he was allowed to keep with him. (Good Samaritan Hospital, Phoenix, Arizona)

pressive factor in interaction remains important. Consider a surgical patient.

Most patients view surgery as a crisis situation. There are many technical tasks involved in preparing a patient for surgery and it is important that they be done correctly; for example, forgetting to remove a patient's dentures could result in serious respiratory complications. However, if during preparation for surgery the nurse neglects the expressive factor in her relationships with the patient, she may allow the patient's fears and anxieties to become intensified and diminishes the chances for satisfactory postoperative relationships.

People are not void of sentiments as they enter into social interaction. In the nurse-patient relationship, both the nurse and the patient bring their sentiments from past experiences to the new relationship. These will be reflected in the new relationship and play a role in the behavior of the participants also.

THERAPEUTIC RELATIONSHIP DESCRIBED

Now that some basic principles of need gratification and of social interaction have been discussed, the idea of a therapeutic nurse-patient relationship can be clarified. A therapeutic relationship is one that aids people in attaining common goals. It is one in which sentiments are positive. From the viewpoint of the patient, he *feels* better as a result of interactions with those serving him, and his improved feelings can often be discerned by observing his behavior. Inflections in the tone of voice, the manner in which he holds his head, the stride of his walk, the movements of his hands, the glimmerings of hope in his eyes, or a smile are examples.

Carl R. Rogers, an eminent psychotherapist, has described what he calls a "helping relationship." For our purposes, this is the same thing as a therapeutic relationship. The author has pointed out several factors that he has found important after years of service to people who have come to him for help.

First, the person offering the help needs to be knowledgeable about himself. The practitioner must be aware of his own needs, feelings, and sentiments. An understanding of self, Dr. Rogers believes, makes one a genuine person, and the patient perceives such a person as dependable and real, characteristics necessary in establishing a helping relationship.

Another factor, according to Dr. Rogers, is that the relationship between practitioner and patient be characterized with feelings of acceptance and with a warm attitude. These characteristics of a helping relationship have been mentioned earlier in this chapter. It is dependent to a large extent on action that is guided by the first basic principle, in relation to man's uniqueness, that is described in Chapter 3.

It is important in the helping relationship that the patient be allowed to be free to explore himself without fear of being judged, according to Dr. Rogers. The relationship will usually deteriorate when the practitioner sits in judgment or places himself as the authority with all of the right answers.

Dr. Rogers believes that a good helping relationship provides a climate in which the patient can develop motivation to change, to grow, to mature, and to cope with his problems in a more satisfactory manner. It is a climate in which the patient's strengths are used to capitalize on his inner resources.

The reader is referred to the book in which Dr. Rogers describes the helping relationship in a study situation at the end of this chapter.

ADMITTING A PATIENT TO A HEALTH AGENCY

The initial relationship between patient and nurse usually begins when the patient is admitted to a health agency of any type such as a hospital, a clinic, a physician's office, a school health facility, an industrial health facility, or a community health program.

Each health agency has its own procedure for the admission of patients; these will vary from one agency to another. The nurse is expected to assume responsibility for that part of the procedure assigned to nursing personnel. For example, if the agency is a well-baby clinic, the nurse may be expected to start a chart and obtain an initial health history from the parent. If the agency offers home health services to patients discharged from a convalescent unit, the nurse may be responsible for coordinating and obtaining a health history from the patient and from records of the agency from which the patient was discharged. If the agency is a hospital with an admitting suite, the nurse may have little or no responsibility in relation to such procedures as applying an identification band, starting a chart, taking note of the patient's valuables and clothing, and other admitting routines. Her responsibility in such instances may begin when the patient has been escorted to the room he will occupy while hospitalized.

In summary, admission procedures and policies are determined by the agency, and the nurse should familiarize herself with them and with responsibilities she must assume at her employing agency.

Even during the earliest contact with the patient at the time of admission, the nurse will wish to observe the three principles described in Chapter 3. She will take steps to maintain and respect the individuality of the patient, be alert to how well the patient's physiologic and psychological needs are being met, and observe precautions that obtain safety in the admission procedure. In addition, she will be aware of the importance of functional and expressive factors in her relationship with the patient.

From surveys of practice, it appears that neglecting the patient's individuality in the admission procedure is an all too common experience. Psychologists and psychiatrists have found that many children have had severe emotional reactions to the experience of hospitalization beginning with the admission procedure. It is convenient for hospital personnel to separate the child from his parents almost immediately upon admission; in this way, certain preparatory routines can be accomplished quickly with or without the child's cooperation. In rapid succession, the

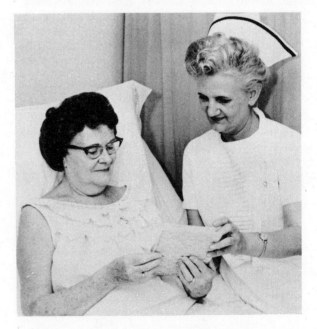

Fig. 11-2. Pictures of loved ones are often a real source of comfort to the patient. Sharing even brief moments with the patient helps the nurse to know the patient and her family better and to understand the patient's needs more adequately. (Photo by Warren R. Vroom)

child is stripped of his own clothing, placed in unfamiliar garb in an unfamiliar bed, and surrounded by unfamiliar children. He is examined; he may have laboratory work done, and then he is given preoperative medications. He may be carried away from his room on an object strange to him, brought to a strange place with furnishings unlike any he has ever seen, and, with little chance to get his bearings.

All patients, adults or children, find it comforting to be greeted pleasantly, as though they were being awaited. Patients like to be called by name and to learn to whom they are talking. It is helpful to the new patient if persons are identified by name pins.

When hospitalization is required, the child is not alone in wanting someone to remain nearby. Adults also find comfort in having a close family member or friend remain until they have the chance to become more adjusted to the new situation. As a matter of fact, talking for even a few minutes with the patient and his family will help the nurse considerably in understanding the patient, and the patient in feeling more comfortable when left alone.

It is best for the patient not to be subjected to a routine which fits no one but is applied to everyone. Admission to a hospital offers examples. Some patients may not wish to be dressed in hospital gowns and placed in bed immediately on admission. If there is no urgency about the patient's admission, the comfort of wearing his own robe and bed clothing means much to him. If not acutely ill, he may wish to be out of bed to explore the place where he is to spend his time. He may want to know who his neighbors are if he is in a unit where there are other patients, for patients very often find companionship, consolation, and reassurance in talking to each other. The new patient should be introduced to his roommates by whoever is admitting him to the unit. He should not be left to do his own socializing, since he may be so concerned for himself that it is not easy for him to approach others.

It is comforting for the patient to have some idea of what to expect concerning what will be done to complete his admission and to start his plan of care. Explanations are easy to give and do much to reduce apprehension. No matter how many details are included in a procedure for admitting a patient, they should be explained to him so that he may be helped to see that they are in his interest. In addition, the thoughtful nurse tells the patient about the call system, where the bathroom is, whether he has bathroom privileges, when he can expect meals to be served, what hours visitors may call, and so on.

Much has been said and written about making the transfer from a normal way of life to that of being a patient easier and more pleasant. Health practitioners who think only in terms of "getting the work done" are contributing little toward developing a therapeutic climate for the patient. Good nursing during the time that a patient is being admitted is largely dependent on the nurse's ability to put herself in another's place, and ask, "What would I like if I were the patient?"

TERMINATING THE NURSE-PATIENT RELATIONSHIP

Dealing with and planning for termination of the nurse-patient relationship is an important part of nursing care. There may be anguish in some instances as a relationship ends, but it can be minimized when termination is anticipated as nursing care progresses. It can also be minimized when there is a mutual setting of goals that serve to reduce misconceptions in expectation of care.

There are a variety of ways in which the termination of nurse-patient relationships can be prepared for. For example, the nurse can assist the patient transferring from one agency to another or from one unit in an agency to another by offering explanations concerning the transfer. In some instances, the nurse may introduce the patient to personnel about to care for him. Termination has been planned for when a teaching program has been used effectively. For instance, the new mother will be less fearful of going home when nursing personnel have taught her how to care for herself and for her newborn baby. The patient will usually feel a sense of effectiveness and competency when he has been included in planning a program of rehabilitation that readies him for adjustments required in his activities of daily living. This is especially true of patients with chronic diseases and permanent physical handicaps.

The thoughtful nurse will include the patient as she plans for turning his care over to another nurse. This may occur, for instance, at change-of-shift time, when a nurse leaves on vacation, or when she departs an agency for employment elsewhere.

Occasionally, termination for some patients produces emotional reactions. The patient may feel angry; he may feel rejected by the nurse; he may deny that a relationship ever really existed; he may feel depressed and helpless. Should reactions such as these occur, the nurse should help and support the

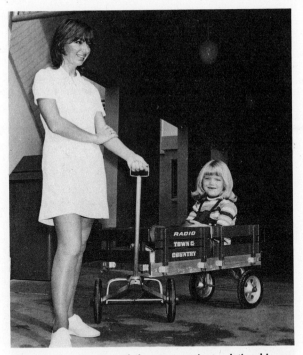

Fig. 11-3. Termination of the nurse-patient relationship can sometimes be difficult. Here, the patient and nurse seem to have had a mutually pleasant experience while the child was hospitalized. The child, being taken to her parents, appears neither fearful nor angry; this is usually a good indication that the nurse-patient relationships have been therapeutic in nature. (Good Samaritan Hospital, Phoenix, Arizona)

patient rather than make him feel guilty or wrong for having these views. However, emotional reactions of this sort are less likely to occur if, during the nurse-patient relationship, the patient has been helped to anticipate termination and has learned that the relationship will end when a particular type of nursing service is no longer required by the patient.

Termination of a relationship has often been said to begin with initiating the relationship. This is especially true when the nurse recognizes that while a particular face-to-face relationship may terminate, care and concern for the patient never do.

PRINCIPLES THAT PROMOTE THERAPEUTIC RELATIONSHIPS

This chapter may be summarized by statements of principles that will guide decision-making and action in the planning and implementation of nursing care in relation to the development of a therapeutic relationship.

Human needs appear on a hierarchy from needs that are high in rank to those that are low in importance.

When needs arise in an individual, attempts are made to meet higher ranking needs before attempting to satisfy lower ranking needs.

Human beings can help each other to meet their needs.

Satisfactory functional and expressive factors aid to attain common goals in social interaction.

Therapeutic relationships are based on a respect for the individuality of the participants.

CONCLUSION

Knowledge from the behavioral sciences serves as a foundation on which to build nurse-patient relationships that are therapeutic in nature. Professional competence is dependent on many factors, certainly one being a commitment to help patients obtain psychosocial as well as physical needs. There are many who feel that the true essense of nursing, and possibly its most important element, lies in the nurse's expressive role in the nurse-patient relationship.

Study Situations

1. In the following reference, the author describes the importance of knowing oneself. How does one become knowledgeable about how one comes to be as one is?

   Rogers, C. R.: This is me. *In* On Becoming a Person: A Therapist's View of Psychotherapy. pp. 3–27. Boston, Houghton Mifflin, 1961.

   Using Dr. Rogers' chapter as a guide, think about how you came to be as you are. Do you know what feelings you have and how they developed?

2. Being nonjudgmental in the nurse-patient relationship is important if the relationship is to be therapeutic. Of significance is not what one feels about others but why one feels that way, according to the following reference:

   Goldsborough, J. D.: On becoming nonjudgmental. **Am. J. Nurs.,** 70:2340–2343, Nov., 1970.

   What three steps does the author suggest to aid one in becoming nonjudgmental? What does the author offer as a suggestion if one cannot handle one's judgmental feelings when caring for a particular patient?

3. Several years ago, a seriously ill nurse wrote of her feelings in this manner: "Help me, care about what happens to me, I am so tired, so lonely and so very

afraid. Talk to me—reach out to me—take my hand. Let what happens to me matter to you."

The author's poem from which the above passage was taken appeared in the following reference:

Johnston, R.: Listen, nurse. **Am. J. Nurs.,** 71:303, Feb., 1971.

Describe how a therapeutic nurse-patient relationship may have helped in meeting psychosocial needs the author expressed in her poignant words.

References

1. Arnold, H. M.: I-thou. **Am. J. Nurs.,** 70:2554–2556, Dec., 1970.

2. Brinling, T.: Tearing down a wall. **Am. J. Nurs.,** 71:1406–1409, July, 1971.

3. Crawford, C. F., and Palm, M. L.: "Can I take my teddy bear?" **Am. J. Nurs.,** 73:286–287, Feb., 1973.

4. Johnson, J. E., et al. Interpersonal relations: the essence of nursing care. **Nurs. Forum,** 6:324–334, No. 3, 1967.

5. Johnson, M. M., and Martin, H. W.: A sociological analysis of the nurse role. **Am. J. Nurs.,** 58:373–377, Mar., 1958.

6. Johnson, M. M., and Martin, H. W.: A sociological analysis of the nurse role. *In* Skipper, J. K., Jr., and Leonard, R. C., eds.: Social Interaction and Patient Care. pp. 29–39. Philadelphia, J. B. Lippincott, 1965.

7. Kelly, H. S.: The sense of an ending. **Am. J. Nurs.,** 69:2378–2381, Nov., 1969.

8. Langlois, P., and Teramoto, V.: Helping patients cope with hospitalization. **Nurs. Outlook,** 19:334–336, May, 1971.

9. Lawrence, M. R.: Relationship control. *In* Carlson, C. E., coordinator: Behavioral Concepts and Nursing Intervention. pp. 331–339. Philadelphia, J. B. Lippincott, 1970.

10. Maslow, A. H.: Motivation and Personality. ed. 2. New York, Harper and Row, 1970.

11. Nalls, S.: Developing a therapeutic relationship. **Am. J. Nurs.,** 65:114–118, Dec., 1965.

12. Newman, M. A.: Identifying and meeting patients' needs in short-span nurse-patient relationships. **Nurs. Forum,** 5:76-86, No. 1, 1966.

13. Orlando, I. J.: The Dynamic Nurse-Patient Relationship. New York, G. P. Putnam's Sons, 1961.

14. Peplau, H. E.: Professional closeness . . . as a special kind of involvement with a patient, client, or family group. **Nurs. Forum,** 8:342–360, No. 4, 1969.

15. Phillips, B. D.: Terminating a nurse-patient relationship. **Am. J. Nurs.,** 68:1941–1942, Sept., 1968.

16. Rodger, B. P.: Therapeutic conversation and post-hypnotic suggestion. **Am. J. Nurs.,** 72:714–717, Apr., 1972.

17. Skipper, J. K., Jr.: The role of the hospital nurse: is it instrumental or expressive? *In* Skipper, J. K., Jr., and Leonard, R. C., eds.: Social Interaction and Patient Care. p. 40–48. Philadelphia, J. B. Lippincott, 1965.

18. Social and psychological aspects of the nurse's role-introduction. *In* Skipper, J. K., Jr., and Leonard, R. C., eds.: Social Interaction and Patient Care. pp. 3–6. Philadelphia, J. B. Lippincott, 1965.

19. Travelbee, J.: The nurse-patient relationship: Part IV—termination. *In* Intervention in Psychiatric Nursing: Process in the One-To-One Relationship. pp. 162–175. Philadelphia, F. A. Davis, 1969.

CHAPTER 12

The Role of the Patient

GLOSSARY

Anger: An emotional pattern characteristically associated with frustration and struggling with a threatening or unpleasant situation.

Anxiety: An emotional pattern characterized by feelings of uneasiness and apprehension of a probable danger or misfortune.

Emotion: A bodily state involving highly motivated feelings and behavior. Associated with visceral changes affecting the circulatory, respiratory, digestive, and glandular systems as well as skeletal muscles.

Fear: An emotional pattern characterized by an expectation of harm or unpleasantness. Usually associated with behavior that attempts to avoid or flee a threatening situation.

Helplessness: An emotional pattern characterized by a "fear of fear" and feelings of being unable to avoid an unpleasant experience.

Hostility: An emotional pattern characterized by feelings of unfriendliness and animosity. May be associated with aggressive action.

Overdependency: An emotional pattern characterized by feelings of helplessness while attempting to search for help and understanding to an extent beyond what is considered normal.

Stress: A state of strain or tension.

Worry: A mild form of anxiety characterized by preoccupation with an unsolved conflict.

INTRODUCTION

In general, persons who seek the services of health practitioners can be expected to experience at least some emotional stress. Even those submitting to a routine physical examination are likely to feel anxiety until assured that their state of health is good. Feelings of anxiety can be expected also in those persons who avail themselves of screening services offered by some health agencies, such as mobile chest x-ray units and diabetes mellitus detection units. When the patient is ill, anxiety can almost certainly be expected to increase.

No matter where the patient may appear to be on a health-illness continuum, perceptions held by the patient and his emotional reactions become important facets in his care. This chapter will discuss some of the implications for nursing when people become patients.

THE PATIENT AS A UNIQUE INDIVIDUAL

Each person is a unique human being, and persons who become patients continue to be just as different from one another as they had been prior to the patient experience. Health practitioners have frequently tended to ignore this and have often behaved with a certain sameness toward all patients. In addition, patients have been expected to be cooperative at all times and to believe without query that all that was being done to them was for their own good. Especially, patients were neither to complain, nor were they to be hostile, anxious, aggressive, or nonconforming. Behavior that was not in line with expectations of health practitioners was likely to be considered as uncooperative behavior, and the patient was often referred to as a difficult patient.

When a person is ill, he assumes a role that is different from the one he had when his health problem was absent. From psychology we learn that behavior is adaptive and purposeful. In other words, all of living is to some degree a process of adapting to one's environment. Behavior is purposeful in that a person acts in a manner that to him has meaning, even when he may not be able to explain the reason for his behavior. Hence, in the process of adapting to the role of the patient, the person's behavior changes, because it is an attempt to adjust to something new. However, the person's uniqueness and his being different from all other persons remain.

Some people adjust to new settings and new experiences with greater ease than others. For example, there are people who move around the country establishing new homes in markedly different surroundings with apparent ease. There are others who feel they cannot live happily except in a familiar environment. So too with patients. Some appear to adjust with ease, while others adjust with greater difficulty as they become patients. This difference in adaptability among patients is another factor in the uniqueness of everyone.

The seriousness of an illness, from a medical viewpoint, may not necessarily be a useful indicator in predicting a person's attitude and reactions when illness occurs. Some patients whose illness may be considered minor in terms of complete recovery may view that illness with great alarm and concern. Other patients experiencing serious illness may appear to show little emotional reaction or concern. However, just as in other behavior, a person's reaction to his illness has meaning and purpose, and no two people are likely to react or behave similarly.

STAGES OF ILLNESS

As just described, adaptation to illness varies among individuals. However, studies have demonstrated that there appears to be a general pattern of adaptation. The phrase "stages of illness" is used here to speak of this pattern. Although investigators have described patterns in the stages of illness somewhat differently and used different terminology to some extent, there is commonality in general behavior characteristics.

Denial or disbelief in being ill is characteristically an early state of illness. Emotional reactions, such as anxiety, fear, irritability, aggressiveness, and the like, often occur. The patient may avoid, refuse, or even forget needed care. As one person said, the patient may appear to flee toward health in attempting to escape illness.

When the person can no longer deny his illness and is aware of what is happening to him, he then tends to move toward a stage of acceptance and turns to professional help for assistance. At first, many patients become dependent on health practitioners and also become symptom- and illness-oriented. Gradually, dependence is likely to lessen as the patient's condition changes and as he is aided to accept more responsibility in helping himself. Nonetheless, it can be expected that at least some patients will continue to deny illness and may even appear to be challenging it. Acceptance for them may not be evident, or at least not until a change in their physical condition occurs at which time they tend finally to accede to illness.

Then follows a period of recovery, rehabilitation, or convalescence. Depending on the patient's illness, this may be a relatively short or long period. If little adaptation is required for a patient to return to a former way of life, convalescence tends to be short. The period will be longer when patients are required to make changes in their life-style. During recovery, without regard to its length, the patient goes through a process of resolving loss or impairment of function. When the period is prolonged due to chronic illness or physical limitations, the patient may experience recurrence of illness requiring efforts to adapt again and again.

A study situation at the end of this chapter will aid the reader in further study of adaptations to illness. Several references direct attention to reports of studies that give support to a stages-of-illness theory.

PHYSIOLOGY OF EMOTIONS

To understand the distress experienced by patients, one needs also to understand the physiology of emotions. This topic is considered in courses in psychology but a brief review will be presented here.

An *emotion* is a bodily state involving highly motivated feelings and behavior. Most responses to emotion operate through the nerve cells and fibers of the autonomic nervous system. This system consists of the sympathetic (thoracolumbar) and the parasympathetic (craniosacral) divisions. The parasympathetic impulses tend to control normal operation of the viscera, such as facilitating smooth muscle contraction, permitting salivation, and slowing the heart rate. Sympathetic impulses increase heart action, inhibit salivation and gastrointestinal activity, raise blood pressure by constricting arterioles, dilate bronchioles, stimulate perspiration, and increase the secretion of adrenalin, which tend to augment the effects of sympathetic innervation. Both the parasympathetic and sympathetic impulses act during emotion. However, the parasympathetic effects usually are masked by the stronger sympathetic effects.

The hypothalamus also plays a part in emotional responses, as does the cerebral cortex. Coordination of responses apparently occurs in part through activity of the hypothalamus, and the cerebral cortex appears to have a restraining or controlling effect on emotional responses.

Physiologic responses to emotion differ from person to person and, also, in the same person from time to time. Nor can one emotion be differentiated from another by physiologic reactions only. However, the physiologic responses to emotions are not disorganized. On the contrary, they are well organized, and even when emotion is strong the body responds harmoniously. What *may* be disorganized is behavior that results from an emotional experience. For example, a person experiencing extreme fear may be so consumed by his emotion that his behavior may become erratic, and, hence, less effective in eliminating or reducing the cause of his fear.

COMMON EMOTIONAL REACTIONS WHEN PEOPLE BECOME PATIENTS

The transition from health to illness is an unpleasant and often a crisis-laden experience for most people. It is the rare person who does not feel afraid and anxious, at least to some degree. Everyone has personal problems; some may very well be exaggerated by illness which adds to the stress of the experience.

Alteration in body image is a fearful possibility to many persons as they become patients. When a threat to usual life patterns exists, the patient may become angry and defiant, or he may minimize the threat in an effort to deny its existence. Many patients suffer anxiety when injured or malfunctioning body parts are involved with the illness. This is more likely to be true when certain emotionally significant organs or parts such as the face, the genitals, the breasts, or the skin, are implicated. Preserving one's

bodily intactness has high priority in one's self-image, and threats to it are usually likely to produce behavior changes.

Some patients may experience feelings of guilt and shame for being ill. Many ill persons feel pessimistic, depressed, and downcast. Men very often consider it an affront to be ill; generally, women are less likely to feel this way, but homemakers may tend to worry and be apprehensive about the care of their families and homes. Breadwinners in the family generally view illness with apprehension if income is threatened. There is often dread of invasion of privacy, with probing questions and detailed physical examinations. There may be fear of pain, which might indeed be a very realistic fear. Young adults may be concerned about interruptions in their education. Children may feel uneasy in strange surroundings as well as fearful of being deserted by their parents. Loneliness and confusion are common reactions, regardless of age.

It is unrealistic to assume that people's emotional reactions can or should be neutralized when they become patients. But there are means by which the nurse can ease mental and physical distress. High quality practice recognizes that a person transformed from an independently functioning individual to that of a dependent and sometimes regressive patient deserves respect.

The literature describing common emotional reactions that may occur as people become patients is voluminous. A wide variety of terms is used, some of which are defined in somewhat different ways. This section will briefly describe a few of the more common emotional reactions. The references and the study situations at the end of this chapter will guide the reader to sources of information for additional discussions.

Fear

Fear is an emotional response characterized by an expectation of harm or unpleasantness. Normally the body reacts by attempting to avoid or withdraw from the threat. When we are afraid, sympathetic innervation, as described earlier, places the body in a state of readiness for action to avoid or escape harm. The person who has fear usually is aware of the danger and has insight into the reasons for his fear. The causes in general are present and real, even though the patient may conceal his fear, as illustrated in an example given below.

Absence of the emotion of fear may seem ideal, but without it life would be infinitely more precarious. We have all experienced fear in our lives, and

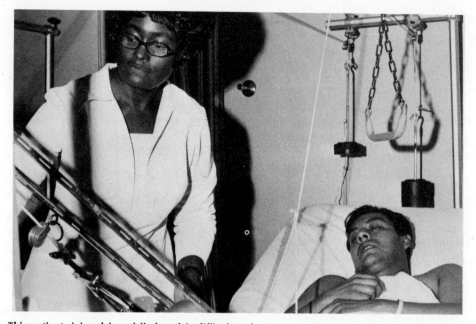

Fig. 12-1. This patient, injured in a fall, found it difficult to be transported many miles from his home to a strange hospital in a strange city. He did not understand the complicated traction; also, a language barrier added to his difficulty. It is easy to appreciate that he experienced much anxiety. (Good Samaritan Hospital, Phoenix, Arizona)

it might be doubted that we could have survived the many dangers had we not been fearful. For example, fear of accidents often results in safer automobile driving. Possibly one of the best lifesaving "devices" for the nonswimmer is his fear of being in water over his head.

Patients with fears may express them rather freely. For example, a patient said he was afraid of receiving oxygen therapy because of the danger of an explosion. A few explanations from the nurse to the patient and to his visitors alleviated the fear readily.

On the other hand, some patients may be reluctant to express fears, believing that they may appear unintelligent and a nuisance if they ask questions. One hospitalized patient, for example, eventually described having marked fear when he did not receive his breakfast when the other patients were served. Instead, a technician came to take a blood sample. The patient was sure his condition had worsened and that he was about to receive some therapy. He was both fearful of what might be happening to him and fearful of asking anyone for an explanation. When one reads in the literature what patients have described as fearful experiences, it is easy to see that many of them could have been avoided or minimized, had someone just taken the time to give some explanations to these people.

Fears may be camouflaged by other behavior. For example, a patient, awakened postoperatively, saw that she was in a bed with siderails in place. She became very angry and told a family member that she "really told off that nurse who put up those railings." When asked why she was upset about having siderails on her bed, the patient said, most indignantly, "I came in here for a simple operation and I don't expect to be treated like someone who is insane. I've heard about how they treat insane people. They put them in beds and fix it so you can't get out. And I'm not crazy!" After the reason for the siderails was explained, the patient's anger quickly subsided, since her fear of being mentally ill was removed.

Anxiety

The dictionary defines *anxiety* as uneasiness of mind caused by apprehension of danger or misfortune. It often is referred to as a persistent, generalized fear of the unknown and is associated with some future event. *Worry* is a mild form of anxiety characterized by preoccupation with an unsolved conflict. Unlike the anxious person, the worried person usually is able to communicate the cause of the concern. Anxiety is characterized by a lack of awareness of the cause of fear. Although pervasive, it is vaguely organized in the mind of the person; hence, he feels helpless and uncertain concerning appropriate action to take.

Anxiety is more difficult to handle than fear. Should one be afraid of a dog, he can try to get away from the situation. But when anxiety is present, the person lacking insight as to its cause feels defeated and has dread of what will happen.

The physiologic reactions to anxiety result from sympathetic innervation. However, because of the nature of anxiety, the responses of the organs to stimulation are not usually as dramatic as when fear, for example, is present.

Because lack of insight is commonly present, an anxious person often directs his attention to the physiologic symptoms of anxiety. Common ones are fatigue, insomnia, diarrhea, urgency of voiding, nausea, anorexia, and excessive perspiration. "Nervous heart" is a common symptom of the anxious person. Or the patient may say he thinks his heart "stands still" at times. When anxiety becomes chronic and persistent, the services of a psychiatrist may be necessary.

Although anxiety can be destructive in nature, it also may be used constructively. This is especially true when the anxiety is not overwhelming. In fact, some persons believe that without anxiety, as well as some fear, the human race might not have survived in situations that made constructive action imperative. The anxiety associated with examination periods in school stimulates many students to carry out effective study programs. The anxiety of an elected official whose neglect of slum conditions may threaten his office can serve to stimulate constructive action.

Not only patients experience anxiety. This period in civilization has often been referred to as the Age of Anxiety. True, it is an age with great changes occurring rapidly. Values have changed rapidly and tensions over appropriate behavior are increased. Civilization will have utilized anxiety wisely if action resulting from it can be put to constructive use.

Stress

Stress is defined as strain or tension. It occurs most often in circumstances necessitating an increased and often prolonged effort to adjust. Any factor that disturbs the physical, psychological, or physiologic equilibrium of the body may be stressful. As in the case of fear, the body strives to rid itself of the factor causing the stress.

Stress is a highly individualized experience. Some persons appear to be able to tolerate a great deal more than others. Or a situation that is stressful for one may not be for another person. The important thing is how each individual perceives and meets the situation that causes the stress. It is a rare person who does not experience stress as he assumes the patient role.

Overdependency and Feelings of Helplessness

Overdependency is an emotional response characterized by feelings of helplessness to an extent beyond what is considered normal. *Helplessness* is a "fear of fear" and a feeling of being unable to avoid an unpleasant experience.

Even in health, human beings demonstrate dependence on others. A mother depends on the family physician to help her keep her family well. The student turns to his counselor for help in planning his educational program. The employee looks to his employer for guidelines that determine what he is expected to do on his job. But characteristically during periods of illness, dependence and feelings of helplessness usually increase and, unfortunately, sometimes to the point of being harmful to the patient. Often it is the nurse who first observes overdependency in an ill person and she may be the one who must make decisions concerning whether a patient's dependency has reached an undesirable level for the patient's own good. A convalescing patient who is reluctant to assume responsibility for his personal care, for instance, may well have grown too dependent during acute illness.

It may be that a patient who has grown too dependent on others is a fearful person. A patient recovering from a coronary thrombosis (heart attack) may be afraid, for example, that assuming graduated exercises may precipitate another heart attack. Another overdependent patient may be angry because he has been permanently handicapped by an illness or injury. He may even blame health personnel for his handicap and become defiant of efforts to assist him to use remaining physical potential.

Whatever the reason for overdependency and feelings of helplessness, the nurse should observe and study possible motives for it. Simultaneously, she will want to assist a patient to surmount overdependency in a manner compatible with the patient's capabilities rather than in a manner that satisfies her own aspirations for the patient.

Anger

Anger is an emotion characteristically associated with frustration and struggling with a threatening or unpleasant situation. It is common, for example, when a goal is blocked, when respect for self has been lowered, or when a goal cannot be attained.

Anger can serve useful purposes. For example, when it can be comfortably and safely expressed, anger may act as a relief valve in a highly-charged emotional situation. Often, being able to express anger makes a person feel better, when it serves as a substitute for the uneasy, unpleasant, and powerless feelings of anxiety. The anger may be directed toward the source of the frustration or it may be aimed at someone or something else.

Like other emotions, anger may be camouflaged. This is especially true in a society such as ours that places taboos on most angry behavior. The child with a cough and sore throat who willfully destroys his toys because the physician has kept him home from school may be angry at being ill, with the physician, and with himself. A mother may be frustrated and angered by her teen-ager who refuses to eat what she considers to be a balanced diet; because she is so angry, she enforces a more rigid curfew policy. A person experiencing pain when no cause can be found may express his anger by being impatient and annoyed at other drivers on his way home from the clinic.

Energy is liberated by the body during periods of anger. When this energy can be directed toward constructive ends, the nurse may help an angry patient find more meaningful and useful behavior. To do so, the nurse must accept the patient's feelings of anger and not take them personally even if directed toward her. She will want to assure the patient that his feelings are not unusual and help him find the cause of his anger. Then, she and the patient can work toward solutions to solve situations producing the emotion. Attempts to find the cause of the anger are helpful so that the difficulty can be dealt with realistically.

Hostility

Hostility is an unfriendliness and animosity that is sometimes associated with a desire for aggressive action. It may occur with anger and with the wish to hurt or humiliate others. Almost all adults experience at least some of it when ill, especially when confined to periods of hospitalization.

The intensity of hostility cannot be judged safely by the intensity of the behavior overtly associated with it. Nor is it always easy to recognize the focus or cause of the hostility for there is a tendency to displace feelings of hostility onto others. For example, a quiet, almost uncommunicative patient may be extremely hostile but may present the behavior he does because expressing his hostility outwardly may be too upsetting for him. He may display his behavior to health practitioners working with him but feel hostile primarily toward relatives who, he feels, have deserted him during his illness.

Sarcasm and abusive remarks are often expressions of hostility. The overdemanding, unreasonable, and argumentative patient may also be expressing hostility by his behavior.

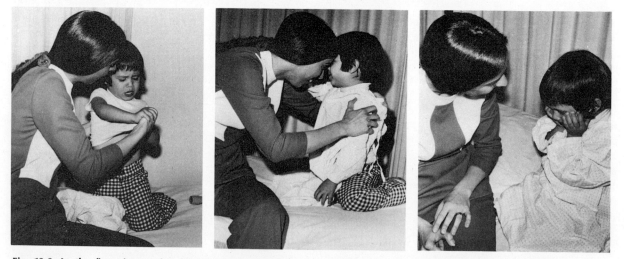

Fig. 12-2. In the first picture, the child shows denial of the nurse and of her efforts to admit him as a patient to the health agency. The nurse remained with the patient and made no attempt to force the child but rather, waited for him to accept her. She demonstrated warmth and understanding for the child, as the second picture illustrates. In the last picture, the child's expression is one of finding the admission procedure not such a bad experience after all. A simple procedure can become a nightmare for any patient, or it can be a pleasant experience when the nurse has insight into her patient's feelings and skill to develop a good nurse-patient relationship. (Good Samaritan Hospital, Phoenix, Arizona)

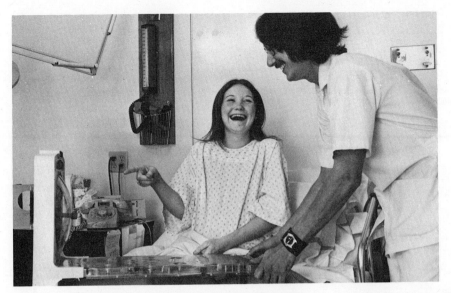

Fig. 12-3. This patient enjoys a few moments of fun playing with a miniature pinball machine. The nurse, who took time out to share the game with the patient, can help to relieve anxiety and stress through incidents such as this, but he is still serious about his work. (Good Samaritan Hospital, Phoenix, Arizona)

As is the case in many situations when patients demonstrate emotional reactions, the nurse most helpful to the patient first demonstrates acceptance of the patient despite his behavior. She will explore situations likely to produce hostility and attempt to help the patient substitute constructive behavior for the hostile behavior he exhibits.

Finally, a word of warning is in order. Human behavior is very complex and no one is likely to be as rational and logical as he thinks he is. A particular type of behavior can rarely be diagnosed in a simple fashion since psychological research has indicated that behavior may be motivated at either the conscious or the unconscious level, or at both levels simultaneously. In addition, behavior is rarely motivated by only one determining agent. Rather, multiple influences may be at work producing a particular kind of behavior.

The danger of oversimplification when attempting to observe and analyze another's behavior is ever-present. Nonetheless, turning away from attempts to understand behavior and failing to respond with warmth and acceptance when patients are communicating via their behavior fall short of professional nursing practice.

WHAT PATIENTS EXPECT OF THE NURSE

When a patient submits to the care of members of the health professions, he has expectations concerning the behavior and abilities of those caring for him. This has been demonstrated by investigation and from what patients have written in articles for professional and lay literature, letters to editors of periodicals, and the like.

Patients expect the nurse to be *professionally competent*. This has been found to be especially true in relation to technical competencies. They are apt to doubt the competence of a nurse who seems unsure of equipment she is using. A casual spoken thought, like "I wonder how this works," or "I can't seem to get this to work," does little for a patient's confidence in the nurse. It is not surprising that a patient questioned his physician about his pulse rate after the nurse who came to take it kept shaking her watch and said she wondered if it was working correctly. But patients are quick to compliment the nurse who carries out a procedure with deftness and self-assurance. One frequently hears patients speak, for example, of the nurse who gives "good shots."

Patients expect nurses to be *serious about their work*. Human emotions can be contagious; hence, patients tend to enjoy having persons who are cheerful, but still obviously sincere, care for them. Patients often enjoy sharing a humorous experience with the nurse (see Fig. 12-3). Humor can often relieve anxiety, stress, and anger and help to develop warm relationships when used appropriately. The give-and-take of humorous incidents can often serve therapeutic ends. However, when a patient overuses humor, he may be using it as a cover-up for stress too great to accept. The alert nurse will wish to learn to recognize humor when used as an escape from reality.

While humor is appreciated, it is the rare patient who accepts frivolity or casualness. Some patients may find it disturbing to see nurses in groups chatting and laughing. Families as well as patients also find it disconcerting when nursing personnel are laughing and talking outside a room in which someone is ill or deeply concerned with his health problem. In situations such as those just mentioned, the nurses might well be serious-minded about their work, but their behavior may cause the patient to be critical.

Patients expect nurses to be *thoughtful, understanding, and accepting* of them. They are critical of behavior that is punitive or judgmental in nature. Calling a patient by his name is a thoughtful and, often, a long-remembered act. It is not that nurses are always expected to *do* or *say* something. Just remaining with the patient for a few minutes to listen to what he has to say, or holding his hand for a few seconds, is a great contribution to his comfort and well-being.

When patients are unable to care for themselves, they expect the nurse to *assist them in meeting their hygienic needs.* Although the nurse may assign other members of the nursing team to this task, the patient still expects the nurse to know about them and what can be done about them. For example, they expect to be bathed when they feel unable to do so for themselves. Placing a basin of water in front of a one-day postoperative patient who has had major surgery and telling him that it is good to be active would be regarded as gross insensitivity, not therapy.

Patients can be made unhappy by having their hair left uncared for when they cannot care for it themselves. Grooming is important to the male patient also, and many express discomfort when not shaven. They do not like visitors to see them in a state that is embarrassing to them. Helping the patient to maintain normal bladder and bowel functions is appreciated, because neglect in these matters usually brings with it many disturbing physiological problems as well as possible psychological ones.

As has been stated earlier, there may be times when there is too much dependence on the nurse. But when a patient needs assistance, he expects the nurse to anticipate and to meet his needs.

Generally patients expect nurses to *orient them to the health care facility.* Nearly everyone is afraid of the unknown, and to be left alone without orientation can be a frightening experience. T. S. Eliot expressed the patient's point of view well in "The Cocktail Party," concerning an impersonal environment, when he wrote:

> All there is of you is your body
> And the "you" is withdrawn.

Courtesies that help patients to feel that they are not just another person aid in developing a desirable therapeutic climate in which to care for them.

Patients expect to receive an *explanation of their care* and they wish to *have their questions answered.* Not knowing and understanding what is being done is a vexing and frightening experience. Apprehension is increased by unfamiliar sounds, medical jargon, and an array of strange equipment. Health practitioners who ignore this aspect of care are often referred to as cruel, unkind, and thoughtless.

Patients wish to be a *partner with health practitioners in planning their care.* This facet of care has been described earlier but its importance can hardly be overstressed. One goal of health care is to help patients attain optimum functioning with the best possible use of capabilities. It can well become an elusive goal if patients are excluded when health care is planned.

Patients expect nurses to *insure their privacy* to the greatest extent possible. While asking personal questions, conducting physical examinations, and carrying out treatments, privacy can still be protected. For example, the nurse who walked into a four-bed hospital unit and loudly asked, "How many of you have had bowel movements today?" demonstrated little respect for the patients' privacy. Families have complained when community health nurses have visited their homes without an appointment. Some persons consider it an invasion of privacy to be called by their first names. Patients are resentful of an invasion of privacy when, during examinations and treatments, nursing personnel have been careless about unnecessary exposure. Patients have also been critical of personnel who invade privacy when they enter closed doors without knocking before entering.

Legal implications when invasion of privacy occurs are discussed in Chapter 4. In the eyes of the law, invasion of privacy may constitute a tort.

Privacy means different things to different people. The patient's age, his sex, the influence of his childhood rearing, the cultural and socioeconomic class of which he is a member, his relationships with health practitioners, all play a role in the concept of privacy held by the patient. Nursing care can be enhanced when various concepts of privacy are respected and when purposeful efforts are made to protect patients from unnecessary invasion of privacy.

PRINCIPLES TO OBSERVE IN AIDING PERSONS TO ADJUST TO THE PATIENT ROLE

There are several principles that the nurse will observe as she aids people to adjust to their roles as patients.

Emotional responses evoke widespread visceral changes affecting the circulatory, respiratory, digestive, and glandular systems as well as the skeletal system.

This principle serves as an aid to the nurse in recognizing when a patient is, for example, anxious or fearful. Not many people admit readily to these emotional responses. This is especially true when patients believe that by so doing, they also are admitting to being unusual or strange. This principle, then, assists the nurse in observing patients for reactions that may have an emotional basis, such as excessive perspiration, frequency in urination, and increased respiratory rates.

Behavior is motivated and there is cause for it.

By observing this principle, the nurse will realize that a patient's emotional behavior has reason or cause. Knowing that the behavior has reason guides the nurse in every approach to the patient. For example, a nurse notes that a patient is crying; the patient tells the nurse, "I'm crying, but for no reason." The nurse knows there is reason despite what the patient has stated. She stays with her, listening for her to express a possible reason. The nurse may feel that she would not handle the situation in the same way, but accepts the patient's right to deal with the situation in a manner that is appropriate for her.

When a stimulus for a particular kind of behavior is annoying, the body responds by attempting to avoid or reduce the stimulus.

Consider the example given previously of the patient found crying. Crying may be a last resort because she knows no way of avoiding an annoying stimulus. Assume this patient is fearful of a diagnosis that will require many subcutaneous injections which she will need to administer herself. Although no one enjoys administering injections to himself, by explanation the nurse might at least alleviate some of the patient's fears and thus diminish the annoying stimulus. Assume instead that this patient is fearful of a certain diagnosis, such as a malignancy, which she associates with death. Fear of death in that case becomes very real. Possibly the most the nurse can do is offer the patient support by listening to her and by being available when her fears become overwhelming. In this case the nearness of a supportive nurse might reduce some of an annoying stimulus.

CONCLUSION

People experience a wide variety of emotions when they become patients. Health practitioners who ignore patients as unique individuals and who fail to consider each patient's point of view are ignoring essential elements in health care. Florence Nightingale stated it well over a century ago when she wrote in her *Notes On Nursing,* "If you knew how unreasonably sick people suffer from reasonable causes of distress, you would take more pains about all these things."

Study Situations
1. The following article discusses how acceptance aids in preventing health practitioners from stripping patients of their individuality:

   Wolff, I. S.: Acceptance. **Am. J. Nurs.,** 72:1412–1415, Aug., 1972.

   Note this sentence which appears on the middle of page 1415: "If he truly 'accepts' the person, the helper then takes him as he is, with a vision of hope about his potential to become."

   What suggestions does the author give to assist one in learning to be more accepting of others?

2. The following article describes three stages in the experience of illness: the transition period from health to illness, the period of "accepted" illness, and convalescence:

   Lederer, H. D.: How the sick view their world. **J. Social Issues,** 8:4–15, 1952. (This article also appears in the following book: Skipper, J. K., Jr., and Leonard, R. C., eds.: Social Interaction and Patient Care. pp. 155–167. Philadelphia, J. B. Lippincott, 1965.)

   Recall patients to whom you have recently given care. Describe the stage of illness you believe each was experiencing, using Dr. Lederer's descriptions of the stages as a guide.

3. What effect can anger and tension have on people? The article given below describes evidence collected by several groups of medical researchers that indicates emotional factors are largely responsible for many chronic illnesses of mankind:

   McQuade, W.: What stress can do to you. **Fortune,** 85:102–107; 134; 136; 141, Jan., 1972.

   Note the description of the physiology of emotions early in the article and the illustration which demonstrates body reactions to anger and tension. According to the author, why has stress become such a problem in a society with innumerable conveniences and comforts and with a life-style considered far easier than it was in previous generations?

4. The following three references, the first two of which were written by patients, describe what patients look for from nursing personnel:

   The art of nursing. Anonymous letter. **Am. J. Nurs.,** 64:66–67, Apr., 1964.

   Note the importance this particular patient placed on the nurse's conveying an interest in the patient's recovery.

Jeffris, J.: The best healing device. **Am. J. Nurs.,** 64:74–77, Sept., 1964.

This patient emphasized the importance of the presence of another human being and the compassion of a nurse when one is ill and handicapped.

Standeven, M.: What the poor dislike about community health nurses. **Nurs. Outlook,** 17:72–75, Sept., 1969.

Note the effects when patients felt deprived of human dignity.

Although the above references were written some time ago, do you believe patients could be likely to make similar comments today about what they wish of nurses?

5. Read the following article:

Kunzman, L.: Some factors influencing a young child's mastery of hospitalization. *In* **The Nursing Clinics of North America.** Philadelphia, W. B. Saunders, 7:13–26, Mar., 1972.

The author notes that a child has fears, anxieties, and fantasies when he becomes a patient, but she reminds her readers a child is not a miniature adult. On page 15 of the article, there is a table that compares a child's situation at home with the situation that exists when hospitalization occurs. Suggest ways that could be used to minimize the trauma a child faces when hospitalized. For example, describe how you believe a child could be helped to master a loss of independence when hospitalization occurs.

6. This chapter referred to emotional reactions when a person's body image is in jeopardy. Read the following article:

Loxley, A. K.: The emotional toll of crippling deformity. **Am. J. Nurs.,** 72:1839–1840, Oct., 1972.

According to quotes from Lowen in the article, how is body image developed? When body image is destroyed, how can the nurse co-build with the patient so that he may renew himself again?

References

1. Abdellah, F. G.: How we look at ourselves. **Nurs. Outlook,** 7:273–275, Mar., 1959.

2. Anxiety—recognition and intervention. Programmed Instruction. **Am. J. Nurs.,** 65:129–152, Sept., 1965.

3. Bloch, D.: Privacy. *In* Carlson, C. E., coordinator: Behavioral Concepts and Nursing Intervention. pp. 251–265. Philadelphia, J. B. Lippincott, 1970.

4. Crate, M. A.: Nursing functions in adaptation to chronic illness. **Am. J. Nurs.,** 65:72–76, Oct., 1965.

5. Davitz, L. J.: Interpersonal Processes in Nursing Case Histories. New York, Springer, 1970.

6. Dittman, L. L.: A child's sense of trust. **Am. J. Nurs.,** 66:91–93, Jan., 1966.

7. Duff, R. S., and Hollingshead, A. B.: Sickness and Society. pp. 291–305. New York, Harper and Row, 1968.

8. Field, W. E., Jr., *et al.*: The senses taker. **Am. J. Nurs.,** 66:2654–2656, Dec., 1966.

9. Graham, L. E., and Conley, E. M.: Evaluation of anxiety and fear in adult surgical patients. **Nurs. Research,** 20:113–122, Mar.–Apr., 1971.

10. Kiening, Sr. M. M.: Denial of illness. *In* Carlson, C. E., coordinator: Behavioral Concepts and Nursing Intervention. pp. 9–28. Philadelphia, J. B. Lippincott, 1970.

11. ———: Hostility. *In* Carlson, C. E., coordinator: Behavioral Concepts and Nursing Intervention, pp. 187–203. Philadelphia, J. B. Lippincott, 1970.

12. Langlois, P., and Teramoto, V.: Helping patients cope with hospitalization. **Nurs. Outlook,** 19:334–336, May, 1971.

13. Levine, M. E.: The intransigent patient. **Am. J. Nurs.,** 70:2106–2111, Oct., 1970.

14. Levine, S.: Stress and behavior. **Sci. Am.,** 224:26–31, Jan., 1971.

15. Magill, K. A.: How one patient handled fear. **Am. J. Nurs.,** 67:1248–1249, June, 1967.

16. Marram, G. D.: Patients' evaluation of their care: importance to the nurse. **Nurs. Outlook,** 21:322–324, May, 1973.

17. Martin, H. W., and Prange, A. J.: The stages of illness—psychosocial approach. **Nurs. Outlook,** 10:168–171, Mar., 1962.

18. Nehring, V., and Geach, B.: Patients' evaluation of their care: why they don't complain. **Nurs. Outlook,** 21:317–321, May, 1973.

19. Peterson, M. H.: Understanding defense mechanisms. Programmed Instruction. **Am. J. Nurs.,** 72:1651–1674, Sept., 1972.

20. Powers, M. E., and Storlie, F.: The apprehensive patient. **Am. J. Nurs.,** 67:58–63, Jan., 1967.

21. Robinson, L.: Psychological Aspects of the Care of Hospitalized Patients. Philadelphia, F. A. Davis, 1968.

22. Robinson, V. M.: Humor in nursing. **Am. J. Nurs.,** 70:1065–1068, May, 1970.

23. Sarosi, G. M.: A critical theory: the nurse as a fully human person. **Nurs. Forum,** 7:349–364, No. 4, 1968.

24. Selye, H.: The stress syndrome. **Am. J. Nurs.,** 65:97–99, Mar., 1965.

25. Sorensen, K. M., and Amis, D. B.: Understanding the world of the chronically ill. **Am. J. Nurs.,** 67:811–817, Apr., 1967.

26. Suchman, E. A.: Stages of illness and medical care. **J. Health and Human Behavior,** 6:114–128, Fall (No. 3), 1965.

27. Thomas, M. D., *et al.*: Anger: a tool for developing self-awareness. **Am. J. Nurs.,** 70:2586–2590, Dec., 1970.

28. Understanding hostility. Programmed Instruction. **Am. J. Nurs.,** 67:2131–2150, Oct., 1967.

29. Weiss, J. M.: Psychological factors in stress and disease. **Sci. Am.,** 226:104–113, June, 1972.

30. Wilkiemeyer, D. S.: Affection: key to the care for the elderly. **Am. J. Nurs.,** 72:2166–2168, Dec., 1972.

CHAPTER 13

Using Communication Skills

GLOSSARY

Cliché: Trite, stereotyped phrase.

Communication: An interchange of information.

Interview: To talk over something special with a person, usually in a face-to-face meeting.

Language: Prescribed way of using words; a means of expressing thoughts or feelings.

Listen: To give heed with the ear while attending closely to what is heard.

Nonverbal Communication: An exchange of information without the utilization of words.

Observe: To see, or notice, while attending closely so as to interpret what is seen.

Open-ended Comment: A response that gives a general lead or broad opening to communication.

Reflective Comment: A response that repeats what a person has said or what a person appears to be feeling.

Semantics: The study of the meaning of words.

Symbol: A sign that represents an idea or concept.

Touch: The tactile sense.

Validate: To confirm.

Verbal Communication: An exchange of information using words.

INTRODUCTION

Communication is the interchange of information between at least two persons. The information is exchanged through hearing, seeing, tasting, smelling, and touching. Everything one does or uses has communicative value—one's work, the house one lives in, the food one eats, the clothes one wears. All that impinges on our senses—a glance, a wink of the eye, a touch, the spoken word, a gesture, the fragrance of one's cologne—communicates something. In other words, we communicate in a variety of ways through talking, signaling, writing, gesturing, drawing, singing, and dancing.

Whenever one person becomes aware of another, the world expands from self to others. The process of communication begins when one person begins a relationship with another. Hence, communication is basic to human relationships. Unless people communicate, no sort of relationship develops between them. The example of two strangers sitting next to each other in a theater demonstrates physical closeness without any type of relationship necessarily developing between them. However, if during the movie these two people exchange words or glances, that is, communicate, a relationship comes into existence. It matters not whether the communication is verbal (one makes a comment to the other) or nonverbal (one frowns at the other for eating popcorn loudly), hostile or friendly, a human relationship is there. Hence, communication is behavior. It involves both physical and mental activity and provides for an exchange of ideas, attitudes, thoughts, and feelings.

ESSENTIALS IN THE PROCESS OF COMMUNICATION

In the process of communication, there *must be a message delivered from one person to another.* A gesture indicating where a visitor may find a particular patient may not be seen. A letter may be lost in the mail. A child playing too far from home may not hear his mother's call. These illustrations demonstrate a breakdown in communication: a message was sent but not delivered to the intended receiver.

If one mumbles while talking, speaks too softly or too rapidly, if there are noises in the room, if the intended receiver is not listening, and so on, any of these may prevent what has been said being heard. Sometimes, patients have been reprimanded because they failed to follow instructions for taking medications at home when they probably did not clearly hear the instructions. For many people, especially the very ill or the elderly, it may be necessary to ask, "Did you hear me?" or "Was that clear?"

When a message is sent, *it must get the attention of the receiver.* A letter that has arrived at its destination must be read. Commercials on television and radio often are sent at a higher decibel level than the programs they interrupt. This device is intended to catch the attention of the audience. The patient's call light is a signal for a nurse, but the communication fails if the light does not catch the nurse's attention. Preoccupation with other thoughts may divert attention. For example, a patient may be so afraid of giving himself injections that his attention is diverted when the nurse attempts to teach him the procedure. Without an attentive receiver, effective communication is not possible.

The sending and the receiving of messages usually cannot be separated distinctly, since both often go on simultaneously. For example, assume that a nurse is talking with a patient who is describing his headache. While the patient talks, the nurse listens and receives the message. But at the same time, she may be sending messages to the patient by the expression on her face and her actions as the patient speaks (such as drumming her fingers impatiently). The patient and the nurse receive messages while transmitting them. Stop for a moment and consider any conversation with another person. One soon realizes that the interchange of messages is constant and simultaneous. Hence, communication is a reciprocal process, and an experience in which both the sender and the receiver of messages participate simultaneously.

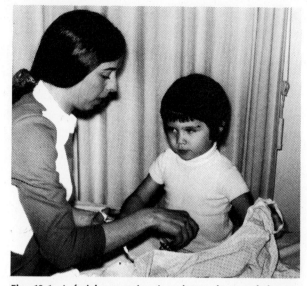

Fig. 13-1. A facial expression is a form of nonverbal communication. While the nurse explains, the patient appears to be very suspicious, possibly also fearful. (Good Samaritan Hospital, Phoenix, Arizona)

Once a message has been sent and received, it *must be interpreted.* Interpretation by the receiver is based on his past experience. If the sender and receiver have had different experiences in terms of the message being sent, a breakdown in communication can result. The sign language of the deaf cannot be interpreted by one inexperienced in this form of communication. A person listening to a message spoken in a language unfamiliar to him cannot interpret the sender's message. Pain means one thing to a person who has suffered a great deal, but it may mean something quite different to one who has experienced little. The grief of death may have relatively little meaning to a person who has not experienced the loss of a loved one.

Consider many of the adjectives used commonly in everyday conversations. What is a *big* car? A *small* child? A *good* meal? A *poor* movie? An *expensive* garment? A *high* temperature? A *rapid* pulse rate? Unless the sender's and receiver's past experiences are similar in relation to the manner in which these adjectives are used, effective communication is impossible.

It is of utmost importance for the nurse to use words that the patient can understand. A nurse speaking to a patient who is to have a blood test would not be of much help if she said, "You are fasting this A.M., since you'll have a V.P. for a B.U.N." She is more likely to convey a clearer message to the patient if she tells him that his breakfast will be delayed until after a blood sample has been taken, that the doctor wishes a study of his blood and that taking food may alter the blood findings. Often, nurses tend to forget that most patients are not familiar with medical and nursing jargon.

The message *must be stated in words having a common meaning to the sender and the receiver.* The study of the meaning of words is referred to as *semantics.* To persons speaking the same language, identical words may have entirely different meanings. For example, the word "democracy" means one thing to most people in the Western world but something quite different in the Eastern world, even when a common language is being used. Communication using such words as liberty, freedom, fraternity, love, and hate will fail unless the sender and receiver attach common meanings to these words. A 45-year-old will be lost in a conversation with a teen-ager unless he knows current teen-ager jargon.

VERBAL AND NONVERBAL COMMUNICATIONS

Communications are described as being either verbal or nonverbal. *Verbal communication* uses the spoken word. (Technically, reading and writing may be considered forms of verbal communication but this chapter will pertain to the spoken word.)

Verbal communication is dependent upon language. *Language* is a prescribed way of using words so that people can share information effectively. Language includes a common definition of words being used, as well as a method of arranging words in a certain order to convey the message. The development of language represented a great step forward in the history of communication, for then everyone using the same language could share information more readily.

Nonverbal communication is the exchange of messages without the utilization of words. It is what is *not* said. Individuals communicate through the use of facial expressions, body movements, tone of voice, gait, and the like. Crying and moaning are oral, but not verbal, communications.

Nonverbal communications are more likely to be involuntary and therefore less under the control of the person conveying the message than is verbal communication. Hence, nonverbal communication is generally considered as being a more nearly accurate expression of true feelings. How many times have we asked or been asked, "What's wrong?",

when obvious appearance and behavior showed that all was not well. The great pantomimist Marcel Marceau and many of the stars of silent motion pictures illustrate in their performances that the power of the body in action and facial expressions can carry innumerable messages and in very dramatic ways.

Nonverbal communication occurs concurrently with verbal communication. There is a proverb that goes: "What you do speaks so loud I cannot hear what you say." For example, the words "hello" and "goodbye" can be said in ways that imply another's presence is either the best or the worst thing that could have happened.

As another example, a patient may joke about his preoperative tests and be casual about his impending surgery, but his expressions do not fool the observant nurse who notes that he is in and out of bed, is unable to sit and read, smokes one cigarette after another, makes frequent trips to the telephone booth, and gets out of the corridor whenever he sees a stretcher coming along.

There are several forms of communication, usually considered nonverbal, that are sometimes used in nursing. A *symbol* is a sign that represents an idea. For example, the national flag of a country is a well-known symbol. The symbol ♀ means female while the symbol ♂ means male. Doodlings have been demonstrated to have communicative value with some patients.

Signals can carry information. For example, most hospitals use a light as a signal when the patient wishes a nurse. A study situation at the end of this chapter calls attention to how a game was used by a child to signal certain messages to his nurses. Most health agencies have a fire alarm system, such as a siren or a bell, to alert everyone to the danger of fire.

The messages of communication cannot always be assumed to mean what the receiver, upon first glance, believes them to be. True meanings may be camouflaged. For example, a person may say he is ill and wishes to leave a meeting; he may be simply bored but uses illness as an excuse to leave. A patient may say he does not wish to eat because he has no appetite; the real meaning of his behavior may be that he is seeking attention. In other words, things may not always be what they appear to be.

Validation is important in order that true feelings and meanings can be discerned. A study situation at the end of this chapter directs the reader to two references that illustrate the importance of validating communication in order to be sure of un-

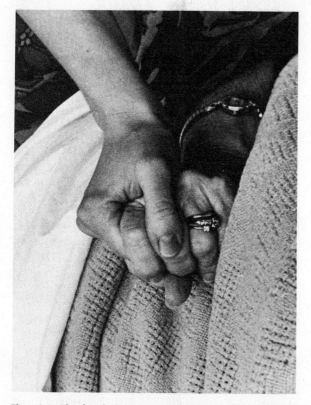

Fig. 13-2. The hand clasp is an example of communicating through touch. The hands of the patient and nurse in this picture illustrate the exchange of feelings subtly but still very positively. (Good Samaritan Hospital, Phoenix, Arizona)

derstanding its true meaning. Validation is a two-way street. The nurse will wish to validate what she believes the patient is communicating to her as well as validate that the patient is receiving accurate messages from her.

TOUCH AS A MEANS OF COMMUNICATION

Touch, the tactile sense, has been studied seriously as a form of nonverbal communication only within the last three decades or so. Anthropologists have been largely responsible for sparking interest in the sense of touch after learning that it has played and continues to play an important role in the various cultures of mankind. Their investigations have further shown that tactile experiences are largely shaped by familial, regional, class, and cultural influences. Such factors as age and sex also play a role in developing meanings that are associated with

touch. These various influences individualize the meaning of touch. In other words, touch expresses very personal behavior and it means different things to different people. Two men embracing upon meeting is usual behavior in some cultures; in others, shaking hands is more common. Tactile experiences between people of different sexes can carry different meanings from tactile experiences between people of the same sex.

Touch can be used to carry a variety of messages: comfort, love, affection, security, anger, frustration, aggression, excitement, and any number of emotional reactions. Figure 13-2 illustrates touch in a nursing situation.

As stated earlier, authorities agree that nonverbal communication is more expressive in conveying the quality and intent of attitudes and feelings than is verbal communication; and touch is one of the most effective nonverbal ways of expressing them. Consider the youngster who defies his parent's verbal admonition and facial expressions to prepare for bed. The message may not be completely grasped until the parent's hand firmly touches his shoulder and steers the youngster to the stairway.

Because of its personal nature, assigning meanings to touch can be complicated and should be done with caution. There can well be differences in interpreting the meaning of touch as much as 50 percent of the time, according to investigations. A patient gloomily told a nurse that his children no longer cared for him because they had not visited him for several weeks. The nurse wished to express comfort and understanding when she patted the patient softly on his shoulder. The patient may have assumed the nurse's gesture meant that she did not consider his complaint to be significant. Anxiety may result when a patient does not know or understand the meaning of a tactile gesture or when he simply dislikes being touched. It must be remembered that specific tactile gestures do not have universal meanings and hence, the use of touch requires care and forethought.

Touch is more highly developed at birth than any of the other sense organs. According to research, tactile experiences of infants and young children appear essential for normal development of self and awareness of others. Many nurses and mothers have been reconsidering and changing child care that minimized body contact and touch. Note the emergence in the popularity of the rocking chair in hospital pediatric units and in many homes.

Physical closeness between patient and nurse is an essential of nursing. There is much use of hands and touching patients when nursing care is given. For example, the nurse who firmly holds the hand of a patient who is anxious and fearful may help to convey understanding and willingness to help. She has transmitted feelings of interest and concern. Dexterity and sureness in the use of her hands may aid to assure a patient of the nurse's expertise, as when adminstering an injection, palpating the abdomen, assisting a patient to walk, or giving the patient a bath. One patient remarked that a nurse's hands gave love when the nurse rubbed her back. Holding a crying child securely in her arms offers the child security and affection. Numerous other examples might be cited. However, these few are helpful in illustrating that when nursing intervention includes the judicious use of touch, it can be an important means of communicating in the nurse-patient relationship.

OBJECTIVES OF NURSE-PATIENT COMMUNICATIONS

Communication is the vehicle by which a nurse learns to know her patient, to determine what her patient's needs are, and to meet his needs. It can be seen that communication is not an end unto itself. Rather, it is the means toward attaining the goal of a therapeutic nurse-patient relationship. The need for communication is continuous since patient needs change as one need is met and other needs emerge. Consider the nursing care designed for a pregnant woman. Her nursing care while she is in the prenatal period is quite different from that during labor and delivery. Her needs, and hence, her nursing care, change again during the postpartum period. Continuous communication is the means to attain the constant goal of assisting this woman to attain and maintain optimum physical and psychological functioning during three very distinct and different periods in her life.

PRINCIPLES OF COMMUNICATION

Psychological well-being requires that individuals have an adequate means for communicating with others. Human beings are social creatures as well as biological organisms. Psychologists and sociologists have demonstrated that social interactions among people are required to fulfill some of our most elemental psychosocial needs, examples of which are love, affection, recognition, and desirability. Communication is basic to human relationships and nursing care is dependent on nurse-patient relationships.

Without communication, an individual is in isolation. Without it, nursing intervention to meet patients' needs is meaningless.

Communication is influenced by the patient's age, mental and physical capabilities, socioeconomic class, culture, interests, and other variables. No one approach will fit all patients. Communicating with a hospitalized patient about the importance of nourishment is quite different from communicating with a well person in her home concerning a nourishing diet for her family. The use of certain slang expressions may be acceptable when communicating with an adolescent but quite unacceptable when communicating with a middle-aged executive.

The following description illustrates certain gestures having a cultural basis. A communication problem resulted when the nurse failed to understand these gestures.

A community health nurse visited Mrs. Martinez, wife of a Mexican migrant worker, and her new baby shortly after they were discharged from the hospital. The purpose of the visit was to establish rapport with Mrs. Martinez in order to learn why she had been hostile about participating in hospital routine concerning personal cleanliness. A language barrier existed to a certain extent, because the nurses in the hospital did not understand Spanish sufficiently well to know what the patient said when she spoke rapidly and angrily.

Upon entering the home the nurse was impressed with evidence of good care being given by Mrs. Martinez's mother. The baby, asleep in the arms of his grandmother, appeared well. The grandmother held the baby out slightly to the nurse, who thought the grandmother wanted her to see the baby more easily. The nurse did not touch the baby. The grandmother extended the baby out even further and while the nurse looked more attentively, she felt no need to touch and handle the baby. The hospital report indicated that the baby was normal and well and so it appeared. When the nurse spoke to the mother about her hospital stay, she quickly realized that she was making no progress. The mother barely answered the nurse's questions and often turned her face away. After a few minutes the nurse left, feeling frustrated for having failed in gaining rapport with Mrs. Martinez. When the nurse returned a few days later, the grandmother politely but firmly told the nurse her services were no longer needed.

The nurse discussed the calls with her supervisor, who was familiar with the culture of this family. Mrs. Martinez and her mother believed the nurse was possessed of an "evil eye" because she gazed at the baby but did not touch him. The nurse would then give *mal ojo*, or "evil eye sickness," to the baby. Had the nurse touched the baby, all would have been well.

When the nurse attempted to discuss personal cleanliness with the mother, the patient had said she was clean but became unclean in the hospital because she was forced to wash herself with water. This violated the prescription of *dieta*, a period after childbirth when mothers of this culture must not have water touch them because it makes them "unclean." The supervisor explained that when Mrs. Martinez left the hospital, she no doubt obtained a local remedy that would undo the harm done her in the hospital. In addition, the family would now seek the services of a *curando*, a woman in this culture with powers to cure the "evil eye sickness" the nurse transmitted to the baby.

Silences are a meaningful part of communication. Silence has many meanings. The patient may be rejecting the nurse and refusal to speak may be defiant and mean, "I have nothing to say to you!" It may be that the patient is exploring his feelings, and speaking at that time may disrupt his thoughts. Silence can be used as a retreat and hence, as an escape from a threat. The patient who refuses to discuss a fear may be using silence to avoid emotion. Silence may be a sign of comfort; close friends or a husband and wife may observe silence and yet, be communicating many things. Silence may be discussed in due time with the patient, especially if the nurse wishes to validate her speculation on its meaning.

Fear of silence sometimes leads to too much talking by the nurse. Whatever the cause of silence, too much talking may mean that the patient's problems cannot be identified and explored. Also, excessive talking usually places the focus on the nurse, rather than on the patient where it should be. A verse in the third chapter of the Book of Ecclesiastes in the Bible states this idea well: There "... is a time for every matter under heaven: ... a time to keep silence, and a time to speak; ..."

Listening is an essential part of communication. Listening is an active process involving hearing and interpretation of what is being said. It requires attention and concentration in order to sort out, evaluate, and validate clues that are the aids to understanding real meanings in what the patient is saying. It requires forgetting about one's self and thinking of the speaker.

Listening selectively, or hearing only what one wants to hear, limits communication. All of us, including patients, are guilty at times of hearing only what we want to hear. No one likes to hear bad news;

no one wants to hear that he must give up some of the pleasures of life; nor do we want to hear that there are difficult times ahead.

Pretending to listen and responding impulsively when someone is speaking are barriers to communication. It is a rare speaker who is insensitive to an attitude of apathy, boredom, lack of interest, or feigned attention on the part of a listener.

Observation is an essential part of communication. Observation is an active process involving seeing and interpreting. It is an especially useful validating tool. For example, a nurse was of the opinion that a patient was fearful concerning the results of certain blood tests he had had, but the patient kept saying that the tests were not important. However, the nurse observed the patient pacing back and forth in the corridor while appearing to be in deep thought. Observing the patient's behavior helped validate the nurse's clue that the patient was possibly fearful and his asserting that he was not appeared to be a cover-up for his true feelings.

Information essential to understanding a person and his problems can best be obtained when communication has a purpose and when it focuses on the individual. To illustrate, if a nurse realizes that knowing something about a patient's usual daily activities will aid her in planning his care, she plans her communications with the patient accordingly.

Social conversations are useful as a display of friendliness and politeness, but generally of limited value in understanding the patient.

A common pitfall is to focus communication on an activity of the nurse rather than on the patient. A nurse missed an important clue concerning the patient's feelings in this conversation:

PATIENT: I don't know why these injections scare me but they do.

NURSE: Let's hurry and get your shot done. Then you won't have time to worry.

Had the nurse posed this question, "You are afraid of these injections?", after the patient made the remark, she would have been focusing on the patient rather than on the procedure.

While being attentive to the patient, the nurse will wish to keep her own feelings to herself. Also, questions that tend to make the patient feel his answers must fit the nurse's expectations are of little value in attempting to understand the patient.

The above principle can be further elaborated by adding that effective nurse-patient communications depend on attitudes of sincere interest in and concern for the patient. Patients are quick to ascertain when personnel are going through the motions of appearing to care. Failure to listen is failure to be concerned. The attribute of *caring* in nursing has been discussed earlier in this text. It is an essential in promoting effective nurse-patient communications.

Still another elaboration of the above principle is that effective communication is promoted when the nurse remains *nonjudgmental*. Patients tend to feel safe when they are allowed to express their feelings without being judged and condemned. A patient was heard to say, "I think I have a right to be afraid of this operation." The nurse would be nonjudgmental and respect that right by responding to the comment by saying, for example, "Tell me what you think has made you afraid."

Consider the nurse who noted that a young woman was crying. The nurse's comment was, "You aren't acting very grown-up. How do you think your husband would feel if he saw you crying like that?" The nurse judged the patient as being immature and the hostility she seemed to be displaying could end effective communication.

A *variety of techniques have been observed to promote effective communication*. Here are some of those techniques.

A comfortable environment promotes effective communication. This is one in which both the patient and the nurse are at ease. Such items as suitable furniture, proper lighting, and moderate temperature are important. Also, effective relationships are enhanced when the atmosphere is relaxed and unhurried in nature. If the nurse seems preoccupied and "on the run," or if the patient is ill at ease for fear of missing visitors or an appointment, communication is impaired. When possible the nurse will wish to sit down while speaking with the patient and in a place so that she and the patient can see each other without strain.

Providing for privacy is important. It may not always be possible to carry on conversations with just the patient and the nurse in a room. However, every effort should be made to provide sufficient privacy so that conversations cannot be overheard by others.

Any distracting influence is likely to interfere, such as preoccupation with personal matters, extremes of emotions, intrusions, and the like. Also, as stated earlier in this chapter, communication is dependent on a common understanding of the words and symbols that are being used in the communication process.

Cliché-type statements generally are to be avoided. A *cliché* is a stereotyped, trite, or pat answer. Most of them tend to indicate no cause for anxiety or concern or lack of interest in what has been said. Typical clichés are "Everything will be all right"; "Don't worry, you will be all right"; or "Your doctor knows best." Cliché-type statements fail to respond to what the patient is trying to say and hence, tend to block communication. While often they are used to reassure a patient, they have little or no effect in doing so.

In certain instances, clichés can serve a purpose. For example, occasionally they may be used to break the ice when conversation begins. However, even then, they lose their effectiveness unless the patient feels the nurse is really interested. For example, one of the most common clichés is "How do you feel?" If the patient has any reason to suspect that the nurse is not sincerely interested in how he feels, effective communication is difficult.

Questions that can be answered by simply saying "yes" or "no" and questions containing the words, "why" and "how" generally elicit little information. Questions that can be answered by "yes" or "no" tend to cut off further information, even when the patient might well wish to go on. For example, the question, "Did you have a good day?", almost begs for a noncommittal sort of answer which tells the listener very little.

Questions using "why" and "how" tend to intimidate the patient. For example, the question, "Why were you not tired enough to sleep?", might better be stated by asking, "What were you doing while you were unable to sleep?"

A comment that repeats what a patient has said or what a patient appears to be feeling tends to encourage the patient to talk and describe more. A comment of this nature is referred to as a *reflective comment*. It is among the most common communication tools. Here are examples of a reflective comment:

PATIENT: I surely wish I knew why I feel so blue today.
NURSE: You are saying that you feel blue . . .

or

PATIENT: My children certainly have been pests lately.
NURSE: Your children are annoying you?

The use of the reflective comment can be overdone, obviously. If the patient concludes that the nurse is employing a technique mechanistically, communication will end.

Broad openings or general leads are often helpful to encourage the patients to go on. Comments of this nature are referred to as *open-ended comments*. They often serve as the bridge to continued conversations. Examples are "And after that . . ."; "And then?"; or "You were saying . . ." Sometimes a nod of the head while saying "Yes . . ."; "Uh-huh"; or "Oh . . ." effectively encourages further conversation.

Comments that help to place events into meaningful sequences or to demonstrate cause-and-effect relationships aid in promoting helpful communications. The question, "When did you start feeling bad?" helps to put events into chronological order. The question, "You started feeling bad yesterday after you forgot to take your medicine?" may determine a possible cause-and-effect relationship.

Questions that appear to probe for information tend to cut off communication. Patients who are made to feel as though they are receiving the "third degree" become resentful and will usually clam up and try to avoid further communication. Although the nurse may feel she needs more information, it is better to follow the patient's lead. Letting him take the initiative allows him to delve more deeply at a time when he is ready. The person who says, "Let's get to the bottom of this," is likely to destroy conversation unless the patient feels like facing the real cause of a problem.

Comments that indicate that the nurse might not have understood tend to encourage clarification for both the nurse and the patient. Interrupting the patient may be necessary but should be done with care in order to avoid breaking a train of thought. Also, interrupting should be done politely in order not to offend the speaker. However when opportune moments arrive in the conversation, interrupting for clarification is important, for failing to explore may result in failing to understand. Examples of comments asking for clarification include "I don't follow you"; "About whom are you speaking?"; and "Are you saying that listening to music takes your mind off things?"

Listening and observing for themes in nonverbal and verbal communication aid in understanding the speaker. Following are suggested questions the nurse will wish to keep in mind when communicating with patients. What are the repeated themes in the patient's speech and behavior? What topics does the patient tend to avoid? What subjects tend to make the patient shift the conversation to other topics? What inconsistencies and gaps appear in the patient's conversation? Answers to these questions are useful tools in understanding the patient and in determining his problems.

SPECIAL PROBLEMS OF COMMUNICATION

Nurses can expect to encounter certain communication problems during the course of their practice that will require special attention. Whatever the situation, however, the same principles of communication will apply that have just been discussed.

Communicating with the deaf, the blind, and the mute person are examples. Writing may be used with the deaf person when gestures are insufficient, unless someone is available to interpret if the person uses sign language. The blind person requires adaptations in care when sight ordinarily is used during the communication process. It is often helpful to ask the patient or members of his family what means of communication have been found to be most effective. Nursing care for the deaf, the blind, or the mute patient will also include consideration and respect for how the patient feels about his physical limitation.

Another special problem is communicating with a patient who speaks a language unknown by the nurse. Using an interpreter is a great assist but with effort, a great deal can be accomplished by using various forms of nonverbal communication. Publications with translation of common health-related terms also are available.

An interesting and helpful learning situation is to practice communicating with an associate who role-plays the patient with special communication problems. Some of the references at the end of this chapter will offer suggestions also.

The nurse caring for a patient who is unconscious will want to remember that the patient sometimes still is able to hear and to feel touch. Communicating with the seriously ill patient is further discussed in Chapter 31.

COMMUNICATING WITH GROUPS

Nurses communicate with groups when teaching patients with special interests, such as teaching diabetics, pregnant women, school children, tuberculous patients, patients with colostomies, and so on.

Communicating with groups of people is somewhat different from communicating with just one other person. The same principles discussed earlier in this chapter apply except that instead of thinking in terms of an individual person, one considers a cluster of individuals having certain commonalities, such as a topic of common interest.

Individual differences among group members are

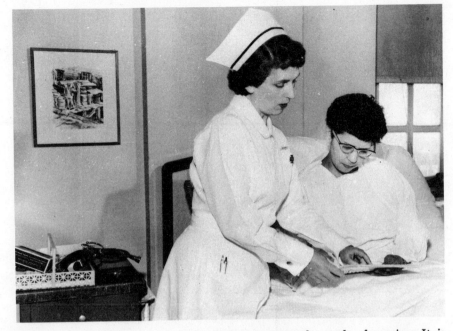

Fig. 13-3. The patient whose communication is handicapped by a language difference can be helped by the use of a language aid. Some health agencies have prepared such aids for their own use, having foreign translations for commonly needed terms, phrases and instructions. Here the nurse is attempting to prepare the patient for a physical examination by using a Spanish-English aid. (Published by Educational Aid, Box 116, Vanderveer Station, Brooklyn, N.Y.)

to be considered, but these usually can best be handled in a one-to-one relationship after a group presentation when a particular problem arises. Using question periods after a general presentation of whatever material is set forth can help also to meet individual differences.

THE INTERVIEW

To *interview* means to talk over something special with a person or persons, usually in a face-to-face meeting. *The interviewee* is the person who is interviewed.

Very often the interview is thought of as a formal type of communication, possibly with a prepared list of questions to ask of the interviewee. However, the word interview need not be limited to such communication only, as the definition above would indicate. Rather, all nurse-patient communication can be considered as interviews.

This text uses the word interview in its broadest sense. Therefore, the principles of communication discussed earlier in this chapter will guide the nurse when she interviews, or talks, with patients.

CONCLUSION

Communication has been viewed as an essential element in establishing the nurse-patient relationship. The nurse is encouraged to strive in a deliberative manner to improve her communication skills in order to aid in attaining the goals of nursing. It is important that she knows what is being communicated and how to assess and validate it as she plans for appropriate nursing intervention.

Effective communication is to learn to know another person for what he is. To be therapeutic, communication avoids attempts to convince or argue someone into submission. It consists of hearing as well as speaking, and especially of hearing what others want to say.

Study Situations

1. Establishing communication with severely burned 11-year-old Stanley required creativity and ingenuity.
   Faulkner, B. L.: From first base to home plate. **Am. J. Nurs.,** 71:2331–2333, Dec., 1971.
   Describe various ways in which the tool described in the above article helped to establish communication between Stanley and the health practitioners caring for him.

2. The following article examines theories of touch as related to nonverbal communication:
   Barnett, K.: A theoretical construct of the concepts of touch as they relate to nursing. **Nurs. Research,** 21:102–110, Mar.–Apr., 1972.
   Note the theoretical construct of touch presented on pages 108 and 109. Also, note the proposals for research on page 109. Recall nursing care you have given recently. Were any of these propositions supported or rejected by your observations in relation to touch?

3. In the following article, the author writes of the adolescent patient:

Tiedt, E.: The adolescent in the hospital: an identity-resolution approach. **Nurs. Forum,** 11:120–140, No. 2, 1972.

Note the seven dimensions of "identity search," on page 123, with which adolescents are concerned, according to Dr. Erik Erikson. Describe nursing practices you believe could help the adolescent cope with the stress of illness and hospitalization. What role do verbal and nonverbal communications assume in the practices you described?

4. In the following book, the author describes communication that suggests one thing to the listener but may mean something very different to the person who spoke:

Berne, E.: Games People Play: The Psychology of Human Relationships. 192 p. New York, Grove Press, 1964.

Select a game or two the author described. Do you believe you have played any of these games? Do you think any of your patients may have played them? For example, note the game called "Why Don't You —Yes But," beginning on page 116. The author points out that the purpose of the game is not to get suggestions for a solution to a problem, as it at first appears, but to reject solutions.

Read the following article:

Levin, P., and Berne, E.: Games nurses play. **Am. J. Nurs.,** 72:483–487, Mar., 1972.

Do you agree with the authors' last statement in the article on page 487, when they wrote, "If a nurse understands she is playing games, she is then in a position to direct her energies toward identifying and solving the problems which give rise to the games, rather than continuing the game playing." The preceding two references illustrate the importance of validating behavior, verbal or nonverbal, since often things are not really what they appear to be.

5. After reading the following article, identify principles of communication described in this chapter, that the nurse-author used when interviewing patients:

Hardiman, M. A.: Interviewing? Or social chit-chat? **Am. J. Nurs.,** 71:1379–1381, July, 1971.

References

1. Amacher, N. J.: Touch is a way of caring—and a way of communicating with an aphasic patient. **Am. J. Nurs.,** 73:852–854, May, 1973.

2. Bender, R. E.: Communicating with the deaf. **Am. J. Nurs.,** 66:757–760, Apr., 1966.

3. Bernstein, L., and Dana, R. H.: Interviewing and the Health Professions. New York, Appleton-Century-Crofts, 1970.

4. Cuthbert, B. L.: Switch off, tune in, turn on. **Am. J. Nurs.,** 69:1206–1211, June, 1969.

5. Drakeford, J. W.: The Awesome Power of the Listening Ear. Waco, Texas, Word Books, 1967.

6. Durr, C. A.: Hands that help . . . but how? **Nurs. Forum,** 10:392–400, No. 4, 1971.

7. Farro, D.: Mr. W. **Am. J. Nurs.,** 70:824–826, Apr., 1970.

8. Fox, M. J.: Talking with patients who can't answer. **Am. J. Nurs.,** 71:1146–1149, June, 1971.

9. Goldin, P., and Russell, B.: Therapeutic communication. **Am. J. Nurs.,** 69:1928–1930, Sept., 1969.

10. Gould, G. T., guest ed.: Symposium on compassion and communication in nursing. *In* **The Nursing Clinics of North America.** Philadelphia, W. B. Saunders, 4:651–729, Dec., 1969.

11. Haggerty, V. C.: Listening: an experiment in nursing. **Nurs. Forum,** 10:382–391, No. 4, 1971.

12. Jakobson, R.: Verbal communication. **Sci. Am.,** 227:73–80, Sept. 1972.

13. Johnson, B. S.: The meaning of touch in nursing. **Nurs. Outlook,** 13:59–60, Feb., 1965.

14. Johnston, R.: Listen, nurse. **Am. J. Nurs.,** 71:303, Feb., 1971.

15. Kron, T., Communication in Nursing. Philadelphia, W. B. Saunders, 1967.

16. Lewis, G. K.: Nurse-Patient Communication. ed. 2. Dubuque, Iowa, William C. Brown, 1973.

17. Manthey, M. E.: A guide for interviewing. **Am. J. Nurs.,** 67:2088–2090, Oct. 1967.

18. Montagu, A.: Touching: The Human Significance of the Skin. New York, Columbia University Press, 1971.

19. Muecke, M. A.: Overcoming the language barrier. **Nurs. Outlook,** 18:53–54, Apr. 1970.

20. Nelson, A. C.: How can you stand the crying? **Am. J. Nurs.,** 70:66–69, Jan., 1970.

21. Oraftik, N.: Only time to touch. **Nurs. Forum,** 11:205–213, No. 2, 1972.

22. Paynich, M. L.: Cultural barriers to nurse communication. **Am. J. Nurs.,** 64:87–90, Feb., 1964.

23. Robinson, L.: Psychological Aspects of the Care of Hospitalized Patients. Philadelphia, F. A. Davis, 1968.

24. Skipper, J. K., Jr., *et al.*: The importance of communication. *In* Skipper, J. K., Jr., and Leonard, R. C., eds.: Social Interaction and Patient Care. pp. 51–136. Philadelphia, J. B. Lippincott, 1965.

25. Travelbee, J.: Communicating with patients. *In* Intervention in Psychiatric Nursing: Process in the One-To-One Relationship. pp. 67–104. Philadelphia, F. A. Davis, 1969.

26. Underwood, P. R.: Communication through role playing. **Am. J. Nurs.,** 71:1184–1186, June, 1971.

27. Veninga, R.: Communications: a patient's eye view. **Am. J. Nurs.,** 73:320–322, Feb., 1973.

28. Wilson, L. M.: Listening. *In* Carlson, C. E., coordinator: Behavioral Concepts and Nursing Intervention. pp. 153–170. Philadelphia, J. B. Lippincott, 1970.

CHAPTER 14

Contributions to Nursing from Anthropology

GLOSSARY

Acculturation: Process by which a culture changes after contact with a different culture.

Anthropology: Study of man using comparative analyses of his physical and behavioral characteristics.

Culture: All learned and transmitted patterns of behavior, expectations, understandings, values, and the like, that one shares with others in one's group.

Ethnocentrism: Preoccupation with one's own culture that leads one to judge all other cultures as inferior.

Genetic Heredity: Process by which physical traits are passed on from one generation to another.

Holism: A concept based on the assumption that a whole has many parts, each of which is related to every other part.

Social Heredity: Process by which cultural traits are passed from one generation to another.

Subculture: A group in a culture that does not hold all beliefs of the larger culture or gives them different significances.

INTRODUCTION

Man, a very complex creature, lives in increasingly complex societies. The anthropologist attempts to study mankind together with his complexities, wherever he lives. The anthropologist's findings as well as his methods of work are becoming important assists in providing high-quality nursing care today.

The discussion here must necessarily be sketchy. Additional information is provided in other courses of study in the nursing curriculum. Also, the study situations and references at the end of this chapter direct attention to sources of information that will prove helpful in continuing the study of the concepts to be discussed here.

DEFINITION OF ANTHROPOLOGY

Anthropology is the study of man. It is based on comparative investigations of man's behavioral and physical characteristics and concerns itself with man in all places, times, and circumstances. Anthropology is interested in the manner in which man adapts and maintains himself in the many different environments and social settings in which he finds himself in the world.

There are many disciplines interested in man and the way he lives and functions. Examples include psychology, sociology, physiology, history, economics, political science, ecology, biology, archeology, and linguistics. A characteristic of anthropology is that it concerns itself with all these fields and more. Hence, anthropology may be called multifaceted as it uses disparate branches of science and humanities to broaden and deepen its picture of mankind.

Because anthropology has so many areas of concern, anthropologists increasingly select areas for specialized study. For example, the *physical anthropologist* is primarily concerned with man as a biological being. The *cultural anthropologist* studies human behavior. *Psychological anthropologists* are concerned with personality studies. The *linguistic anthropologist* studies language and thought. *Social anthropology* emphasizes interpersonal and inter-group relationships. And so on. However, just as in other disciplines with specialization, there is over-lapping of interests among all anthropologists and the goal of all is essentially the same—to learn more about man.

DEFINITIONS OF CULTURE AND SUBCULTURE

Culture is a fundamental concept to the anthro-pologist. *Culture* is everything that an individual learns from groups of which he is a part and that he transmits to succeeding generations. It is what all men have in common. It includes understandings, values, and mutual expectations. It is made up of certain ways of acting, thinking, feeling, and com-municating. We are born into a culture that, for example, over a period of time teaches us what to eat, how and when to eat, what to wear, how to get along and communicate with others, and how to care for ourselves. It includes such activities as using a language, running a government, rearing our chil-dren, getting married, making a living, and fighting a war.

Even superficial observations illustrate that there is remarkable variation in mankind's cultures. For example, the American teen-ager dresses very un-like the Saudi Arabian teen-ager. There is little re-semblance between food customs in Samoa and Sweden. Although there may be elements of com-monality, the Moslem religion is very different from Christianity. Examples such as these can be cited indefinitely.

The word "cultured" sometimes is applied to certain people who display appreciation of fine litera-ture, art, or music. Those not sharing this appreciation may be referred to as "uncultured" persons. But the word is not used in that connotation in this book.

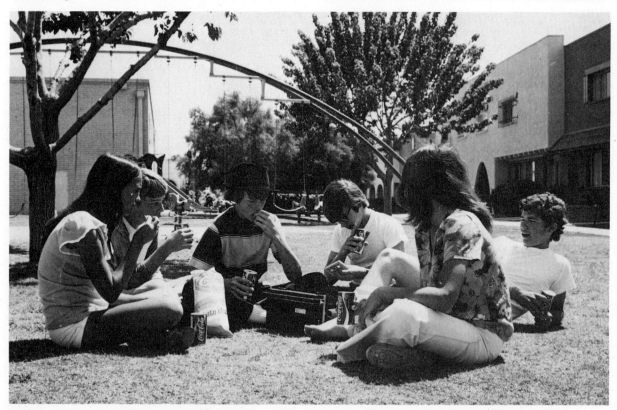

Fig. 14-1. In the American culture, teenagers hold to values and attitudes important to their particular subculture. They tend to hold to their own values and attitudes, for example, in relation to such items as personal groom-ing, eating habits, and types of recreation. They generally prefer socializing with their own age group and often feel uncomfortable when their behavior differs from that of their teenage friends. To ignore their values and atti-tudes would do little to assist the nurse who wishes to establish therapeutic relationships with her teenage patients.

Nor is it so used by social scientists. When we speak of culture here, we are referring to man's behavior and to the ways in which human beings of all social levels carry out their activities of daily living.

A *subculture* is a group within a culture that does not hold all beliefs of the larger culture or gives them different significance. American subcultures, for example, are almost infinitely diversified according to such factors as region, race, education, occupation, income, social class, and so on. Moreover, each individual is the product of a number of subcultures, every one of which will affect his behavior to some degree.

A few examples will illustrate what at least some authorities consider as subcultures in America. There are those who describe a culture of poverty in the United States. Persons living in poverty have been observed often to hold certain common attitudes, as for instance, lack of trust and understanding of individuals from other subcultures. The communes that have sprung up across the country are often thought of as a subculture. Life in a commune is usually very dependent on nature for livelihood and the attitudes its members hold in relation to such things as family life, rearing of children, education, and the like, are very different from other subcultures. There have been descriptions of rural and urban subcultures, the subculture of the industrial worker, and even the subcultures of various types of institutions such as hospitals.

Subcultural points of view are most important for the nurse to keep in mind because they can be very subtle at times and therefore deceiving. If the nurse is caring for a patient whose cultural values are in variance with her own, she will wish to be aware of the differences but respect the patient for what he is.

Recognizing subcultures can aid in removing stereotyped thinking and aid in decreasing prejudices. For example, not all Orientals are stoic, not all English are conservative, not all hippies are dirty, not all city-folks are sophisticated, not all Russians are Communists, and so on.

GENETIC AND SOCIAL HEREDITY

Anthropologists speak of two types of heredity, genetic and social. *Genetic heredity* passes physical traits on from one generation to another through the body's genes. Genetic heredity will be discussed later in this chapter. *Social heredity* passes cultural traits on from one generation to another through teaching its offspring.

Anthropologists have long observed the unrest, the rebellion against authority, and the living in doubt and uncertainty of the American adolescent. These characteristics had been considered to be inevitable behavior resulting from the physiological changes occurring at puberty. Hence, it was theorized that the behavior resulted from genetic heredity. The eminent anthropologist Margaret Mead questioned this theory. She then went to study Polynesian adolescents and noted that adolescent behavior typical of Americans was absent in Samoa. She reported characteristics of the Samoan culture that she theorized made transition from adolescence to adulthood relatively easy. There was a general casualness in Samoan culture; Samoan society tended to be homogeneous and hence, lacked highly competitive groups and widely divergent philosophies of life. Mead's conclusion was that the Samoan culture with its freedom from pressure and the American culture with its many pressures resulted in the difference in the behavior of adolescents.

Attitudes, beliefs, and values learned from a previous generation are generally deeply ingrained. The expressions, "But that is not our (my) custom," or, "We don't do it that way," carry much weight. A woman who has been taught and lived under the rule that "cleanliness is next to godliness" may feel uncomfortable in a slovenly household. She might also be inclined to judge her relatives and friends solely on the basis of their housekeeping. The nurse also finds out that there are a goodly number of well-established attitudes and beliefs (superstitious and otherwise) relating to health. Many of these can interfere with care that is desirable or necessary. For instance, food prejudices may seriously hamper the maintenance of a therapeutic diet. A patient may refuse to have a blood transfusion because he has been taught that this should not be done. He is not necessarily being stubborn; he sincerely believes that this is wrong.

CULTURES ARE SUBJECT TO CHANGE

Anthropologists have shown that mankind's cultures have changed more rapidly and extensively with the emergence of the Western industrial and scientific revolutions. Furthermore, changes are occurring rapidly throughout the world, from the remotest Eskimo village in the Hudson Bay area to Main Street, U. S. A. How do cultures change? There are two common ways.

The first way is by *invention* or innovation. For example, the inventions of the wheel and of fire markedly changed the cultures where they originated. To cite a recent innovation, satellites have brought dramatic change in our communication systems. Western cultures are generally dedicated to progress and therefore tend to value change. Dedication to change and looking to the future rather than clinging to the past are important Western cultural attitudes.

A second way in which cultures change is through acculturation. *Acculturation* is a borrowing process by which cultural elements diffuse among people of different cultures. It results from contacts between societies. For example, the Indian family living on a reservation in New Mexico has a television set which has greatly changed their leisure time activities. The young girl reared on a midwestern farm went off to college in New York City and acquired Eastern mannerisms.

Much diffusion of culture is taking place in the world today, some of it almost instantaneously, as a result of the development of rapid transportation and communication facilities. The airplane, the radio, television, and the printed word have all given modern man access to each other's cultural materials. An American movie may be seen shortly after its making and simultaneously in New York, Cairo, and Tokyo. The length of a fashionable dress shown in Paris becomes a new style almost immediately around the world.

Paradoxically, although change is a law of life, nothing is more natural than the tendency to resist it. It is comforting to be able to preserve some vestiges of the old ways, many of which had been taken for granted and unappreciated until threatened with extinction. However, despite some unwillingness to change, individuals undergo constant modifications of attitude throughout life, changes which may themselves be almost imperceptible until some circumstance brings them into dramatic relief. Consider the person who suddenly embraces a religion different from that which he has always practiced. Although his action may appear abrupt and arbitrary to others, it is likely to be the result of cumulative changes in attitude that have quietly taken place throughout the years. Thus, often we drastically modify our thinking in spite of ourselves.

INFLUENCING CULTURAL CHANGE

Anthropologists have made tremendous contributions to the field of knowledge concerning human cultures. Most of them would agree that their find-

ings are of greater value when they can contribute to a better way of life for their fellow men. However, the question arises—to what extent have we a right to change people's culture or subculture? When we feel a cultural or subcultural characteristic is undesirable for some reason, have we the right to persuade others to accept another cultural or subcultural characteristic "for their own good?"

The question has produced much debate. Some scholars will say that just as we accept the right of man to his own religious beliefs, we must also accept the right of a man to other aspects of his culture. They would add that no one has a right to deliberately change the cultures of others.

Those who feel there is sometimes good reason for attempting to produce cultural change hold that it is justified *under certain circumstances*. They feel that individual rights are not violated when people are given sufficient knowledge concerning alternative behavior so that they can make an intelligent choice. This principle seems to be especially applicable in the field of health.

In a remote Mexican village health workers found that the only local beverage was an alcoholic drink made from the juice of a local plant. There was no safe source of water for drinking. But even when safe water was brought to these people, it was soon learned that they did not fare well. The local drink had been the only source of certain minerals and vitamins essential for health. This example illustrates that although it might well have been desirable for health reasons to change a cultural characteristic, the change became detrimental when consequences had not been ascertained beforehand.

In some instances, a patient's behavior and beliefs may differ from those of the staff and other patients and may seem unacceptable. However, if the nurse applies the principles of cultural change as just described, it may well be that she can transform the situation into a comfortable one for all concerned, as in the following example:

Mike was a young, itinerant farm worker who lived in shacks when he worked and in his battered car the rest of the time. Within a few hours after he was hospitalized, other patients were calling to voice complaints about him. Mike had voided in a wastebasket, and he spat out the window; because he was warm, he threw the top bedcovers over the foot of the bed and lay semiexposed. By the standards of the other patients and the nurses he was committing one social indiscretion after another. Considering what they knew of his background and circumstances, the nurses realized that this young man probably was not aware that there was anything wrong with his behavior. It took a bit of doing to explain the use of a urinal, bathroom facilities, and wipes in which to expectorate, and the inadvisability of letting himself be exposed. Some of Mike's roommates recognized his willingness to "do right" when he knew what to do, and out of kindness and in recognition of his potentialities, they did much to help him.

In this situation, notations were made on his nursing care plan which promoted consistency in the nursing approach to Mike. His illness kept him in the hospital for a while, during which time he expressed a desire to make some changes in his life. With the nurse's help in obtaining a social worker to visit him, possibilities for the future were explored with him. After his discharge he visited the nurses when he came for his clinic appointments. He reported on his progress in learning to read and write, and then on his new job.

This patient was amenable to change. However, he was fortunate in having people about him who showed an interest in him and taught him alternative types of behavior, rather than forcing him to conform to a new culture.

ACQUIRING AN APPRECIATION FOR CULTURAL DIFFERENCES

How does one acquire an appreciation for cultural differences in order that one may better understand one's patients? This section offers some suggestions.

Learning to appreciate cultural differences requires that the nurse make *concerted and conscientious efforts to study different cultures and subcultures.* Schools of nursing include courses in the social sciences in their curricula, which are a good beginning. The literature on culture is voluminous. Library study is an important assist to studying in the classroom. The student of nursing, then, may use course offerings and library study to aid in gaining an understanding of the various cultures of the world and of various subcultures within the society in which she lives.

A study of culture requires an *accepting, nonjudgmental, and objective attitude.* An approach that presumes one's own culture as the best defeats appreciation of others. In every society, people learn, as part of their culture, what is important and what is not, what is moral and what is wrong, and what is good or bad. While these concepts are important to

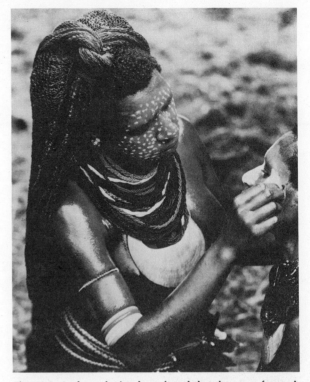

Fig. 14-2. Anthropologists have found that there are few universal cultural characteristics. Body adornment is one, according to students of culture. This photo, taken in New Guinea, shows body adornment in the culture of these people. Tatooing is an example of body adornment practiced by certain subcultures in this country. (Photo by Ray Weiss, Photophile)

persons in every culture, judging people of other cultures by one's own standards leads to failure and inappropriate conclusions in attempting to understand others.

A preoccupation with one's own culture that leads one to judge all but one's own as inferior is called *ethnocentrism.* A certain amount of ethnocentrism is necessary to the survival of a society. Without it, increasing personal conflicts and alienation could result. However, if one is studying other cultures, ethnocentrism defeats the purpose of investigation.

To acquire an appreciation of cultural differences requires that the nurse *conscientiously observe and listen.* Techniques that aid in observing and listening have been discussed earlier in this text. They are important tools when studying different cultures and subcultures.

Many nurses serve a family, a neighborhood, or a community. They can acquire knowledge of subcultural differences as they develop skills in observing and listening during their visits. Nurses employed in schools, clinics, physicians' offices, hospitals, industries, and the like, are well advised to visit the homes whenever possible, and the neighborhoods whence their patients come. The knowledge the nurse gains from such experience is comparable to that acquired by the field work of the anthropologist in studying subcultures first hand.

The participant-observer is one who will study a culture by *living within it* for a period of time. Many nurses choose to live and work in cultures other than their own. This type of experience affords excellent opportunities to compare cultures and to learn to appreciate their differences. A study situation at the end of this chapter refers the reader to articles written by nurses who have been participant-observers in various cultures.

Chapter 1 discussed an interdisciplinary approach to determining and meeting patient needs. This approach, utilizing the skills and knowledge of many occupational groups will promote an appreciation of cultural differences. The anthropologist, the psychologist, the sociologist, as examples, can be important on the health team just as, for example, the nutritionist, the physician, and the nurse.

Recently, a neurological disease was discovered in an isolated part of New Guinea. At first it appeared to be a psychiatric malady. Or possibly, it was thought, it could be the result of eating a narcotic fungus, a common dietary item for these people. Another theory was that it may be a result of long-term inbreeding since linguistic studies illustrated that breeding isolation was typical of the afflicted. After much study, a virus was found to be the culprit. The problem was properly diagnosed only after cultural, linguistic, and botanical evidence was brought into consideration and ruled out. While this example may seem unusually dramatic, it illustrates the importance of the interdisciplinary approach when attempting to identify and meet patient needs.

IMPLICATIONS FOR NURSING

The following discussion summarizes some of the contributions from the field of anthropology that can assist the nurse.

Man's range of behavior is dramatic and diverse, and through many thousands of years, he has survived because of his remarkable ability to adapt to a variety of problems and situations. Man has demonstrated concern for his welfare, health, and for his very existence, and the battle goes on. From anthropology, the nurse can learn appreciation of his long history of survival, his tremendous capabilities for adapting to adversity, and his ability to protect himself from hazards. In her constant striving to understand her patients, this knowledge from anthropology can contribute to her quest.

Anthropology has demonstrated that the study of man requires an open and objective frame of mind. While ethnocentrism has positive uses, it can stand in the way of learning to appreciate the cultures of others. Anthropology may be referred to as a liberating science since it frees one from a judgmental attitude and stimulates creativity and innovation. These requirements for the anthropologist are similar to those required of the nurse interested in promoting high-quality patient care. Effective nursing practice means freeing ourselves of prejudice and bias, accepting the patient as he is, and respecting his potential. Anthropology illustrates that knowing others can teach us that our outlook is not necessarily the only proper one and that there is no room for making hasty judgments concerning the efforts of others.

While not eliminating library and laboratory investigation, anthropological research places heavy reliance on field work by the participant-observer. For the anthropologist, living among the people he studies and conscientiously observing and listening have resulted in learning the rewards, the goals, the frustrations, the strains and stresses, the conflicts, and the satisfactions of others. This approach lends itself well to nursing. It allows one to experience the way others view their world and to determine not necessarily what people say they do but what they actually do. To be an effective participant-observer requires skill. It means gaining the confidence and trust of the persons being studied. A genuine interest and respect for the persons are indispensable. Purposeful efforts to develop these skills are well worth the rewards the nurse can reap in her goal to understanding her patients.

The study of man places reliance on the *holistic* approach. This means looking at man as a whole, from all views and in the context of his total environment, and considering every part as related to every other part. The approach will usually best be accomplished through the use of an interdisciplinary team which takes advantage of the knowledge and skills of various specialists. The holistic approach is utilized in nursing in the concept of comprehensive care, as described in Chapter 2.

The anthropologist utilizes a psychological perspective that pays particular heed to the manner in which children acquire attitudes from their society. For example, many middle class Americans have been observed to have intense drives for achievement and success. They strive for the prestige often associated with the acquisition of money and the goods and services it will buy. This is not a universal drive since not all cultures exhibit it. The peoples of some islands in the South Pacific and the nomads of the Sahara Desert, for instance, do not seem to be so oriented. While the economist looks at the economic structure of American society for an explanation, the psychological anthropologist looks at the same characteristics as a consequence of the way many Americans are reared. Nurses, especially those working with infants and children, are interested in the process of socialization and with the learning of attitudes. Child-rearing differs in cultures and subcultures all over the world. For example, the child-rearing practices of the farm family in rural North Dakota are likely to be quite different from those in suburban Los Angeles. The psychological perspective will help the nurse to better understand her patients when she considers how attitudes are learned and how they come to be.

Cultural factors have been observed to exert strong influences on health and illness and attitudes toward them. In the American culture, health in general holds supreme value and illness is considered unpleasant and undesirable. In some other cultures, illness is sometimes accepted with less concern. For example, in India it is common knowledge that illness and lack of well-being are associated with protein starvation. Yet, because of cultural dietary habits, it has proven difficult to teach mothers to give their babies low-cost high-protein gruels that would aid in preventing malnutrition. Malnutrition is an accepted condition of life for many and is not viewed as a matter of concern.

Here are a few additional examples of other behavior, reflecting cultural differences, frequently seen in nursing: wanting to eat the main meal of the day in the evening rather than at noon; desiring highly spiced and seasoned foods; refusing to undress before a strange person; being upset because it is necessary to sleep in a room with a strange person; avoiding use of a bedpan as much as possible because someone else must care for the contents; keeping a religious object pinned to the bed at all times; re-

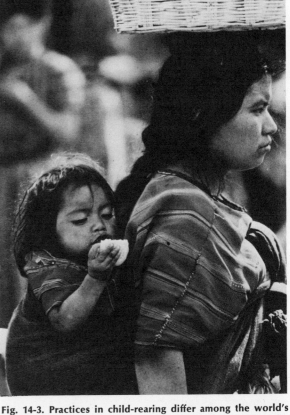

Fig. 14-3. Practices in child-rearing differ among the world's cultures even though they are all aimed at promoting the child's growth and welfare. This photo is of a Guatemalan mother who uses a sling to carry her child, a practice that maximizes body contact. This practice is quite different from child-rearing practices in other cultures. (Photo by Ray Weiss, Photophile)

fusing to take a shower or a bath each day; refusing to have a bath during a menstrual period; refusing to have a vaginal examination done by a male physician; moaning and crying loudly when in pain; unreservedly demonstrating grief when a relative dies.

To change existing patterns of behavior requires taking into account various alternatives and their consequences in order to minimize disruptive effects of change. Anthropologists have learned that attempts to alter behavior without concern for the consequences can be fruitless. Here are two examples described by anthropologists when "better" techniques were unacceptable and too disruptive because they ran counter to established behavior. Hospitals built and staffed at considerable expense were rejected in some places in South America because most people believed a hospital is where "people go to die." Folk beliefs in parts of Africa prevent certain people from giving their children "adult foods" that, if used, would eliminate certain nutritional deficiencies. These findings do not mean that attempts to promote change are better left alone. Rather, as described earlier in this chapter, it teaches us that to bring about effective change requires careful planning.

Man's biological adaptation to differing environments results in changes in the human body through genetic heredity. However, this type of adaptation is a very slow process. In comparing early man with man of today, physiological anthropologists see marked differences in such physical characteristics as size of skull, dentition, muscle and bone structure, and the like. However, they also note an extremely slow process of change. Conditions influencing genetic inheritance are observed today. Nursing with its interest in health and well-being will wish to include the findings from investigation on genetic inheritance as aids to better serve her patients. Examples of disabilities involving genetic heredity include Rh incompatibility, sickle cell anemia, and the lactose deficiency that is seen among some people in the Orient. Another area of study of interest to both anthropologists and nurses is investigation of the relationships between growth rates and nutrition in various cultures today.

As noted, anthropologists have demonstrated that adaptations to environment through genetic changes take place very slowly, possibly too slowly if man is to survive in a civilization based primarily on industry and technology. The human body is engineered to require considerable expenditure of energy. Yet, technology has resulted in a marked decrease in the need to expend energy to live in today's world. While physical work and exercise have decreased, the caloric intake has risen in many cultures, especially of foods high in animal fat. Also, outlets for the release of stress and strain are fewer. Simultaneously, various types of heart disease and atherosclerosis are on the increase.

The cost to the environment of modern day living is seen everywhere. For example, with more people there is less land for recreation, food production, psychological comfort, and the like. Will man run out of the land that he needs to survive? Because of pollution, will he run out of usable air and water? Will the predicted megalopolitan areas create weather that is incompatible with life? Will more

rapid adaptation through cultural heredity be able to substitute for slower adaptability through genetic heredity? Answers to these questions are of interest and concern to everyone, certainly including nurses.

CONCLUSION

From even this brief overview, it can be seen that knowledge from anthropology can assist the nurse in an understanding of and in the use of the three broad principles discussed earlier as basic to nursing. Anthropology has contributed much to an understanding of the uniqueness of man, his complex nature, and the importance of a safe environment. The study of man and his way of life is relevant to all of nursing and fortunately, today many nurses are incorporating cultural and social factors when planning nursing care.

Study Situations

1. The September 1969 issue of **Nurs. Outlook,** volume 17, is devoted primarily to a study of poverty and health care. Select several articles in the issue for reading and then review the sections entitled "Acquiring An Appreciation for Cultural Differences" and "Implications for Nursing" in this chapter. Do you believe that the use of concepts from anthropology might aid us to better understand the poor and as a result, offer them better health care? The editorial, "Is the Question Apathy?", on page 31, reads in part, "The poor have an inbred disinterest in their many physical and societal ills, and a defensive attitude toward those who want to help them. The core of the problem might well be apathy —apathy on the part of those who should seek health care, those who should give it, and those who should assume responsibility for seeing that the exchange takes place." Discuss this quote in relation to the concepts presented in this chapter.

2. The following article reports on a survey of the literature on sociology and its application to public health:

   Mechanic, D.: Sociology and public health: perspectives for application. **Am. J. Public Health,** 62:146–151, Feb., 1972.

   Note early in the article that the author reports the application of knowledge from sociology is often apparently limited by the practitioner's own set of values and the author cites abortion reform to illustrate. What principles of anthropology does using one's own values as a standard of judgment violate? Describe an example from your experience when a *practitioner's values may have stood in the way of effective nursing care.*

This chapter pointed out man's adaptive ability and his motivation to solve his problems. What resulted when a patient's motivation and adaptive ability for mastering his problems were ignored, according to this author's findings?

3. The following two articles describe caring for patients of two very different subcultures in the United States:

Anderson, G., and Tighe, B.: Gypsy culture and health care. **Am. J. Nurs.,** 73:282–285, Feb., 1973.

Steel, J. E.: Soup–soap–salvation. **Nurs. Outlook,** 18:31–34, Aug., 1970.

Note in the first article the recommendations on page 285. List cultural factors that were found to be important in the planning of nursing care for a Gypsy patient. List cultural factors that the author of the second article found to be important in planning nursing care for men who mostly lived on the street.

4. The following articles describe nursing in cultures outside of the United States. As you read them, direct your attention to these questions: What customs of the people tended to interfere with nursing care as practiced in the United States? What behavioral traits of the people described were different from behavioral traits that a nurse would expect to observe of patients from her home town?

Richards, M. A. B.: Cultural characteristics as reflected in Colombian hospitals. **Nurs. Forum,** 11:89–96, No. 1, 1972.

Pinneo, L., and Pinneo, R.: Mystery virus from Lassa. **Am. J. Nurs.,** 71:1352–1355, July, 1971.

Ryan, Sr. L.: Bangla Desh diary. **Am. J. Nurs.,** 71:2158–2161, Nov., 1971.

Weiss, M. O.: Cultural shock. **Nurs. Outlook,** 19:40–43, Jan., 1971.

5. Read the following descriptions of observations made in different cultures:

Deep in the interior of South America, there are people who rarely give their children names until they are two years of age. So many babies die before this age that a child is not really considered an integral part of the family unless he survives the first two years. Hence, he is not named until then. In this South American culture, unlike our own, a high mortality rate is considered inevitable and part of life.

The nurse lives in a world that exists in carefully measured units on the clock. Not hours or even minutes are sufficient to serve as units of time; the second is pressed into service. The routines of health agencies start and end at specified times. The sweep-second hand on the wristwatch is ever-present. Care is often administered in little packages of time labeled "appointments." An appointment has a definite time for beginning and, by inference, a definite minute for termination. Drugs are given to the patient to be taken half an hour before meals, every four hours, once daily at 8 A.M., and so on. Time is an important denominator in the culture of most health workers.

To say the American Indian is not conscious of time is to do him an injustice. He has a wonderful time system that guides his life on the reservation. But it is a clockless world with events to separate time intervals: sunrise, the noonday sun, sunset, full moon. Until the nurse understands a culture in which the clock is a stranger, she is likely to criticize her patients as eternally tardy.

Reread the description of Mrs. Martinez, on pages 123 to 124 of Chapter 13.

Describe how each of the contributions from the field of anthropology, discussed in this chapter in the section "Implications for Nursing," can assist health personnel who worked in the preceding three situations. Some suggestions for acquiring an appreciation for cultural differences were given in this chapter. After reading the three accounts, add additional suggestions you may have.

References

1. Atteberry, M.: West meets east. **Am. J. Nurs.,** 70:1904–1908, Sept., 1970.

2. Bullough, B., and Bullough, V. L.: Poverty, Ethnic Identity, and Health Care. New York, Appleton-Century-Crofts, 1972.

3. Campbell, T., and Chang, B.: Health care of the Chinese in America. **Nurs. Outlook,** 21:245–249, Apr., 1973.

4. Caudle, P.: Found: one person. **Am. J. Nurs.,** 73:310–313, Feb., 1973.

5 Chase, L. G.: The visiting professional. **Nurs. Outlook,** 19:322–324, May, 1971.

6. Chilman, C. S.: Growing Up Poor. Washington, D. C., U. S. Department of Health, Education, and Welfare, Welfare, Division of Research, 1966.

7. Curry, M.: Hungry land—hungry people. **Nurs. Outlook,** 18:32–35, July, 1970.

8. Deregowski, J. B.: Pictorial perception and culture. **Sci. Am.,** 227:82–88, Nov., 1972.

9. Duncan, M. L.: The hospital as a primitive society. **Am. J. Nurs.,** 70:106–107, Jan., 1970.

10. Fleshman, R. P., guest ed.: Symposium on the young adult in today's world. In **The Nursing Clinics of North American.** Philadelphia, W. B. Saunders, 8:1–104, Mar., 1973.

11. Glenn, J. D., and Karels, Sr. R. G.: Pediatric paralysis in Bogota. **Am. J. Nurs.,** 73:299–301, Feb., 1973.

12. Jewell, D. P.: A case of a "Psychotic" Navaho Indian male. In Skipper, J. K., Jr., and Leonard, R. C., eds.: Social Interaction and Patient Care. pp. 184–195. Philadelphia, J. B. Lippincott, 1965.

13. LaFargue, J. P.: Role of prejudice in rejection of health care. **Nurs. Research,** 21:53–58, Jan.–Feb., 1972.

14. Leininger, M.: Nursing and Anthropology: Two Worlds to Blend. New York, John Wiley and Sons, 1970.

15. Leonard, Sr. M. A., and Joyce, Sr. C. A.: Two worlds united. **Am. J. Nurs.,** 71:1152–1155, June, 1971.

16. Macgregor, F. C.: Uncooperative patients: some cultural interpretations. **Am. J. Nurs.,** 67:88–91, Jan., 1967.

17. ———: Social Science In Nursing: Applications for the Improvement of Patient Care. New York, Russell Sage Foundation, 1960.

18. Mead, M.: Culture and Commitment: A Study of the Generation Gap. Garden City, New York, Doubleday, Natural History Press, 1970.

19. Mercy mission to Saigon. **Am. J. Nurs.,** 70:1946–1949, Sept., 1970.

20. Moloney, Sr. M. M.: Some impressions of nursing and nursing education, in the Middle East. **Nurs. Outlook,** 18:56–60, Aug., 1970.

21. Paul, B. D.: Anthropological perspectives on medicine and public health. *In* Skipper, J. K., Jr., and Leonard, R. C., eds.: Social Interaction and Patient Care. pp. 195–219. Philadelphia, J. B. Lippincott, 1965.

22. Schutt, B. G.: Summer reading. Editorial. **Am. J. Nurs.,** 70:1463, July, 1970.

23. Smoyak, S.: Cultural incongruence: the effect on nurses' perceptions. **Nurs. Forum** 7:234–247, No. 3, 1968.

24. Tao-Kim-Hai, A. M.: "Orientals are stoic. *In* Skipper, J. K., Jr., and Leonard, R. C., eds.: Social Interaction and Patient Care, pp. 143–155. Philadelphia, J. B. Lippincott, 1965.

25. Watkins, C.: Peace corps *Parteira.* **Am. J. Nurs.,** 70:2160–2163, Oct. 1970.

CHAPTER 15

Consideration for Religious Beliefs in Nursing Care

INTRODUCTION • RELIGION AND ILLNESS • THE CLERGYMAN'S ROLE
ON THE HEALTH TEAM • JUDAISM • CHRISTIANITY: ROMAN
CATHOLICISM—PROTESTANTISM • OTHER BELIEFS •
STUDY SITUATIONS • REFERENCES

INTRODUCTION

Anthropologists have found that some kind of religion is a part of every culture. *Religion,* in a general sense, may be considered as man's attempt to understand his relationship with the universe about him. It functions to provide orderly relations, more or less, between man and his surroundings.

There are almost countless varieties of religious practices, beliefs, and rituals in the world. This chapter concerns itself primarily with Judaism and Christianity, the most commonly practiced religions in the United States.

RELIGION AND ILLNESS

It is common for most patients to seek support from their religious faith during times of stress. This support is often vital to the acceptance of an illness, especially if the illness brings with it a prolonged period of convalescence or indicates a questionable outcome. Prayer, devotional reading, and other religious practices often do for the patient spiritually what protective exercises do for the body physically.

The values derived from religious faith cannot be enumerated or evaluated easily. However, the effects attributable to faith are in evidence to health workers constantly. Patients have been known to endure extreme physical distress because of strong faith. Patients' families have taken on almost unbelievable rehabilitative tasks because they had faith in the eventual positive results of their effort. Some of the greatest personal triumphs over disease and injury are recorded not in medical or nursing texts but in biographic literature. A health team composed of

every type of expert in medicine can bring the patient only to a certain phase of recovery. The effort to take that which has been "repaired" and to develop it to its fullest must come from the patient. Even though not all patients are faced with major problems because of illness, all are in need of maintaining a constructive and hopeful attitude. Spiritual support often is the key to the hope and determination that helps them and it is a real comfort to many patients to be able to adhere closely to their religious practices during illness.

The presence of a Bible, a prayer book, rosary beads, or other religious objects in the patient's unit is significant. It may well be that the patient spends a portion of each day in devotional reading and prayer. Although some patients may have no objection to do so in the presence of others, other patients may prefer privacy. Inasmuch as patients may feel that a request for privacy may not be understood, it is a thoughtful gesture if the suggestion is initiated by the nurse.

Many hospitals have chapels in which patients may worship, and in some instances regular services are held for various denominations. When regular services are not held, patients are permitted to worship in the chapel at their convenience. Frequently, it is through the consideration of members of the nursing staff that patients are made aware of such facilities.

Although a person's religious faith frequently appears to speed recovery, there are instances in which a religious belief that conflicts with medical aims may hamper a person's adaptation to a health agency or his acceptance of therapy. For example, the doctrine of the Jehovah's Witnesses prohibits blood transfusions. In the Islamic religion, man is regarded as largely helpless in controlling his environment and illness is accepted as his fate rather than as something against which action might be taken. Some Navajo Indians use a lengthy religious ceremony to "cure" certain diseases; tuberculosis is an example. For some people, illness is viewed as punishment for sin, and, therefore, inevitable. Even though concepts such as these may hamper the efforts of health personnel, every attempt should be made to understand them and what they mean to the patient. Only then can cooperation be obtained that may result in the patient's willingness to accept certain therapy. This may very well require the assistance of the patient's religious advisor.

It is important for the nurse to try to gain an understanding of what religion means to the patient. Even within the same faith, people interpret their religion differently. But the sensitive nurse treats the patient's belief with respect in any case. If a particular religious practice presents a problem in relation to the patient's medical regimen, the nurse can turn to the patient, to his family, or to the clergyman for assistance.

THE CLERGYMAN'S ROLE ON THE HEALTH TEAM

Because physical recovery is closely related to mental attitude and emotional stability, the patient's religious counselor plays a key role on the health team. There are instances when he serves as an associate to the physician and the nurse by interpreting therapy and its value to the plan of care. He may very well be the person who helps the patient to accept various phases of care.

The clergyman is equally important to a health team that functions primarily in a health agency, such as a hospital, or to a team in a community setting. As Figure 15-3 illustrates, the patient is receiving pastoral care at home.

In many large hospitals, clergymen of various faiths are available at any time of the day or night. When the patient is in a hospital near his own community, the clergyman from his own church may also visit, and generally this is a satisfying experience for the patient.

The nurse can be helpful to a clergyman by greeting him and helping him to locate his parishioner. If the patient is in a single room with the door closed, the nurse should determine whether the patient is able to receive a call from the clergyman. Having him enter the unit at an inopportune mo-

ment is embarrassing to both clergyman and patient. In other instances, the patient may be located in a unit which has several patients in it. In this situation, too, the clergyman and the patient may be disturbed by a situation which exists in the unit. The patient usually identifies the clergyman as a personal visitor, not as a true member of the health team accustomed to hospital routine and hospital sights. The clergyman, too, recognizes that he does not have the freedom to enter units and be present in situations which a doctor or a nurse may take for granted.

Preparation of the patient's unit for the clergyman's call may vary. The unit should be orderly and free from unnecessary equipment and items. There should be provision for the clergyman to be seated at the bedside or near the patient so that both can be comfortable during the visit. If a sacrament is to be administered, the top of the bedside table should be free of items and covered with a clean white cover. A white paper tray cover is frequently more satisfactory than a towel. If the patient is located in a unit having several patients, he may appreciate having the bed curtains drawn partially so as to provide some degree of privacy. Almost always when a sacrament is to be administered, the entire unit is screened to provide privacy.

JUDAISM

Judaism teaches the unity of God, and God is considered the creator and source of all life. Each person is free to choose between good and evil. Man is considered as a child of God. Unlike Christianity and some religions of the Near East, Judaism does not hold resurrection and immortality as a central concept. One rabbi states that the aim of Judaism is salvation of humanity in history rather than salvation of the soul in the hereafter. Salvation is found by fulfilling social responsibilities. Death is considered part of the continuance of birth, growth, and decay.

The spiritual adviser of the Jewish faith is the rabbi.

There are three forms of Judaism: Reform, Conservative, and Orthodox. Reform Judaism is more liberal than the other two in its thinking, whereas Orthodox Judaism is the most traditional of the three. Conservative Judaism finds its place more or less between Reform and Orthodox Judaism.

The Jewish Sabbath and Holy Days
The Sabbath begins on Friday at sundown and ends on Saturday at sundown. It is a day for rest and

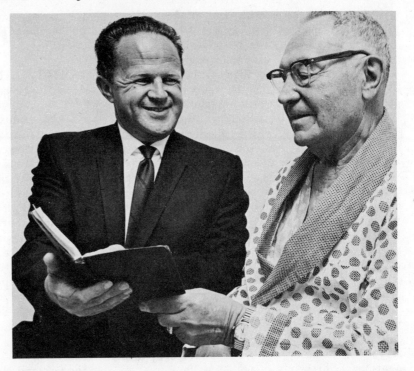

Fig. 15-1. The rabbi's visit and the reading of prayers with him are comforting to the Jewish patient. (Good Samaritan Hospital, Phoenix, Arizona)

worship. For the patient who observes the Sabbath, treatments and procedures should be postponed if postponement will not cause harm to the patient.

In Judaism, New Year's Day is called Rosh Hashanah and usually occurs in September. Rosh Hashanah is the beginning of a ten day period for reflections and consideration of life and its problems. The period ends with the Day of Atonement or Yom Kippur.

Hanukkah usually occurs in December. It is a festival recalling ancient resistance to tyranny and is a time of rejoicing and giving of gifts.

Passover occurs in the spring and is observed for seven days. It is a festival of redemption that recalls the departure of the Jews from Egypt.

There are additional Jewish holy days but the ones just mentioned are observed most commonly by persons of Jewish faith.

Dietary Practices

Dietary practices are important for the nurse to understand, especially when she is caring for patients who observe Conservative or Orthodox Judaism. Reform Judaism does not hold these practices as relevant. Because dietary practices vary in Judaism and also occasionally among Jews practicing the same form of Judaism, the nurse should consult with the patient, a family member, or a rabbi, if questions arise.

Dietary regulations permit the eating of meat of kosher animals and fowl. Animals are considered kosher if they are ruminants and have divided hooves, such as cows, goats, and sheep. Kosher fowl are primarily those that are not birds of prey, such as chickens, ducks, and geese. Fowl and animals are slaughtered, dressed, and prepared in a prescribed manner in order to be considered kosher. Fish are considered kosher if they have both scales and fins, as salmon, tuna, sardines, carp, and the like. Shellfish, such as shrimp and lobster, are not acceptable. Fish do not have to be slaughtered and dressed in a prescribed manner.

Fish and meat products (such as oils and fats), milk and milk products, and eggs are considered kosher if they are from the above-mentioned animals. Plant or vegetable oils are acceptable.

Milk products may not be eaten with or immediately following meat products. An interval of six hours must elapse between eating meat and milk products. Meat products, on the other hand, may be eaten after milk products after an interval of only a few minutes. If a patient is having both meat and milk products during the same meal, serve the products separately, first the milk products and then the meat.

Fish may be eaten with dairy products if prepared with a nonmeat shortening or if broiled.

Kosher foods may not be prepared in utensils used for the preparation of nonkosher foods unless they have been cleansed in a prescribed manner. Fruits and vegetables that have been steamed or cooked in nonkosher utensils are permissible if nonkosher sauce, gravy, or shortening are omitted.

For the patient who is in the hospital and observing dietary practices, the following suggestions are helpful. Use paper dishes for the serving of food; substitute fresh vegetables and fruits for leavened products; if kosher meat or fish is unavailable, use an acceptable protein substitute, such as milk products or eggs.

During the Passover period, leavened products, such as bread, cake, cookies, noodles, or beverages containing grain alcohol, are not used. The nurse may suggest that the family bring matzos (unleavened bread product) for the patient.

If a Jewish patient's observance of dietary practices interferes with his medical regimen, Jewish law permits modifications. Before proceeding with modifications, the nurse should consult with the patient, a member of his family, or a rabbi.

Circumcision

Male Jewish infants are required to be circumcised on the eighth day following their birth. However, the rite may be postponed for as long as necessary if the infant's health does not permit it at that time. The mohel (professional circumciser) may perform it or in some instances, it may be done by a surgeon of Jewish faith while a rabbi attends. A quorum of ten men attends the ceremony, if available. However, such a quorum is not necessary for a religious circumcision.

Death and Preparation for Burial

There are appropriate prayers for the dying patient. Also, if the patient and family so desire, a service of confession and prayer may be observed as death approaches. Preferably the rabbi is present for this—if not the patient's own rabbi, then one associated with the health agency.

A patient who has died may be washed and covered with a clean cloth. Should a Jewish patient who has no kin to claim the body die, a rabbi should be contacted.

Reform and Conservative Judaism do not object to postmortem examination. An autopsy is considered by them to be a means by which medical knowledge learned from the dead can help the living. Either the patient gives consent for autopsy before death or the family grants such permission after death.

CHRISTIANITY: ROMAN CATHOLICISM—PROTESTANTISM

Christianity teaches the trinity of God, that is, there are three persons in one God: God the Father, God the Son, and God the Holy Spirit. God the Father is considered the creator and the source of life. The Son of God is Jesus Christ, who came into the world in human form, suffered and died for the salvation of all men. Christianity holds resurrection and immortality as a central concept. Although social responsibility is important in Christianity, salvation is found through faith in the triune God. However, the two go together—faith and good works.

In the United States, most Christians are Roman Catholics or Protestants. The spiritual adviser in the Roman Catholic faith is the priest. For Protestants the spiritual adviser is called a minister, pastor, or preacher.

Sundays and Holy Days

Most Christians observe Sunday as a day for worship. An example of an exception is the Seventh Day Adventists, who set aside Saturday for worship.

Although many holy days are observed in the various faiths in Christianity, two are held in common and are familiar to almost everyone.

Christmas is observed in most places in the world of Christianity on December 25. It is celebrated as the day on which Christ was born. The day is a joyous one and a time for giving of gifts in memory of Christ's birth.

In the spring, Christians observe Lent and the Easter season. Easter occurs in March or April. The six-week period prior to Easter is called Lent and the Friday before Easter is Good Friday.

Lent is a time for contemplation on the sufferings and death of Christ. Many Christians make personal sacrifices during Lent as a symbol of humility and in memory of Christ's suffering. These sacrifices often involve some kind of fasting, which may need to be taken into account during periods of illness, especially if it interferes with the medical regimen. Good Friday is a day of sorrow when the Christian recalls the agonizing death of Christ on the cross.

Easter marks the end of the Lenten period and is a day of great rejoicing. It commemorates the day when Christ arose from the dead. Belief in His res-

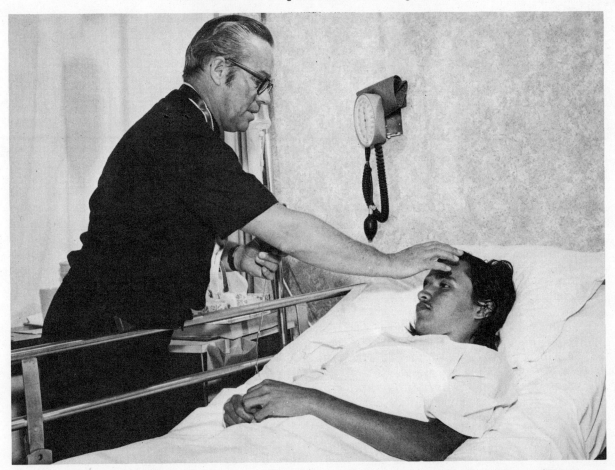

Fig. 15-2. The priest administers the sacrament of the anointing of the sick to this young patient. (St. Joseph's Hospital and Medical Center, Phoenix, Arizona)

urrection confirms the Christian tenet that Christ is the Son of God.

Roman Catholicism

In the care of patients who are of the Catholic faith, the nurse will find it necessary to be acquainted with the following sacraments: baptism, holy communion, and the sacrament of the anointing of the sick. Sacraments in the Catholic faith, by virtue of the fact that they are accepted as having been instituted by Christ, are believed to have the power to produce the effect that each signifies.

BAPTISM: Since a nurse may be present during the delivery of a child or the miscarriage of a living fetus, it is imperative that she understand that, for a Catholic family, any child in danger of death must be baptized. At the time of death all Catholics must be in the state of grace, free from serious sin. It is

mainly by means of the sacraments that sin is absolved and grace given. Baptism is the first sacrament and removes the first, or original, sin deriving from Adam and Eve. To the Catholic, this is absolutely necessary for salvation.

If a priest is not available, the nurse or the doctor should administer the sacrament of baptism. It is preferred that a Catholic nurse or doctor administer the sacrament, but if a Catholic is not available, anyone having the use of reason may do it. It is necessary that the person conferring the sacrament have the intention of doing what the Catholic Church desires and use the proper form. The procedure is as follows: while pouring plain water over the forehead so that it flows upon the skin, say, "I baptize you in the name of the Father, and of the Son, and of the Holy Spirit."

Since baptism may be conferred when there is

possible danger of the child's life, and since the family may not be aware of it, the fact that the sacrament of baptism was conferred should be recorded on the infant's chart and on the chaplain's baptismal roster if there is one in the health agency. If a priest confers the baptism, he will notify the family that it has been done. If the child is baptized by someone other than a priest, the priest should be informed and then he can discuss it with the parents.

Holy Eucharist or Holy Communion: Holy Communion is the most excellent of all sacraments of the Catholic faith because, according to Catholic belief, it contains, under the appearance of bread and wine, the Body, Blood, Soul, and Divinity of Jesus Christ. All Catholics in danger of death should receive communion if possible. As necessary, confession precedes communion. To receive communion, Catholic patients, except those in danger of death, fast; the patient is to fast one hour from solid food. The patient is not required to fast from water and solid or liquid medications.

Prior to communion, the patient should be made comfortable, the unit prepared as described earlier, and the patient given privacy so that he may pray and prepare himself for the sacrament.

Sacrament of the Anointing of the Sick: The sacrament of the anointing of the sick has been changed somewhat since Vatican II. The new rite stresses that it can be administered to ill persons who are not necessarily in immediate danger of death. Also, the new rite emphasizes that any person who must undergo surgery for a reason that has caused the person to be seriously or critically ill may be given the benefit of the sacrament of the sick. In addition, the reception of this sacrament may now be offered to those whose life forces are growing weaker simply because of age, even though death *may* be remote. The sacrament can be administered to groups of persons as well, as for example, a group of hospitalized patients.

When administering the sacrament, the priest anoints the patient's forehead and palms of the hands with holy oil. The prayers used are designed to help the sick endure their suffering, recover their health, and, in case of death, attain salvation.

When the patient appears to be dying, he is obliged to receive communion, if he is conscious and capable of swallowing. If time appears short, communion is given first and then, if still possible, the patient receives the sacrament of the anointing of the sick. Confession before communion is said, if necessary.

The new rite for anointing of the sick eliminates the previous practice of anointing the dead. Instead, the priest offers a prayer of forgiveness for sins and commends the person to the mercy of God. If there is any doubt that the person is dead, then the priest, using his discretion, may anoint the person conditionally. In the case of an unconscious person, the priest may give the anointing of the sick when he has reasonable assurance that the person would desire the benefits of this sacrament, if he were in a position to ask for it.

Protestantism

The Protestant faith embraces a large number of denominations. Some of the religious groups that are active today originated before the Reformation, and others have developed since then apart from the Reformation influence. While certain doctrines are common to most of these denominations, there are individual practices and interpretations which give each a distinct pattern of its own.

While some denominations employ certain sacraments that are similar to those in the Catholic faith, others reject the concept of sacraments and observe baptism and communion as ordinances that are means of grace but not of salvation. Others, such as the Friends (Quakers), reject both ordinances and sacraments.

Baptism: Some Protestant faiths hold that baptism should be performed in infancy. The Baptists, the Disciples, and some others hold that the ordinance of baptism should not be administered before the person reaches the age of accountability. If a child of Protestant parents is in danger of dying, the nurse should ask whether the parents wish to have the child baptized. If the parents wish it and a Protestant minister is not available, the child may be baptized as follows: a baptized nurse who has understanding and belief in the act that she is about to perform may baptize the baby by pouring water continuously over the baby's forehead and saying the following words, "I baptize thee in the name of the Father, and of the Son, and of the Holy Spirit. Amen." The baptism is recorded on the child's chart by the person performing it and the parents are informed as soon as convenient.

Communion: In most Protestant faiths, communion is administered less frequently than in the Catholic faith. However, many Protestant patients request it prior to surgery or during a period of illness. It represents the body and the blood of Christ which were sacrificed for the remission of sin. Before the arrival of the minister, the unit should be prop-

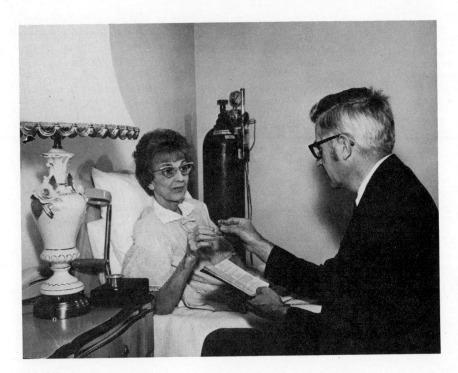

Fig. 15-3. The minister offers Holy Communion to this patient in her home. The clergyman, as a spiritual counselor, is also an important member of the community health team.

erly prepared and the patient given privacy so that he has an opportunity for prayer and self-examination.

OTHER BELIEFS

In the course of her education and working career, the nurse can expect to care for persons holding beliefs less common than those just discussed. Examples include the Jehovah's Witness, Seventh-Day Adventist, Christian Scientist, Moslem, Buddhist, Coptic, and members of the Confucian faiths. It is impractical to discuss all faiths in this text. However, the basic principle remains: in her attempt to understand each patient for whom she cares, the nurse should attempt to understand basic tenets of his faith and how these may influence his therapeutic regimen, his recovery, and his adaptation to the hospital environment. The nurse should never underestimate the power of religion as a part of the patient's recovery.

Some people do not accept any particular religious faith. Nevertheless, they deserve the same respect for what they choose to believe. They have as much a right to believe as they wish as those persons who accept a particular religious creed. Common courtesy demands respect for the beliefs of others.

Study Situations

1. The following article describes a hospital setting in which clergymen were an important part of the health team:
   Morris, K. L., and Foerster, J. D.: Team work: nurse and chaplain. **Am. J. Nurs.,** 72:2197–2199, Dec., 1972. *What conclusions did the authors draw from the experience of having a clergyman as an actively participating member of the health team?*
2. The article given below is an excellent supplement to the section in this chapter describing Judaism. Note the magazine's foreword in italics, which emphasizes that the patient's religious beliefs can color his response to illness.
   Berkowitz, P., and Berkowitz, N. S.: The Jewish patient in the hospital. **Am. J. Nurs.,** 67:2335–2337, Nov., 1967.
3. It will be noted that this chapter did not contain a glossary. Instead, as part of your study, define this sampling of religious terms:

Baptism
Christianity
Holy Eucharist or
    Holy Communion
Judaism
Kosher
Lent
Minister

Priest
Protestantism
Rabbi
Religion
Roman Catholic
Rosh Hashanah
Sacrament
Trinity

References

1. Applebaum, M. M.: What Everyone Should Know About Judaism. New York, Philosophical Library, 1959.

2. Bial, M. D.: Liberal Judaism At Home: The Practices of Modern Reform Judaism. revised ed. Summit, N. J., Temple Sinai, 1971.

3. Hadley, B. J., and Dunlap, M. S.: Autocratic versus democratic beliefs of graduate students in nursing. **Nurs. Research,** 17:19–26, Jan.–Feb., 1968.

4. Inman, K., et al.: If you ask me: what specific assistance has a clergyman given you in helping a patient meet his problems? **Am. J. Nurs.,** 57:737, June, 1957.

5. Jakobovits, I.: Jewish Medical Ethics. New York, Bloch, 1967.

6. McDougall, D. A.: IV.—religious belief and philosophical analysis. **Mind,** 81:519–532, Oct., 1972.

7. Naiman, H. L.: Nursing in Jewish law. **Am. J. Nurs.,** 70:2378–2379, Nov., 1970.

8. Piepgras, R.: The other dimension: spiritual help. **Am. J. Nurs.,** 68:2610–2613, Dec., 1968.

9. Raciappa, J. D.: A total ministry. **Am. J. Nurs.,** 73:645, Apr., 1973.

10. Rosten, L., ed.: Religions in America. New York, Simon and Schuster, 1963.

11. Sacrament for the sick. **Time,** 101:65, Feb. 5, 1973.

12. The Jews: next year in which Jerusalem? **Time,** 99:54–63, Apr. 10, 1972.

13. Westberg, G. E.: Good Grief: A Constructive Approach to the Problem of Loss. Philadelphia, Fortress Press, 1962.

14. ———: Minister and Doctor Meet. New York, Harper and Row, 1961.

CHAPTER 16

The Nurse as a Health Teacher

GLOSSARY · INTRODUCTION · PRINCIPLES OF LEARNING AND
IMPLICATIONS FOR TEACHING · TEACHING OBJECTIVES,
CONTENT, AND EVALUATION · THE TEACHING-LEARNING
ENVIRONMENT · ADAPTING TEACHING TO VARIOUS
SITUATIONS · CONCLUSION · STUDY
SITUATIONS · REFERENCES

GLOSSARY

Affective Learning: Acquiring new attitudes, values, and appreciations.

Cognitive Learning: Acquiring new understandings.

Goal: An aim or end that expresses an unmet need. Effort is exerted to attain the aim and to satisfy the unmet need.

Learn: To add to one's store of knowledge; to have one's behavior change as the result of an experience.

Motivation: Act of giving an inducement or an incentive to action.

Motor Learning: Acquiring new physical skills.

Objective: Synonym for goal.

Operant Theory of Learning: A theory that holds that certain behavior tends to reinforce learning; also referred to as reinforcement theory.

Readiness: Being able or being in due condition to respond only in certain ways.

Teach: To assist another to learn; to impart knowledge.

INTRODUCTION

Health teaching is an essential nursing role. The earliest nursing leaders recognized the importance of health teaching, and through the years, it has grown in significance so that today, health teaching is a preeminent part of nursing.

Various influences have acted to promote health teaching in nursing. For example, the consumer of health services has become more knowledgeable concerning his health. With this awareness, he has come to demand increased information in relation to attaining and maintaining well-being. He feels he has a "right to know" and expects health practitioners to respect that right. Also, with the increase in longevity and in the incidence of chronic diseases, teaching has become especially important in promoting maximum well-being for the chronically ill and aged. Research, too, has promoted the position of teaching in nursing. Studies have shown, for example, that preoperative teaching and encouragement have resulted in fewer complications, less need for pain relievers, smaller changes in physiologic responses, and less anxiety during the postoperative period.

When greater emphasis was placed on patients assuming self-care activities as soon as their physical state permitted, the nurse's role as a health teacher increased steadily. At one time, patients had almost everything done for them by the nurse. Now nurses are helping patients to learn to do as much as possible for themselves. As the values of increased activity and decreased bed rest have been noted, some authorities in physical medicine and rehabilitation concluded that the old approach of too much "tender loving care" was actually harmful.

Man's ability to adapt to adversity has been discussed earlier in this text, and health practitioners are increasingly recognizing and utilizing this ability. Through their teaching efforts, the patient can often gain independence to function effectively in society. Health practices that neglect to assist the patient to a state of independence fall short of what patients expect and are beginning to demand.

Experienced teachers have observed that learning

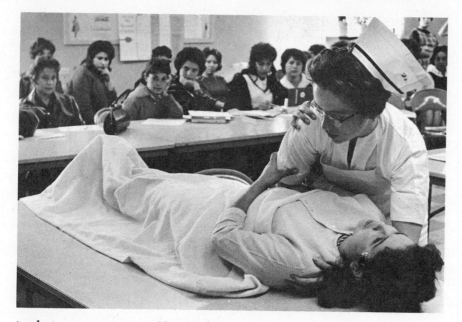

Fig. 16-1. There are many times when the ill person is cared for at home. Here, a nurse is teaching a group of girls how to move a patient while avoiding strain on themselves. (Photo by Mary Ann Gehres of Presbyterian Life)

tends to occur more readily when the student participates actively in the learning experience. This text has placed emphasis on the importance of including the patient in planning his health care and respecting his right to make decisions concerning his life. When the patient is taught and learns alternative behaviors and their consequences, he can then make more intelligent decisions. There is no place in the teaching process for coercing the patient or demanding that he do as he is told. Teaching is dependent upon patient participation as well as imparting knowledge to help him understand the options available to him and to help him overcome attitudes that may stand in the way of changing behavior, if change is his desire.

Obviously, before one can teach, one must have information to share. In this text, there is much information that a nurse will be using when teaching patients. As competency in nursing increases, the nurse will find that opportunities for teaching will increase also. This chapter is intended to assist the nurse to familiarize herself with some of the basic principles of teaching and learning so that she will be better able to teach as she learns.

PRINCIPLES OF LEARNING AND IMPLICATIONS FOR TEACHING

To *learn* is to add to one's knowledge, the word knowledge being used here in its broadest sense. To *teach* is to help someone to learn. Learning is said to have occurred when an experience changes the learner's behavior. This change may be in certain understandings the learner has gained, also referred to as *cognitive learning;* in physical skills he has acquired, also referred to as *motor learning;* or in attitudes, values, and appreciations, also referred to as *affective learning.* When a person provides an experience that results in a change in the learner's behavior, that person has taught and may be called the teacher.

Innumerable opportunities exist for teaching in the practice of nursing. There are times when the nurse plans and participates in formal teaching of an individual or a group of patients. But most often, teaching in nursing occurs more or less spontaneously and in an informal manner. An example occurs when the nurse teaches oral hygiene or care of the skin during the bathing procedure. Even such activities as counseling patients and offering them encouragement and support can be referred to as teaching. When we accept a definition stating that learning has occurred when there is a change in behavior, it can be seen that teaching-learning occurs at many times, in many places, and in many ways.

While teaching may often occur on the spur of the moment, it is still recommended that teaching follow a definite plan. To teach haphazardly and without organization or planning cannot attain success except by sheer accident. Preparing objectives and content for teaching is discussed later in this chapter and will illustrate a plan of action for developing a teaching program. Also, various teaching aids and methods are discussed.

The nurse cannot afford to overlook the fact that many patients learn from observing the examples she sets. For example, the nurse visiting in a home is often teaching when the family observes her covering her mouth and nose, should she sneeze or cough, and washing her hands before beginning her work. On the other hand, the nurse in the clinic is teaching negatively if she displays obvious symptoms of an upper respiratory infection while advising a mother to keep her children at home when they have colds. In teaching, actions and words must be consistent.

How do we learn? Educational psychologists have explored this question for years and while differences of opinions on certain aspects exist, there is general agreement on some principles that guide the learning process. Teaching is dependent on or guided by principles of learning. The examples given in this section will illustrate.

The goal of the learner directs his learning efforts as he strives for a consequence he wishes to attain. A goal is an unmet need. It is the consequence for which the learner is striving. Hence, when learning is in progress, the learner is attempting to satisfy what he sees as his need. For example, a child may desire a cookie that is in a jar outside of his reach; therefore, he needs to learn how to reach the jar. A college football star can remain on the team if his scholastic average is above a certain rating; therefore, to attain his goal he must do well in classes. A bride wishes to please her husband by serving delicious meals; therefore, she learns to cook to attain her goal.

Assume that a nurse wishes to teach a mother the care of her newborn infant. Most new mothers are excited about caring for their babies, and, although they may be somewhat apprehensive, they recognize the need and have the desire to learn. The patient's need to learn this care is one that a nurse can usually discern with ease and capitalize on. However, often an individual's goals cannot be defined clearly, and in some cases the person may even attempt to conceal them. For example, a patient may not seem to be interested in doing certain things for himself or in learning self-care activities. Although he may never admit it, his real goal could be to remain dependent if he has learned to find satisfaction in having things done for him, or continuing in a state of "ill health" helps him remain away from an unsatisfactory work situation.

This concept concerning the goal or need in learning has implications for the teacher. The focus is on the learner's goals, not the teacher's. The goal of the learner may not always be easy to discern, but it is important for the teacher to attempt to identify it. For example, if the nurse wishes to teach a patient measures that will promote normal elimination so that his daily use of laxatives will not be necessary, her efforts will be in vain unless the patient feels he has a need for the teaching. Therefore, it is important for the nurse to discern the patient's goal or help him to develop learning goals that have personal meaning when she begins her teaching program.

Every person has certain capabilities and limitations that determine or set boundaries for what he can do. One aspect of this is what psychologists refer to as *readiness.* Readiness is influenced by many factors, some of the more common ones of which are discussed here.

The stage of illness the patient is experiencing will influence his readiness to learn. Stages of illness are discussed in Chapter 12. For example, a patient who has just learned that he has diabetes is not ready to be taught how to administer his insulin until he has accepted his diagnosis and recognizes the importance of taking insulin. Also, the acutely ill patient is rarely ready for participation in a teaching program.

Consider another example when the stage of illness may influence learning. A woman has had a breast removed, and to insure retaining the best possible function of the arm and the shoulder, exercises are essential. The teaching of the exercise may be ineffective if the patient is still in a period of depression over the loss of this body part. Emotionally, she is almost in a state of mourning, and until she is able to adjust to this change and accept it, the exercises might be carried out better without too much emphasis on teaching. As soon as the patient sees how the exercises are helping her, she usually will want to learn and to practice them.

An individual's intellectual capacity will affect his ability to learn. If he is well-endowed and if he puts his inheritance to good use, the learner can assimilate much in little time. The person who is limited may never learn as much and often needs to spend considerable time in achieving what he does learn.

The degree to which an individual has matured physically and emotionally will influence learning. For example, most children learn to walk at some time between the ages of 12 to 16 months; prior to this period, most children's musculoneurologic maturity is insufficient to permit them to learn to walk, and attempts to teach them to do so result in failure.

Physical maturity is easier to determine than emotional maturity, since the former can be judged, to a large extent, in relation to the individual's chronologic age. Estimating emotional maturity is a different matter; and simply judging it on the basis of chronologic age sometimes leads to false conclusions.

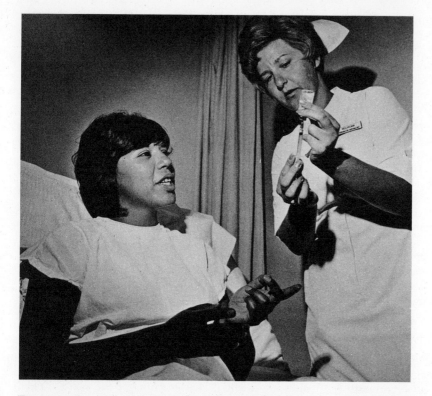

Fig. 16-2. Instruction is given to the patient who will be managing at home. This patient is learning how to prepare and give herself an injection. (Good Samaritan Hospital, Phoenix, Arizona)

For example, a young adult presently dependent on a wheelchair may have sufficient physical maturity to have learned the skills of a mechanic, but he may not demonstrate sufficient emotional maturity to see why he should bother with the rehabilitation that eventually will afford him the ability to earn his own living.

Physical maturity should not be confused with physical ability. For example, a patient may have reached physical maturity, but because of a handicap, say a paralysis of an arm following an injury, he cannot be taught to give himself a subcutaneous injection. This patient may never be physically ready to learn a technique such as giving himself an injection.

An individual's previous experiences will affect the learning process. For example, certain cultures believe that a person is not ill unless he feels and looks ill. Assume that it has been found on a routine examination that a person reared in such a culture has pulmonary tuberculosis and positive sputum but that the disease has not progressed to the point that the patient feels and looks sick. Unless a nurse knows and understands what this patient has learned from his culture, it may be difficult or even impossible to teach him to care for himself in order that he regain health and refrain from exposing his family and friends to the disease.

Consider the patient who practices poor oral hygiene because he has learned an attitude of indifference. As he stated it, "My father never went to a dentist in his life. Anyway, I've never heard of anyone who died because he lost his teeth." This attitude can be expected to block learning of oral hygiene.

Chapter 14 discusses cultural change and points out suggestions to promote attitudinal change, when in the eyes of health practitioners, change seems desirable. But, as indicated, care must be exercised. How much *right* do we have to change a person's choice in the way he wishes to live or die? When a patient's health becomes a menace to others, certain legal implications exist that may involve forcing a patient to do something. For example, states have laws requiring the treatment of persons with active pulmonary tuberculosis who have contact with others because of the communicable implications of disease. But force in this example is different from teaching that offers patients alternatives to present behavior.

A person's previous educational experiences play a vital role in his learning. For example, a patient who is a college graduate with a major in human physiology is ready for information that a patient who is also a college graduate but has a major in English literature may be in no position to understand. Or, consider teaching two patients how to irrigate their wounds; one is a college graduate, the other has reached only the tenth grade. Despite the difference in their educational experiences (and other things being equal), the nurse may teach both in a very similar manner. The amount of formal education that an individual has does not necessarily indicate his ability to learn; some very intelligent people have not had educational opportunities. But the nature of either a formal education or self-teaching to which an individual has been exposed can influence his readiness for learning.

Some patients may find security in having the goal of *not* knowing something. For example, having no apparent interest in learning about his illness may be the result of the patient's experiencing a sense of security in not knowing. He may be refusing or may not be able to recognize a reality that is stressful to him.

Learning in one situation can prepare a learner for a new situation when he recognizes similarities between the two situations. Psychologists have debated transfer of learning for many years. Research has proven that at least some long-held theories were incorrect. For example, investigation showed that although concentration is important in the study of Greek, one's power of concentration is not necessarily improved by studying Greek. However, there are certain situations, as the principle stated above implies, that are considered favorable for learning transfer. For example, assume the nurse is caring for a patient with an amputation who has not lived with or known anyone who has had an amputation. The teaching program for this patient might well be quite different from one used for a patient whose father also had an amputation. In the latter instance, much learning could be transferred.

Consider an example of learning through error. A child began vomiting, had a low-grade fever, and complained of generalized abdominal discomfort. The mother sought medical attention. It so happened that she had had similar symptoms when she was a college student and cared for herself, thinking she had the flu. When she eventually saw a physician, she learned she had appendicitis and emergency surgery was necessary. The mother learned from her illness how *not* to respond to symptoms she now observed in her child. Inappropriate behavior in one situation led to appropriate behavior in another similar situation.

A corollary to the previous principle may be stated as follows: *Learning from previous experiences that is transferred to new situations requires recognizing relationships between the old and the new situations.* A student is about to learn how to do a venipuncture (entering a vein with a needle). In

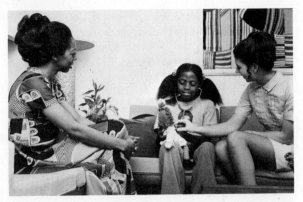

Fig. 16-3. The community health nurse is often called upon to prepare patients for hospitalization. Here, the nurse is helping a child learn about a stethoscope so that she will be better prepared for auscultation. The mother, too, is taught what to expect when her child is hospitalized. (Photo by Ted Hill, Arizona)

previous classes, she has learned how to administer a medication intramuscularly. By being aware of a relationship between intramuscular injections and venipunctures, she can transfer learning. The process begins by directing attention to the past experience of administering an intramuscular injection. Then, relating the past situation to the present one, she notes that there are similarities between the two techniques. Then the *differences* are taught. Thus, the known serves as the springboard for entry into the unknown.

When behavior changes during learning, the learner evaluates the consequences of his behavior by deciding that the new behavior either satisfies or thwarts attainment of his goal. If it is satisfying, he will be motivated to learn more. Evaluation of the response usually is an unconscious experience, i.e., the learner rarely expresses this response nor is he consciously aware of it. For example, the student in nursing usually feels satisfaction and pleasure after being taught to give a patient an injection. However, she may be quite unaware of having evaluated her response.

If the learner decides that his new response is unsatisfactory, one of two things is likely to occur. The learner either will try again and modify his response until he experiences satisfaction, or he may feel thwarted by the unsatisfactory results and become frustrated and discouraged. He may give up further trying, at least temporarily if not permanently.

Assume that a nurse is teaching a patient to use crutches. On his first try he may use the crutches sufficiently well to find satisfaction, even though his skill is far from perfect. He is encouraged to use the crutches again at the earliest opportunity. A second person learning crutch-walking may find little to be happy about in his early trials and become frustrated, but he eagerly attempts it again, until he does learn to use them with satisfaction. But a third patient, unable to use crutches with any success on his first try, becomes frustrated, stating that he is perfectly happy using a wheelchair and refuses further attempts to practice. These three persons all responded to a learning situation, and each evaluated his response in a different way. The first patient experienced sufficient satisfaction to be stimulated to further learning; the second was dissatisfied, but the dissatisfaction became a challenge to try again; and the third was dissatisfied, frustrated, and willing to give up.

Motivation promotes learning. Motivation is the process of stimulating people to act in certain ways. It is highly dependent on the learner's potential interest in learning. A variety of ways have been found useful as assists in motivating or stimulating interest in learning. In general, they are all related to the learner's goal selection, his readiness to learn, and the satisfactions he realizes when he learns. The importance of considering and knowing the patient's goals is discussed earlier. Clarifying goals and directing the learner's attention to what is important, and why, tend to arouse interest by stimulating a need to know.

Readiness for learning is a prime factor in the motivating process. For example, learning is generally stimulated when the educational offering is challenging but not beyond the learner's ability to comprehend. Respect for the learner's previous experiences and building on them when possible tend to stimulate interest and promote learning.

The experience of satisfaction when learning occurs promotes additional learning. Most people enjoy success, and one success encourages another. When the teacher recognizes achievement with a smile and a word of praise, the learner generally responds favorably and continues to learn more. Psychologists refer to this encouragement process as *reinforcement* or *operant theory in learning*.

When learning has not been accomplished and the patient's goal is thwarted, the teacher will wish to take another look at the patient and at the teaching plan. When a person does not learn, there is a reason.

The setting of goals and the readiness of the learner will require further study, and possible adaptation in the teaching program can be made. Repeating attempts to teach a particular thing may prove motivating provided that learning can be expected to succeed on subsequent tries. Possibly failure can be turned to success by improving the conditions for learning. The patient's failure to inject himself successfully may be turned to success when the nurse suggests that the patient try it while sitting on a firm chair rather than on the edge of a bed. Perhaps too much is being taught too fast, and the learner is not experiencing satisfaction by having mastered one thing at a time. Perhaps the goals were unrealistic.

Sometimes, pointing out small degrees of success and giving the patient praise and encouragement help to stimulate him to further learning. It is safer to begin with small segments of relatively easy teaching so that the learner may enjoy satisfaction. Then, the amount and the speed can be geared to the learner's ability and interest.

Additional factors that tend to motivate the learner will be discussed in the section entitled, "The Teaching-Learning Environment."

TEACHING OBJECTIVES, CONTENT, AND EVALUATION

Earlier, the patient's goals in the teaching-learning relationship were discussed. The word *objective* is sometimes used as a synonym for the word goal. This section discusses the objectives (goals) set by the nurse for her patient teaching program. It also discusses selection of content for teaching and evaluation.

The single objective of health teaching is of course to help a patient to attain and maintain optimum well-being. While this broad objective remains, for specific teaching situations, a narrower objective is more useful.

Learning has occurred when behavior changes. Therefore, it is best to state an objective of teaching in behavioral terms so that the nurse and the patient can determine learning progress more accurately. Behaviorally stated objectives were discussed in more detail in Chapter 8.

Assume the nurse wishes to assist a patient to maximum functioning—he has had a heart attack. As a first step, the nurse will probably discuss the patient with his physician. She will wish to become acquainted with the physician's philosophy of care for the patient, as well as with the specific medical regimen. She learns that a low cholesterol diet has been prescribed. Now she can state an objective of teaching more specifically and in behavioral terms: to assist the patient to learn to select and adhere to a diet low in cholesterol content. After teaching, learning success can be evaluated by determining the extent to which the patient observes the diet.

Once an objective has been defined, the nurse will determine content; that is, she will acquire information necessary for the patient to know in order to select and eat the prescribed diet. Answers to questions, such as the following, will assist the nurse to know what content to include in her teaching program. Why is the diet advised? What do words used in a description of the diet mean, such as for example, cholesterol and specifically *low* cholesterol? What is the relationship between the patient's illness and the diet being recommended? Which kinds of food are advised and which are not? What low cholesterol menus are appetizing to the patient and still nutritious? How are the foods prepared? How can the patient adapt his eating habits and still eat away from home with comfort and ease?

While the nurse establishes objectives of the teaching program and selects content, she will wish to keep the principles described in the learning process in mind. As she does, answers to additional questions will become pertinent content as she individualizes her teaching for each patient or each group of patients. A few examples will illustrate, using the patient cited above as the example. What attitudes does this patient hold concerning eating and diet restrictions? Do cultural factors in the patient's background have influence on content? If the patient is a married man, should his wife be included in his teaching program? If so, what adaptations in the content and objectives may be necessary when she also becomes a learner in the situation?

The teaching program can be evaluated when the nurse observes the extent to which the patient follows his diet. If he follows it without fail, the learning goals have been achieved. If he does not, the nurse will then attempt to identify areas where he is unsuccessful and take another look at her teaching program. For example, if the patient follows his diet except when eating out, there are several possibilities the nurse should investigate. Possibly the patient did not understand (learn) how to adapt his diet when eating away from home. Possibly, he did not learn that "at all times" meant at those times when he ate away from home also. Or the patient's attitude may be one of "living it up" while socializing.

In the latter instance, the patient may not be sufficiently impressed with the possible consequences of deviating from the diet. Or, he may be denying them.

To attempt to teach without objectives is like buying an airline ticket without a destination. Even in informal teaching, an objective is important in order to plan and execute a successful teaching program. Once objectives are stated, the content and an evaluation plan can be developed. Several study situations at the end of this chapter describe objectives, content, and evaluation used in particular teaching situations and serve to illustrate well the discussion in this section.

There is important need for recording the progress the patient makes during the teaching program, just as there is need for recording other nursing care activities that have been carried out. If this is not done, there is the possibility that the teaching started by one nurse may never be completed, or that the patient may be taught the same thing by a succession of different personnel—both possibilities irritating to the patient.

THE TEACHING-LEARNING ENVIRONMENT

Learning can occur under adverse conditions, but ideally the environment should help stimulate interest in learning. The following environmental factors should be considered.

Establishing Therapeutic Nurse-Patient Relationships

Teaching can be enhanced when the nurse and the patient have a warm and accepting relationship. The feeling, the tone, and the attitude of the person teaching are more important than many other environmental considerations. If the learner senses that the teacher is interested in him and trying to help him, he will be more receptive and stimulated. However, if he senses urgency or a superior or condescending attitude, the nurse's teaching will have little or no effect.

Providing a Comfortable Environment

The patient as well as the nurse should be comfortable. Suitable chairs, adequate lighting, and good ventilation add to the comfort. Privacy is desirable.

Using Teaching Aids

Many health agencies have audiovisual aids available for patient teaching. In some instances, the agency allows the use of their equipment outside of the agency, as for example, when the nurse is teaching a neighborhood or community group. These aids include film strips and slides. Television and radio offer good teaching programs from time to time that can be used, when convenient, to assist nurses in their patient teaching programs.

Many agencies have a variety of teaching aids

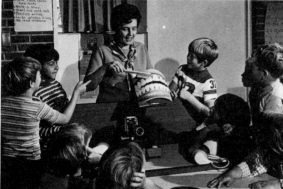

Fig. 16-4. This school nurse has captured her patients' interest. The model of teeth, brush, projector and earphones are audiovisual teaching aids (Paiute Elementary School, Scottsdale, Arizona)

that are free or sold at a low cost. Typical voluntary agencies that offer literature the nurse will often find most helpful are: American Cancer Society, American Heart Association, Kenny Rehabilitation Institute, and the American Foundation for the Blind.

The U.S. Government Printing Office is the source of a large variety of printed material, much of which can aid in patient teaching programs. State and local governmental agencies also often have material available for teaching purposes.

Libraries are another good source of teaching aids. They often have not only books, pamphlets, and periodicals, but also films, slides, and posters for borrowing.

Many companies with health-related products have charts, booklets, and similar material that can be used in teaching programs. In Figure 16-4, the teeth and the brush the school nurse is using to teach a group of children were obtained from a toothpaste manufacturer. Although such material is sometimes prepared primarily to aid in promoting the company's product, most of it is helpful when used judiciously.

Equipment for demonstrations is a helpful teaching aid. For example, if the nurse wishes to teach a mother how to bathe her newborn baby, she should have equipment such as the mother may use at home to demonstrate the procedure.

Programmed instruction has become popular as an aid to teaching. The program offers information and periodically quizzes the learner. If the learner answers questions correctly, he goes on with the program. If he answers incorrectly, he is given additional information before he proceeds. Some of the programmed instruction available on the market can be appropriately used for patient teaching.

Being Free from Distractions

A distracted person rarely is able to utilize learning opportunities to a maximum. Teaching a hospitalized patient during visiting hours can hardly be expected to be beneficial when the patient may have visitors waiting for him. The same is true if he knows that he is to be called to the x-ray department at any moment. The nurse therefore should make sure that no distractions are forthcoming when she attempts to do teaching.

Outside the hospital setting, this principle also holds true. For instance, the housewife who is coping with immediate domestic problems is not able to concentrate on learning.

Using Various Teaching Methods

The stimulating teacher captures the patient's desire to learn when she utilizes a variety of appropriate methods interestingly and with skill. Some settings may limit variety of methods, but almost always, the imaginative nurse can find ways to supplement the spoken word. Examples include the use of audiovisual aids, printed materials, charts, graphs, demonstrations, and so on. Even using the nurse's freehand sketches can make the material come alive. Teaching groups rather than only individuals adds variety. Including a patient with a particular experience as a teacher is often interesting to a group. Using resource people is another method. The nutritionist, for instance, can be included in certain parts of a program designed to teach patients who require special diets. Puppets have been used effectively with children. Using a variety of methods tends to stimulate interest and relieve the monotony of using only "teaching by telling," an approach that sometimes tends to focus more on the nurse than on the patient.

Most persons will agree readily that whatever teaching method is used, the teacher should have her instruction organized. It has been said that learning and bewilderment may differ only in terms of organization. However, organization does not mean rigidity. Flexibility in teaching methods to capture the enthusiasm of the learner is as essential as organization.

ADAPTING TEACHING TO VARIOUS SITUATIONS

When the nurse assumes the role of the health teacher, she finds herself working in a variety of situations. She may be in a hospital, a community health center, a clinic, a physician's office—any place where there are patients to teach. Her patients may be of various ages and may have a variety of backgrounds.

She may be teaching individuals or groups of patients. Health-illness problems differ markedly. Readiness may fall within a wide range, and many different techniques may be necessary to stimulate motivation. The nurse may teach patients with various physical handicaps, such as for example, deafness or blindness. The examples used in this chapter illustrate variety, and many more could have been cited. The reader is referred to additional examples in the study situations and in the articles and books listed in the references at the end of the chapter.

Wherever and whenever the nurse teaches, the principles of learning and their implications for teaching, discussed in this chapter, will apply. The importance of using principles to guide action is discussed in Chapter 3. The nurse as a health teacher will be more effective with less wasted effort if she is guided by basic principles in making adaptations to the myriad of teaching situations she faces.

CONCLUSION

Teaching is a highly individualistic and creative matter. When we recall the outstanding teachers we had, we see that they were often very different from one another, both in their personalities and in their teaching methods. But probably there were at least two factors they had in common: scholarship and enthusiasm.

The good teacher is a scholar, one who constantly seeks out new knowledge in her field and constantly seeks to increase her intellectual growth. While the nursing student is a beginner in the area of intellectual growth and knowledge in her field, an attitude of scholarliness with a sincere interest in her professional development will help her take the first steps toward becoming an effective teacher of her patients.

Good teaching requires the ability to communicate excitement. This is not the excitement we feel when filled with great joy, although elements of it can occur in teaching. More typically, we demonstrate enthusiasm and an interest in the learner. The important person in the teaching-learning situation is the learner. The person who is enthusiastic about her teaching, keeps the learners' needs foremost, and uses principles to guide action generally teaches successfully.

Study Situations

1. The importance of preparing objectives, of having planned content and of evaluation when teaching is described in this chapter. Note the following instructional objectives, stated in behavioral terms, and the content outline, carefully selected to reach the objectives. Note the test items, prepared in relation to the objectives and content, that aid the teacher to determine success or failure of her teaching.

Instructional Objectives:

The student will be able to:

1. List basic reasons regarding the importance of nutrition.
2. Name foods in each of the basic-four food groups.
3. Discriminate between an adequate and an inadequate lunch.
4. Select foods that would comprise an adequate diet for one day.

Content Outline

A. Physical Aspects—nutritional status is related to growth, resistance to infection and recovery from illness.
B. Psychological Aspects—lethargy and/or undesirable emotional reaction may reflect poor nutrition.
C. Adequate Daily Diet—contains a variety of foods from each of the four food groups.
D. Milk Group—(teenagers approximately 4 cups)—cartoned milk, dry milk, cottage cheese, evaporated milk, cheese, puddings, soup made with milk.
E. Meat Group—(2 servings)—liver, beef, pork, fish, poultry, beans, peanut butter, eggs.
F. Vegetable-Fruit Group—(4 servings)—green and yellow vegetables, citrus and tomatoes, potatoes, peppers, dried fruits.
G. Bread-Cereal Group—(4 servings)—rice, ready-to-eat cereal, flour, bread, oats, macaroni.

Test Items

1. Name two (2) basic reasons for eating a balanced diet.
2. Name three (3) examples of foods from the basic-four food groups.
3. Identify the best lunch:

a. hamburger	b. coke	c. macaroni
french fries	cheese-	bread-butter
pear halves	crackers	cake
milk	candy bar	Kool-Ade
	ice cream	

4. Hypothetical situation (mother not home: older sister instructed you to "fix" your own meals). Select from a variety of simulated foods, those you would have during the day.

These three outlines appeared on pages 816 and 817 in the following references:

Dennison, D.: Social class variables related to health instruction. **Am. J. Public Health,** 62:814–819, June, 1972. (Quoted material reprinted by permission of the American Public Health Association, Inc.)

Note also the manner in which a cultural group in

the United States, the low social class, has been found to be disadvantaged in the area of health, according to the author.

2. Read the following article:

    Nickerson, D.: Teaching the hospitalized diabetic. **Am. J. Nurs.,** 72:935–938, May, 1972.

    On page 937, there is a Urine Testing Procedure Check List. This check list serves as an evaluation tool to determine the success or failure of a teaching program. Note that in each item, the teacher is looking to see whether or not behavior has changed as a result of her teaching.

3. In the following article, note the preteaching test on page 524, used to determine levels of knowledge prior to instruction. Upon which principle of learning is this preteaching technique based?

    Kos, B., and Culbert, P.: Teaching patients about pacemakers. **Am. J. Nurs.,** 71:523–527, Mar., 1971.

    On page 525, there is a description of a teaching aid that the authors found useful when instructing patients with pacemakers. What advantages do take-home booklets have, according to the authors?

4. The following articles describe the investigation results when different teaching methods were used:

    Lindeman, C. A.: Nursing intervention with the pre-surgical patient: effectiveness and efficiency of groups and individual preoperative teaching—phase two. **Nurs. Research,** 21:196–209, May-June, 1972.

    Lindeman, C. A., and Van Aernam, B.: The effects of structured and unstructured preoperative teaching. **Nurs. Research,** 20:319–332, July-Aug., 1971.

    In each of these studies, which teaching method proved more effective?

5. The author of the following article stresses the importance of giving people alternatives in behavior in order that they can make intelligent decisions:

    Vincent, P. A.: Do we want patients to conform? **Nurs. Outlook,** 18:54–55, Jan., 1970.

    Note the unfortunate results when patients were not taught how to carry out medical orders when they were away from home.

6. The tremendous needs of some of the Salvation Army's clients are described in the following article:

    Steel, J. E.: Soup-soap-salvation. **Nurs. Outlook,** 18:31–34, Aug., 1970.

    Describe how the nurse used principles of learning when teaching these clients of the Salvation Army. How did she evaluate the results of her teaching? What did the author mean when she said the men were not hard "to reach" but difficult to locate?

References

1. Afek, L. B., and Hickey, J.: Health classes for migrant workers' families. **Am. J. Nurs.,** 72:1296–1298, July, 1972.

2. Agrafiotis, P. C.: Teaching parents about Pierre Robin syndrome. **Am. J. Nurs.,** 72:2040–2041, Nov., 1972.

3. Aiken, L. H.: Patient problems are problems in learning. **Am. J. Nurs.,** 70:1916–1918, Sept., 1970.

4. Barnard, K.: Teaching the retarded child is a family affair. **Am. J. Nurs.,** 68:305–311, Feb., 1968.

5. Berni, R., et al.: Reinforcing behavior. **Am. J. Nurs.,** 71:2180–2183, Nov., 1971.

6. Burke, E. L.: Training program in diabetes care. **Nurs. Outlook,** 19:548–549, Aug., 1971.

7. Copp, L. A.: The waiting room—a health teaching site. **Nurs. Outlook,** 19:481–483, July, 1971.

8. Cross, J. E., and Parsons, C. R.: Nurse-teaching and goal-directed nurse-teaching to motivate change in food selection behavior of hospitalized patients. **Nurs. Research,** 20:454–458, Sept.–Oct., 1971.

9. Davis, E. D.: Give a bath? **Am. J. Nurs.,** 70:2366–2367, Nov., 1970.

10. Dodge, J. S.: What patients should be told: patients' and nurses' beliefs. **Am. J. Nurs.,** 72:1852–1854, Oct., 1972.

11. Grim, R. A.: Mr. Edwards' triumph. **Am. J. Nurs.,** 72:480–481, Mar., 1972.

12. Haferkorn, V.: Assessing individual learning needs as a basis for patient teaching. *In* **The Nursing Clinics of North America.** Philadelphia, W. B. Saunders, 6:199–209, Mar., 1971.

13. Hallburg, J. C.: Teaching patients self-care. *In* **The Nursing Clinics of North American.** Philadelphia, W. B. Saunders, 5:223–231, June, 1970.

14. Healy, K. M.: Does preoperative instruction make a difference? **Am. J. Nurs.,** 68:62–67, Jan., 1968.

15. Kibler, R. J., et al.: Behavioral Objectives and Instruction. Boston, Allyn and Bacon, 1970.

16. Mager, R. F.: Preparing Instructional Objectives. Palo Alto, Calif., Fearon Publishers, 1962.

17. Pohl, M. L.: The Teaching Function of the Nursing Practitioner. ed. 2. Dubuque, Ia., William C. Brown, 1973.

18. Redman, B. K.: The Process of Patient Teaching in Nursing. ed. 2. St. Louis, C. V. Mosby, 1972.

19. Rubin, F. E. et al.: Seminar process—an aid to learning. **Nurs. Outlook,** 19:37–39, Jan., 1971.

20. Sather, M. A.: Volunteer teachers for prospective parents. **Am. J. Nurs.,** 70:1700–1702, Aug., 1970.

21. Scahill, M.: Preparing children for procedures and operations. **Nurs. Outlook,** 17:36–38, June, 1969.

22. Smyth, Sr. K., guest ed.: Symposium on teaching patients. *In* **The Nursing Clinics of North America.** Philadelphia, W. B. Saunders, 6:571–690, Dec., 1971.

23. Storlie, F.: A philosophy of patient teaching. **Nurs. Outlook,** 19:387–389, June, 1971.

24. Trayser, L. M.: A teaching program for diabetics. **Am. J. Nurs.,** 73:92–93, Jan., 1973.

25. Valentine, L. R.: Self-care through group learning. **Am. J. Nurs.,** 70:2140–2142, Oct., 1970.

26. Wolf, V. C.: Some implications of short-term, long-term memory theory. **Nurs. Forum,** 10:150–165, No. 2, 1971.

27. Zimbra, C., and Ladensack, V.: Teaching in silence. **Am. J. Nurs.,** 70:1525–1526, July, 1970.

UNIT 4

The Environment and Health

CHAPTER 17

The Community Environment

GLOSSARY · INTRODUCTION · THE COMMUNITY DESCRIBED ·
TYPICAL COMMUNITY ACTIVITIES AND HOW THEY INFLUENCE
WELL-BEING · IMPLICATIONS FOR NURSING · CONCLUSION ·
STUDY SITUATIONS · REFERENCES

GLOSSARY

Community: Aggregate of people living in the same place and sharing common values and beliefs.

Ergonomics: Study of relationships among individuals and their work and working environment.

INTRODUCTION

It was pointed out in Chapter 3 that environmental influences will tend either to interfere with or to promote well-being and that the nurse is often looked to for leadership in working for the kind of environment that promotes high-level wellness. This unit focuses primarily on environmental factors that may influence health and on the practitioner's interest in an environment that promotes well-being. It discusses implications for nursing action directed toward a healthful environment.

The first chapter in this unit is concerned with the environment of the patient in his community. The last two chapters of the unit direct attention more specifically to practices that promote a healthful environment in the home and in health agencies.

THE COMMUNITY DESCRIBED

The dictionary defines a *community* as an aggregate of people living in the same place and sharing common values and beliefs. Communities are of various sizes, both in terms of number of members and of the area involved. A family is a community and is as old as mankind. A neighborhood, city, county, state, and country are communities. In recent times, the world has been described as an international community. In the context of this definition, it can be seen that everyone belongs to several expanding communities beginning with the family and extending

outward to the community of mankind, as Figure 17-1 illustrates.

Observations of a community illustrate several rather typical characteristics. A community is generally made up of people who have similar values and beliefs. These people live within a rather well-defined geographic area. The community has certain policies and laws and has certain institutions that serve it. A common language is typical. Also, the problems of a community often become the common concern of its members.

A wide variety of activities can be observed within any community. It is the rare activity that is without influence on an individual's state of well-being. Some influences will be positive in nature (tend to promote well-being). While others will be negative in nature (have the opposite effect). The following discussion illustrates.

TYPICAL COMMUNITY ACTIVITIES AND HOW THEY INFLUENCE WELL-BEING

Common activities observed within a community may be classified in a variety of ways. Seven categories have been selected here: values and beliefs; production of services and goods; education and recreation; transportation and communication; protection, safety, and aesthetics; nonofficial agencies; and official or governmental agencies.

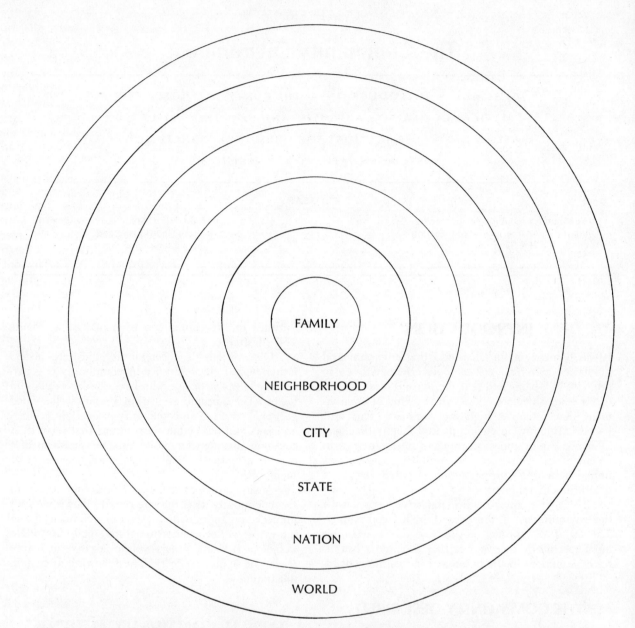

Fig. 17-1. Everyone belongs to several communities and as the community expands, all peoples of the world are included. Environmental concerns are the concerns of all communities and hence, of all mankind.

Communities tend to hold to certain common values and beliefs. While in general, community members tend to hold to similar values and beliefs, they may not always be identical in nature. However, those held in common tend to be reinforced and strengthened within the community. Here are some examples that show how values and beliefs may influence well-being.

When a community places value on recreational activities for all age groups, facilities are usually easily available and enjoy the support and interest of community members. Institutions such as churches, schools, YMCA's, and YWCA's generally are observed to lend a hand to support and encourage healthful activities for all. When a community places little value or interest in this type of activity, facilities and the support they need may be at a minimum. As a result, common leisure-time activities may be of a nature less likely to promote physical and mental well-being.

When community members tend to hold to the belief that mothers should be in the home, child care facilities are likely to be a rarity. On the other hand, those communities whose members feel that mothers have the right to work if they so desire tend to support child care facilities.

Fear and distrust of health practitioners may result in people avoiding care except in crisis situations. It has been observed that such attitudes tend to occur more frequently in isolated rural and in poverty-stricken communities. Individuals living in higher socio-economic communities tend to seek out preventive care. Hence, they tend to have fewer preventable health-related problems than those living in lower socio-economic areas.

Belief in assisting others in times of need can be of great value for many health-related community action programs. On the other hand, a general feeling that every person is responsible for helping himself can result in minimal community service to others.

As Chapter 15 points out, most people hold to religious beliefs, and their implications for health are discussed. Common religious beliefs in a community are important to know since they may serve as important aids in the promotion of well-being.

People in the community produce services and goods to sustain livelihood. When a community's job opportunities are scarce and unemployment rates are high, the results of having limited resources to purchase the necessities for daily living become apparent. Health problems among the unemployed and unemployable are numerous and well described in lay and professional literature. For example, when money is scarce, diets often lack sufficient nutrition, the annual physical examination is omitted, dental care is postponed, and so on. Joblessness has many psychological implications also that tend to erode mental well-being through loss of self-respect, financial independence, and control over certain decisions.

Communities have educational and recreational programs. Education and recreation begin in the home. In addition, most communities have a wide variety of educational programs available to their members. Basic education for children from kindergarten through twelfth grade is typical in this country. There are several trends evident in relation to educational programs in the United States. More facilities and services are becoming available for exceptional persons, that is, those with above average and those with below average mental and physical abilities. Opportunities for learning experiences for children under five years of age are on the increase in many communities. Vocational education is on the increase, as are educational programs for adults, including programs for those with or without benefit of earlier educational opportunities. Health education for all ages is on the increase, both in formally organized and in informal programs. In addition to increasing the learner's areas of knowledge, enriched educational programs tend to enhance a person's independence, opportunities for employment, and his self-concept—factors that in turn tend to promote an individual's psychological well-being.

Consider the following examples of individuals having different kinds of educational experiences, and think about the effects these experiences may have had on their well-being: the children of migrant farm workers whose parents move so frequently in order to follow the harvesting of crops that the children are unable to complete an academic year in any one school; a child with a progressive muscle-deteriorating disease but with an unimpaired intellect who has been able to graduate from high school through a homebound educational program; the teen-agers in a neighborhood who are high school dropouts without vocational skills and who do not have the benefit of health teaching in relation to the use of illicit drugs and the prevention of venereal diseases; children who live in a neighborhood where a language other than English is usually spoken but who attend schools where teaching is done in English and is also the language commonly spoken in the neighborhood. These examples have implications, both positive and negative, in relation to mental and physical well-being.

As mentioned earlier, recreational facilities can help to promote healthful mental and physical activities for all ages. Usually too, community cohesiveness, camaraderie, and morale are increased through the social contacts afforded by the availability of recreational facilities.

Recreational facilities require supervision in order to prevent accidents. For example, swimming facilities without adequate safety features often lead to tragedy. Injuries occurring when recreational equipment is improperly used or maintained is another example of a dangerous condition. When adequate recreational facilities are lacking in a community, destructive activities tend to be more common, and delinquency and crime tend to increase.

Communities rich in opportunities for those interested in the arts, as the dance, music, literature, and art, enrich life and add to the fun and enjoyment of living for most people. These in turn help to promote the community's well-being.

Communities are concerned with transportation

and communication. A variety of transportation facilities are generally available in some communities; in most, local transportation is almost entirely by automobile. Generally, increased mobility has provided ways for people to leave and return to their homes regularly and with ease. This means people are exposed to expanding communities, and as a result, often develop interests and attachments outside their immediate neighborhoods. The "bedroom" communities surrounding a metropolitan area are examples of areas where residents often have loyalties and commitments to communities in which they work as well as to those in which they live.

The marked increase in the use of the automobile for transportation in our society has created many health problems related to pollution from auto exhausts. There are times when the fumes contribute heavily to a blanket of smog around a community with harmful results. In 1952, a week's period of smog in London resulted in approximately 5,000 deaths, according to physicians who studied the disaster. The amount of respiratory damage due to auto pollution is unknown but believed to be extensive, serious, and on the increase.

Man is working to decrease smog and thereby its related problems. Improved highway construction that moves traffic more quickly, experts say, results in less exhaust fumes than when there is much stop-and-go, slow traffic. Automobile manufacturers are faced with increasingly rigid standards designed to decrease the amount of unburned hydrocarbons and carbon monoxide in exhaust fumes. Communities are looking more and more to public transportation to ease the use of the auto. Some communities are considering banning the use of the private car in areas where traffic is particularly troublesome. All these efforts will hopefully decrease smog and the health problems associated with it.

Availability of public transportation influences accessibility of health care services. For example, the mother without a car and with young children will seek only essential or crisis care, as a rule, if no ready means of getting to health services is available to her. It has been observed in communities with limited public transportation that neighborhoods immediately surrounding a health agency, such as a hospital, generally have many elderly residents who chose the location in order to be within easy walking distance of health care facilities.

The size of the community may be said to decrease with improved communications. While the family and neighborhood members may communicate mainly by word of mouth, they are in almost constant contact with the larger communities as well.

With improved communication media, values and beliefs change. There is less solidarity in the family and neighborhood as communities exchange ideas. There is less contentment with status quo and more interest in acculturation as communities view each other through the communication media.

As Chapter 2 pointed out, there is little value in providing a particular health service if the community fails to inform people of its availability. Communication media have been helpful in disseminating information in relation to health and to health services. One result has been mounting consumer demands for better and more health services.

Communities are concerned with protection, safety, and aesthetics. Activities in relation to the conservation of health, life, resources, and property are observed in the community in innumerable ways. Many dangers that previous generations were exposed to have disappeared. For example, the provision of safe drinking water has practically eliminated certain diseases, such as typhoid fever, in many parts of the world. However, as some dangers have been overcome, new perils have appeared. The automobile, for instance, built to serve man so that he would enjoy a better way of life, also kills upwards of 50,000 individuals, and maims countless others each year in the United States.

Auto safety research continues its efforts to make cars safer. Examples of auto safety features, which reportedly are helping to decrease injury and death, include the use of safety belts, stronger bumpers, the elimination of sharp projecting parts, and the use of parts that "give" or collapse upon impact.

Protection from danger and the development of safety and aesthetic measures that will promote well-being require engineering, enforcement of laws, and consumer education. Here are a few examples.

The disposal of wastes has brought about the development of sewage disposal plants that replace the emptying of raw wastes in our lakes and streams. It is now an illegal act in most places to dispose of raw wastes indiscriminately. The consumer is becoming increasingly knowledgeable about the implications of water pollution and is demanding laws and law enforcement that help to prevent it.

As in the case of water pollution, the public has been made equally aware of air pollution and its threat to health and well-being. Engineering and legislation aimed at preventing air pollution from industrial sources is also on the increase.

Indiscriminate use of our natural resources has propelled the role of the environmentalist from a status of relative insignificance to that of a powerful and persuasive voice in our society. Those using or destroying natural resources without consideration for the effects are often viewed as enemies of the public. Increasingly, legislation in relation to the use of natural resources reflects the people's demands for considering ecological balance in the world among plants, animals, and matter.

Space, as an entity, has taken on increasing importance in recent years as the result of concern about progressive limitations on the available space in the world. Because of the vastness of this country, only within the past several decades has space as a factor in healthful living even been considered. It is now an accepted concept that the amount and quality of space available to man can influence him both physically and psychologically. While there are no definitive answers as to the amount of space which is desirable, ongoing studies by social and physical scientists are bringing us new information. For example, the influence of both confinement and vast surrounding space on the astronauts is being thoroughly investigated. The amount and kind of space available is influenced by many factors, including climatic conditions, land usage and control, and building regulations. More attention will undoubtedly be focused on man's need for, and use of, space in the generations to come.

The appearance of our environment has been found to be important in relation to morale and psychological well-being. Slogans such as Keep America Beautiful have caught on and assisted in efforts to improve environmental beauty. Tastes differ among individuals but orderliness and cleanliness are generally recognized aesthetic values in human life. Concern with beauty in our environment can be seen in efforts used to eliminate littering and cluttering of our landscape with neon signs and billboards. Engineering and building of new communities and reclaiming the old are examples of planning that considers both space and beauty as important factors in promoting a healthful way of life. Communities that show little interest in space and beauty tend to have disintegrating neighborhoods, citizen dissatisfaction or apathy, and little motivation to improve the quality of life.

The increase in concern for safety at home, school, and play is evident all about us. Here are just a few examples. Poisonous substances are clearly labeled; containers for medications have caps that children cannot readily open; clearly marked exits, fire escapes, and emergency equipment are a part of schools as well as other buildings open to the public; attention-getting color in clothing is used to promote safety for the hunter; unsafe toys and clothing are removed from the market place; driver education,

examinations, and licenses are aimed at promoting safety in public and private transportation; and those interested in boating find Coast Guard safety education programs easily available throughout the United States.

As a result of increased attention to the problems of man and his work, a new field of study has evolved—*ergonomics*, which deals with the relationship between individuals and their work and working environment. It is especially concerned with fitting jobs to the needs and abilities of the worker. In ergonomics, attention is focused on health-illness factors the employee brings with him to the work setting as well as the injuries and illnesses acquired while employed. Extensive health programs in many industries focus on disease detection, prevention, and treatment. There is evidence of programs concerned with cardiac and respiratory diseases, alcoholism, drug addiction, mental health, and cancer detection and treatment, to name a few.

As a result of increased awareness of relationships between work and health, the federal Occupational Safety and Health Act was passed in 1970. Its purpose is to insure safe and healthful working conditions for employees by promoting the enforcement of standards for the maintenance of safe and healthful work environments, reduction of work hazards, research in occupational safety and health, and the investigation of relationships between disease and illness and the working environment.

It has been observed that most accidents occur at midday or near the end of the work day—the times when the body is at its lowest biological efficiency. These findings correlate with the body's biologic or circadian rhythms which are discussed in Chapter 20. Industry has put this knowledge to work by providing rest breaks at appropriate intervals to promote work efficiency and to reduce accidents.

The long-range effects of noise have been found to influence physical and psychological well-being. Noise abatement efforts have influenced the engineering and construction of jet engines and industrial equipment. As another example, the location of airports is being carefully considered in order to decrease air traffic noises in populated areas. Health practitioners often observe physical and psychological damage in people who have had prolonged exposure to loud noise.

There are various miscellaneous measures that are of community concern in efforts to eliminate environmental hazards. Examples of these efforts include the control of insects and rodents; disposing of abandoned refrigerators and automobiles; and appropriate protection of "attractive nuisances" such as swimming pools and wells, and cisterns not in use.

These examples are but a few of many that could be cited to illustrate the community's concern with protection, safety, and aesthetics. When communities fall short in their efforts, physical and psychological well-being suffer. Certainly, it appears, there is much more work to be done and there is ample opportunity for health practitioners to lead the way. As the citizens of communities have become aware of potential dangers in their environments, their general support and interest in attempts to decrease and eliminate them are evident.

Most communities have nonofficial or voluntary agencies dedicated to serving their citizens. Examples are numerous but here are a few to illustrate: voluntary hospitals; visiting nurse services; clinics; the Red Cross; United Fund; scouting organizations; service clubs; day care centers; and associations concerned with specific disease entities such as heart disease, cancer, and multiple sclerosis. The role of these voluntary agencies and the importance of their contributions in promoting physical and psychological health are well-documented.

Communities have official or governmental agencies dedicated to serving their citizens. Groups of people have governments, ranging from very informal types to highly complex structures. The family, headed by the father or mother or both on a cooperative basis, has its source of rules and customs to which members turn for direction in family affairs. The neighborhood, as in the case of the family, has a very informal government of sorts, but with observation one can usually discern the leaders and those who exert implied authority and offer guidance in neighborhood matters. Communities extending beyond the neighborhood have governments that are clearly discernible and specific in terms of responsibilities and authority.

The primary purpose of government is to promote the general welfare of the governed. In a democracy, the government represents the people through elected officials and the people hold its government accountable for legislation, law enforcement, and services that promote general welfare.

There is hardly a law in existence that is without at least some influence on health and well-being. A few examples of laws with fairly obvious influence on health and well-being include those dealing with pet control, pet disease detection, traffic control, the use and dispensing of narcotics and other dangerous drugs, and food handling and service.

Typical services provided by governmental agencies that influence health and well-being are fire control, sewage and garbage disposal, and public health education. Most communities also have official social service agencies that assist individuals to supplement their own resources. Examples include financial assistance, psychological and legal counseling, and provisions for low-cost housing. In addition, governments typically maintain various health services. Examples include publicly supported hospitals, clinics, and health departments. Official as well as nonofficial health agencies, once devoted primarily to the care of the ill, have increasingly expanded to offer services related to health promotion, health education, early disease detection, and rehabilitation. Both types of agencies have contributed heavily to health-related research as well.

IMPLICATIONS FOR NURSING

The discussion in this chapter has offered a broad overview of environmental influences in community living. Hopefully, it has stimulated the reader to think of the patient's environment outside of his home or health agency, and to realize the tremendous influence environmental factors have on well-being. To summarize, what implications for nursing can be seen from this discussion?

Everyone is constantly reacting to environmental influences in the community of which he is a member. No one lives alone or is isolated from community influences. It is of little value, for example, to rehabilitate a drug addict and then return him to a community environment in which illicit drug use is a common way of life.

The nurse has a wide variety of community resources available to her that can assist her in meeting patient needs. There will be times when simply referring a patient for assistance to another agency may be insufficient. The nurse may need to work as the patient's advocate in obtaining a necessary service. For example, it may be necessary to interpret a patient's need for homemaker services to an agency offering such services. The reader is referred to Study Situation 7 on pages 11 and 12 which describes how one nurse worked as the patient's advocate in the community in which she was employed.

As a responsible citizen in the communities in which she lives, the nurse can assume leadership and actively participate in supporting activities that promote the public welfare. The role of the nurse as a responsible citizen was mentioned in Chapter 1. Several examples in this chapter pointed out that health practitioners are often looked to for assistance when communities face problems in relation to health and

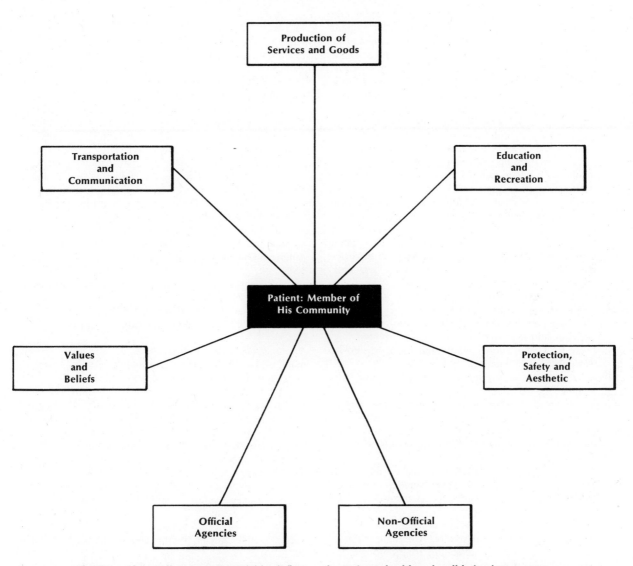

Fig.17-2.   Almost all community activities influence the patient's health and well-being in some way.

well-being. The responsible nurse will assist in effecting change that promotes high-level wellness, both for her own and for her patient's health. She will assist in helping to eliminate environmental hazards to health and support activities that promote well-being.

CONCLUSION

Environmental influences are ever-present and no one exists without them. Some may tend to promote well-being; others are inimical to it. The nurse often functions as an applied ecologist and epidemiologist as she seeks out data and determines clues that will help her in working with patients in the total context of their environments. The nurse can find strengths in the patient's environment and build on them, such as the availability of agencies that may offer assistance in a particular area in which the patient has needs. She may also function as a change agent as she becomes aware of environmental influences (for example, air and water pollution) that stand in the way of promoting health for the patients she cares for and for herself as well.

Study Situations

1. Read the following article:
   Moses, M.: "Viva la causa!" **Am. J. Nurs.,** 73:842–848, May, 1973.

Review the characteristics of a typical community given in this chapter. Did the community of migrant farm workers described in this article display any or all of these characteristics? Now review the categories that this chapter used to discuss common community activities. List common activities in the migrant farm workers' community under each of these categories and indicate which tended to promote well-being. What environmental factors tended to work toward deterioration of well-being? Note the method the author described to gather data concerning what the farm workers most wanted in their health care when financial resources were limited.

2. Most popular periodicals and many newspapers carry articles regularly on environmental issues making the news. Review several of these articles. Describe how the issues being discussed influence health and how solutions to community problems are being sought. For example, read the section on environment in several issues of *Time* magazine and look for implications for health practitioners.

3. In the following article, in the section "Unresolved Problems," note the description of the effects of poor cooperation among official and nonofficial agencies and organizations in the community:

Loeb, B.: United funds, health, and the urban crisis. **Nurs. Outlook,** 17:36–38, Sept., 1969.

How does the author suggest nursing can best help to meet the community's health problems?

4. The group of articles below identify some typical health problems unique to young adults because of their common attitudes and values. Read several of the articles and identify underlying beliefs that you believe influence well-being:

Fleshman, R. P., guest ed.: Symposium on the young adult in today's world. *In* **The Nursing Clinics of North Amercia.** Philadelphia, W. B. Saunders, 8:1–104, Mar., 1973.

5. The community in which we live influences our health. Consider your own community. Are there circumstances which need modification to promote high-level wellness of the residents?

Using the guidelines for developing objectives given in Chapter 8, state the nursing objectives you would use as your goals in relation to the environment if you were a new health nurse assigned to work in your community.

References

1. Diekema, A. J.: The changing environment: some implications for health. **Occup. Health Nurs.,** 17:20–22, July, 1970.

2. Fischer, L. R., guest ed.: Symposium on the nurse in community mental health. *In* **The Nursing Clinics of North America.** Philadelphia, W. B. Saunders, 5:631–712, Dec., 1970.

3. Foley, M. F.: Air travel for patients. **Am. J. Nurs.,** 73:1020–1023, June, 1973.

4. Goldstein, D. H.: The occupational safety and health act of 1970. **Am. J. Nurs.,** 71:1535–1538, Aug., 1971.

5. Hall, E. T.: The Silent Language, pp. 187–209. Garden City, N. Y., Doubleday, 1959.

6. Hamilton, V.: Preventing hearing loss in industry. **The Canadian Nurse,** 66:37–40, Sept., 1970.

7. Jamann, J. S.: Health is a function of ecology. **Am. J. Nurs.,** 71:970–973, May, 1971.

8. Johnson, K. G., et al.: Survey of adolescent drug use: social and environmental factors. **Am. J. Public Health,** 62:164–166, Feb., 1972.

9. Kaplan, M.: Environmental hazards for human health. **World Health,** pp. 4–11, May, 1972.

10. Kenneth, H. Y., guest ed.: Symposium on the ambulatory patient. *In* **The Nursing Clinics of North America.** Philadelphia, W. B. Saunders, 5:195–275, June, 1970.

11. Kramer, M.: The consumer's influence on health care. **Nurs. Outlook,** 20:574–578, Sept., 1972.

12. Kryter, K. D.: Non-auditory effects of environmental noise. **Am. J. Public Health,** 62:389–398, Mar., 1972.

13. Lave, L. B., and Seskin, E. P.: Air pollution, climate, and home heating: their effects on U. S. mortality rates. **Am. J. Public Health,** 62:909–916, July, 1972.

14. Litsky, W. et al.: Solid waste: a hospital dilemma. **Am. J. Nurs.,** 72:1841–1847, Oct., 1972.

15. Maas, R. B.: Personal hearing protection: the occupational health nurse's challenge and opportunity. **Occup. Health Nurs.,** 17:25–27, May, 1969.

16. Pluckhan, M. L.: Space: the silent language . . . **Nurs. Forum,** 7:386–397, No. 4, 1968.

17. Rummerfield, P. S., and Rummerfield, M. J.: Noise induced health loss. **Occup. Health Nurs.,** 17:23–29, 43–46, Nov., 1969.

18. Sargent, F. II: Man—environment—problems for public health. **Am. J. Public Health,** 62:628–633, May, 1972.

19. Shumway, S. M., and Wisehart, D. E.: How to know a community. **Nurs. Outlook,** 17:63–64, Sept., 1969.

20. Stephens, G. J.: Clinical research in human ecology. pp. 76–88. *In* Bergerson, B. S., et al., eds.: Current Concepts in Clinical Nursing. St. Louis, C. V. Mosby, 1967.

21. Swan, J. A.: The environment, the citizen, and the environmental health professional. **Am. J. Public Health,** 62:639–641, May, 1972.

22. Tschirley, F. H.: Pesticides: relation to environmental quality. **JAMA,** 224:1157–1159, May 21, 1973.

23. Wheeler, E. T.: No hospital is an island. **Hospitals, J. Am. Hosp. Assoc.,** 46:113–116; 170, Oct. 16, 1972.

24. Yoder, F.: Implications of the changing environment to occupational health. **Occup. Health Nurs.,** 17:23–25, July, 1970.

CHAPTER 18

The Patient's Immediate Environment

INTRODUCTION

This chapter is concerned with the patient's immediate environment, that is, the one in which the nurse will be carrying out most personal care services. The immediate environment includes, for example, the patient's hospital unit, the area in the home where care is administered, and the nurse's office in an industrial, school, or clinic setting.

Examples from everyday living illustrate how influential our immediate environment is. For example, we react happily or adversely to color, sound, noise, odor, aesthetic factors, and so on. The producers of movies and television programs are well aware of environmental influences when they use music, lighting, sound effects, color, and costuming to influence the effects they wish to create.

It is relatively safe to say that there is no ideal physical environment for everyone. However, an environment that promotes well-being will take at least these factors into consideration: provisions for space, safety, comfort, and ease in accomplishing common activities of daily living.

PROVISIONS FOR SPACE

Each individual has a need for space in his immediate environment. Cultures vary in relation to spatial needs and values. Here are a few examples of behavior in relation to space commonly observed in this country.

Siblings who share a common bed or room usually have an imaginary line that separates one child's side from the other. Classroom chairs and desks have implied ownership. It is common practice to apologize, even in crowded areas, when one person touches another unintentionally. The space one has while waiting in line at the supermarket or at the movie ticket window is considered one's own. In the home, the kitchen is usually mother's territory, the living room has father's favorite chair. In industry, the worker has his designated work area. In a clinic or office, a patient is usually assigned to a chair or a cubicle and the hospitalized patient has a room or unit which he calls his own.

Usually, the larger the space occupied by an individual the more prestige it conveys. For example, in industry the larger the office the higher the status of its occupant. Research in relation to territorial rights has demonstrated that while people tend to defend whatever space they have, the less they have the more vigorously they tend to defend it.

The nurse should consider the patient's need for space when administering nursing care. She should respect the control an individual shows over whatever space he claims. She should recognize the patient's desire to express himself within that space and respect his wish to have his own personal items with him; for example, showing interest and respect for pictures of loved ones, a favorite piece of handicraft or art, a religious object, or a child's favorite toy acknowledges the importance of space and its personal uses.

People need space to grow, that is, space that stimulates and permits them to develop, to change and to mature, both physically and mentally. Growth occurs in all environments and at all ages, irrespective of an individual's position on the health-illness continuum. A healthful environment is one with the space and opportunities to promote that growth.

Health agencies are increasingly aware of the need for space as well as the facilities for growth and most now make appropriate provisions. Examples include a children's play area, a library for patient use, a chapel or "quiet room" for thought and con-

FUNDAMENTALS OF NURSING

Fig. 18-1. These Photos illustrate some of the most common causes of accidents in the home: clutter on a stairway, an overloaded electrical socket, open and unlocked medicine closet, a cooking pot with handle extending over the edge of stove, standing precariously on a chair. (Photos by Ted Hill, Arizona)

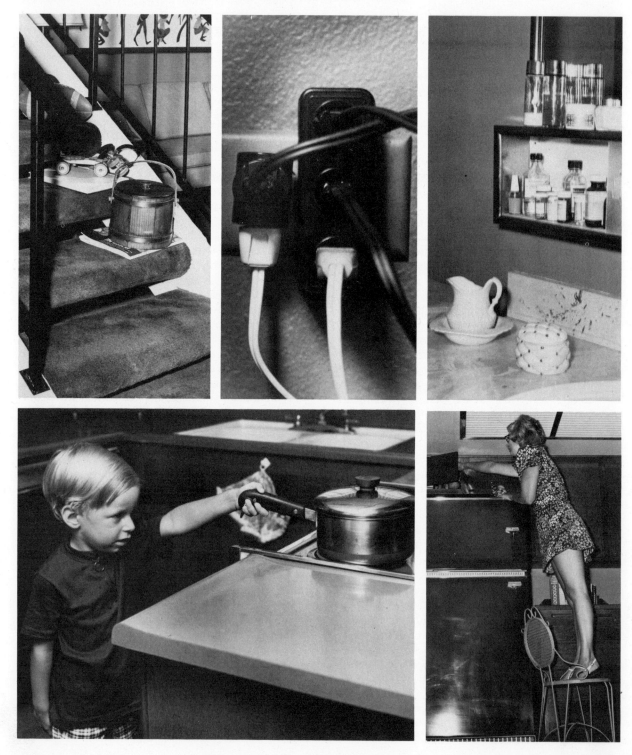

templation, units for recreational and occupational activities, and lounges for visiting. Comparable facilities and the necessary space can usually be made available in the home. Wherever the nurse is administering care, she will wish to consider needs for growth and take steps, as possible, to arrange for an environment that fosters it.

PROVISIONS FOR SAFETY

Safety in the Home

A safe environment is one that is free of harm and danger. It is unrealistic to think in terms of an environment entirely free of hazards. However, there are ways in which hazardous elements in the environment can be at least minimized if not eliminated.

A modification in the design of an item, for example, can reduce a hazard. Sealing drug bottles with caps that are difficult to open, the "child proof" cap, has helped to reduce incidences of young children accidentally swallowing drugs.

Hazards can be reduced when items in the environment are used with care and forethought. Acting hastily and without thinking is a common cause of accidents. For example, ceramic tile and enamel bath tubs have practical and attractive features but they tend to become slippery when wet. "I knew the tub was slippery but I was in a hurry" often explains an accident. Nonskid mats can prevent falls in tubs.

Using equipment for its intended purpose and maintaining equipment properly also help to minimize hazards, as examples given later in this chapter will show.

Most people tend to think of the home as a safe place, and yet, according to the National Safety Council, it is one of the most dangerous places of all. About one-half of accidental injuries and approximately one-third of accidental deaths occur in the home.

FALLS: Falls account for nearly half of the accidental deaths that occur in the home. Major causes include slippery floors, poor lighting, worn rugs, misplaced furniture, and objects littered about. The young, the old, and the physically handicapped are especially susceptible to falls. Measures as simple as guard rails in bathrooms and on stairs, good lighting, and discarding or repairing broken equipment about the home will decrease accidents.

SCALDS AND BURNS: These rank second to falls as the cause of accidental death occurring in the home. Examples of common causes include carelessness in the use of matches, cigarettes, stoves, fireplaces, and barbecues.

POISONING: This causes many deaths in the home each year. It has been reported that more than half a million children under age five are poisoned annually and more than half of these accidents are caused by drugs, with aspirin being the chief cause of death. Analgesics, iron preparations, household cleaning solutions and supplies, insecticides, and paints are also commonly ingested with disastrous results.

ASPHYXIATION: Asphyxiation results in many accidental deaths each year. Persons die of gas inhalation from auto exhausts and gas-fueled appliances, and many choke to death on food and small objects.

ELECTRICAL SHOCKS: Many injuries and accidental deaths from electrical shock occur in the home. Overload of electrical circuits, faulty appliances, frayed wires, handling of electrical devices and cords when shoes and hands are wet are examples of conditions often resulting in injury or death.

INJURIES: While scratches, bruises, and cuts usually are considered minor injuries, they may be serious if not cared for properly. For example, bleeding that persists or wounds that become infected and do not heal require prompt attention.

Increasingly, nurses are offering services to patients in their homes. Also, more and more, nurses are expected to prepare teaching programs that include measures to prevent accidents in the home. As illustrated in Figure 3-4 on page 35, the nurse will wish to be aware of environmental factors that present hazards to her patients and to assist in promoting a safe home environment.

Safety in Health Agencies

As is true in the home, a health agency entirely free of hazards is an unlikely situation. However, as in the home, measures can be taken to help reduce common hazards.

PREVENTING SPREAD OF MICROORGANISMS: A major concern of health practitioners is the danger of spreading microorganisms from person to person and from place to place. Health agencies have policies in relation to practices that limit the spread of microorganisms.

PREVENTING FALLS: The high incidence of falls occurring when patients move from place to place in health agencies is of concern to every health practitioner. The rate tends to increase in agencies caring for patients who have physical limitations and poor coordination and who are debilitated due to illness. There are a variety of safety measures recommended to reduce the number of falls. Examples include handrails, bed siderails, ramps and elevators for

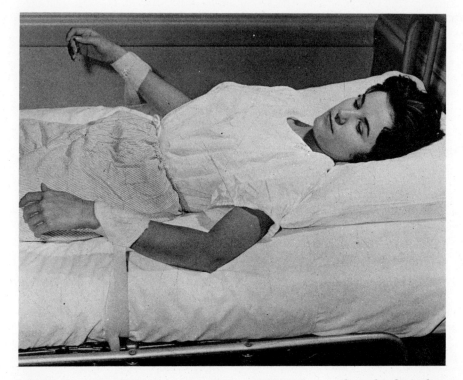

Fig. 18-2. Hand restraints should not immobilize the patient's arms. If they are needed to prevent the patient from pulling out a catheter, a nasal tube, an infusion, or from touching a dressing, they should be applied to serve this purpose. These restraints allow the patient to turn his arms and to lift his arms to some extent.

patient use, nonskid floor coverings, well-lighted corridors that are free of extra equipment and furniture, and nonskid and supportive footwear for patients.

Siderails are a common piece of equipment on agency beds. Agency policy usually guides the practitioner in their use. They are especially important for the safety of patients who are likely to be disoriented, restless, confused, or unconscious. When in doubt about the patient's mental status, it is better to err in the overuse of siderails than to contribute to a situation that results in a patient's falling out of bed.

RESTRAINING PATIENTS: More and more, health personnel are looking for ways and means to minimize the practice of restraining patients. In the care of the mentally ill, for example, psychiatric therapy that includes the use of drugs has greatly reduced the need for the use of restraints. Nevertheless, the nurse in the course of her practice will encounter situations which, in her opinion, require restraint of the patient as a safety measure. For example, she may have reason to believe that the patient will crawl over siderails and fall out of bed or that he will disturb equipment, dressings, or wounds. Figures 18-2 and 18-3 illustrate two types of restraints. If friends or relatives ask to remain with a patient who, in the nurse's opinion, needs some type of restraint or side-

rails on his bed, the nurse should explain the responsibility carefully and use good judgment since it is her responsibility to protect the patient from harm.

PREVENTING EQUIPMENT-RELATED ACCIDENTS: Accidents in health agencies, as in the home, frequently result from using malfunctioning or poorly maintained equipment. With the marked increase in the use of highly sophisticated equipment, it is especially important for health practitioners to learn to use it properly and then know how to recognize signs that indicate the equipment is not functioning correctly. Examples of equipment-related accidents include those occurring as a result of using suction devices with inadequate vacuum and rate regulators on infusion equipment that deliver erratic amounts of solution. Additional examples of common hazardous situations include using improperly grounded electrical equipment, drugs and solutions with expired dates, broken electrical wiring and plugs, and electrical equipment that has been allowed to become wet. There have been claims, albeit unconfirmed, that as many as 1,200 persons die annually as a result of electrical shocks in hospitals. Whether or not these statistics are exaggerated, the increase in the use of electrical equipment in health agencies increases the chances of injury to both patients and health practitioners when safety measures are ignored.

To summarize this section, here are a few guides

that, when observed, will help to decrease equipment-related accidents in health agencies. Use equipment for the use for which it was intended. Do not operate equipment with which you are unfamiliar. Handle all equipment with care. Three-prong electrical plugs that provide for grounding of equipment are recommended. Do not twist or sharply bend electrical cords because you may break the wires inside the cord. Report signs of trouble immediately. Be alert to signs that indicate faulty equipment such as breaks in electrical cords, sparks, smoke, electrical shocks, loose or missing parts, and unusual noises or odors.

MEANS OF IDENTIFYING PATIENTS: It is of extreme importance that each patient receive the care and therapy intended for him. In order to avoid accidents, an accurate, easy-to-use, and reliable way of identifying patients being cared for in a health agency is essential. Even the alert patient may become temporarily confused in a strange setting; therefore, every effort should be made to assure proper identification wherever care is being given.

Most inpatient health agencies use a waterproof wrist bracelet that cannot be removed without destruction of the band. It is imprinted with the patient's name and certain other identifying information, as for example, the health agency's identifying number, the name of the physician caring for the patient, and the patient's unit or room number. It is

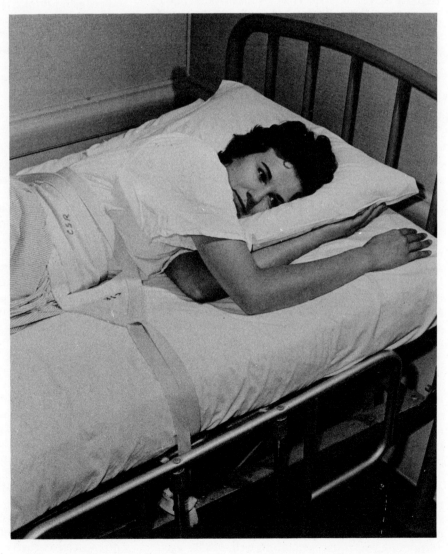

Fig. 18-3. Restraints which can be adjusted to the specific activity limitation desired are more likely to be accepted by the patient and his family. For example, preventing a patient from sitting up, but allowing him to turn from side to side; permitting him to sit up and to turn from side to side, but preventing him from climbing over the siderails or from getting out of bed; or preventing a patient from turning on one side or the other. The purpose of restraints is to help to prevent the patient from harm. They should not interfere with physiologic functioning, such as impairing circulation, limiting muscular activity to the point of immobilization or interfering with respiration.

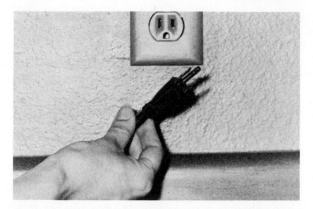

Fig. 18-4. A patient's environment has been referred to as an electrical environment because of the extensive use of electrical equipment. Safety experts recommend the use of a three-prong plug as illustrated in this figure. The grounding wire is connected to the electrical device and, via a U-shaped prong, to the ground so that the electrical current is bypassed when a fault in equipment occurs. (Photo by Ted Hill, Arizona)

also helpful to have the patient's name on his bed but this is not considered sufficiently safe for accurate patient identification purposes.

In delivery rooms, it is common practice to place a wrist or ankle bracelet on the newborn with information corresponding to that on the mother's bracelet. In addition, immediately after birth, infants are often footprinted to prevent identification errors. Footprints are distinctive and easier to secure than prints of the infant's clenched fingers.

Safety Education and First Aid

Instruction in safety assumes an important place in life today. Safety education along with safety engineering and safety enforcement have helped immeasurably to reduce accidents.

Safety education begins in the home. From infancy on, children are exposed to teaching in relation to accident prevention. Many states now require safety instruction in their school systems. For example, safety receives emphasis in such courses as physical education, health education, vocational education, and driver education.

The communications media have given much assistance in teaching safety. Special educational programs are commonly offered in most communities to promote safety. Examples include programs in relation to safe boating, swimming, driving, camping, and hunting. Safety education is included in curricula in schools of nursing and is a part of most continuing education programs as well. Health agencies, too, offer safety education, as for example, in

relation to measures to prevent fire and practices to follow when fire occurs. Certainly, also, the nurse will include safety education in her teaching of patients.

First aid or emergency care is that given a victim of an accident. Training in first aid measures has demonstrated that effective care will be given more promptly at the time of the accident, and the person familiar with first aid care will be less likely to have accidents himself.

Immediate and effective care at the time of an accident has resulted in saving many lives and in reducing complications following accidents. The state of Illinois has gained national acclaim, for example, on its statewide emergency care system that has reportedly improved greatly the chances of saving lives and reducing the frequency of complications following injury.

First aid and emergency care are an important part of the nurse's education. As a responsible member of the health team, she is expected to be able to assist effectively during emergency situations.

PROVISIONS FOR COMFORT

Comfort measures in the environment are not only desirable in themselves but also may be closely associated with safety measures, for example adequate lighting. The comfort measures discussed here apply to the home as well as to the health agency.

Decor

It is no longer considered necessary for a health agency room to be bare and "sterile-looking." White walls and white equipment are being replaced by more colorful furnishings and tastefully decorated walls. However, there is still need for careful planning in the use of color and design. It is best to use combinations that are attractive in an unobtrusive way, because unusual decor may appeal to relatively few people.

It has been found to be unsatisfactory to use wallpaper with a distinct design such as large flowers in rooms serving the ill. Some patients have been disturbed by design, seeing faces and other objects in them. Pictures, bedspreads, and curtains may have the same effect if not selected carefully. Color in ceiling coverings can be pleasant for patients who are confined to long periods on their backs.

Considerable attention also is being given to floor coverings. The cold, bare look is being replaced with attractive coverings. These, too, must be selected with care since parallel lines, tiny squares, and some geometric designs cause some persons to feel dizzy when they look at them. Floor coverings should be able to withstand frequent cleaning. The floor is considered highly contaminated, and hence, solutions with germicidal properties are commonly used for routine floor cleaning.

In recent years carpeting has become more popular in hospitals. Patients and personnel in general find it aesthetically pleasing and comfortable. While opinions vary, many experts tend to believe that carpeting can be cleansed sufficiently so as to eliminate the danger of its becoming a haven for microorganisms.

Lighting

Good lighting is lighting that is adequate for persons to see clearly and without strain for the task at hand. It should be without glare and produce a minimum of shadowing. Good lighting, both natural and artificial, is important for patients and workers. While it is true that the nurse cannot alter windows or some lighting fixtures, certain modifications can often be made. Light bulbs, shades, or lamps can be changed with relative ease.

Adequate lighting for work and reading is essential for the preservation of sight. Lighting has also been observed to affect mood. Some lighting not only helps a person to feel cheerful, it also helps him look better. Other types of lighting, particularly "daylight" fluorescent bulbs, can do the reverse. Many architects use large, almost full-length windows that can be shaded as required for both home and health agencies. In addition to providing much more natural light, they make it more pleasant for patients who enjoy looking out-of-doors.

Usually health personnel need more light to work effectively than do the patients. The glare from overhead lights or from windows that do not have shades partially drawn and the reflection from light objects such as white uniforms and bed linen can become uncomfortable for the worker as well as the patient. Older patients are particularly disturbed by lighting irregularities. While diffuse light in the room may be easier for personnel, it still may not be appropriate for the patient if he wishes to read. The light may be coming from such an undesirable angle that it is almost impossible for the patient to see comfortably close at hand. Ideally, a light at the patient's bed should be sufficiently adjustable so that it can serve the patient and also be used by health personnel when needed for treatment of the patient.

A dim light is valuable as a comfort and a safety measure at night both in homes and in health agencies. The light should be situated so that it does not shine into the patient's eyes, no matter in what position he may wish to sleep. It should give sufficient lighting to the floor around the bed so that if the patient wishes to get up, he can do so with safety. Elderly persons are in particular need of some light at night, since this helps them to orient themselves should they awaken and be confused as to their whereabouts.

Temperature, Humidity, and Ventilation

Most well people are comfortable in a temperature range of 68°F. to 74°F. and with a humidity range of 30 to 60 percent. When the humidity is low, the rate at which body moisture evaporates is increased, and hence, a higher environmental temperature is comfortable. Comfort is also influenced by a person's activity, age, and physical condition. For example, very young, older, sedentary, and ill persons tend to be more comfortable when environmental temperatures are in the high average range.

Most modern health agencies and many homes have air conditioning that maintains comfortable temperatures and humidity. In climates or buildings in which the humidity is very low, humidifiers are often used. Steam from boiling water will accomplish the same objective. When humidity is very high, dehumidifiers are available that remove excess moisture from the air.

Ventilation can be maintained with relative ease when the climate is temperate and when air conditioners are used. Air exchange is especially important when there are many persons in one room or when one person is in a relatively small room for prolonged periods of time. Ventilation is also important when there are odorous or toxic substances in the air. Attention to the patient's covering and clothing is necessary when ventilation creates drafts, especially to older persons who tend to be sensitive to drafts.

Furnishings

Furnishings commonly used in health agencies is often as attractive as any for the home. A trend which makes it more comfortable and safe for patients is to furnish units according to the type of care required by the patient. For example, self-care units for the ambulatory patient have low beds, desks, comfortable chairs and reading lamps, television sets, and other homelike items. Nurses may be required to help arrange a functional unit in the home. This can be a challenge when it involves using the available furniture so as not to incur additional expenses. Both the patient's problems and the family's activities have to be considered in such planning.

Modern health facilities are planned with an eye

for efficiency, orderliness, and cleanliness—all certainly worthwhile objectives. However, one questions whether furniture has to be firmly placed so that, as one hospitalized patient stated, "From my bed I could see only the midriff of a telephone pole through a window. I later learned that it overlooked a beautifully landscaped area." A little ingenuity at home or in a health care facility can usually result in a furniture arrangement which is both convenient and pleasant.

BED: Design of the patient's bed is often a critical factor in his care. For the convenience of health personnel caring for the patient, health agencies have beds that are considerably higher than those found in the home. Early ambulation and encouragement of patients in self-care activities have led health agencies to purchase beds that can be lowered easily so that the patient can get in and out of bed more safely. If the height of the bed is not adjustable, a step stool should be provided for the patient's use. If a patient is to remain in bed for a long period of time at home, a hospital bed may be bought or rented; or a bed can be raised on solid objects such as blocks of wood, for the convenience of those caring for him.

Most health agency beds have an adjustable headrest capable of being raised or lowered electrically or by means of a hand crank. The patient's knees may be flexed by means of another mechanism. The entire lower portion of the bed also may be raised so that both legs may be elevated at the same time. Many beds for home use also now have electrically operated mechanisms that raise or lower the upper and lower portions of the bed.

Most health agency beds are constructed with small wheels, usually with locks on them to prevent unintentional rolling. Some agencies transport patients in their beds to other departments, eliminating the need for stretchers.

MATTRESS: There is no one type of mattress recognized as being best for all situations and circumstances. A good mattress adjusts to body contours to the degree that it permits good alignment. A "soft" mattress which permits the body to sag at points of heaviest weight is not conducive to rest; in fact, such a mattress may cause fatigue and backache. If springs are a part of the mattress, they should be of superior construction and strength so that they will not break or lose their resilience easily. Broken springs are uncomfortable for the patient.

The covering of the mattress should be a quality material that will not tear easily or separate at the seams. It is not general practice to sterilize a mattress after each patient use. Since mattresses have filling,

like horsehair, cotton, or kapok, it is best to keep the mattress protected.

Mattresses with plasticized covering or plastic covers are also in use. Contamination of the mattress filling is reduced, and the mattress may be cleaned after use by washing. However, plastic covers have a disadvantage in that the smooth surface causes the linens to slip, especially when the head of the bed is elevated, and a contour sheet is not used.

A type of mattress on the market has a coil spring and a two-piece zippered cover. According to manufacturers' claims, the cover can be laundered or sterilized—an important factor in infection control. It is also waterproof and fire-retardant.

Foam rubber mattresses are useful in situations where pressure from a more rigid mattress may be harmful to the patient.

PILLOWS: Pillows are usually filled with feathers, horsehair, or kapok. Foam rubber pillows are in limited use, except by some persons who have allergies. A disadvantage is that they cannot be molded as easily as other pillows. Another disadvantage is that the rubber pillow, like the rubber mattress, is inclined to absorb and retain body heat.

In addition to the comfort that most persons derive from having a pillow under the head, pillows are extremely valuable in maintaining good posture for the bed patient. That is why variation in pillow sizes and type of filling is desirable.

Since pillows are used for all areas of the body for support and comfort, it is important that they be protected when there is a possibility of their becoming contaminated by secretions or drainage.

OVERBED TABLE: An overbed table is a great convenience, especially for the bedridden patient. It enables him to eat, read, write, or work more comfortably. The overbed table also makes it possible for him to change his position by leaning forward and resting on it. It has conveniences for the nurse during the administration of care also. The type of overbed table which is supported by a wide foot piece that fits under the bed and has only one post has advantages when bed siderails are in place or when other cumbersome equipment is being used at the bedside. Most overbed tables are designed so that they can be lowered for the patient while he is in a chair and tilted to support a newspaper or a book. Some have mirrors underneath the tilt portion for use when patients comb their hair, shave, or apply make-up. Some also have space for storage of items such as make-up or shaving materials.

Small bed tables placed directly in the bed over the patient's thighs are used in some instances. They are less expensive and particularly helpful in the home. In the care of children who are in cribs, such bed tables are very practical and useful.

BEDSIDE STAND: In most health agencies, a bedside table for storing patient care equipment and personal items is provided. Tables designed without doors require less space than stands with doors. If the stand has three closed sides, the opened end of the table should be designed to be out of sight. The patient is able to manage the stand easily if it is mounted on wheels. A drawer in the table usually is used by the patient for his personal possessions; therefore, it should be placed so that it opens toward his bed. Most stands have provisions for towels and a washcloth to hang on a rod.

There are additions which may be found on some stands such as a hook for the patient's urinal, a paper-bag frame and a "catchall" which a patient may use for various purposes, such as holding occupational therapy projects, newspapers, or magazines.

The bedridden patient at home finds a bedside table a great convenience also.

LAMPS: Floor lamps and bed lamps are a part of most patient units. The lamps should be so arranged that the patient can control them by himself. As mentioned previously, light intensity should vary with the work or the activity of the user. A lamp that has more than one bulb or a three-way light bulb is ideal, since proper intensity is more likely to be obtained.

CHAIRS: Usually, a chair is included as an integral part of the patient's immediate environment. A straight chair with good arm and back support usually is comfortable for the majority of patients. Leg heights of a chair can be managed for the very short patient by placing some suitable object underneath his feet.

Generally, chairs with arms are more comfortable for the patient, but it is also desirable to have chairs without arms available because they are more suitable when a patient must be lifted out of a bed into a chair. The arms do not get in the way of those lifting.

An upholstered chair has disadvantages for older patients and for patients who have some limitation of movement, because more effort is required to raise oneself out of it.

Personal Care Items

The following are basic personal care items: basin, soap dish, mouthwash cup, emesis basin, bedpan, a urinal for the male patient, and a water container and drinking glass.

Manufacturers provide wide selections of equipment for personal care that are both attractive and safe to use. Disposable equipment is available in increasing varieties. This is an important factor in infection control. These disposable items also greatly reduce the work load of cleaning and sterilizing. If only nondisposable care items are available, sterilization between use by different patients is recommended.

Privacy and Quiet

Anyone who is being interviewed, examined, or cared for deserves and appreciates the comfort of privacy. It is very easy for nurses and for others to feel that anything routine to them is also accepted as routine by the patient. Many patients are reluctant to protest the lack of privacy. Persons caring for patients, whether in a clinic, an office, a home, or a hospital, should try to provide as much privacy as possible. They will also wish to be well aware of the legal implications of invasion of privacy, as discussed in Chapter 4.

These are some of the noises that patients complain about most frequently: careless handling of equipment in service areas and of dishes and trays on serving carts and in the kitchen; loud talking on the telephone, in the nurses' station, and during rounds; calling down the corridors; talking by visitors who gather near patients or in the corridors; loud radios, television, and the call system. Many if not all of these noises can be controlled to a great extent, but it takes constant awareness on the part of the nurse to see that they are.

There are various ways to decrease the problems associated with noise. Many buildings use acoustic materials on walls, ceilings, and floors. Carpeting, wall hangings, and draperies absorb noise. Many health agencies have found that special efforts to remind people of ways to reduce noise have been helpful. Considerable ingenuity has gone into designing posters and signs for use in health agency corridors and waiting rooms to help reduce noise.

Quiet background music has been shown to have a calming effect. Many health agencies use piped in music with good results.

The nurse should consider noise factors when planning care since environmental noise can work for or against the patient's well-being.

PROVISIONS FOR EASE IN ACCOMPLISHING COMMON ACTIVITIES OF DAILY LIVING

Using environmental resources is important to promote maximum mobility and independence—

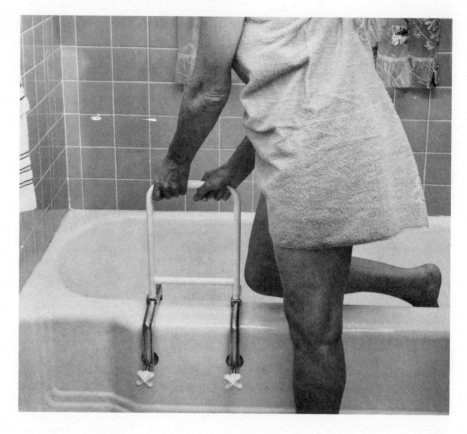

Fig. 18-5. An aid which helps the patient to get into and out of the bathtub offers considerable security to the aged or the physically limited patient. (Bollen Products Co., East Cleveland, Ohio)

for example, for the young who are still learning how to become independent; for the elderly and handicapped who may have to learn new skills to replace those they no longer have; and for the ill who are being helped to a state of wellness. Here are some examples of measures nurses have found helpful when patients are learning to develop, regain, or maintain independence.

For patients required to remain in bed, an overhead trapeze enables them to move about in bed with relative ease. It is a helpful device to assist in toileting, changing linen, and eating, and for providing exercise.

Most health agencies are now constructed to accommodate patients who use wheelchairs, canes, crutches, and braces. Ramps and elevators have already been mentioned. Wide doorways and halls to accommodate wheelchairs also are important. For patients in the home using similar aids to mobility, it is recommended that adjustments be made to accommodate the patient to the extent that it is possible. For example, in many instances, ramps can be built that eliminate steps. Elevator chairs can now be installed in homes for those who cannot use stairways.

Any aid that keeps a patient mobile usually also helps him to remain independent.

Environmental aids to facilitate social interaction are desirable. For example, having the space and comfortable chairs for people to enjoy each other's company helps in meeting a patient's psychosocial needs. The bedridden patient at home may be in a living room or some area where he can more easily participate in family matters and offer his contributions as far as is possible.

The nurse will wish to be aware of environmental factors that promote ease and independence in the management of personal hygiene. Devices such as shower heads that can be adjusted to various levels, tub chairs, foot basins, handrails, and supports on tubs are all helpful. Figure 18-5 illustrates a good device that makes bathing possible and safe for certain patients.

Readily available facilities and space for recreational and occupational activities are discussed earlier. Using such facilities, both in health agencies and in the home, tends to promote mobility as well as offer activity that stimulates the patient mentally and physically. It has been observed that even infants respond to environmental stimulation favorably. Colored mobiles, recorded voices of mother, swings to change the baby's position in his crib, and much holding and cuddling, for example, have been found stimulating for even the tiniest patients.

Environmental factors that maintain independence in relation to elimination are recommended. For example, it is helpful to have appropriately sized toilet facilities for children or a step stool and a removable child's seat to facilitate comfort and safety. Handbars help a patient to move himself from a wheelchair to a toilet.

Many other ways of using the patient's physical environment to promote his independence could be cited. The reader may wish to add examples from her own experience. From the accounts of health practitioners and patients, provisions that help the patient in accomplishing activities of daily living for himself promote well-being and high-level wellness.

CONCLUSION

The patient's immediate environment can either promote or hinder well-being. To assist the patient most effectively, the nurse will wish to make whatever provisions she can to provide a safe and comfortable environment and one that promotes optimum independence for the patient. There will be times when ingenuity is required to overcome problems related to undesirable factors in the patient's environment. However, nursing care is incomplete and less than professional when environmental factors are ignored.

Study Situations

1. The following article discusses examples of environmental aids that can be used easily in the home and clinic for ease of caring for the elderly patient. How many of them are or could be used in situations where you see older patients?
   Schwartz, D.: Problems of self-care and travel among elderly ambulatory patients. **Am. J. Nurs.,** 66:2678–2681, Dec., 1966.
2. The legal responsibility of nurses to provide for the safety of patients is discussed in Chapter 4. Read the following articles and consider the environmental hazards for these patients. Can you think of ways, in addition to those described, by which these patients might have been better protected?
   Hershey, N.: The patient doesn't always win. **Am. J. Nurs.,** 71:967–969, May, 1971.

Hershey, N.: Safety of the difficult patient. **Am. J. Nurs.,** 71:1766–1767, Sept., 1971.
3. The author of the following article reported that 315 persons are killed and 140,000 are injured daily in the United States. Read the article to see what he means by a "management approach" to accident prevention. What role can nurses play in this?
   Schaplowsky, A. F.: Community injury control—a management approach. **Am. J. Public Health,** 63:252–254, Mar., 1973.
4. The following article discusses some of the common potential dangers in the hospital environment. After reading the article, investigate a hospital where you have had clinical experience and see how the hospital controls these hazards.
   Wilkinson, T. K.: Control of physical and chemical agents. **Hospitals,** 46:95–102, Oct. 16, 1972.
5. Many environmental factors influence us daily. The following two references discuss the effects of color and noise on patients. After reading the articles, list ways you could use color and sound as more positive influences in your nursing care.
   Bartholet, M. N.: Effects of color on the dynamics of patient care. **Nurs. Outlook,** 16:51–53, Oct., 1968.
   Haslam, P.: Noise in hospitals: its effect on the patient. In **The Nursing Clinics of North America.** Philadelphia, W. B. Saunders, 5:715–724, Dec., 1970.
6. There are periodicals concerned with hospitals, their structure, furnishings, and services. Browsing through them will be valuable for the nurse to see what is new, what changes other agencies are making, and the effect that some of the new items or proposed changes might have on patient care.
   Look through recent issues of the periodicals listed below for evidence of trends in furnishings, equipment, and so on. Note also how authors and advertisers stress safety factors in the patient environment.
   Hospitals, Journal of the
       American Hospital Association
   The Modern Hospital
   Hospital Topics
   Hospital Management
7. Consider the immediate environment of the next patient with whom you have contact. Using the data-gathering guidelines from Chapter 6, collect information about his environment in relation to space, safety, comfort, and ease of carrying out his activities of daily living. After you have gathered and validated the data, indicate whether or not his environment promotes high-level wellness.

References

1. Allain-Regnault, M.: The decibel inferno. **World Health,** pp. 12–15, May, 1972.
2. Amburgey, P. I.: Environmental aids for the aged patient. **Am. J. Nurs.,** 66:2017–2018, Sept., 1966.

3. Bloch, D.: Privacy. *In* Carlson, C. E., coordinator: Behavioral Concepts and Nursing Intervention. pp. 251–267. Philadelphia, J. B. Lippincott, 1970.

4. Boucher, M. L.: Personal space and chronicity in the mental hospital. **Perspect. Psychiat. Care,** 9:206–210, Sept.–Oct., 1971.

5. Brown, E. L.: Newer Dimensions of Patient Care: Part 1: The Use of the Physical and Social Environment of the General Hospital for Therapeutic Purposes. New York, Russell Sage Foundation, 1961.

6. Burns, W.: Noise and Man. pp. 99–205. London, John Murray, 1968.

7. Carnevali, D., and Brueckner, S.: Immobilization —reassessment of a concept. **Am. J. Nurs.,** 70:1502–1507, July, 1970.

8. Davis, A. J.: Micro-ecology: interactional dimensions of space. **J. Psychiat. Nurs. and Mental Health,** 10:19–21, Jan.–Feb., 1972.

9. Feerick, J. P.: Fire! What do you do first? **Am. J. Nurs.,** 70:2578–2580, Dec., 1970.

10. Fischer, V. G., and Connolly, A. F.: Promotion of Physical Comfort and Safety. Dubuque, Ia., William C. Brown, 1970.

11. Freeman, R. B.: Community Health Nursing Practice. pp. 325–342. Philadelphia, W. B. Saunders, 1970.

12. Gilbert, G.: Electrical hazards in the use of monitors and defibrillators. *In* **The Nursing Clinics of North America.** Philadelphia, W. B. Saunders, 4:615–619, Dec., 1969.

13. Hagerman, C. W., and Moore, V B.: Handbook of bed positions and guide to electrically operated beds. **Nurs. '72,** 2:19–26, Mar., 1972.

14. Hall, E. T.: The Hidden Dimension. Garden City, N.Y., Doubleday, 1966.

15. Hall, E. T.: The Silent Language, pp. 187–209. Garden City, N.Y., Doubleday, 1959.

16 Henley, E. S.: *et al.*: Fire protection systems tested. **Hospitals, J. Am. Hosp. Assoc.,** 47:69–75, Jan. 1, 1973.

17. How electricity comes, goes, and wanders. **RN,** 35:41–42, June, 1972.

18. Hymovich, D. P.: ABC's of pediatric safety. **Am. J. Nurs.,** 66:1768–1770, Aug., 1966.

19. Kamenetz, H. L.: Selecting a wheelchair. **Am. J. Nurs.,** 72:100–101, Jan., 1972.

20. McGuire, M. C.: Preventive measures to minimize accidents among the elderly. **Occup. Health Nurs.,** 19:13–18, Apr., 1971.

21. Miller, R. R., and Johnson, S. R.: Poison control now and in the future. **Am. J. Nurs.,** 66, Sept., 1966.

22. Newman, D. S.: The role of the occupational health nurse in epidemiologic research and education. *In* **The Nursing Clinics of North America.** Philadelphia, W. B. Saunders, 7:153–162, Mar., 1972.

23. Ornstein, S.: A nursing home is not a hospital. **Nurs. Outlook,** 21:28–31, Jan., 1973.

24. Pluckhan, M. L.: Space: the silent language . . . **Nurs. Forum,** 7:386–397, No. 4, 1968.

25. Reed, A. J.: Lead poisoning—silent epidemic and social crime. **Am. J. Nurs.,** 72:2180–2184, Dec., 1972.

26. Rockwell, S. M.: Electricity: it doesn't need to be a problem. **RN,** 35:35–40, June, 1972.

27. Schwartz, B.: The social psychology of privacy. **Am. J. Sociology,** 73:741–752, May, 1968.

28. Skellenger, W. S.: Treatment of poisoning in children. **Am. J. Nurs.,** 65:108–112, Nov., 1965.

29. Snook, I. D., Jr.: Noise that annoys. **Nurs. Outlook,** 12:33–35, July, 1964.

30. Sommer, R.: Studies in personal space. **Sociometry,** 22:247–260, Sept., 1959.

31. Sovie, M. D., and Fruehan, C. T.: Protecting the patient from electrical hazards. *In* **The Nursing Clinics of North America.** Philadelphia, W. B. Saunders, 7:469–480, Sept., 1972.

32. Streufert, H., and Streufert, C.: How color affects patients' responses. **Hosp. Progr.,** 51:28–34, Apr., 1970.

33. Trought, E. A.: Equipment hazards. **Am. J. Nurs.,** 73:858–862, May, 1973.

34. Westaby, J. R.: *et al.*: Integrating accident prevention in total patient care. **Nurs. Outlook,** 11:600–603, Aug., 1963.

CHAPTER 19

Infection Control

GLOSSARY

Antiseptic: Substance that inhibits the growth of bacteria.

Asepsis: Absence of disease-producing microorganisms.

Bactericidal Agent: Substance capable of destroying bacteria but not their spores.

Bacteriostatic Agent: Substance that prevents the growth of bacteria.

Blood Isolation: Practices to prevent the transmission of pathogens by contact with blood.

Carrier: A person or animal who is without signs of illness but who has pathogens on or within his body which can be transferred to others.

Clean Technique: Synonym for medical asepsis.

Communicable Disease Technique: Synonym for isolation technique.

Concurrent Disinfection: Ongoing practices which are observed in the care of a patient to limit or control a pathogenic organism.

Contagious Disease: A disease conveyed easily to others.

Contamination: Process by which something is rendered unclean or unsterile.

Discharge Isolation: Practices to prevent the transmission of pathogens by direct contact with body secretions.

Disinfectant: Substance used to destroy pathogens.

Disinfection: Process by which pathogens but not spores are destroyed.

Enteric Isolation: Practices to prevent transmission of pathogens through contact with fecal matter.

Entry Portal: Entry route for microorganisms into new host.

Fungicide: Substance that kills fungi.

Germicide: Synonym for bactericide.

Host: Animal or person upon which or within which microorganisms live.

Infection: Disease state resulting from pathogens in or on the body.

Isolation Technique: Practices to prevent transfer of microorganisms. Also called communicable disease technique.

Medical Asepsis: Practices to reduce the number and transfer of pathogens. Also referred to as clean technique.

Nonpathogen: Microorganism which does not normally cause disease.

Nosocomial Infection: A hospital-acquired infection.

Pathogen: Disease-producing microorganism.

Physical Sterilization and Disinfection: Use of heat to achieve sterilization and disinfection.

Protective Isolation: Practices to prevent contact between potential pathogens and a highly susceptible person.

Reservoir: Natural habitat for growth and multiplication of a microorganism.

Resident Flora or Bacteria: Microorganisms that normally live on the skin of an individual.

Respiratory Isolation: Practices to prevent the transmission of pathogens by droplet or droplet nuclei.

Reverse Isolation: Synonym for protective isolation.

Sterile Technique: Synonym for surgical asepsis.

Sterilization: Process by which all microorganisms, including spores, are destroyed.

Strict Isolation: Practices to prevent transmission of highly communicable diseases spread by contact and airborne routes.

Surgical Asepsis: Practices that render and keep objects and areas free from all microorganisms.

Susceptibility: Degree of resistance of host to a pathogen.

Terminal Disinfection: Practices used in caring for a patient's environment and belongings after his illness is no longer communicable.

Transient Flora or Bacteria: Microorganisms picked up on skin as a result of normal activities and that can be removed readily.

Virucide: Substance that kills viruses.

Wound and Skin Isolation: Practices to prevent transmission of pathogens by direct contact with wounds.

INTRODUCTION

Microorganisms are naturally present in the environment. Some of these organisms are beneficial and some are not. Some are harmless to most people and others are harmful to many persons. Still others are harmless except in certain circumstances.

The efforts of many persons are involved in maintaining a microorganism-safe environment. Governmental agencies at the international, national, state, and local levels, health personnel, citizens from every walk of life, and family members are all involved in making and keeping the environment as free from harmful organisms as possible. Such efforts include mass immunization programs; laws concerning safe sewage disposal; regulations for the control of certain communicable diseases such as tuberculosis, hepatitis, and venereal diseases; hospital infection surveillance programs; and so on.

STERILIZATION AND DISINFECTION

Definitions

Asepsis is the absence of disease-producing microorganisms, called *pathogens*. *Nonpathogens,* constantly present in the environment or on the host, are microorganisms that do not normally cause disease. The *host* is an animal or a person upon which or within which microorganisms live.

Asepsis generally is divided into two descriptive forms: medical asepsis and surgical asepsis. Concepts of medical and surgical asepsis and related terms as used in this text are based on the following definitions.

Medical asepsis refers to practices which help to reduce the number and hinder the transfer of disease-producing microorganisms from one person or place to another. These practices are sometimes referred to as *clean technique.* The reason for observing medical aseptic practices is that there are always microorganisms in the environment which in some individuals and under certain circumstances can cause illness. Therefore, reducing their number and hindering their transfer increase the safety of the environment. Any number of methods may be used to help to achieve this aim: dusting, vacuuming, washing, boiling, sterilizing, and disinfecting are a few examples.

Generally speaking, medical asepsis practices are followed at all times because it is assumed that pathogens are likely to be present, the exact kind being undetermined. For example, public drinking cups are unsanitary, because pathogens may be present on the cup after use by someone harboring the organisms. On the other hand, there are times when a specific pathogen is known to be present in the environment; for instance, the German measles virus is known to be present in and on the patient having the disease, and also in his environment. In such instances, additional precautions are taken to prevent further spread of this particular organism, a procedure generally referred to as *isolation or communicable disease technique.* Isolation technique includes the use of specific measures related to the way the microorganism is transmitted and to ordinary medical aseptic practices. An example of a specific measure is the use of a gown worn by personnel caring for the patient. Isolation technique is discussed more fully later in this chapter.

Surgical asepsis refers to practices which render and keep objects and areas free from *all* microorganisms. These practices are also referred to as *sterile technique.* Surgical asepsis is concerned with the handling of objects and areas which must be kept sterile. It is used extensively in operating and delivery rooms. For example, the sterile gown and the sterile gloves that the surgeon wears during an operation protect the patient from being contaminated by the surgeon; the forceps used in handling sterile dressings protect the patient from contamination by the fingers.

Contamination refers to the process by which something is rendered unclean or unsterile. In medical asepsis, areas are considered to be contaminated if they bear, or are suspected of bearing, pathogens. In surgical asepsis, areas are considered to be contaminated if they are touched by *any* object which is not also sterile. In medical asepsis, the gown worn by the nurse or the coverall apron worn by a mother when caring for a child who has measles is to protect the nurse and the mother from contamination by the child.

Disinfection is the process by which pathogenic organisms, but not their spores, are destroyed. A *disinfectant* is a substance used to destroy pathogens. It is not usually intended to be used for destroying pathogens in or on the living person.

An *antiseptic* is a substance which inhibits the growth of bacteria. Certain antiseptics can be used safely on the living person.

A *bacteriostatic agent* prevents the growth of bacteria. A *bactericidal agent* is one that is capable of destroying bacteria but not their spores. The term *germicide* is used interchangeably with bactericide. A *fungicide* kills fungi, and a *virucide* inactivates viruses.

Sterilization refers to the process by which all

microorganisms, including spores, are destroyed. It usually refers to methods involving the use of heat, such as boiling, steam under pressure, and dry heat, but chemicals and germicidal gases may be used also. Chemical methods of sterilization are not considered as reliable as physical methods.

While sterilization is an integral part of surgical asepsis, there are innumerable instances when it is also an integral part of medical asepsis. When working against unknown pathogens, there are occasions when it is best to use measures which can be relied on to destroy all microorganisms in order to be safe. For example, in the hospital, personal-care items which are reused by patients are sterilized by boiling or steam under pressure before being offered to another patient. It is possible that the items could be made safe by washing with soap and water and rinsing well. However, since the exact nature of the contaminants is not known, it is safer to use additional precautionary measures.

One of the most important things to remember about surgical or medical asepsis is that their effectiveness is dependent on the faithfulness and the conscientiousness of those carrying them out. The failure to be exact and meticulous cannot be detected in many instances. For example, an article such as a glass, a comb, a syringe, or a needle can be cleaned superficially or not even disinfected, and no one except the person responsible would really know.

Handling and Caring for Supplies and Equipment

CENTRAL SUPPLY UNITS: Most larger health care facilities in the United States maintain a central supply unit where a major portion of the equipment used in patient care is cleansed, kept in good working order, and sterilized. Safety measures for the patient have increased as hospitals have found it economically feasible to centrally purchase, care for, and distribute equipment and supplies. More nursing time is available for patient care when responsibility for cleaning and sterilizing equipment and for preparing trays for procedures, as well as purchasing and distributing supplies, has been delegated to personnel in central supply units. Also, equipment usually receives better care from persons especially taught and employed to care for it.

DISPOSABLE EQUIPMENT: In recent years, health agencies have been using more disposable items that are sterile and ready for use. Certain items such as syringes, needles, instruments for changing dressings, and linens are used only once and then discarded. Other items such as bedpans may be used repeatedly but by one patient only and then dis-

carded upon his discharge. Almost monthly, hospital periodicals report new disposable equipment as it appears on the market. The use of such equipment has not only greatly decreased the amount of time involved in cleaning, repairing, and sterilizing equipment but has also reduced problems in relation to cross-transmission infections. Regardless of whether equipment is sterilized by the agency or sterile when purchased, the responsibility for assuring and maintaining its sterility through proper storage and appropriate checks rests with the agency personnel. Widespread use of disposable supplies in recent years, however, has created one problem, that is, the disposing of these supplies after use. Many agency administrators continue to work on ways to dispose of the tons of solid wastes that accumulate each year.

Trends toward the development of central supply units and the manufacturing of disposable items have changed many responsibilities once assumed by nurses. However, in some situations such as small clinics, offices, and homes, nurses are responsible for the care, disinfection, and sterilization of equipment and supplies or for teaching others to do so. Therefore, it remains important for the nurse to have a good knowledge of sterilization and disinfection techniques.

Procedures for sterilizing and disinfecting equipment and supplies are based largely on principles of microbiology. Certain of those which affect the choice of sterilization and disinfection procedures will be reviewed briefly.

The Selection of Sterilization and Disinfection Methods

NATURE OF ORGANISMS PRESENT: Some microorganisms are destroyed with considerable ease, while others are able to withstand certain commonly used sterilization and disinfection techniques. The tubercle bacillus is an example of an organism that is relatively resistant to most disinfection processes, especially by chemical means. The gonococcus and meningococcus are examples of very fragile organisms that are susceptible to common means of destruction. Bacterial spores are particularly resistant and can withstand many germicides that readily destroy other types of organisms.

Although not a great deal is known about transferring viruses by means of contaminated supplies and equipment, there are two notable exceptions: it is agreed generally that homologous serum hepatitis and infectious hepatitis viruses can be spread by contaminated needles and syringes. The organisms causing the diseases can be spread with such ease that a simple prick of the skin with a contaminated needle may result in illness. Studies indicate also that the viruses causing these conditions are destroyed with certainty only by autoclaving (steam under pressure).

If the nature of the organisms on equipment and supplies is known, the selection of a safe sterilization or disinfection procedure becomes relatively easy. Unfortunately, however, in most situations where many patients with various illnesses are being cared for, the nature of organisms contaminating equipment and supplies frequently is unknown; and it would be an exceedingly difficult and impractical procedure to determine the nature of all contaminating organisms present. Therefore, when medical asepsis is being practiced, the safest method is one that can be assumed to be capable of destroying the pathogenic microorganisms. If surgical asepsis is being practiced, the only safe procedure is one that has been proved capable of destroying all organisms, regardless of their nature. It is unwise to decrease the period of time that has been considered safe for sterilizing or disinfecting equipment and supplies on the assumption that the contaminating organisms present are destroyed easily. *Time* is a key factor in sterilization or in disinfection. Anyone who fails to allow sufficient time for sterilization or disinfection is guilty of gross negligence!

In the home, where the nature of contaminating organisms occasionally may be ascertained with some certainty and where the patient may have developed immunities to certain organisms commonly found in his environment, sterilization and disinfection procedures can be modified more safely than they can in a health agency.

NUMBER OF ORGANISMS PRESENT: The more organisms that are present on an article, the longer it takes to destroy them. For example, an instrument that is contaminated with relatively few organisms can be rendered sterile more quickly than one contaminated with large numbers of organisms. If organisms are protected by coagulated proteins or harbor under a layer of grease or oil, it will also take longer to sterilize or disinfect the article. Articles that are cleansed thoroughly prior to sterilization or disinfection therefore will be made sterile or clean more easily and more quickly than an article that has not been cleansed.

Bacteriologists have found that bacteria exposed to sterilization procedures die in a uniform and consistent manner. The rate of death has been found to be governed by definite laws, so that computation of death rates of bacteria is possible. Theoretically, 90 percent of the bacteria are killed each minute of exposure. Table 19-1 illustrates a theoretical example of the order of death of a bacterial population; the order of death is said to be logarithmic in nature.

Knowledge of bacterial death has important practical implications, and some bacteriologists maintain that this knowledge is applicable for heat sterilization, chemical disinfection, and pasteurization.

TYPE OF EQUIPMENT: Equipment with small lumens, crevices, or joints that are difficult to cleanse and to expose requires special care. For example, if catheters are being placed in a chemical solution, disinfection will be ineffectual if the solution does not fill the lumen of the catheters. It also must be kept in mind that certain pieces of equipment are destroyed by various sterilization and disinfection methods. For example, certain chemical solutions will dull the cutting edge of a knife blade. In using any disinfectant for such a purpose, the student should read the directions carefully. Most common sterilization and

TABLE 19-1: Theoretical example of the order of death of a bacterial population *

Minute	Bacteria living at beginning of new minute	Bacteria killed in 1 minute		Bacteria surviving at end of 1 minute
First	1,000,000	90% =	900,000	100,000
Second	100,000	=	90,000	10,000
Third	10,000	=	9,000	1,000
Fourth	1,000	=	900	100
Fifth	100	=	90	10
Sixth	10	=	9	1
Seventh	1	=	0.9	0.1
Eighth	0.1	=	0.09	0.01
Ninth	0.01	=	0.009	0.001
Tenth	0.001	=	0.0009	0.0001
Eleventh	0.0001	=	0.00009	0.00001
Twelfth	0.00001	=	0.000009	0.000001

* From Perkins, J. J.: Principles and Methods of Sterilization. p. 35. Springfield, Ill., Thomas, 1956.

disinfection methods will ruin lens mountings in instruments such as cystoscopes. Such equipment requires special handling in order to keep it in good condition.

INTENDED USE OF EQUIPMENT: If equipment and supplies are being used when medical asepsis is practiced, it is sufficiently safe for them to be free of pathogenic organisms. But when surgical asepsis is required, equipment and supplies must be free of *all* organisms. Therefore, the intended use of equipment and supplies will influence the selection of a particular procedure for rendering the equipment safe.

In most health care agencies today, in order to insure safety for the patient, almost all articles used for patient care are sterilized prior to use. The nature of contamination is not always certain, as has been pointed out, and, even though in some instances it may be safe to use equipment that is clean, most agencies follow a policy of using, whenever possible, only sterilized equipment and supplies for patient care.

AVAILABLE MEANS FOR STERILIZATION AND DISINFECTION: Sterilization and disinfection may be accomplished by several methods. Chemical sterilization (or disinfection) is accomplished by using solutions or gases (vapors) that destroy bacteria by chemical processes. Physical sterilization (or disinfection) usually is accomplished by the use of dry or moist heat.

Within recent years cold sterilization and disinfection through the use of ionization radiation have been investigated, but the extent to which they can be used has not yet been determined thoroughly. While considerable and encouraging advances have been made in this field, especially since World War II, much research remains to be done. Sterilizing by ionizing radiation holds great promise for the cold sterilization of heat-resistant pharmaceuticals and foods.

Ultraviolet radiation has been found to have germicidal results. It can be used as an effective agent for disinfecting indoor air and working surfaces. Ultraviolet irradiation has been especially recommended as an additive to operating room technique. It also has been used for disinfecting working counters in laboratories, hospital rooms, and elevators. Sunlight is a good and inexpensive source of ultraviolet rays, especially for use in home situations.

Chemical Means for Sterilization and Disinfection

Chemical sterilization employs liquid solutions or gases. Objects to be sterilized are immersed in a solution or exposed to fumes in a chamber or oven

for a specified period of time. Various studies have found serious shortcomings in the use of chemicals for sterilizing purposes. In fact, some authorities state that no chemical solution can be considered completely safe for sterilization. Hence, their use ordinarily is limited to items that are heat-labile or to situations where a more reliable method is not available.

A chemical commonly used for sterilization is ethylene oxide gas. The gas destroys microorganisms by interfering with metabolic processes in cells and it has been found to effect lethal action on spores as well as vegetative cells. Optimal action can be attained at relatively low temperatures (130° to 150° F.) when humidity in the sterilizer is held between approximately 30 to 60 percent. Its penetrating qualities are excellent. Although heat is a reliable and economical sterilizing agent, ethylene oxide has been found by institutions using it to be excellent for any heat-labile item, including rubber, plastic, and paper.

Chemical disinfectants on the market are numerous and new ones are added almost daily. One must be especially careful with substances sold as "all-purpose" disinfectants for home use. Before depending on advertisements, one should be certain that the solution has been adequately tested and is recommended for its safety and effectiveness by a reliable source.

In large health care agencies, the selection of chemical disinfectants is generally not made by the nurse, but in smaller facilities and in the home, she may be called upon to make the decision. When selecting a disinfectant, the nurse should follow the principles discussed in the previous section of this chapter.

Disinfectants are generally used for instrument and equipment disinfection and for housekeeping disinfection. While it was stated earlier that the term disinfectant referred to substances used on inanimate objects, because of their mildness, *some* disinfectants are also used as antiseptics on human tissue.

Disinfectants destroy organisms by disturbing their structure or their metabolic processes through coagulation and alterations of the cell membrane and cell protein. Because of the vast number of available disinfectants, the reader is advised to seek information relative to specific disinfectants in recent chemistry and microbiology texts and current periodicals. A brief description of the major classes of disinfectants used in health settings follows.

PHENOLIC COMPOUNDS: Phenolic compounds are good substances for housekeeping disinfectants. Beside their bactericidal action, they have the property of stability which means they remain active even after exposure to mild heat and prolonged drying.

QUATERNARY AMMONIUM COMPOUNDS: The "quats" are used both as disinfectants and antiseptics because of their mild but effective bactericidal effect. However, they are inactivated by being used with hard water and soap.

CHLORINE COMPOUNDS: The chlorines are useful for the disinfection of water and for house-keeping disinfectants. They should not be used on metals because of their tendency to cause corrosion.

IODINE AND IODOPHORS: Iodine has an effective bactericidal effect but also has an undesirable staining quality. This characteristic is reduced when a detergent is added to the solution. The combination is distributed as iodophors. Iodophors are frequently used as antiseptics because of their fairly rapid germicidal effect and because they are relatively nontoxic.

FORMALDEHYDE: Aqueous solutions of formaldehyde are known as Formalin. They are very effective bactericides. Unfortunately, however, they also have highly irritating fumes and are toxic to human tissue. Therefore, articles disinfected in Formalin must be rinsed thoroughly before coming in contact with human tissue.

GLUTARALDEHYDE: This substance is a newer member of the same chemical family as formaldehyde and is an even more effective bactericidal disinfectant.

ALCOHOLS: Ethyl (grain) and isopropyl (rubbing) alcohols are most commonly used as antiseptics although occasionally they are also used as disinfectants. They act rapidly as germicidals but the effectiveness of ethyl alcohol is sometimes reduced because it is not as good a fat solvent as is isopropyl alcohol. Long-term exposure to the alcohols can damage plastics.

MERCURIALS: These substances have been used in the past, but because they are relatively slow acting and bacteriostatic only, they are not considered as satisfactory disinfectants.

Table 19-2 illustrates the uses of these classes of chemicals.

Physical Means for Sterilization and Disinfection

Physical sterilization and disinfection usually are accomplished by using heat, the most common methods being steam under pressure, boiling water, free-flowing steam, or dry heat.

Dry heat kills organisms by an oxidation process, while moist heat coagulates protein within the cell. Sterilization and disinfection occur when heat is suf-

TABLE 19-2: Classes of chemicals commonly used for disinfection and antiseptic purposes in health care settings

Class	Disinfectant	Antiseptic
Phenolic compounds	X	
Quaternary ammonium compounds	X	X
Chlorine compounds	X	
Iodine and iodophors	X	X
Formaldehyde	X	
Glutaraldehyde	X	
Alcohols	X	X

ficient to destroy organisms, and, the higher the temperature, the more quickly organisms will die. Therefore, an essential factor for heat sterilization and disinfection is that equipment and supplies be exposed to the heat properly. Overloading a sterilizer or packing it in such a manner that equipment and supplies are not exposed to the heat defeats the effectiveness of the process. In the following discussion of various types of heat sterilizers, the recommended times for sterilization are based on the assumption that the packages are prepared properly and sterilizers loaded properly so that the contents are exposed to heat adequately.

STEAM UNDER PRESSURE: Moist heat in the form of saturated steam under pressure is the most dependable means known for the destruction of all forms of microbial life. Steam is water vapor, and in the saturated state it can exist only at a definite pressure corresponding to a given temperature. The amount of pressure has nothing to do with the destruction of bacteria. It is the higher temperature resulting from higher pressure that destroys bacteria.

The autoclave is a pressure steam sterilizer. Most hospitals and many clinics and offices are equipped with pressure steam sterilizers today. Texts dealing with sterilization describe their operation in detail.

Many homes today have pressure cookers that operate on the same principle as pressure steam sterilizers. Foods cooked in a pressure cooker can be prepared more quickly because of the higher temperature attained by steam under pressure. Pressure cookers can be used for sterilizing equipment in the home by placing articles for sterilization on a rack or a screen above the level of water in the cooker.

The amount of time necessary to expose equipment and supplies in a pressure steam sterilizer in order to assure sterility depends on several factors: the type of equipment or supplies to be sterilized, the manner in which they are wrapped or packaged, the way in which the sterilizer is packed, and the temperature and the pressure maintained.

It will be recalled that the temperature and not the pressure is the factor responsible for destruction of microbes. As altitude increases, a higher gauge pressure is needed in order to reach a specific temperature; and in mountainous areas persons operating pressure steam sterilizers must take this fact into consideration in order to secure sterilization.

Table 19-3 illustrates the effect of altitude on the boiling point of water and on steam pressure. Housewives who live in mountainous areas are aware of this difference when they find that they must cook foods longer than is necessary at sea level. Consideration for altitude becomes an important factor in sterilization procedures, as Table 19-3 clearly illustrates.

DRY HEAT: Dry heat or hot-air sterilization is accomplished by using equipment similarr to an ordinary baking oven. Electrically heated hot-air sterilizers are preferred, since they are more reliable and more nearly accurate than other types of dry-heat ovens. Dry heat is a good method of sterilizing sharp instruments and syringes, since moist heat damages the cutting edges of sharp instruments and the ground surfaces of glass syringes. It is also the preferred method for sterilizing reusable needles, since the needles remain dry, and stylets, if they are used, may be left in place safely. Altitude does not affect hot-air sterilizers.

The nature of the articles, the manner in which articles are wrapped or packaged, and the way in which a hot-air sterilizer is loaded will influence the time required for sterilization. Many authorities agree that, for most articles, sterilization occurs when a temperature of 160° C. (320° F.) is maintained for 1 hour or preferably 2 hours.

For equipment and supplies that will not tolerate a temperature of 160° C. (320° F.), a longer period of time at lower temperature is required.

BOILING WATER: Placing equipment in boiling water for a period of time is a common method of sterilization and disinfection, especially in home settings. However, if spores are present on equipment, boiling water is not a practical method of sterilization, since the temperature of the water cannot rise above 100° C. (212° F.). Some spores are exceedingly resistant, and time required to kill susceptible spores is too long and too unspecific. Also, some viruses are resistant to boiling. Therefore, the nature of the organism determines the length of time required for boiling.

Clean equipment can be sterilized in boiling water in a matter of several minutes, while dirty equipment will take longer. Most authorities agree that equipment contaminated with vegetative forms of bacteria can be sterilized if submerged in boiling water for 10 to 20 minutes. These recommended periods of time are based on the assumptions that the equipment is immersed, the sterilizer is loaded properly, and the time is determined from the moment the water begins to boil.

Sometimes trisodium phosphate or sodium car-

TABLE 19-3: Atmospheric pressure, boiling point of water, gauge pressure at 121° C. (250° F.) and temperature when pressure is 15.12 pounds per square inch, at various altitudes*

Height above sea level (feet)	Atmospheric pressure (lbs. per sq. in.)	Boiling point of water ° F.	Gauge pressure at 250° F.	Autoclave temperature with gauge at 15.12 pounds	Time factor †
0000	14.70	212.0	15.12	250.0	1.000
1,000	14.24	210.2	15.58	249.1	1.118
2,000	13.78	208.5	16.04	248.1	1.248
3,000	13.32	206.8	16.50	247.4	1.395
4,000	12.86	205.0	16.96	246.4	1.560
5,000	12.40	203.2	17.42	245.4	1.742
6,000	11.94	201.5	17.88	244.5	1.950
8,000	11.08	198.0	18.74	242.6	2.440
10,000	10.28	194.5	19.54	241.0	3.050
12,000	9.48	191.0	20.34	239.2	3.800
14,000	8.68	185.5	21.14	237.4	4.780

* Adapted from Beckett, J. S., and Berman, P.: Sterilization and Disinfection: With Special Emphasis on Autoclave Sterilization: A Handbook for Nurses. pp. A3–2C. North Hollywood, Calif., A.T.I. Pub. Div. 1953.

† Amount of time required for sterilization at sea level multiplied by time factor compensates for the difference, depending on altitude, in the temperature of the boiling point of water and the temperature within steam pressure sterilizers when the pressure gauge is at 15.12 pounds. For example, if at sea level it takes 10 minutes to sterilize an article, at 5,000 feet above sea level it will take 10 minutes × 1.742 or 17.42 minutes.

bonate is added to water in which equipment is to be boiled. These chemicals help to remove grease under which organisms may harbor and also decrease the time needed for sterilization and disinfection by increasing the "wetting power" of water. When an alkali is added to water, 15 minutes usually is considered to be a sufficient period for boiling.

Equipment that will rust in water can be damaged easily by this method of sterilization and disinfection. Rusting can be minimized if the equipment is placed in the water only after it has boiled briskly for a few minutes. Boiling the water drives off dissolved oxygen; therefore, rusting, which is the result of oxidation, is minimized in boiled water.

Altitude must be taken into consideration when equipment and supplies are sterilized or disinfected by boiling. Table 19-3 indicates the boiling point of water at various levels. In higher altitudes, the boiling time must be increased, since the temperature necessary to boil water is lower as altitude increases.

FREE-FLOWING STEAM: The temperature of free-flowing steam is 100° C. (212° F.) at sea level. Therefore, free-flowing steam for sterilization and disinfection should be used for the same period of time as boiling water. The free-flowing steam method has limited practical use, since it is difficult to load a free-flowing steam sterilizer in such a way that all equipment is exposed fully to the steam.

EMERGENCY STERILIZATION: There are occasions, as in an emergency, when there is insufficient time to wait the prescribed length of time for the sterilization or disinfection method. The usual procedure is to shorten the recommended period of time for sterilization or disinfection. Some persons call this an "emergency sterilization procedure." When the sterilization or disinfection time is shortened, the persons responsible for the decision must understand that a risk has been taken, that sterilization may not have been accomplished, but that the nature of the emergency warrants it.

Cleaning Supplies and Equipment

In the previous discussion, mention was made several times concerning the cleansing of equipment and supplies prior to sterilization and disinfection. Proper cleansing is important, since organisms embedded in organic material or protected under a layer of fat or grease are difficult to destroy. Furthermore, cleansing reduces the number of organisms present, and, as has been pointed out, the fewer the organisms present the easier it is to sterilize or disinfect equipment.

Persons cleaning equipment should wear waterproof gloves if the articles are contaminated with highly pathogenic materials or if there are skin abrasions on the hands. A brush with stiff bristles is an important aid for cleaning equipment, which should be done in water with soap or with a detergent.[1] If equipment is contaminated with organic materials such as blood, wound drainage, or fecal material, soaking in cold water with a detergent prior to washing will help to make the cleansing procedure easier. The brush, the gloves if used, and the basin in which the equipment is cleaned should be considered as being contaminated and treated and cleansed accordingly.

Following thorough cleansing, equipment should be rinsed well and that which will rust should be dried carefully. At the same time, equipment should be examined to see that each piece is in good working order. Cleansing equipment should be done as soon after use as possible, since organic materials that are allowed to dry increase the difficulty with which equipment is cleansed and increases the likelihood of transfer of organisms by air currents.

When equipment has been cleansed thoroughly, it is ready for sterilization or disinfection.

MONEL AND ENAMELWARE: Steam under pressure is the preferred method of sterilizing monel and enamelware. Dry heat also may be used. Boiling is satisfactory.

Some bedpans and urinals are made of monel or enamelware, and, after the contents have been removed and the equipment rinsed, they should be washed and handled in the same manner as other similar ware.

Many hospitals provide equipment designed specifically to clean bedpans and urinals. A common misconception is that all bedpan flushers are sterilizers. In some instances the manufacturer has labeled them as such. The mechanism flushes the contents and then releases free-flowing steam on the bedpans for a period of 1 to 2 minutes. Such equipment has been found to be satisfactory for the care of bedpans and urinals when sterilization is not necessary. However, with current concern for means by which some virus infections are transmitted, it seems that this method of caring for bedpans requires scrutiny. If the flusher is used for bedpans from many patients, cross-infection may occur, since certain viruses are not destroyed by short periods of exposure to live steam.

GLASSWARE: Brushes especially designed to clean lumens and barrels are particularly desirable.

[1] Except for equipment contaminated by organisms in body secretions containing proteins which are coagulated by heat, warm water is more effective than cold water as a cleaning agent because of its lower surface tension.

It is important to disassemble reusable syringes immediately after use in order to prevent the barrel and the plunger from locking. Syringes should be rinsed thoroughly and soaked so that contents will not dry in the barrel and make cleansing difficult. Steam under pressure is recommended for sterilizing glassware. Boiling is the usual method in the home, as, for example, the syringe used by a diabetic patient.

INSTRUMENTS: Great care should be taken to cleanse grooves, crevices, and serrated surfaces where organisms frequently harbor. Following cleansing, instruments should be dried carefully to prevent rusting.

Instruments that do not have a cutting edge should be sterilized in a pressure steam sterilizer. Instruments with a cutting edge should be sterilized by using dry heat. For certain purposes, chemicals are used.

NEEDLES (OTHER THAN SUTURE NEEDLES): Because of their small lumen, reusable needles present a cleansing problem. Immediately after use, cold water should be forced through the needle with a syringe in order to rinse out contents in the lumen. Forcing isopropyl alcohol or ether through the lumen will aid to remove fatty or oily substances.

Dry heat is the preferred method of sterilizing needles. Steam under pressure is also a satisfactory method. Boiling is used when the other methods are not available.

RUBBER AND PLASTIC GOODS: Reusable catheters should be rinsed thoroughly immediately following use; soaking for short periods of time also will aid in cleaning them. A soap or detergent solution should be forced through the lumen until the lumen has been cleansed thoroughly. The transparent plastic catheters make it easier to determine when the catheter is clean of gross soilage. Rubbber or plastic tubing should be rinsed immediately following use.

Steam under pressure is preferred for sterilizing rubber goods. Dry heat may be used for certain types. If chemicals are used, care should be taken so that the solution fills the lumen in order that the lumen will be disinfected. Ethylene oxide gas, where available, may be used for rubber and plastic items.

MEDICAL AND SURGICAL ASEPSIS

Principles Used in Practices of Medical and Surgical Asepsis

There are three basic principles underlying practices of medical and surgical asepsis.

Certain microorganisms are capable of causing illness in man.

Microorganisms harmful to man can be transmitted by means of his direct or indirect contact with them.

Illness caused by microorganisms can be prevented when there is an interruption of the infectious process cycle.

The presence of a pathogenic microorganism does not in itself insure that a disease will occur. When a disease state, called an *infection*, does result from the presence of pathogenic microorganisms in or on the body, it occurs as the result of a cyclical process. The essential components of the process are: the reservoir for the growth and reproduction of infectious agents; a means of exit from the reservoir for the infectious agent; vehicle(s) for the transmission of the agent; entry portal for the agent into a host; and a susceptible host. The susceptible host becomes the new reservoir and the cycle continues. Figure 19-1 illustrates the infectious process cycle and a brief discussion of its components follows.

The *reservoir for growth and multiplication* of the causative microorganism is the natural habitat of the organism. Reservoirs which support organisms pathogenic to man are other humans, animals, or the soil. Tuberculosis bacillus, measles virus, and syphilis spirochete, for example, grow in man. Viruses suspected of causing some types of encephalitis thrive in wild birds, and the rabies virus grows in many types of animals. Bacteria that cause gas gangrene, tetanus, and anthrax grow in the soil. Man and animals can harbor pathogens yet not demonstrate an illness. Persons and animals who have no indications of illness but who have disease-causing organisms on or within their bodies which can be transferred to others are called *carriers*.

The *exit* refers to a means of escape for the microorganism from the reservoir. The organism cannot extend its influence unless it moves away from its original source. While there may be more than one means of exit, most often there is a primary exit route for each type of microorganism. Common escape routes in man are the respiratory, gastrointestinal and genitourinary tracts, and breaks in the skin.

The pathogens must have a means of mobility. Various *vehicles* act as a means to transmit microorganisms. The means can include water and food. For example, water can be the vehicle for the typhoid bacillus; shellfish that live in the contaminated water can also carry this microorganism. Insects, ticks, and mites can transmit organisms causing malaria, encephalitis, bacillary dysentery, and typhus. Air currents can serve as a vehicle, particularly for droplet nuclei which, for example, may contain the causative

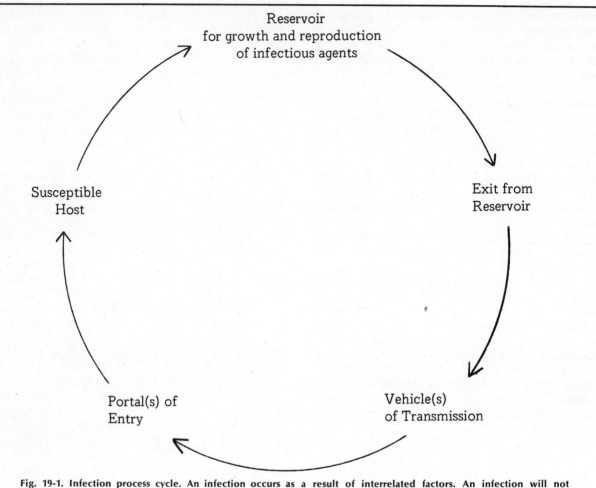

Fig. 19-1. Infection process cycle. An infection occurs as a result of interrelated factors. An infection will not develop if the sequence is interrupted. Hence, efforts to control infections are directed toward interrupting the sequence.

organisms for tuberculosis, chicken pox, smallpox, and measles. Inanimate objects (books being one example) can sometimes serve as vehicles for transmitting pathogens, though much less frequently than once was thought to be true.

The microorganism must now find a *portal of entry* on a new host. The entry route is often, though not exclusively, the same as the exit route. The respiratory and gastrointestinal tracts and the skin are common entry points.

In order for the microorganism to continue to exist, it must find a source which will accept and support it. *Susceptibility* refers to the degree of resistance the potential host has against the pathogen. Many factors, including nature's protections such as intact skin and mucous membranes, gastric secre-

tions, genitourinary system pH level, phagocytes, and hormones influence the resistance of a person to a pathogen. Such factors as age, sex, and race have been shown to be influential also even though the reasons are not entirely clear. Fatigue, climatic conditions, general health status, presence of preexisting illnesses, previous or current treatment with ionizing radiation, and some kinds of medications also may play a part in determining the degree of susceptibility of the potential host.

Because the cyclical process just discussed must exist for infections to spread, breaking the cycle can control infections. Complete elimination of the cyclical process for all pathogens is impossible, but breaking the cycle as frequently as possible is the never-ending goal of infection control. Attempts to eliminate the pathogen reservoirs, to prevent or control the escape and transmission of microorganisms, to prevent new entry sites, and to increase resistance of potential hosts are ongoing infection control activities.

Because there is usually a larger number of persons whose bodies harbor pathogens in hospitals than in other places, patients frequently come in contact with harmful microorganisms and some develop infections while hospitalized. An increased awareness of such occurrences has resulted in a recently coined term, *nosocomial infections*, to describe hospital-acquired infections. Because of concern about this problem, great efforts are being put into hospital infection surveillance and prevention programs.

The role of sterilization and disinfection in relation to asepsis has been discussed. Additional methods of preventing the transmission of pathogens in the practice of medical and surgical asepsis will be discussed in the remainder of this chapter. Attention will also be drawn to other aseptic practices, as appropriate, throughout this text.

Bacterial Flora of the Hands

In 1938, Price, a noted researcher in the area of skin bacteriology, published a summary of studies conducted to determine the bacterial flora normally found on the hands. He pointed out two types—one called *transient* flora or bacteria, the other called *resident* flora or bacteria.

Transient bacteria are relatively few on clean and exposed areas of the skin. Usually, they are picked up by the hands in the normal activities of living and working; therefore, the type and the nature of the organisms will depend largely on the nature of work in which each individual is engaged. For example, a librarian may have many organisms on his hands that also can be found readily on books and papers. Similarly, one who has handled a dressing soaked with drainage may find organisms on her hands similar to those found in the drainage of the wound. Transient bacteria are attached loosely to the skin, usually in grease, fats, and dirt, and are found in greater numbers under the fingernails. Transient bacteria, pathogenic as well as nonpathogenic, can be removed with relative ease by washing the hands thoroughly and frequently.

Resident bacteria are relatively stable in number and type. They are found in the creases and the crevices of the skin, and it is believed that they cling to the skin by adhesion and adsorption. Resident flora cannot be removed easily from the skin by washing with soap and water unless considerable friction also is applied with a brush, and they are less susceptible to the action of antiseptics than are transient flora. Some of them are embedded so deeply in the skin that they do not appear in washings until the skin has been scrubbed for 15 minutes or longer. For practical purposes, it is not considered possible to cleanse the skin of all bacteria.

It was found also that transient flora may adjust to the environment of the skin if the flora are present in large numbers over a long enough period of time; they then become resident flora. For example, if one handles contaminated materials over a period of time, the organisms in the materials, although originally transient in nature, may become resident flora on the hands. If such flora contain pathogenic organisms, the hands may become carriers of the particular organisms. To prevent transient flora from becoming resident flora, it is important that the hands be cleansed promptly after each contact with contaminated materials, and especially if the materials contain pathogenic organisms. Since nurses in the course of their work often handle materials contaminated with pathogenic organisms, the importance of frequent and thorough hand washing becomes evident.

Soap and Detergents and Water as Cleansing Agents

Because soap and detergents lower the surface tension and act as emulsifying agents, they are good cleansing agents when used with water.

Soaps that are made with sodium salts are hard soaps, while soft soaps are made with potassium salts. Glycerol is removed in the process of making hard soaps but is retained in soft soaps.

When soap is used in hard water, an insoluble flaky precipitate is formed when the salts of soap react with the salts found in hard water, and the reaction of the two salts makes the soap ineffectual as a cleansing agent. However, soap used with soft water is an invaluable cleansing agent.

Detergents are popular and effective as cleansing agents because of their surface-tension reducing power. Such representative household products as Dreft, Cheer, and Tide, and Electro-Sol for automatic dishwashers have effective cleansing and emulsifying properties. Detergents do not react unfavorably with the salts in hard water, and therefore, they lather readily in any water of any temperature. Few if any household detergents, however, are effective disinfectants.

Price used various types of soap in his studies on skin cleansing. He experimented with green soap, institutional soap, castile soap, and several popular toilet soaps. None of these soaps had a germicidal agent added. His studies, and other studies also, have found that all the soaps cleansed the hands equally well, and that, although certain toilet soaps may leave a pleasing odor on the skin, their cleansing effect is enhanced neither by the perfumes added nor by their cost.

Since hospital-acquired infections have become a problem, it is often recommended that soaps and detergents containing a germicide be used in the hand-washing technique. The recommendation is made most frequently for operating rooms, nurseries, delivery rooms, and isolation units, although some persons suggest these soaps and detergents for all hospital units.

Substances containing hexachlorophene were used extensively for this purpose in health care settings and had also become very popular for home use to control microorganisms. In 1972, the Federal Drug Administration ruled that hexachlorophene products would no longer be generally available on the commercial market and recommended that such routine practices as bathing newborns, hand washing, and surgical scrubbing with agents containing hexachlorophene be reconsidered. Restrictions came about as a result of experimental studies which showed potential toxic hazards through absorption of hexachlorophene. While the antibacterial effectiveness of hexachlorophene was well-documented and although no recorded incidents of toxicity exist in this country, the hazards of routine use were judged to be too high. Cleansers containing hexachlorophene are available with a physician's prescription and are used in health care agencies with more discrimination. New products containing other antibacterials are in the process of being developed and are coming onto the market.

A rather widely used quaternary ammonium detergent—benzalkonium chloride (Zephiran)—is reported to be a good disinfectant and detergent when the alcoholic tincture preparation is used, but it is not particularly effective in the presence of organic materials such as blood and serum or of soap, nor does it have the residual effects that the phenolic compounds do. Another detergent-germicide combination with widespread and effective use is povidone-iodine (Betadine). Its staining characteristics is being minimized.

Tap water is as effective as sterile water for skin cleansing. The few nonpathogens in tap water are not implanted on the skin during washing and therefore they rinse or wipe off with ease.

Suggested Hand Washing Technique

Studies in relation to hand washing techniques have been reported in the literature since well before the end of the last century. Admonitions concerning the importance of clean hands date back even further, to the time of the ancient Hebrews as reported in the Old Testament. In spite of much evidence to support the importance of careful and frequent hand washing, contaminated hands are considered by many authorities to be the prime factor in cross-infections to this day. Hands in health settings and homes are in constant use: the nurse giving an injection, the physician examining a patient, the maid folding linen, the volunteer helping a patient select reading material, the aide making a patient's bed, the engineer repairing a television control switch, children playing with toys, and mothers carrying out household tasks. Still, much hand washing appears to be more ritualistic than realistic, even though the role of hands in cross-infection is no longer debatable.

Cleansing the hands prior to performing certain procedures using surgical asepsis, such as prior to surgery or the delivery of a baby, is taught when the student learns to assist with these procedures. The suggested technique described herein is intended for use when *medical asepsis* is being practiced.

Many researchers have illustrated the value of certain antiseptics for cleansing the hands. However, if there is no reason to believe that the hands harbor pathogenic organisms in the resident flora of the skin, there would appear to be no need to use antiseptics for medical asepsis practice. Transient bacteria—the type that hands accumulate in everyday living and working—are removed easily by thorough washing with soap or a detergent and water. From a half to one minute is recommended. If the hands have been contaminated with blood, purulent materials, mucus, saliva, or secretions from wounds, washing should be done for two to three minutes. Regardless of the type of soil, friction and a lather are essential to emulsify and mechanically remove the microorganisms. *A sterile brush may be used,* if the hands are contaminated grossly, but it should be used with great care, since it is easy to brush organisms into hair follicles and skin crevices, which may lead to infection and harboring of organisms. The subungual areas should be cleansed with a sterile nail file or an orange stick, and again caution should be exercised to prevent breaking the skin. If good nail hygiene is maintained, it may not be necessary to clean the subungual areas with a stick or file with every washing, but the procedure should be followed if special circumstances warrant it.

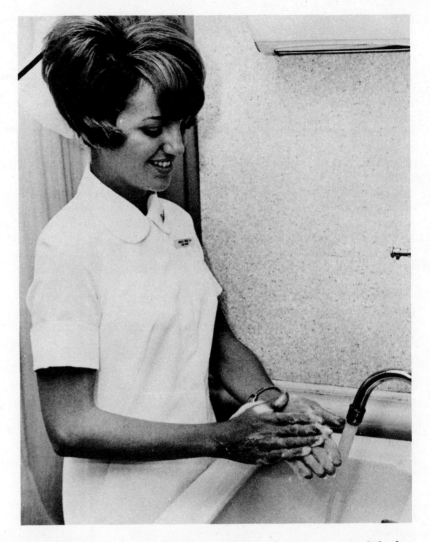

Fig. 19-2. As innumerable studies will bear out, the single most important factor in the prevention of hospital infections is good hand washing technic. It applies to all contacts of health personnel with patients. Its importance cannot be overemphasized. (Photo by Warren R. Vroom)

It is preferable to wash the hands under running water at a sink with foot- or knee-controlled faucets. If the faucets are hand-controlled, a policy should be observed concerning whether they are considered to be clean or contaminated. A paper towel should be used to *open* the faucets before washing if the policy is to keep them clean; a paper towel should be used to *close* the faucets if the policy is to consider them as being contaminated. If it is necessary to use a basin, the water should be changed frequently while washing and after each person's use. The inside of a sink or a basin should be considered as being contaminated.

If bar soap is used for cleansing, the bar should be picked up at the beginning of the washing period and held in the hands during the entire washing period. Following washing, the bar should be rinsed and then dropped onto the soap dish. A soap dish that allows water to drain from the soap is preferable in order to keep the soap firm and dry between uses. It has been found that jelly-like soap can harbor pathogens that transfer from user to user. If a brush is being used, the bar of soap may be held on the back of the brush while using the brush. Simpler techniques use liquid soap dispensed with a foot or knee lever or single-use bar soaps.

The hands and the forearms should be held lower than the elbows during the washing period in order that soiled water will not run up the arms. Following washing and rinsing, the hands should be dried on an individual linen or paper towel. Laundry problems when using linen, and disposal problems when using paper, have increased the use of forced hot air for hand drying in many agencies. It is suggested that a lotion or a cream be used following washing in order to keep the skin soft and pliable. Chapped and rough skin is difficult to keep clean and will break more easily with repeated washing.

If at any time during the washing period the hands accidentally brush along the inside of the sink or the basin or on the soap dish, the entire washing period should be repeated. It is suggested that a timer be placed near the sink so that the washing period can be determined with accuracy.

The technique just described may need to be taught to patients or family members dealing with infections in the home.

Keeping hands clean, regardless of the particular technique followed, is no more reliable than the individual, whose conscientiousness, concern for cleansing all areas thoroughly and respect for his own health, as well as for the health of others, will determine to a great extent the effectiveness of hand washing. For aesthetic reasons as well, persons caring for the ill should practice washing their hands immediately after caring for each patient or after handling equipment used in his care.

Examples of Common Practices of Medical Asepsis

The following examples help to illustrate the fact that medical asepsis is in constant practice:

Paper towels are used in situations where a large number of persons share common wash facilities; paper drinking cups (instead of a common drinking glass) are required by public health regulations in instances where safe drinking fountains are not available; paper straws, such as are used at soda fountains, are wrapped individually so that they are not contaminated by constant handling; cafeterias frequently provide tongs for customers to use when taking rolls or bread; pillows and mattresses must be sterilized before they are sold, and they must have a label attached at the time of sale indicating that they have been sterilized; hairdressers and barbers are required to sterilize combs and other items after use on each customer. These are only a few examples which in every sense represent the practice of medical asepsis in daily living.

Examples from the home include the following: The homemaker washes her hands before beginning any food preparation; she roasts some meats to a higher temperature in order to insure their safety; she washes fruits and uncooked vegetables before serving them; she teaches the children to wash their hands before eating and after going to the toilet; she provides individual items for personal care for each member of the home, such as washcloths, towels, and toothbrushes.

Because certain diseases may be transmitted insidiously, there are many regulations enforced by law in most communities which aim to prevent their spread. Some of these regulations have to do with the examination of food handlers, the management of eating establishments, the disposal of garbage, the construction of sewage systems and public building ventilation, and sanitation requirements. In every sense, these regulations constitute medical asepsis practices. They are defenses against the occasions when contamination may be present.

Most patients practice habits of medical asepsis which they do not recognize by such terms, but they are there. These patients have an understanding of the need for protecting themselves and the means by which it can be done. Never underestimate the patient's ability to evaluate practices of asepsis in a hospital. He is as capable of doing this as he is in judging the practices he sees in a restaurant, a food store, or a motel in the light of how they may affect him. Since patients have some "know-how" in this area, it is only natural that they would expect the nurse to exemplify good health practices in all that she does. Even such activities as stripping the linen from the bed occupied by a patient, carrying linen, washing an item, visiting with a patient, or holding a child provide opportunities for good health teaching.

The following examples illustrate actions which a nurse carries out, based on the fact that appropriate precautionary measures applied to daily activities and personal care aid in preventing the transmission of microorganisms and disease.

Wash the hands frequently but especially before handling foods, before eating, after using a handkerchief, after going to the toilet, and after each patient contact. Clean underneath the fingernails frequently to keep the areas clean and free from contaminated materials.

Keep soiled items and equipment from touching the clothing. Carry soiled linens or other used articles so that they do not touch the uniform. When stooping or bending, hold the uniform so that it does not touch the floor, a grossly contaminated area.

Avoid having patients cough, sneeze, or breathe directly on others by providing them with disposable wipes to hold over their mouths when close contact is necessary, as during an examination.

Clean away from yourself, especially when brushing, dusting, or scrubbing articles. This helps to prevent the dust particles from settling on the hair, the face, or the uniform.

Avoid raising dust. Use a specially treated cloth or a dampened cloth. Do not shake linens. Dust particles constitute a means by which bacteria may be transported from one area to another.

Clean the least soiled areas first and then the more soiled ones. This helps to prevent having the cleaner areas soiled by the dirtier ones.

Dispose of soiled or used items directly into appropriate containers or holders. Wrap items which are moist from body discharge or drainage carefully before discarding into the refuse holder so that handlers will not come in contact with them.

Pour liquids which are to be discarded, such as bath water, mouthcare rinsings, and the like, directly into the drain so as to avoid splattering in the sink. Most agencies caring for the sick have sinks or hoppers which are used primarily for disposing of contaminated liquids and washings.

Sterilize items which are suspected of having pathogens on them. Following sterilization, they are managed as clean items.

Handling Sterile Transfer Forceps

Practices of surgical asepsis are directed toward the elimination of all microorganisms by sterilization and toward preventing microorganisms from contaminating sterile areas. Inasmuch as hands are not sterile, it is obvious that they must not come in contact with sterile items. Sterile gloves or sterile forceps (or clamps) are used when sterility is necessary.

The practice of keeping transfer forceps in containers of disinfectant solution leaves much to be desired. Many agencies have recognized the potential danger of this practice and have discontinued its use. Only forceps taken from wrappers in which they have been sterilized can be considered safe. They are dry and not exposed to possible contamination until the wrapper is opened.

If forceps kept in a disinfectant solution are used, the container should be sterilized and fresh solution used at least daily. There is no scientific justification for only daily care; actually the more frequently this is done, the safer the forceps are likely to be. The opportunity for contamination by means of air currents, personnel, and technique in handling is tremendous.

When transfer forceps are used, these principles should be observed:

A sterile object becomes contaminated when in contact with an unsterile object. If the forceps touch an unsterile item or the sides of the container not in solution, they should not be returned to the container until sterilized.

Liquids flow in the direction of gravitational pull. If the forceps are held so that disinfectant solution will touch the unsterile part of the forceps and flow back to the sterile part, the forceps are contaminated. Therefore, the forceps should always be held so that the blades are lower than the handle.

Examples of Common Practices of Surgical Asepsis

The examples given below illustrate common practices of surgical asepsis. Some practices require extreme caution. It is far better to err on the side of safety than to take the slightest chance on possible contamination.

All items brought into contact with broken skin surfaces of the body, or used to penetrate the skin surface in order to inject substances into the body, or to enter normally sterile body cavities, should be sterile. Examples of such items are dressings used to cover wounds and incisions, needles for injection, and tubes (catheters) used to drain urine from the bladder.

Never walk away from or turn your back on a sterile field. This will prevent possible contamination while the field is out of the worker's view.

Avoid talking, coughing, sneezing, or reaching over a sterile field or object. This will help to prevent contamination by droplets from the nose and the mouth or by particles dropping from the worker's arm.

Hold sterile objects above the level of the waist. This will help to insure keeping the object within sight, thus avoiding accidental contamination.

Avoid spilling any solution on a cloth or a paper sterile set-up. The moisture will penetrate through the sterile field, and capillary action could make the field unsafe. A wet sterile field is always considered to be contaminated if the surface immediately below it is not sterile.

Open sterile packages so that the edges of the wrapper are directed away from the worker, in order to avoid the possibility of a sterile surface touching the unsterile clothing.

COMMUNICABLE DISEASE CONTROL

While all phases of medicine have undergone radical changes in recent years, one of the most dramatic and encouraging is the control and the management of many communicable diseases in the United States. There are several reasons for the marked reduction in communicable diseases. The foremost probably is the discovery of immunizing agents. Helping individuals to build up a resistance to many of the common communicable diseases has become almost a routine aspect of child care in this country. The results of immunization include reducing the mortality rate in infancy and childhood, preventing serious physical limitations which frequently resulted from such illnesses, and helping to improve the health of immunized individuals and to increase their life expectancy.

A word of caution must be issued here lest success result in a careless attitude regarding routine immunizations on the part of the general public and health personnel. Some health practitioners are expressing concern that a false sense of security may result in neglect of immunizations and in an increased incidence of preventable communicable diseases in this country in the future.

Of equal importance in communicable disease control is the discovery of drugs that are specifically effective against the causative organisms. While many people still become ill with some of the communicable diseases, chemotherapy not only brings the infection under control rapidly but also reduces the period of communicability—in some instances, to a matter of hours. Many of the drugs being used make it possible for patients such as those with pneumonia and streptococcic sore throat and tuberculosis to require special transmission precautions for much shorter periods of time than previously was true.

Changes in communicable diseases in recent years have also resulted in other approaches to infection control. Most hospitals now have some type of infection surveillance and prevention program to detect and limit the transmission of nosocomial infections. Specially trained nurses are frequently the key surveillance officers in the day-to-day implementation of the prevention program. They conduct epidemiologic investigations to determine specific pathogen sources, transmission modes, incidence of infections, and means of control. They also institute specific methods to prevent pathogen transmissions.

Types of infections acquired in hospitals are changing. Within the past decade or so, reports indicate more gram-negative organisms are causing infections. Examples of the organisms include *Pseudomonas aeruginosa*, *Proteus*, *Escherichia coli*, and *Klebsiella*. Previously the gram-positive *Staphylococcus aureus* was the most common offender.

The most common infection sites vary, depending upon the patient population. However, studies indicate the urinary tract, surgical wounds, respiratory tract, and skin and subcutaneous tissues are most frequently involved in nosocomial infections. Therefore, precautions relating to the prevalent microorganisms and sites have received special attention.

Nurses have developed a more aggressive detection and prevention role regarding infections in the home, industry, school, and office settings, as well as in the hospital. When a brief hospitalization means the patient is discharged before all laboratory results are reported, the practice of having hospital nurses follow up on significant diagnostic tests with appropriate community referral agencies is especially important. The nurse in a nonhospital setting also frequently is in a position to make appropriate referrals to other health professionals for assistance. The nurse is often in the best position to detect suspicious body secretions and secure a specimen from which a diagnostic culture can be grown. These specimens may be taken, for example, from nose and throat secretions, surgical wound drainage, and skin lesions.

Nurses in all settings can initiate techniques to prevent transmission of suspected or confirmed pathogens. Extensive teaching about precautionary methods to patients, family members, and community groups is an increasingly important part of the nurse's function. Nurses in community health settings often combine their teaching with data-gathering methods to discover other infection sources.

A mutual interest between health care facilities and the community regarding infections has become more obvious in recent years. Concern about the influence on the community of hospital wastes has increased with the prevalent use of disposable products and the difficulties of disinfecting and destroying them. The increase in the number of persons moving from the community into the health care facility and back to the community such as patients, visitors, volunteers, health personnel, repair servicemen, and vendors has greatly increased the potential both for pathogens to be brought into the health care facility and for them to be taken back to the community. Supplies prepared commercially outside the health agency also increase the opportunities for pathogen introduction to the agency, as for example, via laundry, food, and equipment. Much private and federal effort is being put into the problem of infection control. The Center for Disease Control of the U.S. Public Health Service in Atlanta, Georgia, is especially active in working toward improved control and prevention of infections in our communities and health care facilities.

While the incidence of some communicable diseases has been decreased, the prevalence of others remain or has increased. Special techniques and methods the nurse can use to prevent the transfer of communicable diseases are described in the remainder of this chapter.

General Principles for Controlling the Spread of Communicable Diseases

Communicable disease control techniques are based on two general principles:

The transfer of pathogens from person to person can be decreased when dissemination of pathogens is limited. The most practical means of controlling the dissemination is to develop barriers for the common vehicles of microorganism transmission.

Methods to limit the dissemination of specific pathogens are based on the manner in which the pathogen leaves the source (patient), its portal of entry, and its ability to survive outside the host.

Using these principles indicates that communicable disease control techniques can safely vary, depending on the specific organism and its means of transfer. For example, *Mycobacterium tuberculosis*, the organism responsible for pulmonary tuberculosis, leaves the patient via the exhalation phase of respiration and is spread by droplet nuclei. It enters the host's respiratory tract via the droplets in order to cause an infection. Although the pathogen can survive outside the body, current research shows the larger nuclei fall to the surface and are not resuspended easily. Therefore, such particles are not considered especially hazardous. The vehicle for the tuberculosis pathogen is the droplet nuclei. Therefore, the barriers against transmission must focus on keeping the air free of the droplets. As another example, *Treponema pallidum*, the causative agent of syphilis, is found on the mucosa of the genitourinary tract of the male host. The microorganism is very fragile and can live outside of the host only for a short time. Direct contact is the vehicle and therefore, avoidance of sexual relations or use of a mechanical barrier such as a condom is necessary to prevent spreading the pathogen.

Definition of Terms

Communicable disease or *isolation technique* refers to practices that limit the spread of a communicable pathogen. It involves separating infected persons and their pathogens from the unafflicted and rendering contaminated items used in their care safe for reuse or disposal.

A *contagious disease* is a disease that is conveyed rather easily from the sick to the well either by direct contact through an intermediary host or by other indirect means.

It is not uncommon for the terms contagious and infectious to be used interchangeably. However, they are not synonymous. An infectious disease or illness is caused by a pathogen, but it is not always contagious.

Concurrent disinfection is the term used to refer to ongoing practices which are observed in the care of the patient, his supplies, and his immediate environment. Their purpose is to limit or control a pathogenic organism. Concurrent disinfection includes caring for items used by the patient, his body secretions and excretions, and other possibly contaminated items. Specific practices are determined on the basis of knowledge of the involved pathogen.

It may be appropriate to repeat that all practices concerning the care of equipment and other items that are observed routinely as a part of medical asepsis also are considered as concurrent disinfection in that they help to control the spread of pathogens.

Terminal disinfection refers to practices to remove pathogens from the patient's immediate environment and belongings once his illness is no longer communicable. All equipment and supplies and the environment in contact with the patient should be thoroughly cleaned with a germicidal detergent solution or other means of disinfection. If the pathogen can be transmitted via air currents, airing the room is advised; specific measures are dependent on the causative organism. In some instances, measures are prescribed by the sanitary codes of the community which have been more demanding in the past when knowledge of pathogens was less extensive.

Variations in Communicable Disease Practices

Because isolation techniques vary among health agencies, nurses working in one situation may be observing practices that are not followed in a similar agency in the same city or even across the street. Oddly enough, the results in many instances appear to be about the same.

The combined efforts of experts in microbiology, medicine, nursing, and sanitary engineering are necessary to study communicable diseases that are still posing problems and to arrive at flexible and workable techniques to prevent their spread. Thus, all the facts about the illness, the causative organism, the existing facilities of the community and the problems of nursing care can be presented and evaluated. For example, some communities have sewage disposal systems which are inadequate to destroy all disease-producing organisms; therefore, action must be taken to disinfect waste materials before disposing of them in the sewage system; or if the causative agent exists only in the patient's blood, the only items that would be managed with additional care would be those that come into direct contact with the patient's blood; or, if the patient's respiratory secretions contain the causative organism, it may well be that a gown should be worn when coming in close contact with the patient and his bedding; or, if the organism is destroyed easily, the dishes may be safe if washed with hot soapy water. Knowledge of such factors is an important part when making the decision as to whether a person with an infectious disease can safely be cared for at home or must be hospitalized.

Psychological Implications When Using Communicable Disease Control Techniques

Regardless of the specific technique that is used and whether the patient is at home or in a health care facility, one need in his care does not change: attention to the psychological effects of the necessary restrictions. The implications of this are great whether the patient is strictly separated from others or whether he merely needs to observe simple precautions. The feeling of being undesirable to others is great for the patient. He often feels frightened, lonely, "unclean," guilty, and rejected. Because the person responds as a total being, his emotional state can influence his recovery rate.

Teaching and supportive measures are probably the two biggest contributions the nurse can make to this aspect of a patient's illness. The patient and his family need to have an accurate understanding of the pertinent epidemiological facts of the situation and of how to carry out the specific precautions necessary. Particular emphasis needs to be placed on the idea that it is the pathogenic organism which is unwanted, not the patient. Since misunderstandings can breed distrust, resentment, and fear, it is extremely important for the nurse to validate that the patient and his family have an accurate understanding of the situation. Their feelings often prevent them from asking for clarification or assistance. The nurse may find that she needs to extend her teaching to a patient's fellow employees or classmates. Misunderstandings on the part of a patient's acquaintances can also influence a patient's feelings of rejection, even after he has recovered.

Both the patient and his family may need support and reassurance regarding handling the isolation precautions and the feelings that may evolve. If the patient is being cared for at home, family members may need much help in understanding why the patient's behavior may change extensively and in how to cope with it. The patient who resents and ignores the precautions needs help in being accepted as a person and in constructively expressing his feelings.

Studies have been done which show that the extensive separation of persons from others can be extremely traumatic. The goal now is to minimize the extent of the precautions and the length of time they must exist as much as can safely be done. The problem of striking a balance between what is best for both the patient and for others is a delicate one. The skill and ingenuity of the nurse are often taxed extensively in caring for the patient with a communicable disease.

A well-informed nurse who understands how to protect herself and her patients and a well-informed patient who is cooperating in his care are by far the best combination of communicable disease precautions.

Types of Isolation Practices

As stated previously, there are many variations of specific isolation techniques. In an attempt to organize communicable disease precautions, the Center for Disease Control of the U. S. Public Health Service has epidemiologically categorized isolation procedures into seven groups: strict, respiratory, enteric, wound and skin, discharge, blood, and protective. A patient's particular pathogen and its means of transmission determine which category of precautions is appropriate to institute. The specific techniques are described in the publication, *Isolation Techniques for Use in Hospitals*. The book is listed in the references at the end of this chapter. A brief description of the categories follows.

STRICT ISOLATION: The purpose of strict isolation is to prevent the transmission of all highly communicable diseases spread by both contact and airborne routes. The technique requires that the patient be in a private room and that persons coming in contact with the patient wear gowns and masks and observe rigid precautions. This type of isolation is frequently used with patients who have illnesses such as smallpox, diphtheria, or *Staphylococcus aureus* infections of extensive burns.

RESPIRATORY ISOLATION: The objective of respiratory isolation is to prevent the transmission of pathogens by droplet nuclei. It also requires that the patient be in a private room, that masks be worn, and that particular precautions be taken with respiratory tract secretions. This method may be used for patients with diseases such as pertussis (whooping cough), measles, and active pulmonary tuberculosis.

ENTERIC ISOLATION: The goal of enteric isolation is to prevent diseases which can be transmitted through direct or indirect contact with infected fecal material. Persons can be safely cared for in rooms with others as long as care is taken to avoid fecal contamination. Gowns should be worn by those having direct contact with the patient. It is recommended that persons with serum hepatitis be treated with these precautions even though the most prevalent transmission route of serum hepatitis is via the blood. There have been reported instances of serum hepatitis being communicated in other ways. Cholera and salmonellosis are examples of other diseases that may be cared for using these precautions.

WOUND AND SKIN ISOLATION: Wound and skin isolation is designed to prevent cross-infection from pathogens transmitted by direct contact with wounds. It is preferable that the patient have a private room and that persons in contact with the patient wear gowns. Special care of wound dressings and drainage is essential. Patients with such conditions as gas gangrene, impetigo, and generalized wound infections may warrant these precautions.

DISCHARGE ISOLATION: The purpose of discharge isolation is to prevent cross-infections from pathogens transmitted by direct contact with wound secretions where the likelihood is slight but possible. The primary precautions relate to the handling of lesion drainage and oral and fecal secretions and excretions. Patients with minor wounds and infected burns, anthrax, scarlet fever, and poliomyelitis may require such precautions.

BLOOD ISOLATION: Blood isolation is designed to prevent cross-infections from organisms transmitted by contact with blood. Special care is taken with needles and syringes contaminated with the patient's blood. Hepatitis and malaria are examples of two diseases which may require this care.

PROTECTIVE ISOLATION: The purpose of protective isolation is to prevent contact between potential pathogens and a person with greatly increased susceptibility. These precautions are also known as *reverse* isolation precautions and are discussed later in this chapter.

The patient needs to be located in a physical environment in which it is feasible to carry out the intent of whatever precautions are necessary. Hand washing facilities in the immediate area are vital. Adjoining bathing and toilet facilities are desirable, whenever possible. Adequate space separating the person harboring the pathogen and others helps to decrease the possibility of transmission in all situations. A separate room with a door that can be kept closed is essential in circumstances where the causative organisms are airborne. Ventilation in the area should have a minimum of six air changes per hour. To prevent cross-circulation or recirculation of air between the isolation room and other areas, slight negative pressure in the room in relation to adjoining areas is desirable. Exhaust window fans can be used for this. Facilities to discard excretions, drainage, and other contaminated substances safely are important.

Facilities for diversion may be especially important for persons confined to rooms alone. Selection of the environment for the patient should be based on the patient's needs and availability of facilities to carry out the appropriate techniques to prevent pathogen transmission.

Personal Contact Precautions

Figure 19-3 indicates the most common vehicles of transmission. This section discusses methods used to develop vehicle barriers.

As indicated earlier, personal contacts between the patient with a communicable disease and others is extremely important from a psychological standpoint. Depending on the degree of illness, the patient may need personal contacts for physical assistance also. Important as the contact is, it is probably the contact that is most responsible for pathogen transmission. More specifically, inadequately cleaned hands transmit more microorganisms than any other single transmission vehicle. Hand washing technique has been discussed and can only be emphasized here again as being extremely important.

Patients and family members need to have an explanation of the purposes for using hand washing and wearing apparel as barriers to vehicle transmission of organisms through personal contacts. As stated in Chapter 13, because touch is such an important part of communication, it may be important to the nurse-patient relationship to set up barriers to vehicle transmission so the avoidance of touch is not necessary.

GOWN TECHNIQUE: In those situations where gowns are worn, individual gown technique is recommended. This means gowns are worn only once and then are discarded for disinfection if they are not disposable. Disposable gowns are destroyed in an appropriate manner. *Multiple gown technique,* or the reuse of gowns, has been practiced extensively in the past. This technique required careful removal and donning of the gown to avoid contamination. Since contamination does often occur, the Center

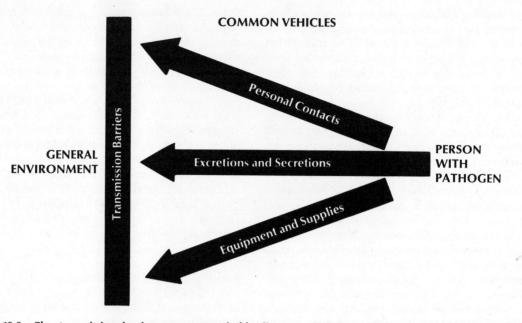

Fig. 19-3. The transmission barriers are communicable disease or isolation techniques. Note that the transmission barriers prevent common vehicles from transporting pathogens from the infected person to the general environment.

for Disease Control recommends this approach be abandoned.

Gowns that are used for isolation technique are made of washable or disposable material; most are made to be worn over the outer garments of the wearer. They are designed with the opening in the back and a tie around the waist to help to keep the gown secure and closed. Some have stockinet at the wrists; others have buttons. They may have buttons or tie strings at the neck. These minor variations do not affect the use or the value of the gown. All have the same purpose of protecting the clothing of those who come in contact with the patient from contamination.

Supplies of gowns should be available outside the immediate patient environment so the wearer can put one on before entering the patient's area. There is no special way in which a clean gown must be put on. However, it should be closed well in the back so that all parts of the wearer's clothing are covered.

When the wearer is ready to leave the unit, the gown is unfastened and removed so that the wearer turns it inside out. In other words, the wearer takes off the gown and rolls it up so that the contaminated part is inside. Then the gown is discarded in a special hamper provided for it. The wearer now washes her hands thoroughly, making certain that special precautions are taken to prevent contaminating the

faucets if foot- or knee-controlled faucets are not available.

MASKS: A variety of practices is observed in the use of the *mask* as a barrier in caring for a patient who has a communicable disease which can be transmitted via the respiratory tract. In some instances, all personnel and visitors to the patient wear masks; in other situations personnel, visitors, and also the patient wear a mask. On the other hand, it may be that only the patient wears the mask; and in certain techniques, neither the patient nor the personnel wears a mask.

Theoretically, the mask is intended to filter inspired and expired air in order to trap the organisms in its meshes. The purpose of the mask should be understood by the wearer; for example, if a patient has active pulmonary tuberculosis, it is recommended that he wear the mask to provide a barrier for the pathogens he may exhale. In situations where the patient is unable to cooperate by wearing the mask, persons coming in contact with him then may need to wear masks. In the newborn nursery or other situations when protective techniques are used, the purpose is to protect the infants or the patient from the air expired by the workers and hence, personnel wear masks.

If masks are worn by persons coming in contact with the patient, they should be stored with the gowns outside the patient area and put on before entering the room. Masks should cover both the nose and mouth and be worn only once. Moisture makes masks ineffective and so they should be removed and appropriately discarded as frequently as necessary to keep them dry. The actual length of time a mask can be worn safely, which is partly determined by the type of mask, is a debatable question. Newer high-efficiency, disposable masks are more effective than reusable cotton gauze masks and are preferred for preventing airborne and droplet-spread infections.

GLOVES: Gloves may be worn in some situations during certain phases of patient care. They may be used as a barrier when handling wound dressings or when carrying out treatments if drainage is present. Sterile gloves may also be worn at times to protect a particularly susceptible patient from the introduction of organisms when caring for an open wound. Gloves are worn only once and then discarded appropriately. Gloves should be changed after direct handling of potentially contaminated drainage and before completing the patient's care. Both reusable and disposable gloves are available commercially.

HAIR AND SHOE COVERS: Hair and shoe covers are not used generally except in some protective precautions. When they are worn, all hair on the head should be covered, and the shoe covers should also protect the open ends of trouser legs.

Excretion and Secretion Precautions

Organisms can escape from the host through body secretions and excretions. Urine and feces and respiratory, oral, vaginal, and wound drainage may require special precautions.

Urine and feces may need to be treated before disposal into the sewage system. As mentioned previously, this precaution is unnecessary in those communities in which the sewage disposal techniques are adequate to destroy organisms. Home sewage systems may make disinfection necessary in some situations.

The problems that the disinfection of excreta brings to any nursing service usually are numerous. The psychological implications as well as the hazards of handling several pails or bedpans of excreta make it an unpopular procedure. Therefore, efforts should be made to ascertain the absolute necessity for disinfecting excreta before it is done.

The disadvantages of the usual health agency bedpan flusher have been discussed. The safest practice is to empty the bedpan, rinse it thoroughly with cold water, wash it with soap or detergent and water if necessary, and then sterilize it with steam under pressure before reuse.

If there is drainage, tissues and other items may be contaminated by wound, mouth, nose, or vaginal drainage, and they may be considered as pathogen vehicles and must be handled carefully. The usual technique is to place the contaminated materials in an impervious bag and close it tightly. When the bag is removed from the patient area, it should be placed in a larger, clean disposable bag or container, keeping the outer surface uncontaminated to protect persons handling refuse. The entire container then is discarded by incineration or other methods deemed appropriate by the agency.

Specimens of body secretions or excretions may need to be collected for laboratory analysis. As with the dressings and other items, it is important that the outside of the container not be contaminated with the pathogens for the protection of laboratory personnel. A second larger, clean bag or container is also often used in these situations to provide a barrier between the pathogens and the persons handling the container.

Equipment and Supplies Precautions

Equipment and supplies contaminated by pathogens can become vehicles for infection transmission if effective barriers are not developed. Common equipment used in providing patient care, such as the sphygmomanometer, stethoscope, and other physical examination equipment, should be left in the patient's room whenever possible for his exclusive use until the illness has subsided. Disinfection of the equipment should be in the manner appropriate to the causative organisms and situation. A thermometer should also be left at the patient's bedside in a container of disinfectant. Cleaning the thermometer before placing it in the disinfectant and appropriate changing of the disinfectant solution are important points to remember. Needles and syringes must be handled carefully, especially if contaminated by the hepatitis virus. Nondisposable syringes and needles should be rinsed thoroughly in cold water and then disinfected before they are prepared for reuse. The extensive availability of disposable equipment in today's world makes the safe handling of contaminated supplies much easier. Disposable thermometers, physical examination equipment, and needles and syringes can be merely prepared for destruction after use.

If linen and personal laundry are contaminated with pathogens, they should be removed from the patient's immediate environment using the double bag technique described earlier. The outer bag's external surface should always remain clean and the bag's contents should be clearly marked to indicate

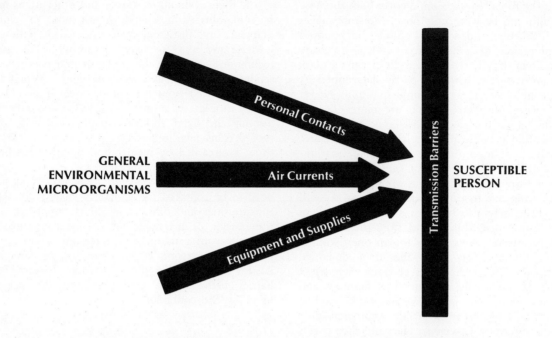

Fig. 19-4. This diagram illustrates protective or reverse isolation. Note that the susceptible person is protected from common vehicles transporting microorganisms from the general environment by transmission barriers.

they are contaminated. Vigorous movements when changing bed linen should be avoided to prevent air movement and spread of microorganisms.

Modern hospital laundering processes make it possible for almost all linens of patients with communicable diseases to be handled in the usual manner. There are some exceptions, as when linens are contaminated with organisms that are spore-forming, as the bacilli of tetanus, gas gangrene, and anthrax. For such causative organisms, the linens should be sterilized by steam under pressure before they are handled by laundry workers.

For items of clothing or apparel that are not washed easily in a machine, airing in sunlight for six to eight hours is effective against organisms in vegetative forms. This would be suitable procedure for such items as blankets, decorative bed jackets, and the like. Also, gas sterilizers, discussed earlier in this chapter, may be used.

Home laundering can generally be safely accomplished with sufficiently hot water or boiling the items and using an appropriate germicidal detergent.

Most health agencies use mechanical dishwashers that leave dishes free of pathogens. If this is not the case, it then becomes necessary to take special precautions when a patient has a communicable disease, especially one that is transmitted via secretions from the mouth. In some agencies, after rinsing the dishes they are boiled. Other agencies use disposable dishes so that only the silverware needs boiling. The technique of placing soiled dishes in a container of water and boiling them before being washed is a questionable practice. The heat of the water often coagulates the food particles remaining on the dishes. If the organism is contained within these solids and is particularly resistive, it may survive the washing process. Therefore, the dishes should be rinsed thoroughly first before being washed and subjected to heat. Many mechanical dishwashers used in restaurants and hospitals provide for rinsing the dishes before they are washed. Rubber gloves should be worn if the dishes are rinsed by hand.

If contaminated, leftover food should be wrapped and discarded along with other wastes from the patient's room. Liquids should be poured down the drain or the toilet if a satisfactory sewage system is available. If not, they may be disinfected before discarding.

Protective (Reverse) Isolation

Protective isolation comprises those practices designed to prevent a highly susceptible person from coming in contact with pathogens. Protective isolation is also referred to as *reverse isolation*, because its goal is the opposite of the usual isolation process. The purpose of protective isolation is to protect a *specific* person against encounter with *any* pathogens in contrast to the usual isolation goal of keeping a *known* microorganism away from any person. The barriers for protective isolation must be designed to prevent vehicles from conveying organisms to the patient. Figure 19-4 demonstrates the goal and common pathogen vehicles.

As indicated earlier, some persons are highly susceptible to infections, even from microorganisms they could normally resist. Persons with certain diseases (leukemia, agammaglobulinemia, and lymphomas) or those receiving certain treatments (total body irradiation) or certain medications (steroids, antimetabolites, or immunosuppressives) need to be protected from as many microorganisms as possible.

Specially constructed rooms or commercial devices can be used to provide an environment as free from organisms as possible. The special space should be under slight positive pressure with respect to adjacent rooms so air flow from the protected room or area moves to the adjoining spaces. Persons caring for the patient do so by wearing a sterile "space suit" type of apparel or by working through special sealed openings in the "plastic walls" of the area. All substances coming in contact with the patient are sterilized, that is, air, linen, food, medications, equipment, and supplies. This is a highly sophisticated and complex type of technique to implement.

Modifications of protective isolation may merely provide for sterilization of all supplies entering the patient's room, plus sterilization of clothing worn by health care personnel.

CONCLUSION

Disinfection, sterilization, and isolation techniques vary. They should be based on knowledge of the causative pathogen, its reservoir, exit mode, transmission vehicles, entry portals, and susceptibility of new hosts. Barriers to prevent transmission of pathogens are the most realistic means of preventing microorganism transmission. The nurse must use her knowledge judiciously in order to provide safe patient care when dealing with infections and communicable diseases.

Study Situations

1. The following articles describe nurses' roles in infection control in the hospital and community:
   Wenzel, K.: The role of the infection control nurse. *In* **The Nursing Clinics of North America,** Philadelphia, W. B. Saunders, 5:89–98, Mar., 1970.
   Lentz, J. F.: The nurse's role in extending infection control to the community. *In* **The Nursing Clinics of North America,** Philadelphia, W. B. Saunders, 5:165–174, Mar., 1970.
   After reading them, describe nurses in the clinical area where you are practicing who are carrying out these functions.
2. The following article describes the author's views about a decreasing focus of attention on communicable disease control in this country:
   Jekel, J. F.: Communicable disease control and public policy in the 1970's—hot war, cold war, or peaceful coexistence? **Am. J. Public Health,** 62:1578–1585, Dec., 1972.
   What are the reasons the author gives for being concerned?
3. Views regarding immunizations change as knowledge advances. The following article describes prevailing ideas in 1973. Read it and then evaluate yourself and your family to see if your immunization protection is considered to be adequate.
   Francis, B. J.: Current concepts in immunization. **Am. J. Nurs.,** 73:646–649, Apr., 1973.
4. The treatment of diseases has also changed. Read the following articles for examples of newer approaches in the treatment of tuberculosis and venereal disease:
   Brown, M. A.: Adolescents and VD. **Nurs. Outlook,** 21:99–103, Feb., 1973.
   Mushlin, I., and Nayer, H. R.: Big city approach to tuberculosis control. **Am. J. Nurs.,** 71:2342–2345, Dec., 1971.
   Weg, J. G.: Tuberculosis and the generation gap. **Am. J. Nurs.,** 71:495–500, Mar., 1971.
5. The following articles describe implementation of protective isolation in two settings. After reading the articles, see how many barriers to pathogen-carrying vehicles you can enumerate in these situations:
   Laduke, M. M., et al.: Germfree isolators. **Am. J. Nurs.,** 67:72–79, Jan., 1967.
   Seidler, F. M.: Adapting nursing procedures for reverse isolation. **Am. J. Nurs.,** 65:108–111, June, 1965.
6. Nurses must frequently initiate action in relation to the control of infectious diseases. These actions should be based on sound assessments. Implement the assessment process described in Chapter 7 to determine the appropriate precautionary measures in the following situations:
   • A mother is concerned about preventing her two- and three-year-old children from acquiring German measles from their six-year-old brother who has just begun to develop the rash.
   • A young man has just entered the hospital with an infected leg injury acquired from an accident involving a piece of farm equipment. As he removes his trousers, you note that purulent drainage has soaked through his dressing.
   • A woman hospitalized for observation begins to

have symptoms of diarrhea and vomiting. This occurred after her husband has been diagnosed as having salmonella food poisoning from some food they ate.

References

1. Burgess, R. E.: Aseptic management of disposables. **Hosp. Top.,** 48:95–98; 113, Jan., 1970.

2. Burke, J. F.: Bacteria-free nursing unit—a new approach to isolation procedures. **Hospitals, J. Am. Hosp. Assoc.,** 43:86–91, Jan. 16, 1969.

3. Chapman, J. S.: The atypical mycobacteria: their significance in human disease. **Am. J. Nurs.,** 67:1031–1033, May, 1967.

4. Dineen, P.: Studying effectiveness of scrubbing, preparation of patient's skin. **Hosp. Top.,** 49:74–75, May, 1971.

5. Dyer, E. D., and Peterson, D. E.: Safe care of IPPB machines. **Am. J. Nurs.,** 71:2163–2166, Nov., 1971.

6. Engley, F. B., Jr.: Biological interrelationships. **Hospitals, J. Am. Hosp. Assoc.,** 46:83–92, Oct. 16, 1972.

7. Engley, F. B., Jr.: Proper use of ethylene oxide discussed in sterilization and disinfection session. **Hosp. Top.,** 49:67–73, May, 1971.

8. Evans, M. J.: Some contributions to prevention of infections. *In* **The Nursing Clinics of North America.** Philadelphia, W. B. Saunders, 3:641–648, Dec. 1968.

9. Feeney, R.: Preventing rheumatic fever in school children. **Am. J. Nurs.,** 73:265, Feb., 1973.

10. French, J. G.: Students study cross-contamination. **Am. J. Nurs.,** 67:2104–2106, Oct., 1967.

11. Garner, J. S., and Kaiser, A. B.: How often is isolation needed? **Am. J. Nurs.,** 72:733–737, Apr., 1972.

12. Ginsberg, F., and Clarke, B.: When to use disinfectants and which ones not to use. **Mod. Hosp.,** 119:110, Aug., 1972.

13. Golden, D. L.: Constant monitoring guarantees sterility. **Hospitals, J. Am. Hosp. Assoc.,** 46:79–85, Sept. 16, 1972.

14. Greene, V. W.: Microbiological contamination control in hospitals. **Hospitals, J. Am. Hosp. Assoc.**

Part 1—perspectives. 43:78–83, 87–88, Oct. 16, 1969.
Part 2—role of the engineer. 43:83–89, Nov. 1, 1969.
Part 3—role of nursing service. 43:71–75, 78, Nov. 16, 1969.
Part 4—role of housekeeping. 43:69–80, Dec. 1, 1969.*
Part 5—role of administration. 43:74–78; 118, Dec. 16, 1969.
Part 6—roles of central service and the laundry. 44:98–103, Jan. 1, 1970.

* V. W. Green and D. Vesey, co-authors.

Part 7—role of the laboratory. 44:66–70, Jan. 16, 1970.
Part 8—role of the medical staff. 44:124–129, Feb. 1, 1970.

15. Herrmann, J., and Light, I. J.: Infection control in the newborn nursery. *In* **The Nursing Clinics of North America.** Philadelphia, W. B. Saunders, 6:55–65, Mar., 1971.

16. Himmelsbach, C. K.: Nosocomial infections. **Hospitals, J. Am. Hosp. Assoc.,** 44:84, 88–92, Feb. 16, 1970.

17. Hohle, B. M.: The atypical mycobacteria: patient care at home. **Am. J. Nurs.,** 67:1033–1036, May, 1967.

18. Isolation Techniques For Use In Hospitals. Washington, D. C., U. S. Department of Health, Education, and Welfare, Public Health Service, 1970.

19. Keusch, G.: Bacterial diarrheas. **Am. J. Nurs.,** 73:1028–1032, June, 1973.

20. Kicklighter, L.: The nurse epidemiologist. **Hospitals, J. Am. Hosp. Assoc.,** 47:48–56, Jan. 1, 1973.

21. Litsky, W., et al.: Solid waste: a hospital dilemma. **Am. J. Nurs.,** 72:1841–1847, Oct., 1972.

22. Lloyd, R. S., et al.: Sterilization of clinical oral thermometers with ethylene oxide. **Hosp. Manage.,** 109:16–21, Jan., 1970.

23. Mangan, H. M.: Care, coordination and communication in the life island setting. **Nurs. Outlook,** 17:40–44, Jan., 1969.

24. Marinaro, A.: Rationale of sterility, sterlization and sterility testing. **Hosp. Top.,** 49:118–120, Jan., 1971.

25. Marples, M. J.: Life on the human skin. **Sci. Am.,** 220:108–115, Jan., 1969.

26. Murphy, P. R.: Tuberculosis control in San Francisco's Chinatown. **Am. J. Nurs.,** 70:1044–1046, May, 1970.

27. Nordmark, M. T., and Rohweder, A. W.: Scientific Foundations of Nursing. ed. 2, pp. 240–258. Philadelphia, J. B. Lippincott, 1967.

28. Perkins, J. J.: Principles and Methods of Sterilization in Health Sciences. ed. 2. Springfield, Ill., Charles C Thomas, 1969.

29. Rendell-Baker, L., and Roberts, R. B.: Gas versus steam sterilization: when to use which. **Hosp. Top.,** 48:81–83, 86–88, Nov., 1970.

30. Schuman, L. M.: Epidemiology—the problem defined and principles. *In* Corrigan, M. J., and Corcoran, L. E., eds.: Epidemiology In Nursing. pp. 3–61. Washington, D. C., The Catholic University of America Press, 1961.

31. Streeter, S., et al.: Hospital infection—a necessary risk? **Am. J. Nurs.,** 67:526–533, Mar., 1967.

32. Symposium on infection and the nurse. *In* **The Nursing Clinics of North America.** Philadelphia, W. B. Saunders, 5:85–177, Mar., 1970.

33. Wright, N.: Methods and principles of sterilization. **Hosp. Manage.,** 109:65–67, May, 1970.

UNIT 5

Common Nursing Intervention Measures

CHAPTER 20

Gathering Data in Relation to the Patient's Physical Health Status

GLOSSARY

Antipyretic: A fever-reducing agent.

Apnea: Absence of breathing.

Arrhythmia: Irregular pulse rhythm.

Atrioventricular or Auriculoventricular Node: Tissue at base of atrial septum that normally picks up electrical current from S-A node, abbreviated A-V node.

Auscultation: Procedure to examine organs by listening to sound within the body.

Bradycardia: Slow heartbeat.

Cardinal Signs: Synonym for vital signs.

Cheyne-Stokes Respiration: Gradual increase and then gradual decrease in depth of respiration followed by period of apnea.

Circadian Rhythm: A biological or behavioral process that recurs in approximately every 24-hour cycle.

Confusion: Condition of mental bewilderment.

Constitutional Symptom: A sign due to the effect of a disease on the whole body.

Crisis: Rapid drop of body temperature to normal.

Cyanosis: Bluish coloring of skin and mucous membrane.

Dehydration: Depletion of body fluids, causing skin to be loose and wrinkled and to feel dry.

Depolarize: To destroy polarity.

Diaphoresis: Excessive perspiration.

Diastole: Period when least amount of pressure is exerted on aterial walls during heartbeat.

Dicrotic Pulse: Exaggerated ending of pulse wave which feels as a double pulse to touch.

Disoriented: Being unaware of time, place, and/or one's surroundings.

Distention: Swelling or expansion.

Dorsal Position: Patient lies flat on his back, legs together.

Dorsal Recumbent Position: Patient on back is brought close to edge of bed, legs separated, and knees flexed.

Dyspnea: Difficult breathing.

Ecchymosis: A collection of blood in subcutaneous tissues, causing purplish discoloration.

Ectopic Pacemaker: Areas where heart impulse may originate other than at S-A node.

Edema: Retention of fluid in tissues with consequent swelling.

Electrocardiogram: Graphic record produced by electrocardiograph, abbreviated EKG.

Electrocardiograph: Instrument that measures and records electrical impulses of heart.

Exhalation: Synonym of expiration.

Expiration: Act of breathing out.

External Respiration: Act of lung ventilation, oxygen absorption, and carbon dioxide elimination.

Fast: Abstinence from food and fluids.

Gastric Analysis: Laboratory examination of gastric contents.

Genupectoral Position: Synonym for knee-chest position.

Homeokinesis: Synonym of homeostasis.

Homeostasis: Maintenance of uniformity or stability.

Homeothermal: Maintaining same body temperature irrespective of environmental temperature.

Hyperpnea: Increased depth of respiration.

Hyperpyrexia: High fever, above 41°C. (105.8°F.).

Hypertension: Abnormally high blood pressure.

Hypotension: Abnormally low blood pressure.

Hypothermia: Body temperature that is below average normal range.

Hypoxia: Low oxygen content.

Incoherent: Disconnected thought or speech.

Inhalation: Synonym of inspiration.

Inspiration: Act of breathing in.

Intermittent Pulse: Period of normal pulse rhythm broken by periods of irregular rhythm.

Intermittent Temperature: Alternating temperature between a period of pyrexia and a period of normal or subnormal temperature.

Internal Respiration: Act of using oxygen by body cells.

Jaundice: Yellowness of the skin.

Knee-Chest Position: Patient rests on his knees and chest with body flexed approximately 90° at hips.

Korotkoff Sounds: Sounds that indicate systolic and diastolic pressure when determining blood pressure.

Lead: Placement pattern of sensors used in electrocardiography.

Lithotomy Position: Same as dorsal recumbent position except feet are placed in stirrups and buttocks are at edge of examining table.

Lumbar Puncture: Insertion of a needle into the subarachnoid space.

Lysis: Gradual return of body temperature to normal.

Meniscus: The curved surface at the top of a column of liquid in a tube.

Mucus: Viscid watery-appearing secretion produced by mucous membrane.

Objective Symptom: A manifestation presented by one person that can be directly observed by another.

Oriented: Being aware of time, place, and one's surroundings.

Orthopnea: A type of dyspnea in which breathing is easier when patient sits or stands up.

Palpation: Procedure designed to feel a part with the fingers or hand.

Paracentesis: Withdrawal of fluid from a body cavity; usually, term used to refer to removal of fluid from abdominal cavity.

Parallax: Apparent change of position of an object when seen from two different angles.

Percussion: Procedure designed to determine the density of a part by means of tapping the surface.

Poikilothermal: Maintaining same body temperature as environmental temperature.

Polarity: To have an electrical charge.

Polypnea: Respiratory rate above average normal range.

Prodromal Symptoms: A manifestation that precedes the development of a disease.

Prosthesis: An appliance or artificial part used for a natural part of the body.

Pulse: A wave set up in walls of artery with each beat of the heart.

Pulse Pressure: The difference between systolic and diastolic pressure.

Purkinje System: Interlacing network in ventricles that carry electrical currents through the ventricles.

Purulent Drainage: Discharge containing pus.

Pyrexia: Elevation of body temperature.

Rash: An eruption on the skin.

Recrudescent Temperature: After pyrexia, temperature returns to normal, but then temperature elevation returns.

Remittent Temperature: Above normal fluctuating temperature.

Repolarize: To restore polarity.

Respiration: Act of breathing and of using oxygen in body cells.

Responsive: Answers with word and/or gesture.

Sanguineous Drainage: Discharge containing blood.

Serosanguineous Drainage: Discharge containing serum and blood.

Serous Drainage: Light-colored discharge containing serum.

Sim's Position, Right or Left: Patient is on his side with top knee flexed sharply onto abdomen and lower knee less sharply flexed.

Sinoatrial or Sinoauricular Node: Tissue in upper part of right atrium where heartbeat originates, abbreviated S-A node. Also called heart's pacemaker.

Spinal Tap: Synonym for lumbar puncture.

Sputum: Substance from respiratory tract ejected from mouth.

Stentorous Respiration: Noisy breathing.

Subjective Symptom: A manifestation felt or perceived by one person that cannot be detected directly by others.

Systole: Period when maximum pressure is exerted on arterial walls during heartbeat.

Tachycardia: Rapid heartbeat.

Thoracentesis: Entrance and aspiration of fluid from the pleural cavity.

Tidal Air: Volume of air exchanged with each respiration in a state of rest.

Tissue Respiration: Synonym of internal respiration.

Unconscious: Lacking capacity for sensory perception.

Unresponsive: Unable to answer when spoken to.

Urinalysis: Laboratory examination of a urine specimen.

Vasoconstriction: Condition in which arterioles are in a state of contraction to a greater than usual degree.

Vasodilation: Condition in which arterioles are in a state of enlargement to a greater than usual degree.

Vital Signs: Measurements in relation to body temperature, pulse, respirations, and blood pressure.

Wound: Break in continuity of skin.

INTRODUCTION

This unit describes information the nurse will use in order to assist patients to meet certain requirements of daily living. Many nursing intervention measures will be discussed. But data are essential before nursing services can be rendered, as Unit 2 indicates. This chapter presents common methods used in gathering data about the patient's physical health status, an important part of the health state profile.

The word physical, according to the dictionary, refers to the body as distinguished from the mind. As this text has stated earlier, it is almost impossible to separate the mind and body; rather, they function interdependently and as a whole. Although the primary focus of this chapter is related to and discusses the physical examination, the patient's mental and emotional status are not to be ignored.

The expanded role of the nurse is discussed in Chapter 1. In some schools of nursing, students are being taught to assume more responsibility in relation to conducting the physical examination than once was the case. Also, in many health agencies, graduate nurses are taking increased responsibility for the physical examination. In some settings now, for example, the nurse is often expected to conduct the entire initial physical examination. The reader will be expected to observe the policy in her school of nursing or in the health agency in which she practices concerning the exact responsibility she will assume when a physical examination is done.

Agency policy will also be observed in relation to attendance during a physical examination. For example, it is the policy of some agencies to require a female nurse to be present when a male physician is examining a female patient. This is for the psychological comfort of the patient as well as protection for the physician and the agency.

Details of some specific techniques and the interpretation of the findings of a physical examination are not described here. These techniques and their interpretations are more appropriately discussed in texts dealing with more advanced clinical nursing practice.

SELECTING AND ORGANIZING APPROPRIATE DATA

When a patient has a physical examination, decisions must be made in relation to selecting appropriate data, and the guidelines offered in Chapter 6 are applicable here. For example, three questions offered to assist the nurse in selecting relevant data are helpful: Who is the patient? For what reason is the patient being considered for receiving care? What factors in this patient's life are playing a part in his present situation?

There is no one correct method of organizing data gathered during a physical examination. Health agencies generally have forms to serve as guides that will assist the nurse in selecting as well as in organizing the data. The importance of accurately re-cording the data gathered cannot be overemphasized, as Chapter 10 indicates. The forms are used according to health agency policy.

SELECTING METHODS TO GATHER DATA

As Chapter 6 indicates, health practitioners will use observation, interviewing, and inspection most commonly during the physical examination. This chapter will focus primarily on inspection and observation. The eyes of the examiner are used to observe and inspect the patient. Sight is also used when instruments such as the thermometer and sphygmomanometer are employed. The sense of touch often reveals information, as when the examiner feels the temperature of the skin. Hearing is used, for example, when listening to a patient's breathing.

Percussion involves striking a particular area of the body, either with the fingertips or with a percussion hammer, in order that the examiner may listen for sounds to determine density of the tissue. Percussion is used when the examiner taps the patient's chest wall in order to determine the sound created. If fluid, secretions, or a solid mass are present, the sound will be dull; when the level of fluid or obstruction is passed, a hollow sound will be heard.

Palpation uses the sense of touch as the examiner feels or presses on the body. For example, palpation is used when the abdomen is examined to feel the various abdominal organs.

Auscultation uses the sense of hearing for interpreting sounds in the body and usually is performed with the aid of the stethoscope. Auscultation is used when the examiner listens to the patient's heart sounds with the stethoscope.

When the patient has records from other health agencies, the examiner will want to use them for information. However, parts of the examination may be repeated. This will be especially true when the data are not sufficiently up to date and when validation of information is indicated.

GATHERING DATA DURING THE PHYSICAL EXAMINATION

The physical examination may be said to begin when the patient is admitted to a health agency. Certain basic information gathered on admission will be useful during the examination proper such as the

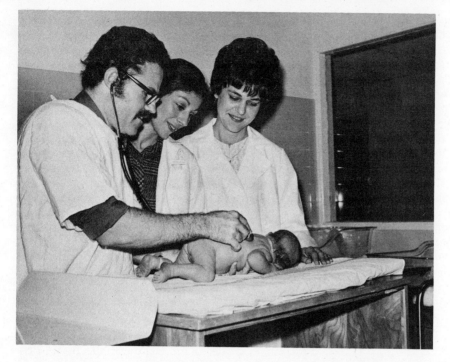

Fig. 20-1. The physician uses the stethoscope to listen to the infant's chest sounds. He is instructing the nurses in the use of auscultation. (Good Samaritan Hospital, Phoenix, Arizona)

patient's name, address, age, sex, primary complaint if any, and the like. This type of baseline information is discussed in Chapter 10.

A health history is then obtained, generally from the patient. When this is not possible, a member of the patient's family will usually assist. History taking is discussed in Chapter 6 and illustrated in Figure 6-3.

The patient's physician may obtain a medical history prior to the nurse's first contact with the patient. However, if this is not the case and if time and circumstances permit, attending the physician's history-taking interview is a good way to get to know the patient better. In either case, the nurse will still wish to obtain a nursing history of her own.

There are certain common terms used to describe the signs or symptoms manifested by the patient. A *subjective symptom* is a manifestation that is felt or perceived by one person but cannot be detected directly by others. For example, pain is a subjective symptom; it can be felt and described by only one person but it cannot be observed directly by another. An *objective symptom* is a manifestation presented by one person that can be directly observed by another. Swelling of the ankles and a skin rash are examples of objective symptoms.

Constitutional symptoms are produced by the effect of the disease on the whole body, as a fever. *Local symptoms* are noted in some special area or part of the body, such as a swollen jaw. *Prodromal symptoms* precede the development of disease, such as an "achy feeling" before an acute infectious disease develops.

Using accurate and objective descriptions of signs or symptoms is important to assist the health and the nursing teams to meet a patient's needs. For example, a patient may say he has a "bellyache." The nurse should describe the area of the abdomen where the pain is experienced and the nature of the pain. Or, the patient may say he "threw up." The nurse would record when vomiting occurred, what type of vomitus it was, and how much there was.

Preparation for the Physical Examination

The physical examination may be done in an examining or a treatment room or in the patient's room if he is hospitalized. Most health agencies have a tray or basket for holding the necessary equipment. The following items are usually kept in readiness: ophthalmoscope (for examining the eyes), otoscope (for examining the ears), ear speculum, nose speculum, head mirror, flashlight, stethoscope, sphygmomanometer, tape measure, tongue depressors, tuning fork, skin pencil, percussion hammer, tissue wipes and waste container, safety pins, cotton, and test tubes for hot and cold water. For rectal and vaginal examinations, the following items are necessary: bivalve vaginal speculum, sterile or clean gloves, powder, and lubricant.

As part of a physical examination, several laboratory tests are done. Each agency has its own procedure or laboratory manual concerning the type of container in which to collect the specimen, the amount of specimen needed, preparation of the specimen, the laboratory to which the specimen is sent, and the like. The nurse's responsibilities will vary, depending on the agency's procedure. Necessary items for laboratory examinations should be readily available, such as specimen containers, slides, and cotton applicators. The collection of specimens and common laboratory findings are discussed later.

The nurse will wish to have material available for draping. Some agencies have disposable paper drapes, but the same purpose can be achieved with a bath blanket, a draw sheet, or the top bedcovers if the patient is examined in a bed. The purpose of the draping is to avoid exposing the patient except for the part being examined. In some instances, it may be necessary to provide an extra cover to prevent the patient from drafts or being chilled. This is particularly true when the patient is very ill or elderly.

The patient may need assistance in assuming and retaining proper positions for examining. While the examination is being conducted, the nurse keeps the patient draped properly, exposing areas of the body as indicated. The legal implications when a patient is exposed unnecessarily are discussed in Chapter 4 in the section dealing with invasion of privacy.

Positioning the Patient

There are several common positions used when a physical examination is done. The *erect* position is the normal standing position. The patient wears slippers, or the floor is protected. The draping is arranged so that body contours, posture, muscles, and extremities can be inspected conveniently.

In the *dorsal* or *horizontal recumbent position*, the patient lies flat on his back with his legs together, in bed or on the examining table. His head may be supported with a pillow and his legs extended or slightly flexed at the knees to relax the abdominal wall. He is covered with a drape. Parts of the drape are folded back to expose the area being examined. The dorsal position is assumed most commonly for examination of the abdomen, the chest anteriorly, the breasts, the reflexes, the extremities, the head, the neck, the eyes, the ears, the nose, and the throat.

In the *dorsal recumbent position*, the patient is brought close to the edge of the bed while lying on his back with the legs separated and the knees flexed; the soles of the feet rest flat on the bed or table. One pillow may be placed under the head. A drape is placed diagonally over the patient with opposite corners protecting the legs and wrapped around the feet so that the drape will stay in place. The third corner of the drape covers the patient's chest, and the fourth corner is placed between the legs. A disposable pad may be placed under the patient's buttocks to avoid soiling linen. The corner of the drape between the patient's legs is raised and folded back on the abdomen to expose the part being examined. Figure 20-2 illustrates the dorsal recumbent position.

The *lithotomy position* is the same as the dorsal recumbent position except that the patient is usually on a table equipped with foot stirrups. The patient's buttocks are brought to the edge of the table. The knees are flexed, and the feet are supported in the stirrups. A disposable pad may be placed under the patient's buttocks, and draping is the same as for the dorsal recumbent position. The position is assumed usually for digital examination of the rectum or instrument examination of the vagina. Figure 20-3 illustrates the lithotomy position.

In the left *Sim's position*, the patient lies on his left side and rests his left arm behind his body. The right arm is forward with the elbow flexed and the arm resting on a pillow placed under the patient's head. The patient's body inclines slightly forward. The knees are flexed, the right one sharply on the abdomen and the left one less sharply. In the right Sim's position, the placement of the extremities is reversed. The position usually is assumed for a digital examination of the rectum or the vagina. A disposable pad may be used under the buttocks. One corner of the drape is folded back on the patient's hip to expose the area being examined. Figure 20-4 illustrates the Sim's position.

In the *knee-chest or genupectoral position*, the patient rests on his knees and chest with his body flexed approximately 90° at the hips. The head, turned to one side, rests on a small pillow. A small pillow also may be placed under the chest. The arms are above the head or they may be flexed at the elbows and rest alongside the patient's head. The lower legs are placed perpendicular to the thighs. The knee-chest position frequently is assumed for an instrument examination of the rectum. The drape is placed so that the patient's back, buttocks, and thighs are covered. Only the area to be examined is exposed. This is a very difficult position for most

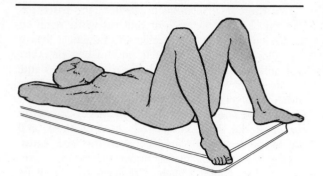

Fig. 20-2. Dorsal recumbent position.

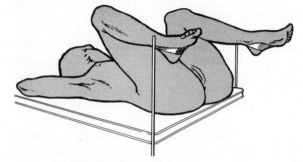

Fig. 20-3. Lithotomy position.

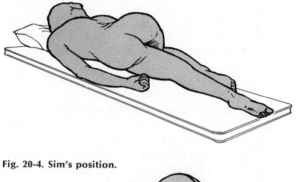

Fig. 20-4. Sim's position.

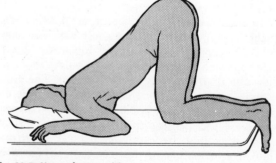

Fig. 20-5. Knee-chest position.

patients to assume, especially for the elderly patient. Therefore, the nurse should have all equipment ready and should not assist the patient into position until the examiner is to commence. Figure 20-5 illustrates the knee-chest position.

The dorsal recumbent, lithotomy, Sim's, and knee-chest positions are used to examine areas of the body which cause embarrassment to some patients. The examinations can be made easier for the patient if the nurse takes every precaution to prevent exposure and to give explanations and directions slowly and carefully. Even when a patient is properly draped for an examination, there may be concern that someone can see into the unit or come into the room. The nurse should make every effort to see that this does not happen.

Observing the Patient's General Mental and Emotional State

While observing the patient, the nurse should become aware of the patient's responsiveness and orientation and of emotions the patient may be experiencing. Below are some common terms used to describe a patient's mental state.

To be *oriented* means being aware of time, place, and one's surroundings; to be *disoriented* is the opposite. The word *confusion* is used to describe a condition of mental bewilderment. A *responsive* patient answers by word, or gesture, or both; the *unresponsive* patient appears to be unaware of his surroundings and unable to answer when spoken to. The word *incoherent* describes disconnected thought or speech. The thoughts are unrelated and the listener is unable to make sense from what is being said. The *unconscious* patient lacks the capacity for sensory perception. When using terms as these, it is helpful to describe what the patient actually says or does, or does not say or do. These are some examples: "Could not answer appropriately when asked current date and city where he was"; or, "Responded appropriately to all questions"; or "Spoke of brother, who has been dead for years, as if he were alive"; or "Speaks in phrases which have no apparent relationship to each other."

Chapter 12 describes common emotions, and the nurse will wish to be alert to behavior that reflects the patient's emotional state. Terms such as anxious, frightened, unconcerned, resentful, uncooperative, and the like are often difficult to define in a precise manner and may be interpreted differently among health and nursing team members. Therefore, it is better to record the behavior observed. Here are examples: "Facial and extremity muscles tense, jaw set, hands clenched, perspiring heavily"; or, "Moves frequently about room, talking rapidly, exaggerated response to sound stimuli."

Measuring the Patient's Height and Weight

It is common practice to measure the patient's height and weight upon admission to a health agency. Even though the patient may have been weighed recently at home, it is preferable to weigh him on admission so that subsequent weights can be taken on the same scale, thus making comparisons more nearly accurate. The patient's height is measured at the same time; he should be asked to remove his shoes for this procedure. It is good medical aseptic technique to place a paper towel on the scale before the patient stands on it with his bare feet and to use a clean towel for each patient.

Weighing the patient and measuring his height may be delayed if he is too ill, unless it is necessary to know the weight for purposes of therapy. To make weighing easier for very ill patients, some agencies have portable or bed scales. The scale can be rolled to the patient's bedside where he can be assisted onto it.

Many factors enter into a consideration of what is normal weight, such as age, body build, height, and sex. Therefore, it is difficult to determine where abnormality begins. Many authorities accept a 10 to 15 percent variation from the average described in weight tables as being within normal limits.

The nurse will wish to be aware of evidence that suggests the patient is experiencing unusual weight losses or gains.

Examining the Skin, Hair, and Nails

Since the skin covers almost the entire surface of the body, it is a good indicator of a person's health status. In addition to its general appearance (smooth, wrinkled, dry, or well hydrated) the nurse also is concerned with evidence of injury or lack of good care. These would be evidenced by bruises, scratches, cuts, insect bites, and sores. The presence of any of these is recorded. Treat all lesions on a patient with great care to avoid possible contamination of objects and transfer of infection to other persons. Because of the danger of infections, newly admitted patients with open lesions or draining ones are checked carefully. In many agencies, cultures are taken; the patient may be placed on special precautions until the laboratory reports are complete.

Fingernails and toenails also are an indication of the patient's general physical condition. Brittle or dry nails may well be a clue to nutrition or to a state of illness.

Hair is also a clue to the person's state of health. It is not uncommon for the hair to lose its gloss and texture or even fall out during periods of illness.

Some terms used to describe the skin follow.

Flush is a redness of the skin, as in a blush. It is usually associated with an elevated temperature, and the face and the neck are more likely to be affected than the other parts of the body.

Cyanosis is a dusky, bluish color usually seen in the lips, the mucous membranes, and the nail beds. It is caused by lack of oxygen. Cyanosis is often observed when a person is chilled while swimming or immediately upon coming out of the water. Persons with heavily pigmented skin must usually be observed for cyanosis in the nail beds or in the mucous membranes.

Jaundice is a yellowness of the skin. Usually, it affects the entire body, and almost always the whites of the eyes.

Dehydration is a depletion of body fluids causing the skin to be loose and wrinkled and to feel dry. Typically, the lips and the tongue are dry and parched.

A *rash* is an eruption of the skin. Because the descriptive details of a rash are complex, comprising type of spots, size, elevation, coloring, and presence or absence of drainage or itching, they are dealt with more appropriately in a text on skin diseases. The nurse should indicate exactly where on the patient's body a rash is noticed and its general appearance.

Ecchymosis is a collection of blood in subcutaneous tissues, causing purplish discoloration. Note location, size, and coloring, of which the last is an indication of how recently it occurred.

Diaphoresis is an excessive amount of perspiration, as when a person's entire skin is moist and perspiring.

Edema is retention of fluid in the tissues with consequent swelling. It may also occur in body cavities. The skin appears taut over these areas, and if the fingers are pressed gently into the areas, an impression may remain after pressure has been released.

A *wound* is a break in the continuity of the skin. The wound should be described as to size, shape, depth, and location. If drainage is present, it too is described as to amount and character. For example, it could be scant, moderate, or profuse. Common terms for describing its appearance are as follows: (1) serous—containing the serum (clear portion) of the blood; (2) sanguineous—containing a great deal of blood; (3) serosanguineous—containing both serum and blood; (4) purulent—containing or consisting of "pus."

Examining the Head and the Neck

The contour of the skull is examined, and occasionally the examiner may wish to measure the size of the cranium with a tape measure. The physical characteristics and the facial expressions and the condition of the hair and the scalp are noted. The head and the neck are palpated for nodules. The thyroid gland in the neck, the larynx, and the trachea are palpated.

Examining the Eyes

Eyelids and eyeballs are inspected, and movements of the eyes are noted. A flashlight may be used to determine the reaction of the pupils to light. The interior of the eyeball is inspected from the corneal surface to the eyegrounds with the aid of an ophthalmoscope. Sight and field of vision are examined with the aid of a reading test chart and a perimeter chart. Unless there is reason for a detailed examination of sight and field of vision, test charts and perimeter are not used for the routine physical examination. A tonometer is used to test pressure within the eye.

If a patient's sight is limited, this should be noted since it will be an important consideration in planning nursing care. For example, the patient may need assistance with eating, personal hygiene, meal preparation at home, or even returning for follow-up care.

Examining the Ears

The general contour is noted. The external auditory canal and the eardrum are observed with the aid of an otoscope or an ear speculum and head mirror. The mastoid area is palpated and inspected. Tuning forks are sometimes used to test acuity of hearing. The most accurate way to test hearing is with an audiometer, an instrument for gauging and recording the power of hearing. Unless there is indication for careful study of hearing, an audiometer is not used for most routine physical examinations. The nurse will wish to note if a patient with limited hearing uses a hearing aid.

When speaking to a person who has difficulty in hearing, it is helpful to speak distinctly, face him, and make certain that what has been said is understood. Shouting is to be avoided unless it is absolutely necessary. Many persons learn to read lips. At night, in order to avoid disturbing others, directing a flash-light on one's face so that the patient may watch mouth and facial expressions when a patient is hospitalized, is helpful. Another measure that is helpful with some types of hearing loss is to place the ear tips of a stethoscope in the patient's ears and to speak into the bell portion.

Examining the Nose

The nose is inspected and palpated. A flashlight or a head mirror and a nasal speculum are used to inspect the nostrils and the septum. Sense of smell is determined by having the patient smell commonly recognized substances.

Examining the Lips, the Mouth, and the Throat

Examining the lips is usually by inspection. A tongue depressor and a light are used for inspecting the mouth, teeth, gums, tongue, hard and soft palate, tonsils, pharynx, and larynx.

Examining the Breasts

The breasts are examined for symmetry, position, and size. Palpation is used to determine the presence of tumors. The nipples are examined by inspection and palpation.

Examining the Chest and Respiratory Tract

Contour, size, and shape of the chest are inspected, and respiratory movements are noted. Percussion is used to set up vibrations in underlying tissue; the type of sound produced is significant to the examiner, since certain sounds over air-containing and airless tissue are characteristic of health and others are characteristic of disease. Auscultation with a stethoscope is used to hear and evaluate breath sounds. During auscultation of the chest, the patient may be asked to cough, and he should be provided with tissue wipes to cover his mouth when so doing.

Most authorities agree that a physical examination is incomplete without a chest x-ray. Some health agencies have a policy that patients have a chest x-ray made on admission. Routine chest x-ray is helpful in early lung cancer detection and has aided immeasurably in diagnosing tuberculosis long before the patient might have become aware of having the disease. X-rays also aid in determining the contour and the size of other organs in the chest, and of the ribs.

If the patient has a cough, it is described as non-productive if no matter or discharge from the respiratory tract is produced. If there is expectoration, it is called a productive cough, and the expectoration is described. *Mucus* or *sputum* can be a viscid watery-appearing secretion of the mucous membranes or it can be of greater viscosity and color, depending upon its cause and origin. It can be expectorated with or without a cough. If a patient has a cough, the nurse should determine whether the patient understands how to protect others when he coughs and how to dispose of tissues safely.

Observations in relation to the patient's respiratory rate are described later in this chapter.

Examining the Abdomen and the Back

Inspection will determine the general contour of the abdomen, the condition of the skin, and the distribution of pubic hair. By palpation, normal organs or abnormal masses may be noted. Percussion is used to detect fluids. Auscultation of the abdomen is used to examine the pregnant woman to determine the fetal heart rate or to detect peristaltic movements of the intestinal tract.

In order to describe the location of signs and symptoms of the abdomen, systematic areas of the abdomen have been defined. The most common method of subdividing the abdomen is by describing four quadrants. A line drawn from the tip of the sternum to the pubic bone through the umbilicus and a horizontal line crossing the other at the um-

bilicus divides the abdominal area into four quadrants. These quadrants are called the right and the left upper quadrants and the right and the left lower quadrants. They are frequently abbreviated RUQ, LUQ, RLQ, and LLQ, respectively. Figure 20-6 illustrates these four divisions.

Distention is a swelling or expansion. Abdominal distention often occurs in illness, as for example, when a mass is present in the gastrointestinal tract, or when a person has eaten foods that are particularly irritating to the tract. Tapping gently on the area usually will produce a hollow, drumlike sound; if a mass is present, no hollow sound is present.

The back is inspected and palpated to determine its contour and the position of the spine.

Thorough examinations of the abdomen, the pelvis and the back usually include x-ray examinations, but x-rays are used infrequently unless a pathologic condition appears to exist. Contrast media, such as dyes and barium, are used for x-ray examinations of abdominal and pelvic organs. X-ray of the spine is scheduled when detailed examination of the spine is indicated. The nurse is often responsible for preparing or instructing the patient about preparation for radiological examinations.

Observations in relation to gastrointestinal elimination are discussed in Chapter 26. Observations in relation to nausea and vomiting are discussed in Chapter 25.

Examining the Cardiovascular System

Inspection, palpation, percussion, auscultation, and roentgenography are used to determine the size and the shape of the heart, abnormal pulsations, heart sounds, murmurs, and so on. A study of heart function can be done with the use of an electrocardiograph, described later in this chapter. Also described later are methods to determine the pulse rate and the blood pressure.

Examining the Musculoskeletal System

Inspection and palpation are used to examine the musculoskeletal system. General contour is noted, and joints are inspected. Occasionally, the extremities are measured with a tape measure. X-rays frequently are used as an aid in examining the skeletal system.

The Neurologic Examination

During the neurologic examination, the reflexes and the various senses are examined. Usually, the percussion hammer is used to test reflexes. A skin pencil is employed frequently to mark certain neuro-

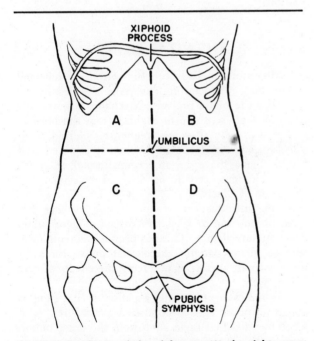

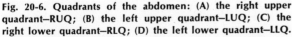

Fig. 20-6. Quadrants of the abdomen: (A) the right upper quadrant—RUQ; (B) the left upper quadrant—LUQ; (C) the right lower quadrant—RLQ; (D) the left lower quadrant—LLQ.

logic as well as musculoskeletal findings on the patient's body. The senses of touch and pain are examined with cotton and with a pin. Placing test tubes containing hot and cold water on the skin may be used to test heat and cold receptors.

Examining the Genitalia, the Perineum, the Anus, and the Rectum

These areas are examined by inspection and palpation. Rectal and vaginal examinations rarely are done on children and young adults unless specific complaints are referred to these areas. A bivalve vaginal speculum is used to examine the vagina and the cervix. Gloves are used for this part of the examination.

Physicians usually recommend that men over 40 years of age have a digital rectal examination at least on an annual basis. The examination aids in early detection of cancer of the prostate gland.

Observing for Pain

Pain is a subjective phenomenon; one person cannot accurately assess the type and intensity of pain that another person is experiencing. The nurse will interview and observe the patient to arrive at objective descriptions of pain. Pain and common terms used to describe it are discussed in Chapter 23.

Noting Physical Limitations

A specific notation is made of a patient's physical limitations. Observing for limited vision or hearing have been discussed earlier. Other examples include patients with various types of amputations; with loss of function in a body part; or with artificial orifices, such as a colostomy. Some of these patients may use a *prosthesis*, which is an artificial part of the body. Examples include an artificial eye, an artificial limb, or an artificial breast. Others may use a crutch, a cane, braces, or girdles. Still others may use items such as a colostomy belt and bag, elastic hose, or moistureproof underpants. Some patients have cardiac pacemakers. A high anterior chest scar with some protrusion is a clue of a pacemaker although most patients having a pacemaker are likely to indicate voluntarily that they have one. Any such items are clues to possible limitations and the nurse will wish to note their presence and reasons for using them.

Some patients may speak freely about such items just described, even warning all to be careful of them and possibly not wanting them out of their sight. Other patients may not feel as free to talk about their problem, and with them a cautious approach is

necessary. It is not a matter of ignoring the presence of such items, but rather one of asking the patient what can be done to make it easier to manage his activities of daily living.

It is important to ask the patient if he has any allergies to drugs or other agents. An allergic reaction can be a serious manifestation. When patients have allergy problems, the information should be clearly and conspicuously stated in the patient's record.

Following the physical examination, the nurse assists the patient as necessary. For safety and courtesy reasons, the patient should be assisted off an examining table. He may also need assistance with dressing.

The nurse will follow the agency's policy in relation to the care of equipment used during the physical examination. This includes cleansing and returning items to their proper place and discarding disposable items carefully and as specified by the agency.

A physical examination generally includes observation of the patient's body temperature, pulse, respirations, and blood pressure. Also an electrocardiogram is commonly included in a physical examination. The next sections of this chapter will discuss observations in relation to these parts of an examination.

THE VITAL SIGNS

Alterations in body function often are reflected in the body temperature, the pulse and respiratory rate, and the blood pressure. Mechanisms governing them are very sensitive to changes from the normal, and that is why they are frequently referred to as *vital signs* or *cardinal signs.* When it is noted that the vital signs have deviated from normal, it means that the patient needs to be observed for evidence of cause and of effects.

The introduction of monitoring devices has made it possible to keep patients' vital signs under constant surveillance. This has been a lifesaving measure for many patients, because it makes for a far more accurate means of observing the effects of care being given.

As indicated, obtaining a patient's vital signs is a part of most agency admission procedures. It is recommended that upon admission, the nurse obtain these signs whenever possible rather than to assign the task to members of the nursing team who may have less knowledge concerning the meaning of deviations from normal.

Most adult patients are familiar with the procedures for obtaining body temperature, pulse and respiratory rates, and blood pressure. However, an explanation of the procedures by the nurse will help put the patient at ease. Explanations should be given to children also for the same reason.

Body Temperature

A phenomenon known as the "24-hour" or *circadian rhythm* has been observed in many animals, including man. Certain daily events in biological man appear to recur every 24 hours and therefore, the word circadian, meaning "nearly every 24 hours," is often used to describe the rhythm. The rhythm can be observed in relation to biological functioning that involves, for example, body temperature, sleep, and blood pressure. Body temperature, for instance, is usually 1° to 2°F. lower in the early morning than in late afternoon. This variation tends to be somewhat higher in infants and young children.

Man is *homoiothermic* (also spelled homeothermic); that is, he is warm-blooded and maintains body temperature independently of his environment. Cold-blooded animals are called *poikilothermic*, meaning their body temperature is the same as their environment. Fish, frogs, and reptiles are examples of poikilothermic animals.

TEMPERATURE REGULATION: There are various factors that influence body temperature regulation or control. Temperature is maintained through a balance between heat loss and heat production. This balance is influenced by physical and chemical means and through nervous system stimulation.

The body produces heat chemically through the metabolism of food. Body metabolism will increase in order to produce more heat for the body as necessary. In cold weather, a diet high in protein which stimulates metabolism aids in heat production. During hot weather, a high protein diet will place added work upon mechanisms that produce heat dissipation. Heat production is increased also by epinephrine, norepinephrine, and thyroxin.

Physically, the body gains heat from its environment, but this is of lesser significance than heat produced chemically. For example, clothing, sun, and the ingestion of hot foods may increase body temperature.

The body "stokes its furnace" to produce heat through stimulants to metabolism. This is generally brought about by increased muscular tone. The contraction of smooth muscles when "gooseflesh" occurs is an example. Shivering is movement of skeletal muscles by involuntary nervous control which stimulates metabolism Exercising, often found comforting when one is cold, increases muscle tone and stimulates metabolism which in turn increases heat production.

Heat is dissipated from the body primarily through physical processes. As much as 95 percent is lost through radiation and convection and through evaporation of water from the lungs and skin. Most of the remaining amount is lost through excreta (urine and feces) and in raising the temperature of inspired air to body temperature. A negligible amount is normally lost through conduction except when the body is in contact with cold surfaces for prolonged periods of time, as when lying on cold surfaces or when immersed in water that is below body temperature.

Temperature regulation is an example of *homeostasis,* which is the maintenance of uniformity or stability in the body within narrow limits. A synonym is *homeokinesis.* Homeostatis is also observed in the body's ability to maintain water and pH equilibrium of body fluids. To maintain constancy of temperature, the hypothalamus in the central nervous system, located at the base of the brain, plays an important role as the body's thermostat. The hypothalamus has two parts: the anterior hypothalamus is concerned with heat dissipation and the posterior hypothalamus governs heat conservation efforts.

What happens when body temperature is elevated? It is generally theorized that the thermostat in the temperature-regulating center is at a higher level and heat dissipation is decreased. The regulation of the temperature has not broken down; rather, the thermostat has been set at a higher degree. When fever begins, the skin is often pale and dry while metabolism is normal. Once fever reaches a certain level, then balance begins again. The thermostat theory is also supported when one observes the action of *antipyretic,* or fever-reducing, drugs; they are believed to reset the heat-regulating center since these same drugs do not affect body temperature when the person's temperature is within normal range.

To summarize, thermal balance is maintained through heat production and loss. Heat is produced primarily through metabolic activity and through exercise. Heat is lost to the environment through radiation, convection, evaporation, and conduction. Changes in the vascularity of the skin modify body temperature; when blood is directed to the skin through vasodilation, heat loss is increased, and when the skin vessels contract, heat is conserved. Perspiration protects the body from overheating because the body is cooled by evaporation.

TABLE 20-1: Equivalent centigrade and Fahrenheit temperatures and directions for converting temperatures from one measure to another*

Centigrade	Fahrenheit	Centigrade	Fahrenheit
34.0	93.2	38.5	101.3
35.0	95.0	39.0	102.2
36.0	96.8	40.0	104.0
36.5	97.7	41.0	105.8
37.0	98.6	42.0	107.6
37.5	99.5	43.0	109.4
38.0	100.4	44.0	111.2

* To convert centigrade to Fahrenheit, multiply by 9/5 and add 32. To change Fahrenheit to centigrade, subtract 32 and multiply by 5/9.

NORMAL BODY TEMPERATURE: Body temperature is recorded either in degrees of centigrade or degrees of Fahrenheit, abbreviated °C. or °F., respectively. Table 20-1 illustrates comparable centigrade and Fahrenheit temperatures and explains how temperatures are converted from one system to another. The thermometer is placed in the mouth to obtain an *oral* temperature, in the anal canal to obtain a *rectal* temperature, or in the axilla to obtain an *axillary* temperature.

The average normal oral temperature for adults is considered to be 37° C. (98.6° F.); the average normal rectal temperature is 37.5° C. (99.5° F.); and the average normal axillary temperature is 36.7° C. (98° F.). Variations occur in each individual and a range of 0.3° to 0.6° C. (0.5° to 1.0° F.) from the average normal temperature is considered to be within normal limits. However, wider variations from the average temperature have been found to be normal for certain individuals.

The body temperature has been observed to be lowest during the early morning hours and highest during the late afternoon or early evening hours. An inversion of this cycle has been observed in persons who work at night and sleep during the day hours. Exercise, manner of living, amount and kind of food ingested, and external cold also may influence body temperature. Newborns and young children normally have a higher body temperature than adults.

ELEVATED BODY TEMPERATURE: An elevation in normal body temperature is known as *pyrexia*. The lay term for pyrexia is *fever*. *Hyperpyrexia* is high fever, usually above 41° C. (105.8° F.). Pyrexia is a common symptom of illness, and there is sufficient evidence to believe that an elevation in body temperature aids the body in fighting disease. For example, in an infectious disease, when the causative organisms are destroyed by a total body response, the elevated temperature apparently helps to destroy bacteria as well as to mobilize the body's defenses.

The physiologic reason for pyrexia is not understood clearly, but it is believed commonly that it is the result of a direct action on the temperature-regulating center in the hypothalamus. Heat loss is decreased or heat production is increased or both occur when body temperature rises above normal. Cells in the central nervous system may be impaired when the body temperature surpasses 41° C. (105.8° F.), and survival is rare when it reaches 43° C. (109.4° F.). When high body temperature occurs, death usually is due to failure of the respiratory center, but may be due also to inactivation of body enzymes and destruction of tissue proteins.

Pyrexia may take a variety of courses, usually depending on the pathologic process occurring in the body. Several terms are used to describe the course of an elevated body temperature. The *onset* or *invasion* is the period when pyrexia begins; it may be either sudden or gradual in nature. When the temperature alternates regularly between a period of pyrexia and a period of normal or subnormal temperature, it is called an *intermittent* temperature. A *remittent* temperature is one that fluctuates several degrees above normal but does not reach normal between fluctuations. A *continued* temperature is one that remains consistently elevated and fluctuates very little. When pyrexia subsides suddenly, the drop to normal is called a *crisis*; a gradual return to normal temperature is called *lysis*. In certain instances, when body temperature has returned to normal following pyrexia, a patient may experience a temporary *recrudescence* or *recurrence* of temperature. This may be due to increased activity or exertion, in which case there is usually little cause for alarm. However, a recurring temperature may also be a sign of relapse; therefore, the temperature warrants frequent checking.

When pyrexia occurs, body metabolism is elevated above normal, and the respiratory rate and the pulse rate will also increase, as a rule proportionately with increased body temperature. The patient usually experiences loss of appetite, headaches, general malaise, depression, and occasionally periods of delirium. Observing for other signs as body temperature rises is important, such as urinary output, color of skin, and condition of tongue and mouth.

LOWERED BODY TEMPERATURE: A body temperature below the average normal range is called *hypothermia*. Death usually occurs when the temperature falls below approximately 34° C. (93.2° F.), but exceptional cases of survival have been reported when body temperatures have fallen considerably lower. There are a few illnesses associated with hypothermia, especially those producing unconsciousness; therefore, it is important to observe a patient closely when body temperature falls below normal.

While an elevated body temperature is a protective device for the body, a lowered body temperature is also beneficial in some instances. Rates of chemical reactions in the body are slowed, thereby decreasing the metabolic demands for oxygen. Hypothermia as a form of therapy is discussed in clinical texts. Figure 20-7 illustrates the range of human body temperature.

The Thermometer: The glass thermometer most commonly used to measure body temperature has two parts: the bulb and the stem. Mercury is in the bulb and, being a metal, will expand when exposed to heat and rise in the stem. The stem is calibrated in degrees and tenths of a degree. The range is from about 34° C. (93° F.) to about 42.2° C. (108° F.). A wider range of temperature is not necessary, since human life rarely exists above or below these temperatures.

Fractions of a degree usually are recorded in even numbers, as 0.2 or 0.6 or 0.8. If the mercury appears to be a bit more or less than an even tenth, it is common practice to report the nearest tenth.

Some oral thermometers have a long slender mercury bulb, and others have a blunt bulb similar to that used on almost all rectal thermometers. The blunt bulb on the rectal thermometer is to help to prevent injury when it is inserted. The long slender bulb on the oral thermometer is thought to give a larger surface area for contact. When using a thermometer in the home or in a different agency, check to see whether it is an oral or a rectal thermometer. Some thermometers have this printed on them; others do not.

There are electric thermometers now available on the market that measure body temperature in a matter of seconds, according to their manufacturers. There are two temperature sensors, one for oral and one for rectal use. They are equipped with disposable covers, a feature that aids to eliminate chances of cross-infection and to decrease cleaning chores. There are various models available; some are hand held, others are desk models, and still others fasten to clipboards.

Another device for measuring temperature is a disposable patch or tape which is applied to the abdomen. The temperature-sensitive tape changes color at different temperature ranges. It is generally

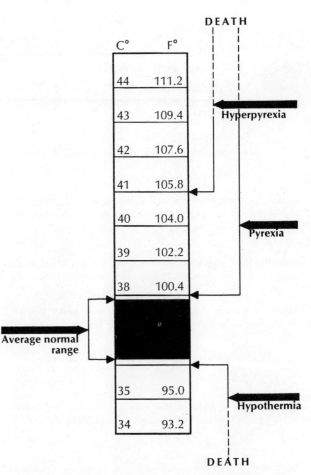

Fig. 20-7. The range of human body temperature, as measured orally.

recommended for well infants born at term. A rectal temperature should be used if the color on the tape illustrates that the temperature is either above or below normal average range.

There are also measurement devices which provide for a constant monitoring of a patient's temperature. These are generally used in situations when the patient is critically ill. The thermometer probe is attached to an alarm device that indicates when the patient's temperature moves beyond a specific range.

Some agencies have adopted the procedure of using one thermometer only for each patient. The thermometer is kept in the patient's unit and is disposed of when he is discharged, or, the thermometer

RATIONALE GUIDING ACTION IN OBTAINING BODY TEMPERATURE

The purpose is to measure body temperature.

ORAL METHOD

SUGGESTED ACTION	RATIONALE
If the thermometer has been stored in a chemical solution, wipe it dry with a firm twisting motion, using clean soft tissue.	Chemical solutions may irritate mucous membranes and may have an objectionable odor or taste. Soft tissue will approximate the surface, and twisting helps to contact the entire surface.
Wipe once from the bulb toward the fingers with each tissue.	Wiping from an area where there are few or no organisms to an area where organisms may be present minimizes the spread of organisms to cleaner areas.
Grasp the thermometer firmly with thumb and forefinger, and with strong wrist movements shake the thermometer until the mercury line reaches the lowest marking.	A constriction in the mercury line near the bulb of the thermometer prevents the mercury from dropping below the last temperature reading unless it is shaken down forcefully.
Read the thermometer by holding it horizontally at eye level, and rotate it between the fingers until the mercury line can be seen clearly.	Holding the thermometer at eye level facilitates reading. Rotating the thermometer will aid in placing the mercury line in a position where it can be read best.
Place the mercury bulb of the thermometer under the patient's tongue and instruct him to close his lips tightly.	When the bulb rests against the superficial blood vessels under the tongue and the mouth is closed, a measurement of body temperature can be obtained.
Leave the thermometer in place for 7 to 10 minutes.	Allowing sufficient time for the oral thermometer to reach its maximum temperature results in a more accurate measurement of body temperature.
Remove the thermometer and wipe it once from the fingers down to the mercury bulb, using a firm twisting motion.	Cleansing from an area where there are few organisms to an area where there are numerous organisms minimizes the spread of organisms to cleaner areas. Friction helps to loosen matter from a surface.
Read the thermometer and shake it down as described above.	
Dispose of wipe in a receptacle used for contaminated items.	Confining contaminated articles helps to reduce the spread of pathogens.

RECTAL METHOD

SUGGESTED ACTION	RATIONALE
Wipe, read, and shake the rectal thermometer as the suggested procedure for obtaining an oral temperature indicates.	
Lubricate the mercury bulb and an area approximately 1 inch above the bulb.	Lubrication reduces friction and thereby facilitates insertion of the thermometer and minimizes irritation of the mucous membrane of the anal canal.
With the patient on his side, fold back the bed linen and separate the buttocks so that the anal sphincter is seen clearly. Insert the thermometer for approximately 1½ inches. Permit buttocks to fall in place.	If not placed directly into the anal opening the bulb of the thermometer may injure the sphincter, or hemorrhoids if present.

SUGGESTED ACTION	RATIONALE
Leave the thermometer in place for 2 to 3 minutes. Hold the thermometer in place if the patient is irrational or is a restless child or infant.	Allowing sufficient time for the thermometer to register results in a more accurate measurement of body temperature.
Remove the thermometer and wipe it once from the fingers to the mercury bulb, using a firm twisting motion.	Cleansing from an area where there are few organisms to an area where there are numerous organisms minimizes the spread of organisms. Friction helps to loosen matter from a surface.
Read and shake the thermometer and dispose of wipe in a receptacle used for contaminated items.	

AXILLARY METHOD

SUGGESTED ACTION	RATIONALE
If the thermometer has been stored in a chemical solution, wipe it dry with a firm twisting motion, using a clean tissue.	Chemical solutions may irritate the skin. The presence of solution may alter the skin temperature. Soft tissue with the aid of friction aids in removing the solution.
Read and shake the thermometer as the suggested procedure for obtaining an oral temperature indicates.	
Place the thermometer well into the axilla with the bulb directed toward the patient's head. Bring the patient's arm down close to his body and place his forearm over his chest.	When the bulb rests against the superficial blood vessels in the axilla and the skin surfaces are brought together to reduce the amount of air surrounding the bulb, a reasonably reliable measurement of body temperature can be obtained.
Leave the thermometer in place for 10 minutes or more.	Allowing sufficient time for the axillary thermometer to reach its maximum temperature results in a reasonably accurate measurement of body temperature.
Remove, read, and shake the thermometer and dispose of wipe.	

is sent home with the patient. It has been recommended that thermometers used for patients having hepatitis be discarded when the patient is discharged.

Thermometers have not escaped the trend toward disposables, and there are disposable ones available also on the market.

SELECTING A SITE FOR OBTAINING BODY TEMPERATURE: Most agency policies specify the site to be used for obtaining the temperature. However, the nurse must make modifications under certain circumstances.

Oral Temperature: Oral temperatures are contraindicated for unconscious and irrational patients and for infants because of the danger of breaking the thermometer in the mouth. Oral temperatures are also contraindicated for patients who breathe through their mouths, those with diseases of the oral cavity or surgery of the nose or the mouth, and those receiving nasal oxygen therapy.

If the patient has had either hot or cold food or

fluids, it is generally recommended that a period of approximately 30 minutes should elapse before obtaining an oral temperature to allow time for the oral tissues to return to normal temperature.

Rectal Temperature: A rectal temperature is more accurate than an oral or an axillary temperature. If a patient having an oral temperature taken routinely shows a considerable change in his temperature, it is good practice to check it rectally. Some hospitals require rectal readings on patients having an elevated temperature. It is usual procedure to obtain rectal temperatures for infants, for unconscious, and for irrational patients. Rectal temperatures are contraindicated for patients having rectal surgery, diarrhea, or diseases of the rectum.

Axillary Temperature: Obtaining an axillary temperature is rare and is used only when both oral and rectal temperatures are contraindicated or the sites are not usable or accessible. Unless the patient is capable of cooperating, the nurse will need to re-

RATIONALE GUIDING ACTION IN DISINFECTING CLINICAL THERMOMETERS

The purpose is to disinfect a thermometer that has been used for obtaining a patient's temperature.

SUGGESTED ACTION	RATIONALE
Use a soft tissue for cleansing the thermometer.	Adhered organic matter interferes with disinfection.
Use a clean, soft tissue each time the thermometer must be wiped.	Soft tissue comes into close contact with all surfaces of the thermometer.
Hold the tissue at the end of the thermometer near the fingers.	Cleansing an area from where there are few organisms to an area where there are numerous organisms minimizes the spread of organisms to cleaner areas.
Wipe down toward the bulb, using a twisting motion.	Friction helps to loosen matter from a surface.
After the thermometer has been wiped, cleanse it with soap or detergent solution, again using friction.	Soap or detergent solutions loosen adhered matter.
Rinse the thermometer under cold running water.	Rinsing with water helps to remove organisms and foreign material loosened by washing. Also, certain chemical solutions are rendered ineffective in the presence of soap—for example, benzalkonium chloride (Zephiran Chloride).
Dry the thermometer after it has been rinsed.	The strength of a chemical solution is decreased when water is added to the solution.
Immerse the thermometer in the chemical solution specified.	Chemical solutions must be used in proper strength for the proper length of time in order to be effective.
Rinse the thermometer with water after disinfection and before reuse.	Chemical solutions may irritate the mucous membrane of the mouth or the rectum. Also, they may have an objectionable odor and taste.
Return the thermometer to the storage receptacle.	

main in attendance to hold the thermometer. The axillary temperature is the least accurate way of obtaining body temperature, since the axilla is easily influenced by environmental conditions and because it is often difficult to approximate skin surfaces while the bulb of the thermometer is held in place. If the axilla has just been washed, taking the temperature should be delayed, since the temperature of the water and the friction created by drying the skin will influence the temperature.

CLEANSING CLINICAL THERMOMETERS: Making a glass clinical thermometer safe for use with another person presents a problem. Heat sufficient to kill pathogenic organisms will ruin thermometers by causing the mercury to expand beyond the column within the thermometer. Therefore, the method of choice is to disinfect thermometers in a chemical solution.

The suggested action and the underlying rationale in the procedure on this page apply to either oral or rectal thermometers. However, since a lubricant is used on a rectal thermometer, cleansing to remove the lubricant thoroughly prior to disinfection is essential. If the lubricant is not removed thoroughly, organisms may harbor in a film of lubricant, and the disinfection procedure becomes ineffective. Detergents are particularly effective for emulsifying oils and fats even in cool and hard water; therefore, it is preferable to use a detergent rather than soap.

In many agencies, it is common practice to have thermometers issued from a central supply unit. After being used, one thermometer for each patient, they are returned for cleansing and disinfection. The central supply unit may have a machine for shaking down the mercury in many thermometers simultaneously.

In the home, thermometers should be cleansed with soap and water and then stored for reuse by the same person. If the thermometer is to be used by more than one person or if the person has a known or suspected infection transmitted by oral secretions, it should be disinfected with an appropriate bactericide following the cleansing.

Pulse

The stimulus for contraction of the heart starts in the *sinoauricular* or *sinoatrial node*, which is in the upper part of the right atrium. Because the node sets the pace of the beat, it is often referred to as the pacemaker. The contraction stimulus, a type of electrical current, passes as a wave through the rest of the heart.

The heart is indeed a remarkable organ. In the average life-span, it beats millions of times and pumps millions of gallons of blood. It rests for only part of a second between each beat and except for a malfunctioning heart, seldom is there a beat misplaced. About 5 liters of blood are estimated to be pumped from the heart every minute.

Each time the left ventricle of the heart contracts to eject blood into an already full aorta, the arterial walls in the blood system expand (distend) to compensate for the increase in pressure. This expansion of the aorta sends a wave through the walls of the arterial system which, on touch, can be felt as an impact or light tap. The sensation of the impact or tap is called the *pulse*.

PULSE RATE: On awakening in the morning, the pulse rate of the average healthy adult male is approximately 60 to 65 beats per minute. The pulse rate for women is slightly faster—about seven to eight beats per minute more than for men. Pulse varies with age, gradually diminishing from birth to adulthood and then increasing somewhat in very old age. It has been noted also that body size and build of an individual may affect the pulse rate. Tall, slender persons often have a slower rate than short, stout ones. Very wide variations in pulse rates have been noted in normal healthy adults. The American Heart Association accepts as normal for adults a pulse rate of between 50 and 100 beats per minute.

There are numerous causes for changes in the pulse rate. The rate of the heartbeat responds readily to impulses conducted along the sympathetic and the parasympathetic nervous systems. Stimulation of the sympathetic system increases the heart rate and, therefore, the pulse rate. This system responds quickly to emotions; consequently, the pulse rate increases when a person experiences fear, anger, surprise, worry, and the like. The sympathetic system also receives impulses from internal organs of the body. For example, pain in the abdomen will cause the pulse rate to quicken, usually due to sympathetic stimulation. The rate also increases with exercise as the heart compensates for the increased need for blood circulation.

Prolonged application of heat to the skin will stimulate the heartbeat and increase the pulse rate. The pulse rate increases when blood pressure decreases as the heart attempts to increase the output of blood. When blood pressure returns to normal, the pulse rate usually will decrease. Elevated body temperature is accompanied by an increase in pulse rate—usually an increase of about seven to ten beats per minute for each 0.6° C. (1° F.) of elevation above normal.

When the pulse rate is over 100 beats per minute, the condition is referred to as *tachycardia*. The word comes from two Greek words meaning quick and heart.

Stimulation of the parasympathetic system decreases pulse rate. The drug digitalis, commonly taken by patients having heart ailments, is an example of an agent that decreases the pulse rate by stimulating the vagus nerves of the parasympathetic system.

The term used to describe the pulse rate when it falls below approximately 50 beats per minute is *bradycardia*. A slow pulse rate is less common during illness than a rapid pulse rate. Therefore, when bradycardia does occur, it should be reported to the physician immediately.

RHYTHM OF THE PULSE: Normally, the pulse rhythm is regular, and the time interval between beats is equal. The force of the normal pulse is equal with each beat. Irregular pulse rhythm is called *arrhythmia*. An *intermittent pulse* is one that has a period of normal rhythm broken by periods of irregular rhythm. An intermittent rhythm may be a serious sign, as in certain heart diseases, or it may be a temporary condition due to emotional upset or fright. If the ending of the pulse wave is exaggerated, the pulse wave feels double to touch, and the pulse is said to be a *dicrotic pulse*.

VOLUME OF THE PULSE: Under normal conditions, the volume of each pulse beat is equal. The pulse can be obliterated with relative ease, by exerting pressure over the artery, but it remains perceptible with moderate pressure. When blood volume makes it difficult to obliterate the artery, the pulse is called *bounding*. If the volume is small and the artery can be obliterated readily, the pulse is called *feeble, weak*, or *thready*. A thready pulse usually is associated with a rapid pulse rate.

THE ARTERIAL WALL: When the fingertips are placed over an artery, the sense of touch will determine certain characteristics of the arterial wall. Normally, it is elastic, straight (unless the fingertips rest on a normally tortuous artery), smooth and round. With advancing age, the arteries become less elastic and smooth, and a normally straight artery may feel tortuous to touch.

COMMON SITES FOR OBTAINING THE PULSE: Usually, the radial artery at the wrist is used for obtaining the pulse rate, since it is easily accessible and it can be pressed against the radius. If it is not possible to obtain the pulse at the wrist, other superficial arteries of the body may be used. Figure 20-8 illustrates common sites. It is possible to obtain the pulse rate easily and with little disturbance to the patient if the nurse understands how to use alternative sites. A site should be used that does not produce exertion or discomfort for the patient, since this could alter the pulse rate.

Occasionally, a patient has a radial pulse that is difficult to count. It may be so irregular and the force of the beats so uneven that it is difficult to de-

termine an accurate count. Using alternative sites may not provide any more accuracy. Two nurses checking the pulse may have different counts. A more accurate estimate of the heartbeats per minute can be obtained by placing a stethoscope over the apex of the heart. The impulse of the heart against the chest wall can be heard in the space between the fifth and the sixth ribs about 3 inches (8 cm.) to the left of the median line and slightly below the nipple.

There are times when the *apical-radial pulse* rate may be taken; that is, the pulse rate is counted at the apex of the heart and at the radial artery simultaneously. This requires two persons; one listens over the apex of the heart with a stethoscope, and the other counts at the wrist. They use one watch conveniently placed between them. After listening and feeling to be sure that they can get the best possible count, they decide on a time to start counting, for example, when the second hand is at a specified place. At this time, both persons start counting for a full minute.

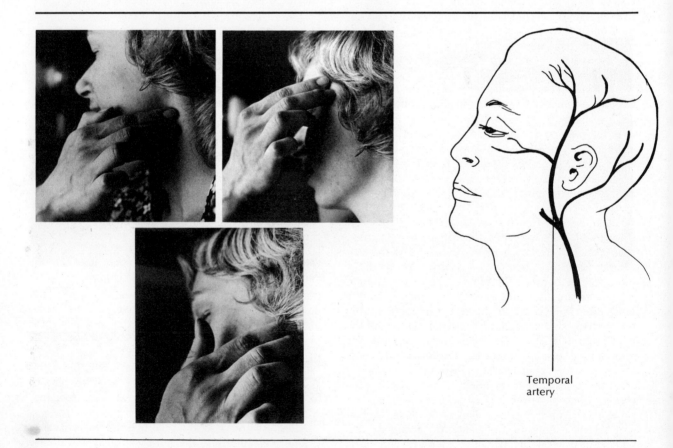

Temporal
artery

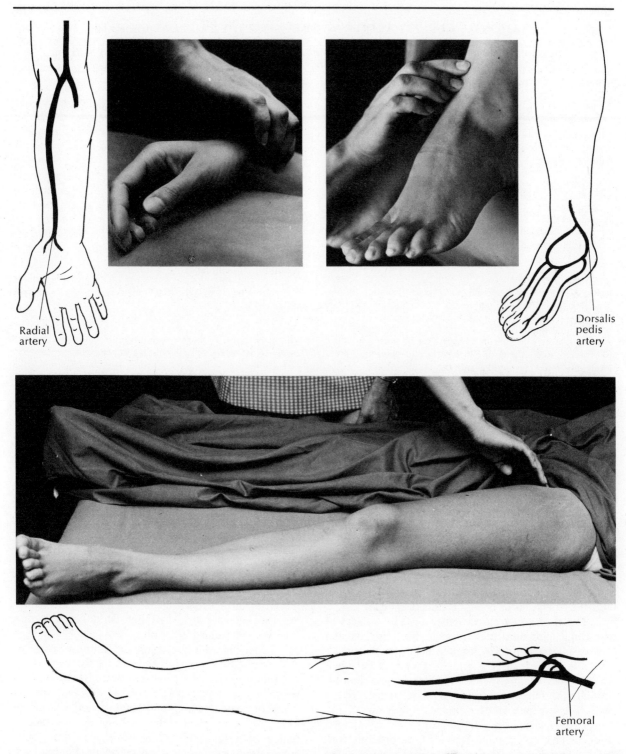

Fig. 20-8. These photos illustrate common sites where the pulse rate can be readily obtained. The artist's sketches illustrate the location of the artery the nurse is palpating in each case.

RATIONALE GUIDING ACTION IN OBTAINING THE RADIAL PULSE RATE

The purpose is to count the number of times the heart beats per minute and to obtain an estimate of the quality of the heart's action.

SUGGESTED ACTION	RATIONALE
In lying position, have patient rest his arm alongside his body with wrist extended and palm of hand downward. In sitting position, have forearm at a 90° angle to his body resting on a support and with wrist extended and palm of hand downward.	These positions are ordinarily comfortable for the patient and convenient for the nurse.
Place the first, second, and third fingers along the radial artery and press gently against the radius; rest the thumb in apposition to fingers on the back of the patient's wrist.	The fingertips, sensitive to touch, will feel pulsation of patient's radial artery. If thumb is used for palpating the patient's pulse the nurse may feel her own pulse.
Apply only enough pressure so that the patient's pulsating artery can be felt distinctly.	Moderate pressure allows nurse to feel the superficial radial artery expand and contract with each heartbeat. Too much pressure will obliterate the pulse. If too little pressure is applied, pulse will be imperceptible.
Using a watch with a second hand, count number of pulsations felt on patient's artery for half a minute. Multiply this number by 2 to obtain rate for 1 minute.	Sufficient time is necessary to study rate, volume, and quality of pulse.
If pulse rate is abnormal in any way, count pulse rate for a full minute. Repeat counting if necessary to determine accurately the rate, the quality, and the volume.	When the pulse is abnormal, full minute countings are necessary to allow for irregular timing between beats.

Respiration

The term *respiration,* in its broadest sense, begins with the act of breathing and includes the body's use of oxygen and the elimination of carbon dioxide. *Inspiration* or *inhalation* is the act of breathing in, and *expiration* or *exhalation* refers to breathing out. *External respiration* includes lung ventilation, the absorption of oxygen, and the elimination of carbon dioxide. *Internal respiration,* sometimes referred to as *tissue respiration,* includes the use of oxygen by body cells for the production of heat through oxidation and the liberation of energy from the food we eat.

The thorax is a closed structure. The air sacs of the lung communicate through the air passages (nose, pharynx, trachea, and bronchi) with the atmosphere. With inspiration, the thorax is enlarged, causing the pressure in the thorax to be less than atmospheric. The atmospheric pressure, being greater than the pressure in the thorax, forces air to the lungs that expand to fill the space of the enlarged thorax. The muscles involved with respiration contract to produce expiration. The diaphragm and the external intercostal muscles are the primary muscles of respiration. Other muscles of the thorax and those of the abdominal wall may play a part; however, when breathing is difficult for any reason, they become important to assist with respiration.

The chemical stimulation of an increased carbon dioxide tension in the blood is an important phenomenon of involuntary respiration. As carbon dioxide accumulates in the blood, the respiratory center is stimulated directly and also indirectly by the carotid and the aortic glomi, and the rate and the depth of respiration are increased. This involuntary chemical stimulation is responsible for the limitation of voluntary control of breathing. A new mother, not realizing this, may panic when her child has a temper tantrum and holds his breath.

When breathing is voluntary, impulses travel to the respiratory center in the medulla oblongata from the motor area of the cerebral cortex. Because of this arrangement, a person can automatically control his breathing when talking and singing, and voluntarily hold his breath until the carbon dioxide tension builds up excessively in the blood. Laughing from amusement or happiness and crying or sobbing from grief or sadness modify respirations by impulses from the brain that are carried to the respiratory center.

The respiratory center responds reflexly from impulses that can be carried over any sensory nerve in the body; for example, excitement, anger, fear, pain, unusual sights and sounds, and the like will reflexly alter respiratory rates and depths. Coughing, sneezing, and hiccuping are modified arts of respirations also largely brought about reflexly. Afferent fibers or the pulmonic vagi also reflexly stimulate the respiratory center. Through this course, impulses from the lungs reflexly end each respiratory act. It is believed that certain centers in the brain also reflexly affect respirations.

RESPIRATORY RATE: Normally, healthy adults breathe approximately 16 to 20 times a minute. Wider variations have been observed in healthy persons. The respiratory rate is more rapid in infants and young children. It has been noted that the relationship between the pulse rate and the respiratory rate is fairly consistent in normal persons, the ratio being one respiration to approximately four heartbeats. Increased rate of respiration is called *polypnea.*

During illness, the respiratory rate may vary from normal. When body temperature is elevated, the respiratory rate increases as the body attempts to rid itself of excess heat. Any condition involving an accumulation of carbon dioxide and a decrease of oxygen in the blood also will tend to increase the rate and the depth of respirations.

There are conditions that characteristically predispose to slow breathing. For example, an increase in intracranial pressure will depress the respiratory center, resulting in irregular and shallow, slow breathing, or both. Certain drugs will also depress respirations.

RESPIRATORY DEPTH: At rest, the depth of each respiration is approximately the same. The volume of air normally exchanged in each respiration, the *tidal air,* varies greatly with individuals, but the average is about 500 c.c. of air. The depth of respirations is described as *deep* or *shallow,* depending on whether the volume of air taken in is above or below normal. Increased depth of respirations is called *hyperpnea.*

NATURE OF RESPIRATION: Ordinarily, breathing is automatic, and respirations are noiseless, regular, even, and without effort. Between each respiration there is normally a short resting period.

Difficult breathing is called *dyspnea.* Dyspneic patients usually appear to be anxious, and their faces are drawn from exertion. Often, the nostrils will dilate as the patient fights for his breath. The abdominal muscles are used to aid in breathing.

Dyspneic patients frequently find relief if they sit up in bed, which places the thorax in a vertical position. This condition is called *orthopnea.* According to one authority,

The improvement in breathing observed in this position has been interpreted as due to the following mechanism: when the thorax is in the orthopneic position (i.e., vertical) the abdominal viscera do not press against the diaphragm, and the negative pleural pressure increases; this causes pulmonary congestion to diminish. The distensibility of the lung and vital capacity increases; this causes the Hering-Breuer reflex to diminish; circulation improves, the pressure of the cerebrospinal fluid diminishes, and the blood supply to the respiratory center also improves.[1]

Cheyne-Stokes respirations refer to breathing consisting of a gradual increase in the depth of respirations followed by a gradual decrease in the depth of respirations and then a period of no breathing or *apnea.* Dyspnea is usually present. Cheyne-Stokes respirations are a serious symptom during illness and very often occur as death approaches.

Breathing that is unusually noisy is referred to as *stertorous.* A snoring sound is common.

There are still other terms that describe various types of respirations. Describing the specific character of the respirations rather than attempting to use an uncommon term that may be misinterpreted is recommended.

OBSERVATION OF THE PATIENT: While the respiratory rate is being obtained, the color of the patient and his act of breathing should be noted. *Hypoxia* is present when the patient is not receiving an adequate supply of oxygen. (Anoxia means no oxygen but the term is commonly used as a synonym for hypoxia.) As a result of hypoxia, the skin and the mucous membranes will appear cyanotic. Both abdominal breathing, involving the diaphragm and the abdominal wall muscles, and costal breathing, involving the intercostal muscles, are present. In certain disease conditions, either one or the other may be exaggerated.

Cyanosis is more marked on the body where numerous small blood vessels lie close to the skin surface, such as the nailbeds, the lips, the lobes of the ears, and the cheeks. When cyanosis is not marked, these may be the only areas appearing cyanotic. In marked cyanosis all areas of the skin may appear bluish. If pallor is present, cyanosis may be masked. If the skin is flushed for any reason, cyanosis

1. Houssay, B. A. *et al.:* Human Physiology. ed. 2, p. 301. New York, McGraw-Hill, 1955.

RATIONALE GUIDING ACTION IN OBTAINING THE RESPIRATORY RATE

The purpose is to obtain the respiratory rate per minute and an estimate of the patient's respiratory status.

SUGGESTED ACTION	RATIONALE
While the fingertips are still in place after counting the pulse rate, observe the patient's respiration.	Counting the respirations while presumably still counting the pulse keeps the patient from becoming conscious of his breathing and possibly altering his usual rate.
Note rise and fall of patient's chest with each inspiration and expiration.	A complete cycle of inspiration and expiration constitutes one act of respiration.
Using a watch with a second hand, count number of respirations for a minimum of half a minute. Multiply this number by 2 to obtain patient's respiratory rate per minute.	Sufficient time is necessary to observe rate, depth, and other characteristics.
If respirations are abnormal in any way, count the respiratory rate for a full minute. Repeat if necessary to determine accurately rate and the characteristics of breathing.	Full minute countings allow for unequal timing between respirations.

may be intensified. In persons with dark skin, cyanosis usually can be detected by examining the color of the mucous membrane of the mouth and under the tongue to see if there is a dusky appearance.

FREQUENCY OF OBTAINING TEMPERATURE AND PULSE AND RESPIRATORY RATES: As indicated earlier, obtaining the patient's temperature and pulse and respiratory rates is a part of the physical examination. At other times, agency policies govern when and how frequently they are to be obtained. Patients having elevated temperatures and those who are in the immediate post-operative period may have observations made as often as every four hours. In some self-care, chronic illness, or psychiatric units, these observations are not made routinely. When a patient's condition is not associated with an elevated temperature, there seems to be little justification for observing these signs several times a day.

Although auxiliary personnel may make temperature, pulse and respiration observations, the nurse responsible for the patient is ultimately responsible for these observations. Should a patient show untoward symptoms or change in pulse and respiratory rates, the nurse should count the pulse and the respirations and if necessary, take the temperature. They are cardinal signs and good clues to what is happening in the body.

Monitoring devices in hospitals make it possible to have a constant measurement of a patient's vital signs. Use of such equipment enhances the nurse's ability to gather such data.

Blood Pressure

From the study of human physiology, it can be recalled that maximum pressure is exerted on the wall of the arteries when the left ventricle of the heart pushes blood through the open aortic valve into the aorta. The highest point of pressure in the arteries is called *systolic pressure*. The lowest point, or pressure which is constantly present on the arterial walls, is called the *diastolic pressure*. The difference between the two is called the *pulse pressure*. Determining systolic and diastolic pressure is an excellent way of determining the work of the heart and the resistance offered by the peripheral vessels. Blood pressure is recorded in millimeters of mercury, abbreviated mm. Hg, and recorded as follows: 120/80, 120 being the systolic pressure and 80 being the diastolic pressure.

Persons whose blood pressures are above normal are in a state of hypertension. When the cause of the hypertension is known, it is called *secondary hypertension. Primary* or *essential hypertension* is hypertension without a known cause. A blood pressure below average is called *hypotension*.

MAINTENANCE OF BLOOD PRESSURE: There are five factors responsible for maintaining blood pressure.

Peripheral resistance: The circulatory system has a high pressure system (arteries) and a low pressure system (capillaries and veins). Between the two are the arterioles, very fine muscular tubes. When the arterioles contract, their caliber become small and less blood flows through to the capillaries. When the arterioles are in a state of overcontraction, the condition is called *vasoconstriction*. In the opposite condition, the arteriole walls are relaxed and increased amounts of blood reach the arterioles. The arterioles are then in a state of dilation, or *vasodilation*. Normally, arterioles are in a state of partial contraction—they are neither fully dilated nor fully relaxed. Constriction greater than normal results in a higher blood pressure; less constriction results in a lower blood pressure. The degree of vasoconstriction affects diastolic pressure and is its chief determinant, all other factors being normal. Persistent diastolic hypertension is the most serious and most common blood pressure disturbance in man.

The pumping action of the heart: When increased amounts of blood are pumped into the arteries (that is, when cardiac output is increased) the arteries will distend more, resulting in an increase in blood pressure. When less blood is pumped into the arteries (that is, when cardiac output is decreased) blood pressure will fall. Hence, a weak pump action results in a lower blood pressure than a strong pump action.

The blood volume: When blood volume is low, for example following a hemorrhage, blood pressure is low because there is decreased pressure on the arteries. Increasing the quantity of blood will increase the pressure because there will be more pressure on the arteries.

The viscosity of the blood: Viscosity is the quality of adhering, that is, having a sticky, glutinous consistency. The viscosity of the blood depends on the number of red blood cells and the plasma protein content. The more viscous the blood, the higher the blood pressure will be; that is, the more viscous the fluid, the more force is required to move it.

The elasticity of the vessel walls: Arteries have a considerable quantity of elastic tissue that allows for their ability to stretch. When the heart rests between each beat, the walls of the arteries recoil although pressure in them does not drop to zero. The state of pressure keeps the blood entering the capillaries and veins in a continuous flow, not in spurts. Simultaneously, the arterioles, normally in a moderate state of contraction, offer certain resistance; therefore, the elasticity of the walls in addition to the resistance at the arterioles helps to maintain normal blood pressure. Vessels that have little elasticity offer more resistance than vessels with great elasticity. As resistance increases, so does the pressure.

NORMAL BLOOD PRESSURE: Studies of healthy persons indicate that blood pressure can fall within a wide range and still be normal. Since individual differences are considerable, it is important to know what is the normal blood pressure for a particular person. If there is a rise or fall of 20 to 30 mm. Hg in that person's pressure, it is significant, even if it is well within the generally accepted range of normal.

The normal newborn infant has a systolic pressure of approximately 20 to 60 mm. Hg. Blood pressure increases gradually until puberty when a more sudden rise occurs. At about 17 or 18 years of age, blood pressure reaches adult level. At 20 or so, a man's average, normal blood pressure is usually given as 120/80 mm. Hg. A steady but not great rise continues from then to old age in healthy individuals. For a young adult, a systolic pressure of 140 may be considered high, but for a person of 60 years of age, it may not arouse great concern. Having a consistently low blood pressure, for example, 90 to 115 mm. Hg in an adult, appears to cause no ill effects. Rather, a lower than average blood pressure is usually associated with longevity.

Average range of pulse pressure is about 30 to 50 mm. Hg. The pulse pressure assumes an important factor in certain illnesses inasmuch as it varies directly with the amount of blood being pumped out during systole.

It has been found that nearly all persons will show normal fluctuations within the course of a day. The blood pressure is usually lowest early in the morning before breakfast and before activity commences. The blood pressure has been noted to rise as much as 5 to 10 mm. Hg by late afternoon, and it will gradually fall again during the sleeping hours.

There are several factors that will influence blood pressure in the normal healthy person. The age factor has already been mentioned. The sex of the person influences blood pressure, females usually having a lower blood pressure than males at the same age. Blood pressure has been observed to rise after the ingestion of food. It will also rise during a period of exercise or strenuous activity. Emotions such as anger, fear, and excitement will generally cause a rise in blood pressure. A person who is lying down will have a lower blood pressure as a rule than when he is in a sitting or a standing position.

MEASURING BLOOD PRESSURE: A sphygmomanometer and a stethoscope are necessary to measure blood pressure by the indirect method.[2] The sphyg-

---

2. The *direct method* of obtaining blood pressure is done by placing a needle in an artery and connecting it with a manometer. This method is used when very precise measurement is needed.

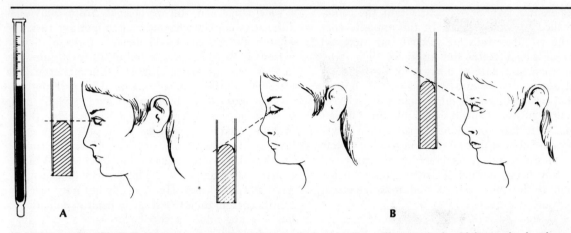

Fig. 20-9. a. This sketch illustrates meniscus, the point at which a reading of pressure should be made. b. These sketches illustrate how blood pressure readings could vary when eye is at different levels in relation to the meniscus. This phenomenon is known as parallax.

momanometer has a cuff which consists of an airtight, flat, rubber bladder covered with cloth. The cloth extends beyond the bladder to various lengths. There are two tubes attached to the bag. One is connected to a manometer. The other is attached to a bulb that is used to inflate the bladder. A needle valve on the bulb allows the operator to permit air to escape while pressure is being read.

One type of manometer is a mercury manometer which has a mercury-filled cylinder or tube calibrated in millimeters. When mercury rises in the tube, the upper or top surface of the mercury is curved convexly. The top most point on the curved surface is call the *meniscus*. It is caused by the cohesive force of the mercury molecules. When determining blood pressure on the mercury manometer, the meniscus indicates the pressure. The meniscus of the mercury is read at eye level. If the meniscus is above eye level, the pressure reading will appear lower than it really is. The apparent change of position of an object when seen from two different angles is referred to as *parallax*. Figure 20-9 illustrates meniscus and how pressure readings may be incorrect when the meniscus is above or below eye level.

Another type of manometer is called the aneroid manometer. It too has a cuff but it is attached to a round calibrated dial with a pointer that indicates pressure. The nurse in Figure 7-6, on page 69, is using an aneroid manometer.

The width of the cuff, that is, the distance the cuff extends up and down the limb (the arm being used most frequently), is a factor in obtaining an accurate blood pressure reading. If the cuff is too small, such as an average cuff used on an obese person, the reading could very well be higher than the actual pressure in the artery. Pressure is not evenly transmitted. If a cuff is too large, as an adult cuff used on the thin arm of a child, the reading may be less than the pressure in the artery. In this instance, pressure is being directed toward a smaller surface area and therefore is more concentrated. It is recommended that the cuff width be 1.2 times the diameter of the limb. The length of the bladder is important also. It should be sufficiently long to completely encircle the arm in order that pressure on the arm is equally applied to all parts.

The stethoscope is needed in order to listen to the sound directly over the artery as the pressure in the cuff is released and the blood is permitted to flow through. The bell or conelike construction in the tip of the stethoscope magnifies the sounds in the artery, and these sound waves are transmitted by means of the tubing to the listener. By listening to the sounds and watching the mercury column or dial, the blood pressure reading is obtained. Make certain that the eartips of the stethoscope are directed into the external canals of the ears and not against the ear itself. Individual differences in persons using a stethoscope will determine if the ear tips should be directed one way or the other into the ears. Every nurse should experiment to determine which method is best for her. If the patient has been active, a short period of rest is indicated before taking the reading.

It is best to take the blood pressure in as short a

RATIONALE GUIDING ACTION IN OBTAINING THE BLOOD PRESSURE WITH A MERCURY MANOMETER

The purpose is to measure the patient's systolic and diastolic blood pressure by an indirect method.

SUGGESTED ACTION	RATIONALE
Have the patient in a comfortable position with the forearm supported and the palm upward.	This position places the brachial artery so that a stethoscope can rest on it conveniently in the antecubital area.
Place yourself so that the meniscus of mercury can be read at eye level, and no more than 3 feet away.	If the eye level is above or below the meniscus, an inaccurate reading occurs. A distance of more than 3 feet will result in an inaccurate reading.
Place the cuff so that the inflatable bag is centered over the brachial artery (it lies midway between the anterior and the medial aspects of the arm) so that the lower edge of cuff is 2 cm. above antecubital fossa.	Pressure applied directly to the artery will yield most accurate readings.
Wrap the cuff smoothly around the arm and tuck end of cuff securely under preceding wrapping.	A twisted cuff and wrapping could produce unequal pressure and thus an inaccurate reading.
Use the fingertips to feel for a strong pulsation in the antecubital space.	Accurate blood pressure readings are possible when the stethoscope is directly over the artery.
Place the stethoscope on the brachial artery in the antecubital space where the pulse was noted.	Sound transmission can be distorted when source and reception are misaligned.
Pump the bulb of the manometer until the mercury rises to approximately 20 to 30 mm. above the point where it is anticipated that systolic pressure should be.	Pressure in the cuff prevents blood from flowing through the brachial artery. Lack of blood causes a numb sensation in patient's lower arm.
Using the valve on the bulb, release air 2 to 3 mm. per heartbeat and note on the manometer the point at which the first sound is heard; record this figure as the systolic pressure.*	Systolic pressure is that point at which the blood in the brachial artery is first able to force its way through, against the pressure exerted on the vessel by the cuff of the manometer.
Continue to release the air in the cuff evenly and gradually. Sounds may become a bit "muffled."	The artery is open, but still partly occluded.
Note the reading on the manometer when the last distinct loud sound is heard. Record this figure as the diastolic pressure.	Diastolic pressure is that point at which blood flows freely in the brachial artery and is equivalent to the amount of pressure normally exerted on the walls of the arteries when the heart is at rest.
Allow the remaining air to escape quickly, remove the cuff, and cleanse the equipment according to agency procedure.	

* Increase drop to 5 to 6 mm. for patients who have a known wide pulse pressure until near the expected diastolic.

time as possible in order to prevent venous congestion. The inflated cuff acts as a tourniquet. Venous congestion in the arm below the cuff will affect the reading.

When necessary to repeat the procedure in order to be certain an accurate blood pressure reading is obtained, allow the venous circulation in the lower arm to return to normal, 20 to 30 seconds or more if necessary.

If a patient is to have frequent blood pressure readings taken and the cuff is left in place, it is necessary to check to see that it has not rotated out of position before taking the next reading. Make certain the cuff cannot be inflated accidentally between readings.

The series of sounds for which the operator listens when taking blood pressure are called the *Korotkoff sounds*. The first clear sound when blood first

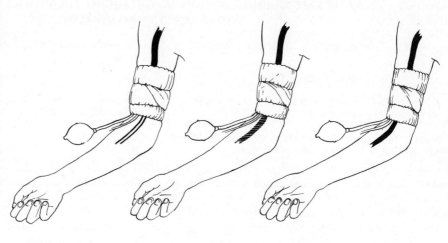

Fig. 20-10. When the cuff has been inflated sufficiently, it will occlude the flow of blood into the forearm (left). No sound will be heard through the stethoscope at this time. When pressure in the cuff is reduced sufficiently for blood to begin flowing through the brachial artery (center), the first sound is recorded as the systolic pressure. As the pressure in the cuff continues to be released, the last distinct sound heard through the stethoscope is the diastolic pressure. At this time, blood flows through the brachial artery freely (right).

flows through the compressed artery is the systolic pressure. The sound then normally becomes louder. The sound next is muffled and then it disappears. Diastolic pressure occurs at the point when sound disappears. Figure 20-10 illustrates this.

There are electronic instruments now available for measuring blood pressure. According to the manufacturers, blood pressure readings are available to the operator in 10 seconds. The inflation and deflation of the cuff is automatic and there is a signaling device on the instrument that monitors systolic and diastolic measurements. These instruments require no stethoscope since a microphone built into the cuff activates circuitry that produces a sign to the operator when systolic and diastolic pressures occur. The manufacturers point out that the electric devices eliminate errors due to hearing acuity, interference of outside sounds, and poor visual and auditory correlation.

FREQUENCY OF MEASURING BLOOD PRESSURE: The patient's blood pressure usually is obtained on admission to a health agency and when a physical examination is done. If the patient has an illness involving the circulatory system or has had surgery, daily or even more frequent readings may be necessary. As with temperature, pulse, and respiration observations, the nurse will exercise judgment. Very ill patients who are hospitalized and in need of almost constant recording of vital signs are usually placed in the intensive care facilities where this can be done by means of monitoring systems.

ELECTROCARDIOGRAPHY

The *electrocardiograph* is an instrument that measures and records electrical impulses of the heart. The findings are important for studying heart function. The graphic record produced by the electrocardiograph is called the *electrocardiogram* and is commonly abbreviated EKG.

The electrical activity in the heart can be picked up through sensitive sensors placed on the skin. These sensors are placed in various places on the body. The placement patterns of sensors are referred to as *leads*. The same cardiac activity is monitored on each lead, but the waves on the electrocardiogram look somewhat different. The trained observer recognizes normal and abnormal findings for each placement of sensors.

Heart muscle cells are electrically charged, or *polarized*, in a state of rest. When cells are electrically stimulated, they *depolarize* and contract. Depolarize means to destroy polarization. The cells repolarize during the resting phase that follows contraction. *Repolarize* means to restore polarity. Depolarization and repolarization are electrical happenings that are recorded by the electrocardiogram.

When atrial depolarization occurs, the atria then contract. Atrial repolarization occurs when the atria are at rest. When ventricular depolarization occurs, the ventricles then contract. Ventricular repolarization occurs during ventricular rest.

The heartbeat originates in the *sinoatrial* or *sino-*

auricular node, commonly abbreviated *S-A node,* which is located in the upper part of the right atrium. It is frequently referred to as the heart's pacemaker. Currents radiate quickly throughout the atria from the S-A node and stimulate their contraction. A second node, the *atrioventricular* or *auriculoventricular node,* commonly abbreviated A-V *node,* picks up the current. The node is situated at the base of the atrial septum. The A-V node divides into two bundle branches and each in turn, gives rise to numerous "twigs" that interlace throughout the ventricles. This interlacing system is called the *Purkinje system.* Figure 20-11a illustrates the structures through which electrical current travels through the heart.

Figure 20-11b shows a drawing of a normal EKG. The waves on the electrocardiogram are lettered, as illustrated. The P wave occurs when elec-

trical charges, originating in the S-A node, cause the atria to depolarize and contract. The wave of Q, R, and S occurs when the electrical charges result in ventricular depolarization and contraction. Wave T represents relaxation of the ventricles during which time ventricular repolarization occurs. Repolarization of the atria occurs during the QRS segment but it is not usually as visible on the electrocardiogram as ventricular repolarization is. The sum total of P, Q, R, S, and T represents the cardiac cycle. Another way of describing the cardiac cycle is that it consists of atrial and ventricular depolarization and repolarization.

Look again at Figure 20-11. It illustrates how each electrical phenomenon occurring in the normal heart appears on the electrocardiogram.

When the S-A node is not functioning properly

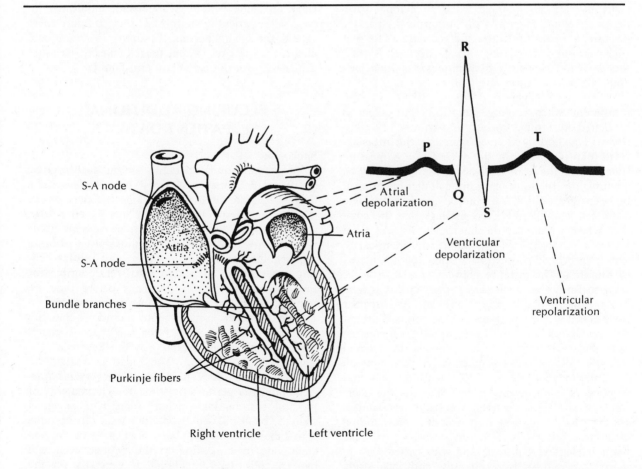

Fig. 20-11. Illustration of how electrical phenomenon occuring in the normal heart appears on the electrocardiogram. (Adapted from illustration in Meehan, M.: EKG Primer. Am. J. Nurs., 71:2201, Nov. 1971)

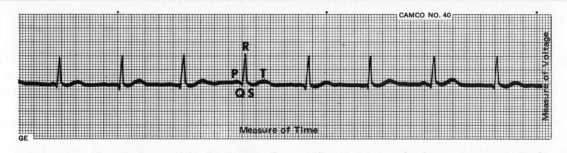

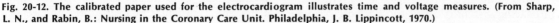

Fig. 20-12. The calibrated paper used for the electrocardiogram illustrates time and voltage measures. (From Sharp, L. N., and Rabin, B.: Nursing in the Coronary Care Unit. Philadelphia, J. B. Lippincott, 1970.)

as the heart's pacemaker, other areas in the heart become potential pacemakers. These pacemakers, referred to as *ectopic pacemakers*, may be in the A-V node, atria, or ventricles. A condition known as heart block is an example when an ectopic pacemaker develops. There is a disruption in the passage of current between the atria and ventricles. The ventricles do not stop beating when this occurs. Rather, they beat independently from impulses of their own and usually at a slower rate than the atria.

The ruled paper used for an EKG aids immeasurably when reading the EKG. The paper is calibrated in 1 mm. squares, as Figure 20-12 illustrates. The horizontal lines represent the measurement of voltage while the vertical lines measure time. When the heart is diseased, the waves may be abnormal in size, form, or position. The time interval between waves also has diagnostic significance. Here are a few examples of EKG findings that are commonly found when certain conditions exist. An atrial flutter is characterized by rapid and identical P waves; an ectopic pacemaker has probably originated in the atria. The distance between similar waves is short in time when tachycardia is present; it is long in time when bradycardia is present. An irregular rhythm is due often to disease in the coronary artery. The drug quinidine tends to retard electrical conduction; the result is that the P waves may be notched and the QRS segment may be wider than normal.

Interpretation of an EKG requires skill and practice. It is an invaluable tool to study the heart function when properly used. More and more, nurses are expected to have at least a basic understanding of electrocardiography. For nurses working with patients having heart diseases and with patients in intensive care and coronary care units, additional study and practice are necessary since understanding EKG readings is critical in the care of these patients.

Patients who are seriously ill frequently have constant monitoring of the heart action including the impulse transmission and myocardial response. Devices which permit the patient to move around and carry on some activity while being monitored increase the patient's comfort. The electronic devices extend the health personnel's ability to secure data about the patient. Their usage generally requires explanation for the patient and his family.

SECURING ADDITIONAL PATIENT DATA

Specimens

Depending on the patient's age and health status, additional data may be secured to compile a more detailed picture of his physical health state. X-ray examinations have already been mentioned as one such method. Analysis of specimens of body fluids and tissues is another way. The nurse often carries a responsibility for instructing the patient and for securing specimens. She is also usually responsible for the correct labeling of specimens before they are transported to the laboratory. An inaccurate or unmarked specimen can be more hazardous than no specimen at all. A request for the type of examination desired should accompany the specimen.

Blood Specimens: The blood is one of the most significant body tissues that conveys information about the person's health state. The majority of physical examinations include some type of blood analysis. Multitudes of laboratory tests can be done with blood specimens. The role of the nurse is generally one of explaining to the patient what will happen and what preparation is necessary for the examination. Many blood specimens are secured while the patient is in the fasting state. *Fasting*

TABLE 20-2:   Normal laboratory values*

Constituents	Normal range
BLOOD	
Bleeding time	1-3 min.
Cholesterol, total (plasma or serum)	150-250 mgm. %
Clot retraction time	begins in 1 hr.—complete in 24 hrs.
Coagulation time	6-12 min.
Erythrocytes	4,500,000-5,000,000/cu. mm.
Glucose	70-120 mgm. %
Hemoglobin (average for both sexes)	14-16 Gm/100 cc.
Hematocrit average for men	47% ± 7%
Hematocrit average for women	42% ± 5%
Icterus index (serum)	4-6 units
Leukocytes	5,000-10,000/cu. mm.
Basophils	0.25-0.5%
Eosinophils	1-3%
Lymphocytes	25-33%
Monocytes	2-6%
Polymorphonuclear neutrophils	60-70%
pH	7.35-7.45
Platelets	200,000-400,000/cu. mm.
Prothrombin time (Quick)	10-15 sec.
Reticulocytes	0.8-1.0%
Sedimentation rate (Westergren) in first hour	
Men	0-12 min.
Women	0-20 min.
Volume	7-9% body wt.
CEREBROSPINAL FLUID	
Cell count	1-7 lymphocytes per cu. mm.
Colloidal gold	negative
Diffusible calcium	4.5—5.5 mg./100 cc.
Pressure (in resting position)	120—200 mm. water
Specific gravity	1.003—1.008
Sugar	40—70 mg./100 cc.
Total protein	20-40 mg./100 cc.
URINE	
Average amount in 24 hrs.	1,000—1,500 cc.
Chlorides (Na)	10—15 Gm. per 24 hrs.
Phenolsulfonphthalein P.S.P.	60—75 percent in 2 hrs.
Urea clearance	54 cc. blood per min.
Urea	20—35 Gm. per 24 hrs.
Uric acid	0.4—1 Gm. per 24 hrs.

* Courtesy of Becton, Dickinson and Company.

means to abstain from food or fluid ingestion. The period of fasting will vary with the tests to be done and laboratory techniques used. Whether patients are in their own homes or in a health agency, they need a careful explanation about the fast period.

Blood specimens are generally collected by laboratory personnel. In some situations, the nurse may be responsible for deciding what laboratory tests are to be done and to take some action, depending on the results of the examinations.

In all situations, the nurse should be sufficiently familiar with the more common normal blood examination values to be able to recognize deviations. Blood examination results are one more factor in the data she collects about the patient in order to provide effective nursing care. Normal adult values for some of the more common laboratory blood tests are given in Table 20-2.

URINE SPECIMENS: A *urinalysis* is the laboratory examination of a urine specimen. Analysis of the urine is another common way of securing data about the health state of an individual. The nurse is often responsible for instructing and/or securing a sample of urine. A cooperative patient can be instructed to put the specimen into a clean or, in some instances, a sterile container. Care should be taken that the outside of the container is not contaminated.

Most laboratories prefer a specimen of several hundred milliliters that is collected soon after arising from sleep. Special urine collection techniques are discussed in Chapter 26.

Like common blood specimens, the nurse should be able to recognize deviations from normal in the urinalysis. Table 20-2 shows normal adult laboratory analysis values for urine.

SECRETION SPECIMENS: Specimens of body secretions are collected for the purpose of microscopic examination or to introduce them into a culture medium to promote growth of microorganisms present. Body secretions from the throat, vagina, rectum, and wounds or lesions are most often collected for these purposes.

A sterile, long-handled applicator and sterile test tubes are generally used. Some agencies also use sterile glass slides.

The sterile cotton-tipped end of the applicator should be placed directly into the area where the specimen is desired and rotated to make certain secretions adhere to the applicator. The applicator is then carefully placed directly into the test tube or onto the slide and handled according to the laboratory policy. Precautions should be taken so that the applicator is not contaminated before or after securing the secretion specimen. Nor should the secretions be allowed to contaminate other surfaces.

Lumbar Puncture

A *lumbar puncture*, or *spinal tap*, is the insertion of a needle into the subarachnoid space in the spinal canal. The procedure is part of the physical examination for some patients. It is generally performed by a physician with the nurse assisting.

INDICATIONS FOR A LUMBAR PUNCTURE: Cerebrospinal fluid normally fills the ventricles of the brain, the subarachnoid space, and the central canal of the spinal cord. The fluid is clear and transparent. It may be necessary to enter the subarachnoid space for several reasons: to obtain a specimen of the fluid for analysis and for culture; to establish any alterations in the usual pressure of the cerebrospinal fluid; to relieve pressure; to inject drugs or to inject dyes for x-ray visualization.

NECESSARY EQUIPMENT: Because the subarachnoid space is a sterile cavity, surgical asepsis is observed. Normally, the cerebrospinal fluid pressure is

greater than atmospheric pressure, and many pathogenic conditions of the central nervous system are characterized by an increase in this normal pressure. Therefore, the lumbar puncture needle contains a carefully and precisely fitted stylet so that fluid will not escape while the needle is in place, except when the physician removes the stylet.

The necessary sterile equipment includes a 20- or 22-gauge lumbar puncture needle, 3 to 5 inches long; a small syringe and a 22- or 25-gauge needle for the injection of local anesthesia at the site of injection; a fenestrated drape, gauze and cotton balls, and gloves for the physician. Many sets include specimen containers and some a manometer for measuring the pressure of the fluid. If not included, they are added at the appropriate time. Commercially prepared disposable spinal tap trays are available also. If the physician wishes to inject a drug into the spinal canal, another sterile syringe of the appropriate size is necessary. The local anesthetic of the physician's choice is brought to the working unit. One percent procaine hydrochloride usually is used. The physician may want a stool so he can be seated during the procedure.

Prior to the procedure, the nurse examines the skin area where the physician will be working. If hair is present, the physician is asked whether he wishes the area to be shaved.

ASSISTING THE PHYSICIAN: The fourth or the fifth lumbar space is the usual site of entry. The needle enters the subarachnoid space by passing between the vertebrae into the canal. In order to spread the vertebrae and to provide the widest possible space for easier insertion of the needle, the patient is positioned on his side and with his back arched. Figure 20-13 illustrates this position. He is brought near the edge of the bed or the treatment table where the physician will work. The patient is asked to flex his knees and bring his head and shoulders down as close as possible to his knees. A small pillow may be placed under the patient's head and between his knees for comfort. Some patients are unable to assume or maintain this position without assistance. This can be done by facing the patient and grasping him behind his knees with one arm and behind his neck with the other arm so that the back remains arched as much as possible. Other patients may have difficulty in understanding or be disoriented. They will need repeated assurances of what is being done. However, the head should not be pulled down or the knees pressed against the abdomen, since this increases intraspinal fluid pressure, leading to a falsely elevated pressure.

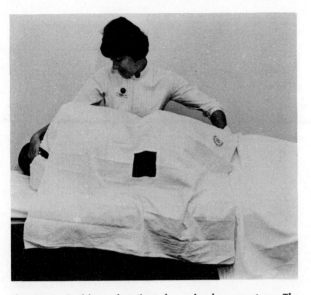

Fig. 20-13. Position of patient for a lumbar puncture. The nurse is helping this patient to assume and maintain the desired position by holding her one arm behind his knees so that they are flexed and bringing his head forward by putting her other arm behind his neck. In this position his back is arched.

The nurse may have to help the patient to maintain the desired position. After helping the physician to get his equipment in order, the nurse returns to the opposite side of the bed to do this. It is important to explain to the patient that he must remain motionless during the procedure. Moving about makes insertion of the needle more difficult and also may cause the needle to break.

Occasionally, the physician may prefer having the patient in the sitting position during the lumbar puncture. The patient sits on the edge of a treatment table, his feet are supported on a chair and his arms are placed over the shoulders of a person who helps to support him in position, or his arms are supported on an overbed table placed in front of him.

The fourth or the fifth lumbar space is located approximately at the same level on the back as the iliac crest. After an antiseptic has been applied to the area, the physician puts the sterile fenestrated drape in place. The opening is over the area that has been cleansed and where the needle will be inserted. Care should be taken so that the drape does not slip about during the procedure and thereby contaminate the working area. The area of the drape surrounding the working area is kept sterile.

The nurse prepares the bottle of anesthetic that the physician has ordered and holds it so that he can

check the label and withdraw some, or the nurse may pour the drug. The physician begins the procedure by anesthetizing the skin and the subcutaneous tissue at the site of injection.

When the anesthesia is effective, the physician inserts the lumbar puncture needle. After the needle is in place, the physician may apply the manometer to the needle to determine the cerebrospinal pressure. The pressure normally is not constant and will be observed to fluctuate somewhat with each pulse beat and each respiration. The normal average range of pressure is about 6 to 12 mm. of mercury or 90 to 150 mm. of water. The physician may ask the nurse to make a notation of the pressure reading. If the lumbar puncture needle is resting freely in the subarachnoid space, pressure usually can be increased when venous compression occurs. The physician may ask the nurse to apply hand pressure to the abdomen. The pressure can also be increased by compressing the jugular vein. This is called the Queckenstedt's test and is used if intraspinal lesions are suspected. The most reliable reading can be obtained by the use of the blood pressure cuff wrapped about the neck. This provides for a more even pressure. The mercury column is elevated to 50 mm. Since there is variation in this practice, the nurse should always understand the physician's procedure if she is to assist in this test.

After pressure has been determined, specimens will be collected if desired. If sterile tubes are provided in the set, the physician may collect the specimens himself and hand them to the nurse for proper labeling and handling.

If not included, the physician may ask the nurse to hold the tubes below the opening of the needle while he regulates the flow of cerebrospinal fluid with the stylet. Care should be observed to prevent touching the needle or the hands of the physician with the collecting tubes. It may also be important to note and mark the order of fluid removed on each specimen container. Table 20-2 indicates normal cerebrospinal fluid values.

During the procedure, the nurse observes the patient's reaction carefully. His color, pulse rate, and respiratory rate are noted and reported to the physician immediately if anything unusual is observed. Care should be exercised to prevent alarming the patient if any report is being given to the physician.

When the procedure is completed, the needle is removed, and compression is applied to the site for a short while. A small sterile piece of gauze may be applied to the site and fastened with adhesive.

Immediately following the procedure, the patient

may be placed in the recumbent position, preferably without a pillow. Fluids usually are offered. This is intended to avoid postspinal headache. It generally is believed that the headache is due to the tear in the dura mater made by the needle, which allows for seepage of small amounts of cerebrospinal fluid. Differences of opinion do exist about the effectiveness of positioning in avoiding the occurrence of the headache. The nurse will want to follow the practice in her area. If a headache does occur, the patient usually is treated symptomatically.

The patient's general physical reaction to the procedure is observed. This is of particular importance if the procedure was carried out to relieve pressure. Any unusual reactions such as twitching, vomiting, or slow pulse are reported to the physician promptly.

Thoracentesis

A *thoracentesis* is the entering and aspirating of fluid from the pleural cavity. The pleural cavity is a potential cavity, since normally it is not distended with fluid or air. Its walls are in approximation, and normal secretions keep them from adhering. The physician generally performs the thoracentesis with the nurse assisting.

INDICATIONS FOR THORACENTESIS: When a thoracentesis is done as a part of a physical examination, the pleural cavity is entered to determine whether fluid is present, if this cannot be established satisfactorily by other means. If fluid is present, specimens usually are obtained and analyzed to assist in diagnosis. If an accumulation of fluid in the pleural cavity causes difficult respiration and discomfort, a thoracentesis may also be done for therapeutic reasons to remove the fluid. This, in turn, relieves respiratory embarrassment.

Fluid in the pleural cavity results from inflammation caused by an infection which increases the normal secretions in the pleural cavity. If the fluid is purulent, the condition is called *empyema*. Fluid may accumulate also in the pleural cavity as a result of impaired circulation. This is common when a tumor is present. Air in the pleural cavity is due almost always to accidents when the chest wall has been punctured.

EQUIPMENT NEEDED: Because the cavity being entered is sterile, surgical technique is used. The basic equipment for entering the pleural cavity includes a small syringe and a 22- or 25-gauge needle for administering a local anesthetic at the site of injection; a blunt 15-gauge needle, 2 to 3 inches long; gauze and cotton; sterile rubber gloves for the

physician; sterile specimen tubes; and a fenestrated drape. A skin antiseptic and a local anesthetic agent are also necessary. Commercially prepared disposable trays containing the equipment are also available.

Normally, the pressure in the pleural cavity is less than atmospheric; therefore, equipment for suction is almost always necessary to remove the fluid. The physician indicates the method that he will use.

One way to remove fluid or air from the pleural cavity is to aspirate it with a syringe. A large syringe —usually 50 c.c.—frequently is used. When this method is employed, a sterile syringe with a three-way stopcock attached is added to the sterile equipment. The physician withdraws the fluid into the syringe and adjusts the stopcock so that he may push the fluid into the collecting container. He readjusts the stopcock and reaspirates the pleural cavity. A hand-operated large volume bellows pump can also be attached to the needle for aspiration. This device eliminates stopcock manipulation.

Another method for removing fluid from the pleural cavity is to drain the fluid into a bottle in which a partial vacuum has been created. The bottle has a stopper on it to which is attached a two-way stopcock. To one opening in the stopcock is attached rubber tubing which connects with the needle in the pleural cavity. Air is removed from the bottle through the other opening in the stopcock with either a motor-driven or a hand-operated suction pump. When this method is used, the tubing which connects the needle and the bottle is sterilized. It is convenient to use a calibrated bottle for the drainage in order to determine readily the amount of fluid that has been removed.

To enhance the safety and the effectiveness of the procedure, a plastic catheter to thread through the needle after it is in the site can be used. Then the needle can be withdrawn. The catheter reduces the possibility of puncturing the lung or doing other damage; also, its flexibility makes it possible to feed it into a pocket of fluid which the needle may not have reached accurately. The catheter is also more comfortable for the patient.

Prior to the procedure, the nurse examines the skin area where the physician will be working. If hair is present, the physician is asked whether he wishes the area shaved.

ASSISTING THE PHYSICIAN: Usually, this procedure is carried out when the patient is in a sitting position on a chair or on the edge of a treatment table or bed with his feet supported on a chair. Figure 20-14 illustrates this position. If the patient cannot sit up, he may lie on his side. Usually, he is

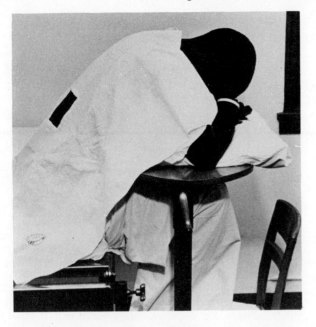

Fig. 20-14. Position of the patient for a throacentesis.

placed on the affected side with the hand of that side resting on the opposite shoulder.

The skin is prepared over the area where the physician indicates that he will insert the needle. The exact location will depend on the area where fluid is present and where the physician can best aspirate it. The needle will be inserted between the ribs through the intercostal muscles, the intercostal fascia and into the pleura. After the skin is prepared, the physician places the drape. The nurse may need to help anchor it in front of the patient's shoulders to prevent its slipping about on the field of work. The nurse prepares the bottle of anesthetic drug and holds it so that the physician can read the label before he withdraws some or she pours some.

The physician begins by anesthetizing the area where the needle is to be inserted. When anesthesia is effective, the physician inserts the needle. The nurse usually is asked to assist with the collection of specimens. The nurse is responsible for having the container ready for the physician to empty the syringe if the syringe method is being used. If a bottle is being used to collect the drainage, the nurse assists by operating either the hand- or the motor-driven pump that creates the partial vacuum in the bottle.

During the procedure, the nurse observes the patient for reactions. The patient's color, pulse rate, and respiratory rate are observed, and anything un-

usual is reported to the physician immediately. Fainting, nausea, and vomiting may occur.

When the procedure is completed, the needle (or plastic catheter) is removed. The nurse assists with placing a small sterile dressing over the site of entry.

Following the procedure, the patient should be observed for changes in his respirations. If fluid is removed, respirations usually will be eased. If the lung has been punctured accidentally (the use of a blunt needle aids in preventing this accident), respiratory embarrassment becomes acute. If present, sputum should be observed, and if blood appears or if the patient has severe coughing, the physician should be notified promptly.

Abdominal Paracentesis

The withdrawal of fluid from the peritoneal cavity is referred to as an abdominal paracentesis. The word *paracentesis* means the withdrawal of fluid from any body cavity, but it is common practice to use the term when referring to the removal of fluid from the peritoneal cavity. The technique is used to secure abdominal fluid for analysis or for the therapeutic value of removing excess fluid. This procedure also is normally performed by a physician with the nurse assisting.

The accumulation of fluid in the peritoneal cavity in called *ascites* and often occurs with certain liver, cardiac, and renal diseases.

INDICATIONS FOR A PARACENTESIS: When used for diagnostic purposes, specimens of the fluid are taken for examination in order to identify certain organisms or cells. For example, the fluid may be analyzed to determine whether or not cells of a malignant tumor are present. A paracentesis will help to relieve symptoms caused by the accumulation of fluid in the peritoneal cavity. The symptoms are caused by the pressure of the fluid. For example, respirations may be embarrassed if the fluid causes pressure on the diaphragm, or frequency of voiding may be increased, since the fluid may make it difficult for the urinary bladder to fill to normal capacity.

EQUIPMENT NEEDED: Since the peritoneal cavity is normally a sterile cavity, surgical asepsis is observed for the procedure. Normally, the pressure in the peritoneal cavity is no greater than atmospheric pressure, but, when fluid is present, pressure is greater than atmospheric. Gravity will aid in the removal of fluid; therefore, the fluid will drain of its own accord until pressure is equalized.

A sterile trocar and cannula are used to enter the peritoneal cavity. This instrument is usually 4 to 5 inches in length with a bore of approximately one-eighth of an inch. In order to introduce the trocar easily, a very small incision is made in the skin which is sutured following the procedure. The sterile items needed include: a small syringe and a 22- or 25-gauge needle for anesthetizing the skin prior to making the incision; a scalpel for making the incision; suture material, small clamps or forceps, a suture needle, and scissors for closing the incision; sterile tubing to be attached directly to the trocar for drainage; a sterile fenestrated drape or towels; gauze and cotton balls and gloves. Skin antiseptic and an anesthetic usually will be needed. Disposable paracentesis trays are also available.

A clean container for drainage, preferably a calibrated bottle, is necessary. The use of a plastic catheter threaded through the trocar once it is in place is a method used by some physicians. It provides for greater safety and comfort to the patient. In addition, its small caliber reduces the rate of flow of the fluid. When the plastic catheter is used, both the physician and the nurse may need to consider available equipment for connecting the catheter to drainage tubing. A large-gauge needle inserted into the plastic tubing and then attached to suitable-sized drainage tubing is one means used.

Prior to the procedure, the nurse examines the patient's abdomen. If hair is present, the physician is asked whether or not he wishes the area to be shaved.

ASSISTING THE PHYSICIAN: Weigh the patient prior to and after the treatment. The patient should be offered a bedpan before the procedure is begun. This is of particular importance when a paracentesis is to be performed because, if the urinary bladder is full, there is danger of puncturing it with the trocar. If the patient is unable to void, the physician should be notified; then he may order the patient to be catheterized.

Since gravity will be used to assist the drainage, the patient is placed in a sitting position. The patient may be supported in the sitting position in bed; he may be placed at the side of the bed or the treatment table with his feet supported on a chair; or he may sit on a chair during the procedure. A chair is most comfortable because it offers good back and arm support. This is important, since the procedure may take quite a while if a large amount of fluid is to be withdrawn. After the patient is in position, with legs slightly separated so that the site of entry is readily accessible, he should be covered adequately for warmth and to prevent unnecessary exposure. A

pair of pajama pants helps to keep the patient's legs covered and also to prevent exposure. Figure 20-15 illustrates positioning and draping. The trocar will be passed through the abdominal wall into the peritoneal cavity near the midline of the abdomen approximately halfway between the umbilicus and the pubis. The skin over this area is cleansed, and the physician places the sterile drape in position. The nurse may need to secure it to prevent its slipping.

The physician then anesthetizes the site of entry, incises the skin, and introduces the trocar and the cannula. When the trocar is in place, the physician will pull back on the cannula to see if fluid will drain; if it does, the drainage tube is attached. The specimens will be obtained and should be carefully labeled. If a plastic catheter is used it is threaded through at this time. The nurse places the distal end of the tubing in the container for drainage. The greater the vertical distance between the trocar and the container for drainage, the greater will be the pull of gravity. If fluid is draining too rapidly, the container should be elevated on a stool. Rapid drainage may produce symptoms of shock.

During the treatment and after, the nurse observes the patient for untoward reactions associated with electrolyte imbalance. His color and respiratory and pulse rates are noted. Signs of fainting are watched for. The patient may begin to experience relief from the pressure of the fluid, and these signs are observed by the nurse also.

The nurse notes the type and the amount of drainage present. After the needle has been withdrawn and the incision sutured, the nurse should place a sterile heavy dressing over the site of incision, since leakage usually occurs. The patient often is more comfortable if an abdominal binder is used for support following the procedure.

Gastric Analysis

Gastric analysis is the laboratory examination of gastric content. The stomach contents are removed by means of aspiration through a tube which has been inserted through the mouth or nose and the esophagus. Removal of the gastric specimens is often the responsibility of the nurse. The tube itself may be inserted by nurses in some health agencies and by physicians in others.

INDICATIONS FOR GASTRIC ANALYSIS: A gastric analysis can be done to examine the volume or constituents of stomach secretions. It is done most commonly when stomach pathology is suspected.

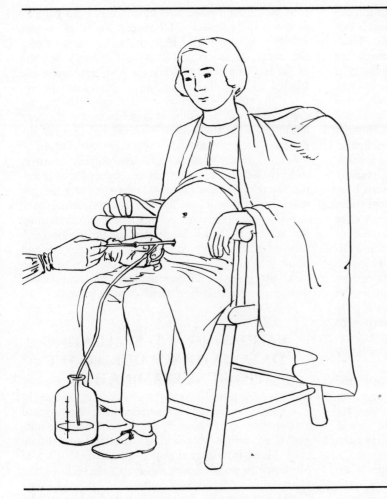

Fig. 20-15. Position of the patient for an abdominal paracentesis.

NECESSARY EQUIPMENT: Since the stomach is not a sterile cavity, the equipment need not be sterile, but medical asepsis is observed. The tube is introduced through one of the nares or the mouth. It is made of rubber or plastic and is 12 to 24 inches longer than the distance from the patient's mouth to his stomach. The tube commonly used is the Levin tube. Either a bulb-type syringe or a plunger-type syringe is used to aspirate the stomach contents. Usually, a 50 c.c. syringe is preferred.

The larger the lumen of the tube, the easier it is to remove thick stomach contents. However, the larger the tube, the more discomfort the patient experiences in swallowing it. When a small tube is used, it is passed through one of the nares; if a larger tube is used, the patient is asked to swallow it through the mouth.

Before the tube is inserted, it may be helpful, especially when using rubber, to place the tube on cracked ice for 15 to 20 minutes. This cooling of the tube makes it less flexible and therefore easier to handle. In addition, a water-soluble lubricant should be available for lubricating the tube.

The number and type of specimen containers will be determined by the tests to be performed and the laboratory procedure.

REMOVING GASTRIC CONTENTS: In most instances, the patient is placed in the sitting position so that gravity aids the passage of the tube. If the patient is unable to sit up, he may lie either on his back or on his side.

The approximate distance to the stomach is determined by measuring the distance from the tip of the sternum to the bridge of the nose. The length should be marked on the tube before initiating insertion. The lubricated tube is introduced through one of the nares or over the top and middle of the tongue. Asking the patient to breathe through his mouth is generally helpful. When the tip of the tube reaches the pharynx, ask the patient to begin swallowing. As the patient swallows, insert the tube until the marked point is reached. Since the delicate mucous membrane can be damaged, insertion through the nasal or oropharyngeal areas should be gentle. Force should not be used. Usually, adequate lubrication and rotation of the tube with gentle pressure will aid ease of movement. Since some persons have nasal septum deviations and other pathological states of the nasopharyngeal area, if one naris cannot be entered readily, the alternate one should be used. If for any reason, the tube cannot be inserted readily, another more experienced practitioner should be secured. If the patient is allowed water, permitting him to take sips while the tube is being passed aids in the ease with which the tube is swallowed.

The gag reflex is stimulated by tube insertion in most patients. However, it should be a temporary reaction. Persistent gagging may mean the tube is being passed too slowly or too rapidly.

In some instances, the tube may enter the trachea rather than the esophagus. Coughing, difficulty with breathing, and the inability to hum are indications of this misplacement. The tube should be immediately removed when the trachea has been entered.

Once the tube has been inserted the appropriate distance, placement within the stomach should be positively ascertained. There are a number of techniques to determine tube placement, but the only completely reliable one is the aspiration of gastric contents through the tube. However, there are situations when the tube may be properly placed and because of the viscosity of the gastric contents, they do not move readily up the tube when suction from the syringe is applied. Holding the end of the tube under water to observe for bubbles can be tried. If the tube is in the lung, air should escape through the tube in the form of bubbles. If there is any doubt about the tube placement, seeking the opinion of another nurse or a physician, or repositioning the tube is essential.

When proper placement is assured, the tube should be taped securely at the nose or cheek. If the tube is not secured, swallowing, coughing, sneezing, and even talking can displace it.

Removal of stomach contents is achieved by aspirating with the syringe. The number of specimens to be taken and the time intervals between them will vary according to the procedure of the laboratories in the various agencies. However, almost all request a fasting specimen and then the administration of a test meal. At intervals following the meal, samples of gastric contents are taken. The specimens are labeled and handled according to the agency policy.

Following completion of the examination, the gastric tube can be removed. After loosening the tape holdings, while the tube is pinched tightly near the patient's face, it should be quickly withdrawn. A towel or similar cloth should be available to cover and remove the tubing from the patient's view immediately. The tube's removal may stimulate the gag reflex but this will usually only last momentarily.

The gastric analysis is usually done to determine the volume of hydrochloric acid in the stomach. A tubeless gastric analysis, involving dye ingestion and urine specimen collection, is also possible to determine the presence of free hydrochloric acid, but it does not determine how much acid is present.

VALIDATING AND EVALUATING DATA GATHERED DURING THE PHYSICAL EXAMINATION

Validation of data gathered during the physical examination is recommended. As Chapter 6 points out, it is neither necessary nor practical to validate every bit of information that is gathered. It is up to the nurse to decide when she feels validation is necessary.

When there are discrepancies in the data, validation is advisable. As one example, if there are discrepancies when the patient's blood pressure is taken upon admission to a hospital and when taken again the next day, the findings should be validated.

Validation is recommended when the nurse has drawn inferences from findings made during the physical examination. For example, she may wish to validate with the patient that he seems to be having difficulty seeing or hearing. Changes in symptoms, such as amount of wound drainage, vital sign characteristics, or discomfort can sometimes be validated by the patient, by his health record, or by another health practitioner.

Doubt in the accuracy of the data calls for validation. For example, a patient's temperature, taken orally, falls within normal range; yet, the patient feels warm to touch and complains of a headache and nausea. The nurse will wish to recheck the patient's temperature since she realizes that an elevated temperature is commonly found with the symptoms the patient presented.

The data are evaluated to determine appropriateness and accuracy. These questions, offered in Chapter 6, will aid the nurse to evaluate data: Do the findings aid to convey the patient's present state of health? Have all relevant factors in the patient's situation been considered? Are the relationships between factors in the patient's situation appropriate and accurate? The reader is encouraged to review Chapter 6 for a more detailed discussion of the entire data-gathering process.

CONCLUSION

The health state profile, developed during the data-gathering process, is an important tool for assessing and planning nursing care and for nursing intervention. This chapter has described the gathering of certain data that are important to have in order to prepare an objective and accurate profile. This text goes on to describe data gathering in remaining chapters also. However, basic data necessary in nearly every situation have been presented here.

Study Situations

1. As a method to review and increase your knowledge in relation to measuring blood pressure and to understanding electrocardiography, the following two references are suggestions for your study:
Correcting common errors in blood pressure measurement. (Programmed Instruction) **Am. J. Nurs.,** 65:133–64, Oct., 1965.
Meehan, M.: EKG primer. (Programmed Instruction) **Am. J. Nurs.,** 71:2195–2202, Nov., 1971.

2. The following article states that the stethoscope, once an instrument used almost entirely by physicians, is now an important part of the nurse's equipment:
Littmann, D.: Stethoscopes and auscultation. **Am. J. Nurs.,** 72:1238–1241, July, 1972.
How does the author describe the typical sound of a heartbeat when the stethoscope is placed over the apex of the heart? How does he describe normal respiratory sounds? What suggestions are offered for the cleaning of a stethoscope?

3. The following two articles describe research findings on determining optimum placement times for oral and rectal thermometers:
Nichols, G. A., et al.: Rectal thermometer placement times for febrile adults. **Nurs. Research,** 21:76–77, Jan.–Feb., 1972.

Nichols, G. A., et al.: Measuring oral and rectal temperatures of febrile children. **Nurs. Research,** 21:261–262, May–June, 1972.
What criterion was used to determine optimum placement time? How does optimum placement time differ from maximum placement time? What suggestions did the authors offer as a reason for optimum placement time taking longer in children?

4. Equipment for automated multiphasic health testing is available and is reported to be a valuable aid when performing a physical examination. The equipment is briefly described in the following reference:
Automated multiphasic health testing. **Am. J. Nurs.,** 73:880, May, 1973.
The manufacturers indicate that their equipment provides an accurate, rapid and efficient means of gathering certain basic data. The data are fed into a computer and then appear in a printout immediately upon completion of the examination. Other than possibly the cost of the equipment, do you see any disadvantages in its use? Is there a health testing system of this type in your area? If so, you may wish to observe the system in operation.

5. For an interesting description of circadian rhythms, the following article is suggested reading:
Aschoff, J.: Circadian rhythms in man. **Science,** 148: 1427–1432, June 11, 1965.
According to the author, how has industry used knowledge of the circadian rhythm in its work and employment practices? How does the periodicity of the body's functions affect the jet traveler?

References

1. Bell, S.: Early morning temperatures? **Am. J. Nurs.,** 69:764–766, Apr., 1969.
2. Betson, C., and Ude, L.: Central venous pressure. **Am. J. Nurs.,** 69:1466–1468, July, 1969.
3. Caffeine and fever. **Time,** 100:56, Oct. 2, 1972.
4. Collen, M. F., and Davis, L. F.: The multitest laboratory in health care. **Occup. Health Nurs.,** 17:13–18, July, 1969.
5. Cononi, G. A., and Siler, M.: Automated multiphasic health testing in the hospital setting. **J. Nurs. Administration,** 2:70–80, Nov.–Dec., 1972.
6. Devney, A. M., and Kingsbury, B. A.: Hypothermia in fact and fantasy. **Am. J. Nurs.,** 72:1424–1425, Aug., 1972.
7. Dubin, D.: Rapid Interpretation of EKG's . . . A Programmed Course. ed. 2. Tampa, Fla., Cover, 1972.
8. Electronic sphygmomanometer. **Am. J. Nurs.,** 72: 131, Jan., 1972.
9. Flynn, E. D.: Barriers to utilization of multiphasic screening—the nurse's role. **Occup. Health Nurs.,** 17: 19–21, July, 1969.

10. Foley, M. F.: Variations in blood pressure in the lateral recumbent position. **Nurs. Research,** 20:64–69, Jan.–Feb., 1971.

11. Folk, G. E. Jr.: Introduction to Environmental Physiology: Environmental Extremes and Mammalian Survival. Philadelphia, Lea and Febiger, 1966.

12. Jackson, E. B. Jr.: In the screening clinic: guidelines to the appraisal of some common problems. **Am. J. Nurs.,** 72:1398–1400, Aug., 1972.

13. Keegan, L. G.: Dispelling the myth of the apical-radial pulse in digitalis therapy. **Am. J. Nurs.,** 72:1434–1435, Aug., 1972.

14. Keough, G., and Niebel, H. N.: Oral cancer detection—a nursing responsibility. **Am. J. Nurs.,** 73:684–686, Apr., 1973.

15. King, G. E.: Taking the blood pressure. **JAMA,** 209:1902–1904, Sept. 22, 1969.

16. Lee, R. V., and Elisha A.: Spurious fever. **Am. J. Nurs.,** 72:1094–1095, June, 1972.

17. Lehmann, Sr. J.: Auscultation of heart sounds. **Am. J. Nurs.,** 72:1242–1246, July, 1972.

18. Moore, V. B.: In-bed weighing. **Nurs. '72,** 2:13–16, July, 1972.

19. Nichols, G. A.: Taking adult temperatures: rectal measurement. **Am. J. Nurs.,** 72:1092–1093, June, 1972.

20. Nichols, G. A., and Kucha, D. H.: Taking adult temperature: oral measurements. **Am. J. Nurs.** 72:1090–1092, June, 1972.

21. Normal blood, plasma, and serum values. *In* **The Nursing Clinics of North America.** Philadelphia, W. B. Saunders, 5:361–367, June, 1970.

22. Oszustowicz, R. J.: Now, just tell the computer what ails you. **Mod. Hosp.,** 119:83–87, Sept., 1972.

23. Purintun, L. R., and Bishop, B. E.: How accurate are clinical thermometers? **Am. J. Nurs.,** 69:99–100, Jan., 1969.

24. Schmidt, A. J.: TPR's: an old habit or a significant routine? **Hospitals, J. Am. Hosp. Assoc.,** 46:57–60, Dec. 16, 1972.

25. Tate, G. V., et al.: Correct use of electric thermometers. **Am. J. Nurs.,** 70:1898–1899, Sept., 1970.

26. Traver, G. A.: Assessment of thorax and lungs. **Am. J. Nurs.,** 73:466–471, Mar., 1973.

27. Walker, E.: Responsibilities of the hospital nurse in the clinical use of radiation. *In* **The Nursing Clinics of North America.** Philadelphia, W. B. Saunders, 2:35–48, Mar., 1967.

28. Weinstock, F. J.: Tonometry screening. **Am. J. Nurs.,** 73:656–657, Apr., 1973.

CHAPTER 21

Providing for Personal Hygiene

GLOSSARY · INTRODUCTION · GENERAL PRINCIPLES FOR CARE OF THE
SKIN AND MUCOUS MEMBRANE · CARE OF THE SKIN ·
BATHING THE PATIENT · CARE OF THE HAIR · ORAL HYGIENE ·
CARE OF THE NAILS · CARE OF THE FEET · CARE OF THE EYES ·
CARE OF THE EARS AND NOSE · PERINEAL CARE · THE DECUBITUS
ULCER · CONCLUSION · STUDY SITUATIONS · REFERENCES

GLOSSARY

Acne: Eruption of skin due to inflammation and infection of sebaceous glands.

Alopecia: Baldness.

Athlete's Foot: A fungus infection on the skin of the feet.

Bedsore: Synonym for decubitus ulcer.

Caries: Cavitation of the teeth.

Ceruminous Gland: One found in the external auditory canal that secretes a substance called cerumen.

Dandruff: Condition characterized by itching and flaking of the scalp.

Decubitus Ulcer (Plural: Decubiti): Lesion of the skin in which surface breaks down with progressive destruction of underlying tissue.

Dermis: Underlying portion of the skin.

Epidermis: Superficial portion of the skin.

Gingivitis: Inflammation of the gums.

Hirsutism: Excessive growth of body hair.

Nits: Lice eggs.

Pediculicides: Preparation for destroying lice.

Pediculosis: Infestation with lice.

Periodontitis: Extensive inflammation of gums and alveolar tissues.

Plaque: A coating on teeth consisting of mucin, carbohydrate, and bacteria.

Pyorrhea: Synonym for periodontitis.

Sebaceous Gland: One found in the skin that secretes an oily substance called sebum.

INTRODUCTION

People differ in personal hygiene practices. Variations in the performance of personal hygiene care certainly are permissible. The time of day for brushing the teeth and for bathing, or the frequency of shampooing the hair and changing bed linens and sleeping garments are relatively unimportant. The important thing is that personal care be carried out conveniently and often enough to promote personal hygiene.

The nurse may assist the well patient to develop personal hygiene habits. During illness, the nurse helps the patient to continue sound hygienic practices. For example, the patient may feel that it is too much bother to brush his teeth while he is feeling ill, and he may neglect to do so without help or an explanation of its importance. If the nurse notes that

the patient is unaware of certain hygienic practices or that he uses an unsound practice, she has an opportunity for teaching. It is important to include family members in this teaching whenever it is appropriate. Including the family is especially important when patients are being cared for at home.

In certain instances, daily hygienic practices may need to be modified because of the patient's condition. For example, the patient who has an elevated temperature may need special mouth care in order that his lips and his tongue and the mucous membrane of his mouth may not become dry and crack. Or the patient who has dry skin may need lotion rubbed into the areas of the elbows and the heels to prevent irritation.

Nurses often are asked about hygienic fads and superstitions, which offers the nurse opportunity for health teaching. Such discussions often help the nurse to understand her patient better and may very well reveal attitudes that affect the patient's health or his recovery from illness.

GENERAL PRINCIPLES FOR CARE OF THE SKIN AND MUCOUS MEMBRANE

Practices concerned with the care of the skin and the mucous membrane are guided by this basic principle: *Unbroken and healthy skin and mucous membrane serve as first lines of defense against harmful agents.* The general functions of the skin include protection, secretion, excretion, heat regulation, and sensation. Mucous membrane lining the body orifices has the same general functions except that it is less important in aiding excretion. When the skin and the mucous membrane are healthy and intact, they function at their optimum.

This chapter is concerned with practices that aid to keep the skin and the mucous membrane healthy and intact and to minimize irritation. For example, in the selection of soaps, detergents, makeup, deodorants, and depilatories, products should be used that minimize chemical irritation on the skin and the mucous membrane in order to prevent injury. Mechanical irritation is minimized when friction is used judiciously, as when rubbing the patient's skin or smoothing the linen on which the patient lies. Patients with sensitive or tender skin, as infants and older patients, are handled very carefully to prevent skin breaks and irritation. Physical irritation is minimized when the nurse applies emollients and avoids drying agents such as alcohol when the skin is already dry. It is also minimized when the nurse keeps the skin dry and cool and the mucous membrane moist. Chemical and mechanical irritation is reduced when body secretions and dirt are removed by bathing. Microbial invasion is reduced by keeping the skin and the mucous membranes intact through prevention of mechanical, physical, and chemical irritation.

Resistance to injury of the skin and the mucous membrane varies among individuals. Individual resistance is influenced by factors such as age, general health of the patient, and the amount of subcutaneous tissue. The very young person and the older person have particularly sensitive skin and mucous membrane. When body cells are poorly nourished or hydrated, as in the emaciated or the dehydrated patient, the skin and the mucous membrane are more susceptible to injury. Very thin and very obese people tend to be more subject to skin irritation and injury.

Body cells adequately nourished and hydrated are more resistant to injury. Chapter 25 discusses the importance of nutrition to good body functioning. Cells in the skin and the mucous membrane need adequate nourishment and hydration. The better nourished the cell, the better its ability to resist injury and disease.

A corollary to adequate nourishment and hydration of cells is that *adequate circulation is necessary in order to maintain cell life.* When circulation is impaired for any reason, the cells involved are nourished inadequately; hence, they are more subject to injury. The importance of this principle will be illustrated more clearly in relation to the prevention of bedsores, discussed later in this chapter.

CARE OF THE SKIN

The skin consists of two distinct layers. The superficial portion is called the *epidermis* and is made up of layers of stratified squamous epithelium. It contains pores of sweat glands and shafts of hair in most parts of the body. The deeper layer is called the *dermis* and consists of smooth muscular tissue, nerves, fat, hair follicles, certain glands and their ducts, arteries, veins and capillaries, and fibrous elastic tissue. The skin covers the entire body and is continuous with mucous membrane at normal body orifices. Figure 21-1 illustrates a cross-section of normal skin.

The skin serves to protect underlying body tissue and organs from injury; it prevents microorganisms from invading the body; water, including nitrogenous wastes, is excreted through the skin; and the skin houses sense organs of touch, pain, heat, cold, and pressure. The skin also plays an important part in the regulation of body temperature. Heat is lost from the body through vasodilatation and evaporation of perspiration, and heat is retained through vasoconstriction and the phenomenon known as "goose pimples," which are formed by the contraction of muscular tissue in the dermis, thus making the hair stand on end.

The cutaneous glands include the *sebaceous,* the *sweat,* the *ceruminous,* and the *mammary* glands. The sebaceous glands secrete an oily substance called sebum which lubricates the skin and the hair and keeps the skin and the scalp pliant. The sweat glands secrete perspiration. The cerumen in the ear canals, consisting of a heavy oil and pigment, is secreted by the ceruminous glands. Milk is secreted during the postpartum period, by the mammary glands.

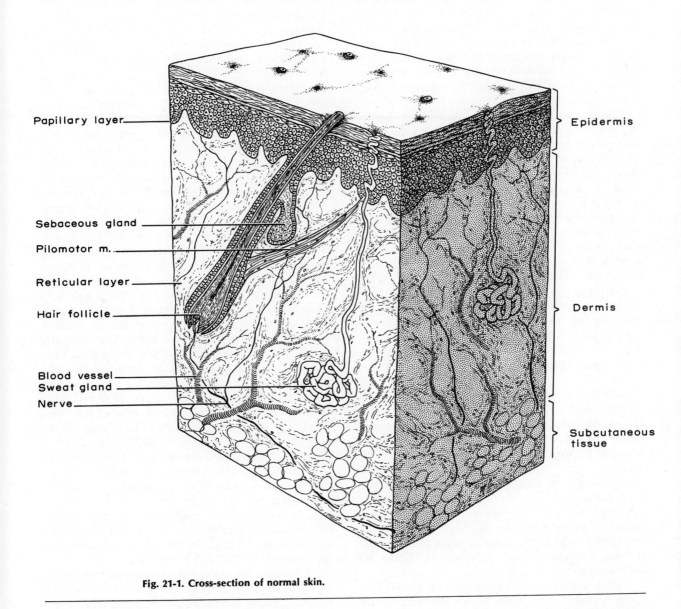

Papillary layer

Sebaceous gland

Pilomotor m.

Reticular layer

Hair follicle

Blood vessel
Sweat gland
Nerve

Epidermis

Dermis

Subcutaneous
tissue

Fig. 21-1. Cross-section of normal skin.

Age is a factor in caring for the skin. Because an infant's skin is injured easily and subject to infection, he should be handled and bathed gently to prevent injury. Young children's skin becomes more resistant to injury and infection but requires frequent cleansing because of toilet and play habits.

During adolescence, the skin should be kept immaculately clean and free from irritation to aid in the control of acne, a common condition during these years. During adolescence and up to approximately 50 years of age, secretions from skin glands are at their maximum. Hence, more frequent bathing is necessary to prevent body odors and the accumulation of secretions and dirt.

As age advances, the skin becomes less elastic and thinner. Subcutaneous fat decreases. Wrinkles appear, most of which are deep in the dermis. Since less oil is secreted from sebaceous glands, the skin becomes dry, often scaly, and rough in appearance. Brown frecklelike spots often appear on the hands, arms, neck, and face. They may begin appearing as early as 35 years of age. They tend to become more numerous and larger with aging. These spots are often referred to as old-age freckles or liver spots. Liver diseases do not cause these spots; rather, they are due to exposure to the wind and the sun. If they become thickened or develop crusts, it is wise to seek medical advice to determine whether any are precancerous lesions. Changes that occur in the skin with aging are irreversible.

Illness very often alters the condition of the skin and makes special care necessary. Severe fluid loss through fever, vomiting, or diarrhea reduces the fluid volume of the body. This condition makes the skin appear loose and very often flabby. The skin can be lifted easily, and it may not spring back as it does when the patient is well. Also, excessive perspiration may present a problem during illness. Some illnesses are accompanied by a change in pigmentation of the skin. The most commonly seen change in the skin color is that of jaundice. This symptom of several pathologic conditions is a yellow to deep green-yellow pigmentation of the skin. Other diseases may produce tiny hemorrhagic spots on the skin or mottled areas, and the skin appears as though the underlying blood vessels are barely covered.

Soaps, Detergents, and Creams

A great variety of soaps and detergents is available on the market today. However, there is very little difference in their quality, despite advertising claims. The expensive ones, with their color, perfume, and endorsements, have not been found to be superior to the less expensive ones as cleansing agents.

Although the skin may be cleansed in various ways, for most people, the best way is with soap or detergent and water. The choice of soap is largely a matter of personal preference. Some contain more oils or fats than others; some contain abrasive substances; still others contain detergents. Nearly all are scented.

Soaps are made from vegetable and animal fats. Most detergents are made from petroleum derivatives. Detergents are especially satisfactory when the water is hard, cold, or salty. Persons who are sensitive to soap often find that they can use detergents without difficulty. Detergent bars are available, but there is no contraindication for using the mild granulated or liquid detergents on the skin. The laundry-type detergents may cause burning and irritation of the skin. Youngsters and elderly people require special attention concerning the selection of an appropriate soap or detergent, since their skin is more subject to injury and to irritation. If the skin at any age

is very dry, creams may be used. Bath oils aid to control the symptoms of dry skin. Alcohol or any other defatting agent should be avoided on dry skin.

When the outdoor temperature and humidity (or both) are low, to prevent drying of the skin, less frequent bathing and using creams more often are recommended. Soaps and detergents should be rinsed off well after bathing. Since wool often acts as an irritant to dry skin, other types of fabric usually are preferable. Some of the chemicals used to produce wrinkle-resistant fabrics are irritating, especially to dry skin. It is recommended that clothing made of these fabrics be washed one or two times before wearing. Adding moisture to the air with a humidifier and increasing fluid intake help to relieve dry skin.

Bath oils are often used when the skin is dry, although most appears to be removed when rubbing the skin dry. These oils make bath tubs slippery, and care must be exercised when oils are used, especially for the elderly, to prevent mishaps. They may help an itchy skin, provided the itching is not due to systemic diseases. Most bath preparations contain chemicals that help to soften water, contain a fragrance, and in some, have bubble ingredients. Bubble bath preparations should be mixed well in the bath water before sitting in the tub. Urinary tract infections have been reported in children when there was direct contact with concentrated solutions.

For those who are sensitive to both soap and detergents, creams may be used. *Cold creams* consist of an oil or wax, water, and perfume. The cream feels cold because the water evaporates, producing a feeling of coolness. The oil or wax liquifies on the skin and loosens or suspends dirt, oily secretions, perspiration, bacteria, makeup, dead cells, and other foreign material on the skin surface. They are then removed with tissue or a soft cloth. The oil in cold cream is a nonvegetable oil that will not become rancid.

Cleansing creams are similar to cold creams except they contain little or no water. Cleansing lotions and foams are essentially cleansing creams prepared in fluid or foam form. A washing cream is also a cleansing cream but so prepared that it can be removed by rinsing it off with water.

Emollient creams are a type of cold cream. They are intended to remain on the skin and to prevent dryness and therefore, usually are less greasy than cold creams. If the oil base has a high melting point, it does not feel greasy and seems to disappear into the skin; hence, creams made of this type of base are often called vanishing creams. Emollient or moisturizing creams do not add moisture to the skin. Rather, the oily film they leave on the skin retards normal moisture evaporation, and the film helps to hold down the scaly skin surfaces. Cocoa butter, petroleum jelly, and lanolin are effective emollients and are used in many cosmetic emollient creams.

Soap and detergents and water are more effective than creams for cleansing the skin. Personal preference, sensitivities, and the amount of moisture in the skin will serve as guides concerning whether to use soap or a detergent and water, or creams, or both.

Deodorants and Antiperspirants

Perspiration, commonly associated with body odor, is essentially odorless. The odor occurs when bacteria, normally present on everyone's skin, act on the skin's normal secretions. When one perspires from a warm environment or from nervous tension, the body is attempting to rid itself of excess heat through evaporation.

Keeping the body and clothing clean is the prime requisite for preventing body odors. Deodorants and antiperspirants may be used *after* the skin is clean. Boric acid or zinc stearate and a fragrance usually are used in deodorants to mask or diminish body odors. Antiperspirants are intended to reduce the amount of perspiration. They contain aluminum chloride, tannic acid, or zinc sulfate.

Body odor is not often a problem with children and the elderly. Hormones that stimulate the growth of sweat glands begin during adolescence and gradually decrease with age.

Antiperspirants and deodorants should be used with care in order to prevent irritation of the skin. There are toilet soaps that, according to manufacturers' claims, kill skin bacteria and therefore eliminate body odors. However, deodorants, medicated soaps, toilet waters, and powder cannot replace the need for bathing.

Deodorants to control odor in the vaginal area have become widely marketed. They may be applied directly to the area or they may be placed on sanitary napkins. Although these deodorants do not contain aluminum salts which are irritating to mucous membrane, they are intended for external use only. They should not be used on tampons. Some have been reported as possibly harmful when sprayed into the vagina. Repeated use is not generally recommended because of reported irritation and rashes, nor should they be used on broken skin areas. No therapeutic benefits from their use have been proven to date. As was true of other deodorants, these special deodorants cannot replace cleanliness of the area.

In normal healthy women, regular daily douching is believed to be both unnecessary and unwise. The practice tends to remove normal bacterial flora, and if the solution is high in acid content, it may irritate or injure normal cells. Many women use douches for personal hygiene reasons after intercourse. The practice is satisfactory when the solution is nonirritating. There are many products on the market that can be used in douching solutions. Personal preference will guide the woman in her selection. Many gynecologists apparently feel that a normal saline or mild white vinegar solution (a tablespoon or two in one quart of water) is just as satisfactory.

The preferred method for douching is to use a bag with tubing and a douche tip or a rubber catheter. While lying in the bathtub, the catheter or tip is inserted gently (never forced), and the bag is held two or three feet above the level of the hips. Contracting the muscles around the vaginal orifice or holding the vulva to close the orifice allows the solution to collect and to distend the vagina, making a thorough cleansing more possible. The solution is allowed to escape, and filling and emptying the vagina continues until all the solution is used.

Medical assistance is recommended when a discharge or irritation and itching about the vaginal orifice persists. Frequent douching to relieve the symptoms may only tend to aggravate the cause of the problem. Before a vaginal examination, a douche is contraindicated because it will remove secretions and any discharge—specimens which are necessary for diagnostic procedures.

Cosmetics

Cosmetics frequently enhance the appearance of a clean and healthy skin, although certain cultural and religious groups would not agree with this opinion. For older people, makeup used judiciously helps to disguise blemishes, improves skin coloring, and makes wrinkles appear less obvious. Creams and lotions made by reputable concerns are safe to use, but it has not been demonstrated that their cost is commensurate with their quality. The choice is chiefly a matter of personal preference.

The skin has absorbent ability but to a limited degree. Nourishment is transported to the skin through the blood; absorption by skin tissue cells is negligible. Claims for creams that nourish and rejuvenate the skin tend to be misleading. Most contain estrogens, but the primary benefit of the creams is their emollient effect. Various exotic ingredients such as mink and turtle oil have been added to creams, but there is still a lack of scientific evidence to support manufacturers' claims for their rejuvenating effects. At present, there appears to be no way in which results of aging on the skin can be reversed.

From time to time, cosmetics containing harmful ingredients have appeared on the market. However, these occasions are rare and usually are discovered promptly. For persons sensitive to one type, the variety is large enough so that often another brand with a different type of base, dye, or perfume can be found. Makeup applicators and puffs should be kept clean.

Medicated Soaps and Cosmetics

Various antiseptics have been incorporated in soaps and cosmetics, but they have not been proven to be as beneficial as most advertisements claim. A danger is that users may develop sensitivities not only to the particular antiseptic, but also to chemically related products. Hexachlorophene was one antibacterial agent commonly used in soaps and powders. As mentioned in Chapter 19, the Food and Drug Administration has banned its use except by prescription.

Shaving Methods and Cosmetics for Men

There does not appear to be evidence that one shaving method is better than another. Individual preferences are based on factors such as type of skin, quality of beard, the frequency with which one shaves, the presence of skin problems, and convenience. Blade shaves tend to give a closer shave than electric shaves, but many men find an electric razor convenient and practical. Electric razors are especially convenient to use for the ill and bedridden patient.

Preparations used prior to shaving are intended to soften the beard for easier shaving. After-shave preparations consist primarily of alcohol, water, and perfume. They tend to make the freshly shaven face feel good and have primarily a cosmetic rather than a therapeutic effect.

An ingrown hair is one that curves back into the skin. The cause is not clearly known, although shaving with the grain of the beard and with a sharp blade and shaving more frequently but less closely help to reduce the problem for many men. Permanently removing ingrowing hairs may be required in severe and persistent cases.

It is recommended that warts that are in the way of shaving be removed to prevent injuring them and to prevent their spread.

Men are tending to use more cosmetics, deodor-

ants, and antiperspirants than previously. They should exercise the same care in their selections and use as do women for their cosmetics.

Hirsutism

Hirsutism is the excessive growth of body hair. Custom dictates what hair on the body is superfluous. In American culture, axillary hair is considered superfluous for women, but it is not so considered, for example, in some European and oriental countries. Hence, superfluous hair has more important psychological implications than physical.

Superfluous hair can be removed by tweezers, waxing, chemical depilation, shaving, or electrolysis. Waxing is usually done by a beautician. A warm wax which imbeds the hair is applied to the skin, allowed to harden, and then removed quickly, plucking the hair in the process.

The safest and the most economical way to remove unwanted hair is to use a razor. It has not been proved that repeated shaving causes excessive growth and coarseness of hair. Depilatories which either destroy hair shafts or mechanically remove hair often irritate the skin and cause infection, although many persons find them safe to use.

The only way to remove hair permanently is by electrolysis, a process by which the hair follicle is destroyed with a mild electric current. This is an expensive and tedious process and requires a careful and experienced operator.

Older people tend to have softer and finer hair. Superfluous hair on the face is common and the nurse can give advice concerning its removal if the patient finds that it is a problem.

A six percent solution of hydrogen peroxide (20 volume peroxide with 20 drops of ammonia added to one ounce of peroxide) may be used as a bleach for superfluous hair, especially on the face. The bleached hair is hardly noticeable and often solves the problem easily and inexpensively.

Excessive body hair is thought to be an inherited characteristic. Hirsutism has been observed to occur at the time of menopause; authorities do not agree on its cause. However, it is a misconception that it results from the overuse of creams. Excessive body hair is commonly associated with the use of certain drugs, corticotropin (ACTH) being one.

Acne

Acne is an eruption of the skin due to inflammation and infection of the sebaceous glands. Medically speaking, acne is not a serious condition, although it can lead to permanent scarring. It occurs most commonly during the teen years when its appearance is especially disturbing from a psychological viewpoint. Acne usually appears on the face, neck, shoulders, and back.

During adolescence, endocrine gland activity increases, and among other things, the hormones cause enlargement of the sebaceous glands and increased glandular secretions. When these secretions become dammed up in the sebaceous ducts and inflammation with infection occurs, blackheads and pustules appear.

There are various ways to control acne and minimize scarring. The infected areas should not be squeezed and picked. Because of oiliness of the skin and hair, typical during adolescence, frequent washing with soap and hot water is recommended. Cosmetics, especially oily ones, should be used sparingly. Some persons find that the sun or ultraviolet exposure helps, but caution to prevent burning is important. If certain foods, usually chocolate and nuts, appear to make the condition worse, they should be eliminated from the diet. Using dietary restrictions indiscriminately usually are of no avail.

In severe cases, the use of drugs may be indicated. There are surgical procedures that aid to eliminate scarring when this is a psychological problem.

BATHING THE PATIENT

An important purpose of the bath is to clean the skin. Some persons may require daily or even more frequent bathing while others may bathe less frequently and still be clean. The condition of the skin, the type of work, the place of work, the type of activities, and the weather conditions are all guiding factors in establishing bathing habits.

In addition to its cleansing purpose, for many patients a bath can be very refreshing when they are feeling restless and uncomfortable. Depending on the situation and the temperature of the water used for the bath, the patient may feel stimulated and ambitious following it, or he may relax to the point that sleep follows soon after. To those who enjoy a bath, the feeling of cleanliness and relaxation that accompanies it is satisfying. Hence, warm water usually is used for bathing, since the warmth tends to relax muscles. The cooling effects of the bath, even when warm water is used, result from evaporation of water from the body surface.

The cleansing bath also affects physiologic activities. Massaging the skin will affect the peripheral

nerve endings and the peripheral circulation. If firm movements are used in stroking the various areas, muscles will be stimulated, and circulation will be aided. This action on the circulation often results in increased kidney function. It is not uncommon for a patient who has been given a bath to void immediately following it.

The activity involved in bathing also can be of great value to the musculoskeletal system as a form of exercise. If the bath is taken or given with this advantage in mind, it is possible to exercise all of the major muscle groups and place almost all joints through full range of joint motion. Chapter 22 describes exercises to accomplish this. As the muscle groups contract, blood within the veins is assisted to return to the heart. The activity of the muscle groups helps to maintain muscle tone.

If, during the bathing process, there is a definite attempt to include some planned exercise, respirations also will be involved. Increasing the rate and the depth of respirations has physiologic advantages, such as increasing the oxygen intake and preventing congestion within the lung tissue.

Whether given by the nurse or taken by the patient, a bath can be so managed that it functions effectively as a conditioning activity for the body. Middle-aged and elderly patients often will say that they are too stiff to reach down and wash their legs while in bed, to get into a bathtub, to brush their hair, to button or tie a bed gown in the back. They may very well be correct, but investigation often will show that there is no pathologic basis for this limitation. Their knees are stiff, and they cannot reach in back because possibly they have not attempted to do so for a long time. Many of these patients can be helped to increased activity by nurses who can explain the values of good body mechanics.

Bathing the patient offers the nurse one of her greatest opportunities for getting to know the patient, for observing his physical and emotional status, and for identifying his needs. It offers an excellent opportunity for health teaching and at a time when the patient often demonstrates readiness for learning. The importance of *caring* in nursing was discussed in Chapter 3. Many patients have expressed the feeling that sincere interest and caring about the patient's welfare are best shown by those who give personal care. While it is possible to have numerous contacts with the patient during the course of the day, few are as prolonged as the time spent in preparation for and assistance with the bath. Therefore, the nurse will consider carefully before delegating the bath to others when the opportunity to use this time with the patient is available to her.

Some people prefer a shower to a tub bath, and vice versa. Some bathe in the morning on arising and others in the evening before retiring. Some bathe daily, others every other day, and still others once a week, or even less frequently. It may be difficult to satisfy all these habits in hospital situations, but, when practical, most patients appreciate when their home bathing habits can be observed. It is helpful to indicate changes in health agency bathing routines for a particular patient on the patient's nursing care plan.

No matter where or when the patient is to be bathed, the nurse still has the responsibility for assisting the patient as needed, seeing that he has his necessary articles and checking to see that safety and privacy measures have been considered. Protecting the patient from possible sources of injury or harm include avoiding drafts; making certain that the water is a safe, comfortable temperature; and providing means for preventing slipping in the tub or the shower. The patient should never be left out of easy calling distance of the nurse, and the doors of bathrooms should not be locked. These precautions apply to patients of all ages.

The Shower Bath

Even if the patient can manage by himself, the nurse should make certain that all is in order before permitting him to use the shower. If the patient is weak, he should be watched closely and every precaution taken to avoid an accident. Health agencies generally have guide rails on the wall both inside and outside the shower stall for safety purposes. These rails are available and relatively easy to install in home showers. It is best if there are two levels of rails in the stall; one placed low enough so that, if a patient prefers to sit on a stool while in the shower, he can assist himself to stand. Sitting in the shower is much safer for the older patient or the patient who is still weak. Also, sitting on a chair or a stool makes it easier for the patient to wash his legs with less likelihood of slipping.

The Tub Bath

For the physically limited person, the advantages of the tub bath are often defeated by the disadvantages of the tub itself. It is not a particularly easy device to get in and out of. In some instances, the addition of an attachment to the tub or a rail on the wall will make it easier to enter and leave. A bathtub hand support was illustrated in Figure 18-5 on page 176. Another arrangement that has helped many patients is the use of a chair alongside the tub. The patient sits on the chair and eases to the edge of the tub. After putting both feet into the tub, it is then easier for him to reach the opposite side of the tub and ease down into the tub. Occasionally, it is easier if the patient has a towel or a mat in the tub and then, instead of easing down directly, to kneel first and then to sit down. In some instances, it is best

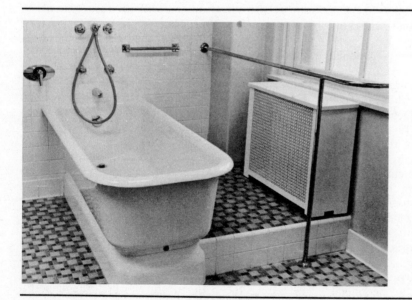

Fig. 21-2. An example of a bathtub that is used in continuing care units. It is situated so that the patient may step up on one side and get into it easily, yet it is on floor level on the other side so that the nurse can stand at a level convenient to her if she must assist the patient. (Courtesy Muhlenberg Hospital, Plainfield, N. J.)

for the bath water to be run after the patient is seated and then drained before the patient attempts to get out of the tub. A hydraulic lift which can be installed in home bath tubs can be used to assist. The person sits on a seat, swings over the tub, and then lowers himself into the tub. The reverse is done for getting out of the tub. A tub installation that makes it easier for a patient to get into a tub and still provides for the nurse assisting the patient is illustrated in Figure 21-2.

The Bath Taken in Bed

Some patients must remain in bed as a part of their regimen, even if they are permitted to care for themselves, feed themselves, read, and possibly do some prescribed exercises. If they have not had a bed bath previously, they may need some suggestions on how to proceed to bathe themselves.

In addition to providing the patient with all of the necessary articles for oral hygiene and for washing, the nurse prepares the unit so that it is more convenient for the patient. This includes removing the top bed linen and replacing it with a bath blanket so that the patient does not get the bedding wet. The necessary articles should be placed conveniently, usually on the bedside or overbed table. Clean clothing should be placed within easy reach. Makeup items for the woman patient should be left where she can obtain them after she has finished her bath. Male patients may wish to shave either before or after they have bathed. This may require providing clean hot water.

Patients in bed will have varying degrees of physical ability to bathe themselves. Some patients will be able to wash only the upper parts of their bodies. The rest of the bath is then completed by nursing personnel. Other patients will be able to wash all but their backs. Some patients are able and are encouraged, as a part of their bed exercises, to wash their backs as well. Washing every area of the body while in bed requires considerable manipulation and exercise. This activity in itself is a good conditioner for someone who is not up and about. With good teaching the nurse can help the patient to understand its values.

The Bath Given in Bed

For patients who are restricted in their activity and for those who are unable to move, the bath is refreshing and physiologically stimulating. For the very ill and inactive patient, bathing with modifications of water temperature and types of strokes used can bring considerable relief from discomfort.

Before starting the bath, it is best to offer the patient the bedpan.

The following description of a bath assumes that the patient is able to be raised or lowered in bed and that, while there is limitation of movement, it is possible for the nurse to manage the patient alone. It also assumes that only routine hygienic care is needed. Bathing procedures vary. The following suggested actions are given as guides.

SUGGESTED PROCEDURE FOR BATHING A PATIENT IN BED

Obtain all articles needed for hygiene and bed making. For the patient's psychological comfort, provide for privacy.

Arrange the articles in order of use for convenience in working.

Remove the top bedding and fold linen to be replaced on the bed so it is ready when needed without being rearranged. Place bath blanket over patient to avoid exposure and to provide warmth.

Assist the patient to the side of the bed for convenience and ease in working.

Elevate the head of the bed slightly while oral hygiene is being done, to avoid having the patient aspirate liquids.

Lower the head of the bed and remove either all pillows or all but one. Assist the patient to raise the head and the shoulders in order to remove the pillows.

Arrange washcloth in a fashion to prevent corners from dragging over the patient's skin. Use firm but gentle strokes.

Wash the patient's face, ears, and neck. When washing the eyes, wipe from the inner canthus outward and use a separate portion of the washcloth for each eye.

Wash and dry the patient's arms. Wash and dry the patient's chest. Then wash and dry the abdomen, including the area of the thighs near the groin.

Drape the bath blanket around the upper thigh to prevent exposure of the patient while washing the leg.

Lift the patient's leg at the bony prominence at the ankle and the heel and then support the leg on your arm until you can place it carefully into the basin of water. Wash each leg separately.

Change the water.

Roll the patient to the side-lying position and bring him close to the edge of the bed.

Place the towel along the back and turn the bath blanket back to expose the patient's back. Wash the back of the neck, the shoulders, the back, the buttocks, and the posterior upper thighs. Use firm, long strokes.

Rub the patient's back with alcohol and then powder or rub with lotion if he prefers or if his skin is dry.

Roll the patient back to the back-lying position.

Wash the genital area. If the patient is able to do this, provide water, soap, and towel within easy reach and leave the unit. Remove equipment which can be cleaned while the patient is busy.

Comb the patient's hair after the bed is made. The old pillow case or towel can be used to protect the bed from combings.

Back Rub

Following the bath, most hospital procedures suggest giving the patient a back rub, either with alcohol or with an emollient preparation. The values are similar to those discussed in relation to a bath. A back rub relaxes the patient, stimulates muscles and peripheral circulation, and acts as a general body conditioner. Agencies differ concerning back rub practices. One of the study situations at the end of this chapter describes one in which the reader will be interested.

Making an Occupied Bed

It is usual procedure to plan to change linens at the time that the bed bath is given, since the top bedding will be already off. The occupied bed is made by rolling the patient over to the far side of the bed and tucking the soiled bottom linens and the rubber or plastic draw sheet toward the center of the bed and well under the patient. The clean linens are then placed so that one half of the bottom of the bed can be made. The patient can then be rolled over onto the freshly made part of the bed. The soiled linens are removed, and the clean linens are pulled through tightly. A smoother bed will be possible if the pull on the clean linen is done directly behind the patient's back. The weight of the patient will then hold the linen in place. The bottom of the bed is then completed. The patient is usually turned back toward the center of the bed, and the top of the bed is made. The use of contour bottom sheets has greatly reduced the amount of time needed to tighten sheets.

There are variations in the procedure for making the occupied bed. However, these small differences have no real effect on the patient's comfort. In some instances, it is necessary for nurses to devise unique ways to change the linens on a patient's bed because of the nature of the patient's condition, orthopedic appliances on the bed, or treatments that may be in progress.

CARE OF THE HAIR

The hair is one of the accessory structures of the skin. As illustrated in Figure 21-1 each hair consists of the shaft, which projects through the dermis beyond the surface of the skin, and the hair follicle, which lies in the dermis. Hair grows in the follicle and receives its nourishment from the blood which circulates through each follicle.

Hair has many cultural overtones and its care and styling are often influenced by one's values. Styles change within a culture. Note, for example, the change from a short-cut style for men to a longer hair style in this country. Black people have favored the "Afro" or "natural" style. Women tend to change hair styles and color more often than men in this country.

Good general health is essential for attractive hair, and like the skin, cleanliness aids in keeping it attractive. Illness affects the hair, especially when endocrine abnormalities, increased body temperature, poor nutrition, or anxiety and worry are present.

The hair is exposed to the same dirt and oil as the skin. It should be washed as often as necessary to keep it clean. For most persons, a weekly shampoo is sufficient, but more often or less frequent shampooing may be indicated for others. Daily brushing of the hair aids in keeping it clean and in distributing oil along the shaft of each hair. Brushing also stimulates the circulation of blood in the scalp.

A comb used for arranging the hair does not replace brushing. Personal preference dictates the selection of a comb, but sharp and irregular teeth which may scratch the scalp should be avoided. A large-tooth comb is recommended for very curly hair, as for example, the hair of a black person. The comb and the brush should be washed each time the hair is washed and as frequently as necessary between shampoos.

If the hair is dry, oils may be used. Pure castor oil, olive oil, or mineral oil are satisfactory, but perfumed preparations may be used with safety if sensitivity of the skin is no problem. The hair of black people tends to be dry, and hence, the use of oil is usually necessary. If the hair is oily, more frequent washing is indicated.

The care of short hair rarely presents problems. However, time and attention to an important part of grooming may be necessary when the hair is long. During the acute phase of illness, the patient may ask to have the hair left undisturbed. To do so, especially if the hair is long, may prove to be disastrous. Hair which becomes entangled is difficult to undo. Hours of careful combing of tiny sections of hair may be necessary if a patient's hair is not combed for even one day. The best way to protect long hair from matting and tangling is to ask the patient for permission to braid it (some patients may not wish to have their hair arranged in braids). Patients usually will consent to such a procedure if it provides them with more comfort during a time when they are unable to manage the arranging of their own hair. Parting the hair in the middle on the back of the head and making two braids, one on either side, prevents the discomfort of lying on one heavy braid on the back of the head. Braiding the hair of a black person is usually the best way to prevent matting and tangling of long hair.

Occasionally, a patient's hair is almost hopelessly matted, and cutting the hair may be necessary. Before a patient's hair is cut, it is usual procedure to have the patient sign a written consent. It is also considered good policy for the nurse to discuss the necessity for cutting the hair with an immediate member of the patient's family.

Nurses should be aware of the fact that most patients have a hair style that is most satisfying to them. If it is necessary to comb and arrange a patient's hair, the nurse should ask the patient how it is to be arranged. Doing so in the fashion the patient considers best is often a big boost to morale.

Hair Loss

Normally, a certain number of hairs are lost and some start growing each day. Some permanent thinning of hair normally accompanies aging. Hair loss from plaiting, excessive back combing and "teasing," or the use of hair rollers is usually temporary, and hair returns when the tension on the hair shaft is halted. Some people experience hair loss due to illness with high fever, certain medications, x-ray therapy of the head, childbirth, and general anesthesia. There appears to be no evidence that hair loss occurs as a result of wearing wigs or excessive shampooing. It is believed by some that an excessive intake of Vitamin A may play a role in hair loss.

Baldness is called *alopecia*. It is rare in women and common in men. There is no known cure for baldness despite the promises of many advertisements. Alopecia is believed to be hereditary and no

amount of external treatment is likely to help. Hairpieces, frequently worn by persons who are bald, require the same care as normal hair, but less frequent washing is necessary since they are not lubricated with oil from the sebaceous glands.

A relatively recent surgical procedure for baldness is the hair transplant. Hair is taken from donor sites, usually from the back or sides of the scalp, and transplanted to areas with no hair. It is a long and expensive procedure but reportedly has decided benefits for persons who find baldness especially disturbing.

Dandruff

Dandruff is a condition characterized by itching and flaking of the scalp. Nearly everyone experiences dandruff at some time. Persistent severe cases usually require medical attention. Although microorganisms play a role in infections often associated with severe dandruff, they apparently are not the cause of it. Proprietary products have not been found to be effective for "curing" dandruff although some help to suppress it temporarily. Daily brushing and shampooing as necessary in most cases will aid in keeping the scalp free of dandruff.

Shampoos and Rinses

A large variety of shampoo products are marketed, many of which are advertised to care for special hair problems. Personal preference guides purchasing, but shampoos that dry the hair excessively or irritate the scalp should be avoided. Certain shampoos on the market, recommended for dry hair, are designed to remove all substances except the natural oils. However, if the hair is dry and unmanageable after washing, a few drops of oil rubbed into the hair produces satisfactory results. Detergents are more effective than soap when used with hard water. Liquid and cream shampoos rinse from the hair with greater ease than does bar soap.

Various rinses may be used following a shampoo, such as antistatic creme rinses, protein rinses, beer rinses, and lemon juice or vinegar rinses. In each case, a film remains on the hair shaft that helps to give the hair body and a glossy appearance. Rinses tend to make freshly shampooed hair more manageable; however, there is no scientific evidence to indicate that they penetrate the hair shaft.

A variety of waterless or dry shampoos are available. They usually consist of an alkali and an absorbent powder. Dry shampoos cannot replace a regular shampoo in terms of cleaning, but they are helpful in removing at least some of the dirt, oils, and odors from the hair. They have been especially helpful for patients too ill or incapacitated to have a water shampoo.

Permanent Waves

Home permanent waves have become very popular with women who have learned how to use them, and they often mean additional comfort for patients confined for long periods of time. In some situations, as in a chronic illness unit, the nurse may be asked to assist a patient with a home permanent wave. If the nurse feels that she has the necessary competence, the procedure could result in considerable satisfaction for the patient.

Pediculosis

Infestation with lice is called *pediculosis*. There are three common types of lice: *Pediculus humanus*, var. *capitis*, which infests hair and scalp; *Pediculus humanus*, var. *corporis*, which infests the body; and *Phthirus pubis*, which infests the shorter hairs on the body, usually the pubic and the axillary hair. Lice lay eggs, called *nits*, on the hair shafts. Nits are white or light gray and look like dandruff, but they cannot be brushed or shaken off the hair. Frequent scratching and scratch marks on the body and the scalp suggest the presence of pediculosis. Although anyone may become infested with lice, the continued presence of pediculosis is usually a result of uncleanliness.

Pediculosis can be spread directly by contact with infested areas or indirectly through clothing, bed linen, brushes, and combs. The linen and the personal care items of patients with pediculosis require separate and careful handling to prevent spreading from person to person.

There are any number of preparations, called *pediculicides*, for the treatment of pediculosis, some of which will destroy the nits as well as the lice. Several treatments are usually necessary before all the nits are destroyed. The procedures and the medications used for the treatment of pediculosis vary from hospital to hospital and with the personal preference of the physician. Shaving off the infested hair is frequently done, especially when pubic and axillary hair are infested. Although shaving is a relatively simple way of handling pediculosis, shaving the scalp is rarely done.

Giving a Shampoo

Many health agencies have beauticians and barbers to assist with the care of the patient's hair, including shampooing it. However, this convenience does not relieve the nurse of her responsibility to see to it that the patient's hair is cared for properly.

If a beautician is not available, shampooing a patient's hair may become a nursing responsibility. If the patient is ambulatory, there is no real problem. If the patient is confined to bed but is able to be moved onto a stretcher, he can be transported to a convenient sink for a shampoo. The hair is washed and rinsed over the sink while the patient remains lying on the stretcher. This is illustrated in Figure 21-3.

For patients who must remain in bed for a shampoo, the patient's head and shoulders are moved to the edge of the bed. A protective device is placed under the head. This may be a Kelly pad or an improvised trough made from a large rubber sheet which has been built up on both sides by rolling a towel into each side. To prevent the bed from getting wet and to insure a thorough cleansing and rinsing of the hair, it is necessary that the patient and the trough or pad be so placed that the water constantly drains. Newer devices for shampooing hair in bed are now available. They have a rigid frame which reduces the likelihood of the water flowing into the bed. Procedures for shampooing a patient's hair in bed depend on the equipment and the facilities available in the agency or the home. Following a shampoo, the patient's hair is dried as quickly as possible to prevent him from becoming chilled.

ORAL HYGIENE

The mouth is the first part of the alimentary canal and an adjunct of the respiratory system. The ducts of the salivary glands open into the vestibule of the mouth. The teeth and the tongue are accessory organs in the mouth and play an important role in beginning digestion by breaking up food particles and mixing them with saliva. The mucous membrane which lines the mouth is not as sturdy as skin; therefore, care is needed while cleaning the mouth to prevent injury.

General good health is as essential as cleanliness for maintaining a healthy mouth and teeth. The relationship, for example, between good teeth and a diet sufficient in calcium and phosphorus along with Vitamin D, which is necessary for the body to utilize these minerals, is well-established.

Dental disease is considered epidemic in the United States. The American Dental Association has estimated that there are about a billion untreated cavities, with the average American having five. Here

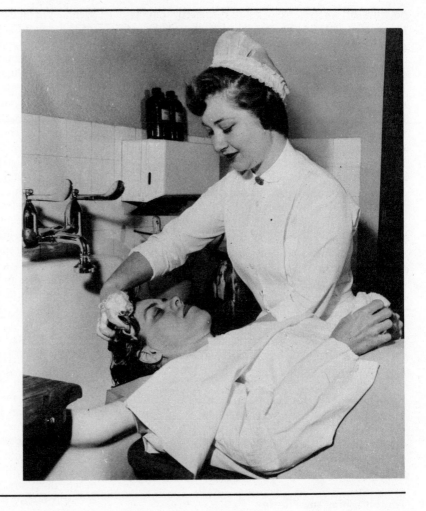

Fig. 21-3. A convenient way for the patient to have her hair shampooed is to place her on the stretcher and move her to a sink or a hopper. The patient's neck is resting on the edge of the hopper, which has a bath towel covered with a small plastic sheet on it. This makes it more comfortable for the patient and also provides for the shampoo and the water to run off easily. A much more thorough washing and rinsing can be done this way, and the entire procedure is easier for both the patient and the nurse.

are additional interesting statistics compiled in mid-1972 and reported in the *Wall Street Journal* (July 28, 1972.):

• By middle age, about half of the population has some form of periodontal disease.

• About 25 million Americans have lost their teeth and about another 25 million have lost about half of their teeth.

• Approximately half of the children two years old have gum disease or tooth decay.

• About 95 percent of school age youngsters have multiple tooth decay.

These are shocking statistics when dental scientists believe that a huge number of these problems could have been prevented. But as many dentists have said, people do little about their teeth until a condition becomes intolerable and many people simply learn to live with dental problems without apparent concern.

The benefits of good oral hygiene and dental care are numerous. There is aesthetic value in having a clean and healthy mouth. Having one's own teeth contributes to an intact body image. When the mouth and teeth are in good condition, gustatory pleasure and the beginning of the digestive process are enhanced.

The decay of the teeth with the formation of cavities is called *caries*. A rather well-defined chain of events appears to foster dental caries. An accumulation of mucin, carbohydrates, and bacteria normally found in the mouth form a coating on the teeth that is called *plaque*. The bacteria act on the carbohydrate to form lactic acid. The plaque prevents acid dilution and neutralization and prevents colonies of bacteria from being dispersed. The acid eventually destroys the enamel of the teeth through decalcification, and caries result.

To prevent decay, the chain must be broken somewhere. Cutting down on carbohydrate intake helps. Sweets are the worst offenders. It is impractical to remove sweets from the diet, but dentists highly recommend that sweet snacks between meals, such as soft drinks, candy, gum, jams, and jellies, be eliminated as much as possible. The mouth cannot be cleansed of its bacteria, but dispersing the bacteria with careful cleansing is helpful. This can best be done by brushing and flossing the teeth.

The major cause of tooth loss in adults over approximately 35 years of age is gum disease. *Gingivitis* is an inflammation of the gums; a common cause is Vincent's angina or trench mouth. *Periodontitis* is a more marked inflammation of the gums and involves the alveolar tissues also; it is commonly called *pyorrhea*. Symptoms include bleeding gums, swollen tissues, receding gum lines with the formation of pockets between the teeth and gums, and loose teeth. If unchecked, tooth tissue and bone tissue are lost. Regular dental care and good oral hygiene are the best preventive measures for periodontal disease.

The old saying, "an ounce of prevention is worth a pound of cure," can be applied very aptly to the care of the teeth. Most dentists recommend a dental examination every six months and preferably every three months, but frequent dental examinations are not a substitute for good oral hygiene.

Toothbrushing and Flossing

The brush should be small enough to reach all teeth. The bristles should be sufficiently firm to cleanse but not so firm that they are likely to injure tooth enamel and gum tissue. Many dentists recommend a soft-textured, multitufted toothbrush with a flat brushing surface. Others recommend brushes with widely spaced tufts. When the tufts are widely spaced, the brush is somewhat easier to keep clean and dry.

There is a difference of opinion concerning the best way to brush one's teeth. Many dentists are recommending that the brush be placed at a 45° angle at the junction between the teeth and the gums with the tufts facing in the direction of the gums. This method is illustrated in Figure 21-4. Other dentists recommend that the brush be placed at the same angle but with the tufts facing in a direction away from the gum line. When assisting and teaching patients, the nurse will wish to follow the preference of the patient's dentist.

Food clearance time helps to determine frequency of brushing. It takes about 15 minutes for decay-producing foods and liquids to be cleared from the teeth after their ingestion. Sticky foods such as candy will adhere longer. It is during this time, directly after eating, that most damage is done by bacteria. Therefore, it is ideal practice to brush one's teeth immediately after eating and drinking. When this is not practical, at least a thorough rinsing of the mouth is helpful and better than nothing. Most children eat frequently between meals, and it is particularly important for them to be taught to brush their teeth and rinse their mouth often. The tongue also should be cleansed with the brush. Many persons are unaware of the need for frequent cleansing and the nurse often finds herself in an excellent position to teach patients and members of their families of its importance.

Automatic toothbrushes (electric or battery-operated) have been found to be simple to use and as good as hand brushes in removing debris and plaque. Water spray units are available to assist with oral hygiene. The unit, attached to a faucet, sprays water under pressure upon areas to which it is directed. If an undue amount of water pressure is used, damage to gum tissue may occur. It is helpful as an aid to brushing because it flushes material from around braces and dental bridges.

Many bacteria in the mouth become lodged between the teeth. The toothbrush cannot effectively reach these areas and hence, flossing several times a day is highly recommended. The practice not only removes what the brush cannot but helps to break up colonies of bacteria. Figure 21-5 illustrates a recommended way to floss teeth.

SUGGESTIONS FOR FLOSSING *

1. The fingers controlling the floss should not be more than ½-inch apart.

2. Do not force the floss between the teeth. Insert it gently by sawing it back and forth at the point where the teeth contact each other. Let it slide gently into place.

3. With **both** fingers move the floss up and down six times on the side of one tooth, and then repeat on the side of the other tooth until the surfaces are "squeaky" clean.

From Effective Oral Hygiene. Developed by USAF School of Aerospace Medicine, Brooks Air Force Base, Texas. Published by The Academy of Periodontology, Chicago.

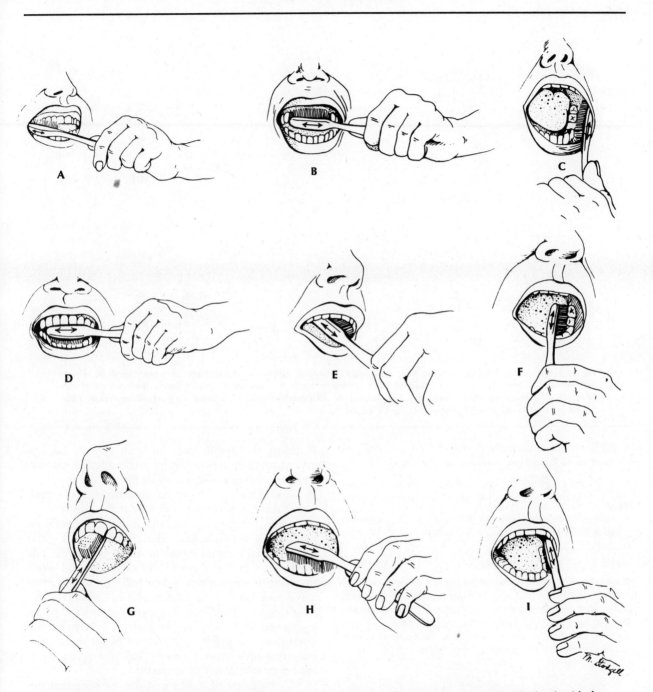

Fig. 21-4. For the outside surfaces of all teeth and the inside surfaces of the back teeth, position the brush with the bristles at the junction between the teeth and gums, as in A; note the exact position of the brush. Then move the brush back and forth with short strokes several times as in Figs. B through F. Study each figure carefully. For the inside surfaces of the upper and lower front teeth, hold the brush vertically, as in Figs. G and H, and make several gentle back and forth strokes over the gum tissue and teeth. To clean the biting surfaces brush back and forth as in Fig. I. (From Effective Oral Hygiene. Developed by USAF School of Aerospace Medicine, Brooks Air Force Base, Texas. Published by The Academy of Periodontology, Chicago.)

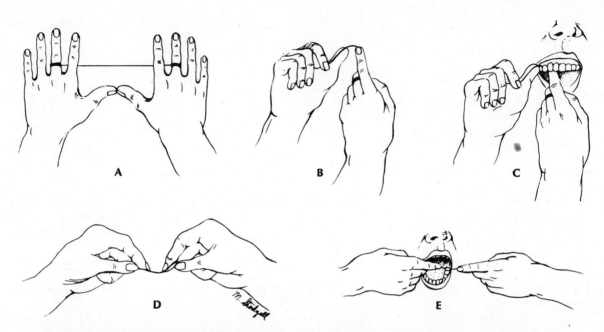

Fig. 21-5. Flossing technique, A. Wrap floss on middle fingers. B. Thumb to the outside for upper teeth. C. Flossing between upper back teeth. D. Holding floss for lower teeth. E. Flossing between lower back teeth. (From Effective Oral Hygiene. Developed by USAF School of Aerospace Medicine, Brooks Air Force Base, Texas. Published by The Academy of Periodontology, Chicago.)

4. Go to the gum tissue with the floss, but not into the gum so as to cause discomfort, soreness, or bleeding.

5. When the floss becomes frayed or soiled, a turn from one middle finger to the other brings up a fresh section.

6. At first flossing may be awkward and slow, but continued practice will increase skill and effectiveness.

Rinsing

Rinse vigorously with water after flossing to remove food particles and plaque that you have cut loose. Also rinse with water after eating when you are unable to floss or brush. Rinsing alone will not remove the bacterial plaque. Water spraying devices alone will not remove the bacterial plaque because of the fatlike material in the plaque.

Toothpastes and powders aid the brushing process, usually have a pleasant taste, and often encourage brushing, especially among children. Most dentrifices are safe to use, but those containing harsh abrasives may scratch the enamel of the teeth and therefore are not recommended. Salt, sodium bicarbonate, or precipitated chalk are just as effective for cleansing the mouth and the teeth and are far less expensive than proprietary products on the market. Dentifrices containing stannous fluoride have proven to be effective in aiding to decrease dental caries, and, hence, are recommended by many dentists.

"Bad breath" or halitosis is often systemic in nature. For example, the odor of onions and garlic on the breath comes from the lungs where the oils are being removed from the bloodstream and eliminated with respiration. When halitosis results from a systemic cause, oral treatment can only mask the odor temporarily at best. Mouthwashes may be pleasant to use, and some persons prefer a mildly flavored mouthwash to a salt or a sodium bicarbonate solution, but they cannot remove halitosis when odors are being eliminated by respiration.

If the cause of halitosis is due to poor oral hygiene, cleansing will reduce the odor. Certain mouthwashes claim antiseptic value which supposedly decreases the bacteria in the mouth. However, such claims are not well-founded; mouthwashes have little more, if any, value than plain water. If they are used in a concentrated form, they may injure oral tissue, and infection and additional odor may result.

Oral hygiene is equally important for persons with dentures. The removable type are removed and cleansed with a brush. There are brushes designed for dentures which are helpful in cleaning in small areas. There also are preparations in which to soak dentures to aid in removing hardened particles. Some dentists recommend that removable dentures remain in place except while they are being cleaned. If the patient has been instructed to remove his dentures while sleeping, a disposable denture cup is convenient and easy to use. From an aesthetic standpoint, dentures should not be placed in cups, glasses or other dishes that are used for eating purposes. Keeping the dentures out for long periods of time permits the gum lines to change, thus affecting the fit of the dentures.

Water Fluoridation

The addition of fluoride compounds to drinking water that is fluoride-deficient, for the prevention of dental caries, has been under study for approximately 25 years. In general, studies have indicated that fluoridation has aided in reducing dental caries and that it is a safe public health measure. Still, in certain areas public opposition has been sufficient to prevent its use.

Some dentists apply a fluoride compound directly to the teeth at regular intervals. Studies indicate that this procedure has reduced tooth decay among children by as much as 40 percent.

Giving Oral Hygiene

While the care of the mouth described earlier is still applicable during illness, there are numerous occasions when it must be modified to meet changes in the mouth. These changes usually are an alteration in the amount of secretion in the mouth and the formation of a coating on the tongue. If the patient is able to assist with his own mouth care, it may very well be a matter of providing him with the materials necessary to cleanse his mouth more frequently. If the patient is helpless, the nurse will help make certain that special attention is given to the patient's mouth as often as necessary to keep it clean and moist. It is not unusual to provide special mouth care as often as every hour, especially for patients who are unable to take fluids or are not permitted fluids by mouth. For those patients who are permitted foods, the mouth should be cleansed before meals so that the patient may enjoy them.

Medicated mouthwashes may be used for special mouth care, especially if the patient likes the taste of an aromatic solution. However, it will be re-

called that plain or salted water will help equally well to loosen mucus particles and to cleanse the mouth mechanically. If the mucus is very tenacious, a solution of half water and half hydrogen peroxide is effective for cleansing.

It may be necessary for the nurse to use some means for opening the patient's mouth for cleansing if the patient is unconscious. A tongue blade usually works satisfactorily. Several methods are possible for cleansing the mucous membrane of the mouth after it is opened, but each has certain limitations. If gauze is wrapped about a tongue blade and secured with adhesive so that it does not come off, the resulting applicator is usually too large to clean all surfaces of the mouth well. If small gauze squares are held with a clamp, it is easier to reach all surfaces, but there is danger of damaging the membrane with the clamp. Large cotton applicators, prepared so that the cotton will not come off the stick, seem to be effective. The cotton is less irritating than gauze, and the size can be varied easily, depending on the situation. The patient's toothbrush may be used, but care must be exercised not to injure the mucous membrane. If the brush is stiff and hard, running hot water over it softens the bristles and there is less tendency to injure gum tissues.

Whenever placing an object such as a toothbrush or an applicator into a patient's mouth, a mouth gag should be used to hold it open if the patient tends to close his mouth. One should not use the fingers to hold a patient's mouth open. The mouth constantly harbors organisms, and a human bite is a potentially dangerous wound.

When introducing fluid into the mouth of an unresponsive patient, keep the head in such a position that even a small amount will not be aspirated by the patient. When dipping the applicator into the solution to be used for cleaning the mouth, make certain that it is moist but not so wet that solution will pool in the mouth.

After cleaning the surfaces of the mouth, clean the teeth, using the patient's toothbrush, and then clean the tongue, using gauze held on a clamp or wrapped over a tongue blade or the patient's toothbrush. The tongue is not as subject to injury as the mucous membrane of the mouth. After the entire mouth has been cleansed, moisten the mucous membrane with water. An emollient may be applied to the lips to help prevent cracking. The skin on the lips is very thin, and evaporation of moisture from them takes place rapidly, especially when the patient has a fever.

If the patient is able to take fluids by mouth, an

excellent aid to oral hygiene and comfort is frequent moistening of lips and mouth with water.

If the patient has removable dentures, they should be cleansed as often as hygiene indicates. If they are kept clean, the patient is more likely to keep them in the mouth. However, if permitted to get coated with mucus, they will annoy the patient, and he will wish to have them removed. Extreme care should be taken when managing a patient's artificial dentures. They represent a considerable financial investment, and damage or loss is not only expensive but embarrassing for the patient.

When artificial dentures are cleansed, they should be held over a basin of water so that should they slip from the person's grasp, they will not drop onto a hard surface. Warm water is used since hot water may warp the plastic material from which most dentures are made. When the patient's teeth are not in the mouth, they should be stored in a suitable container and in a safe place.

To care for the mouth of the acutely ill patient is a well-recognized responsibility of the nurse. While a variety of solutions and moisturizers have been used to cleanse and moisten oral tissue, studies suggest that the procedure appears to be more important than the agent that is used. This finding supports the personal experience of many well persons, that is, that no mouthwash, breath freshener, ointment, or paste replaces a thorough mechanical cleansing of the oral cavity.

CARE OF THE NAILS

Like the hair, the nails are an accessory structure of the skin. They are composed of epithelial tissue. The body of the nail is the exposed portion; the root lies in the skin in the nail groove where the nail grows and is nourished.

The fingernails may be trimmed by filing or cutting in an oval fashion. Trimming the nails too far down on the sides is contraindicated because of possible injury to the cuticle and the skin around the nail. Great care must be exercised if a nail scissors is used to prevent injuring tissue surrounding the nail. Hangnails are broken pieces of cuticle; they should be removed by cutting. Hangnails can be prevented by pushing the cuticle back gently with a blunt instrument or with a towel after washing the hands when the cuticle is soft and pliable. Using emollients help to prevent hangnails. Cleansing under the nails is accomplished best by using a blunt instrument, being careful to prevent injuring the

area where the nail is attached to the underlying tissue.

Splitting and peeling of the nails is usually due to dryness. To decrease the condition, it is helpful to avoid contact with soap and water as much as possible, use a good hand cream frequently and avoid the use of nail polish and polish remover, both of which have a tendency to dry the nails.

There are preparations on the market that are advertised as helping to reduce splitting and peeling of nails. Most of them contain formaldehyde, a chemical that easily irritates skin tissue. These preparations should be used while carefully following the manufacturer's instructions.

CARE OF THE FEET

Proper foot care is important at any age; however, with aging and especially when illness is present, it becomes even more so. Also, in her teaching role, the nurse will wish to assist patients to appreciate the importance of foot care.

Proper care starts with cleanliness. This includes bathing the feet, rinsing off the soap or detergent thoroughly, and drying the feet well, being careful to include the interdigital areas. It is best to place the feet in a basin of water when caring for a bedridden patient during the bath procedure. If the feet tend to perspire freely, frequent bathing and using food powders with deodorant ingredients are helpful. These powders are more absorbent than are regular after-bath powders and often contain menthol which makes the skin feel cool.

The nails are trimmed, but in a manner that avoids digging into or cutting away nail at the lateral corners of the nail and toe. Patients with ingrown nails, especially older people and patients with circulatory disorders or diabetes, may require the services of a physician or podiatrist.

For older patients whose nails can be expected to be brittle and striated, it is recommended that the feet be soaked first to soften the nails for easier trimming. The feet may be placed in a basin of water. Or, they may be wrapped in damp cloths and placed in plastic bags if this procedure is more convenient than soaking in water. Adding an alkali such as Epsom salt or soda bicarbonate to the water helps soften dry scaly skin.

Improperly fitting shoes are a major cause of foot problems and can lead to corns, calluses, bunions, and blisters. The back of the shoe, or the counter, should fit snugly but not tightly. A heel offering safe support is recommended. There should be about three-quarters of an inch of space in the shoe beyond the great toe when standing and the widest part of the shoe. In a good fitting shoe, the arch of the foot will lie comfortably over the arch in the shoes. The soles should be flexible and nonslippery. Shoes with rough ridges, wrinkles, or tears in the linings should be discarded or repaired.

Improperly fitting, worn, or soiled hosiery contribute to foot problems. For some persons with allergies or skin infections, nylon hosiery are contraindicated.

For most people, especially the elderly, going barefoot is not recommended. The practice is likely to result in injuries to the skin. Going barefoot in public rest rooms is especially dangerous because of the likelihood of contracting *athlete's foot,* a common fungus infection that is easily transmitted in showers and tubs.

The nurse will wish to be alert to any symptoms of foot problems. These include infections, inflammations, ingrown nails, breaks in the skin in the interdigital area, fissures or cracks, corns, calluses, bunions, and pressure areas that may result in decubiti.

CARE OF THE EYES

The eyes very frequently reflect the state of health. The nurse will observe that, during illness, the eyes may water more freely and appear glasslike. As health returns, the eyes regain their normal appearance. Secretions from the eyes may adhere to the lashes, dry, and become crusty, or there may be slight discharge from the mucous membrane. If discharge is present, it may accumulate in the corners of the eyes, especially during sleep. Water or physiologic saline should be used to wipe the eyes clean. Wipe from the inner canthus (corner near nose) to the outer canthus. This is to minimize the possibility of forcing the discharge into the area drained by the nasolacrimal duct. Use a clean portion of the patient's washcloth each time the eye is wiped. Soft, disposable tissues may also be used, especially if there is any question about the cleanliness of the washcloth.

Eye Glasses

Most problems with glasses result from losing or misplacing them. Glasses are essential for many persons and represent a considerable financial investment. Hence, the nurse should take precautions to prevent breakage and loss. She should also encourage

patients needing glasses to wear them in order to avoid eyestrain.

In 1972, President Nixon issued a proclamation which read in part ". . . It is never too early, but often may be too late, to take action to preserve our vision . . . Preventive efforts, of course, are the key —we should take all possible steps to prevent eye injuries at home, in the school, at play, or on the job. And regular professional eye examinations for all members of the family are an important part of any effort to preserve sight."

In recognition of the need for safety, the Food and Drug Administration now requires that all eyeglass lenses and sunglass lenses be impact-resistant. Lenses are most often made impact-resistant by heat treatment, chemical treatment, or by making the lenses thicker. Plastic lenses are more impact-resistant than glass on a comparable basis.

Plastic lenses have become popular because they are considerably lighter in weight than glass lenses. A refraction or correction for eye faults is as accurate when using plastic as when using glass. The one decided disadvantage of using plastic is that the material scratches very easily. The nurse will wish to be aware of this when handling and cleaning a patient's glasses.

Contact Lenses

A contact lens is a small disc worn directly on the eyeball. The so-called hard lenses are made of a nonpliable and nonabsorbent plastic material. Soft lenses are of a plastic material that absorbs water to become soft and pliable.

Contact lenses offer several advantages over glasses. Some eye defects such as a misshapen cornea sometimes cannot be corrected as well with ordinary lenses. Contacts cannot be seen when worn which for many people, especially entertainers, is important for cosmetic reasons. Many athletes have found them safer to use than eyeglasses when participating in contact sports events.

It is recommended that persons contemplating the use of contacts consult a physician and study their care and use under the supervision of one who specializes in the fitting and dispensing of contact lenses. Persons wearing contact lenses need to take special precautions to keep them free of microorganisms that may lead to eye infections and to use them in a manner that will not injure or scratch the surface of the eye. They are to be removed before sleeping or swimming and when in the presence of irritating vapors and smoke. The lenses should not be in contact with cosmetics, soaps, and hair sprays

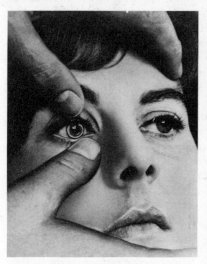

Directly over the cornea: This normal wearing position of a corneal contact lens is also the correct position for removing it. If the lens cannot be removed, however, slide it onto the sclera.

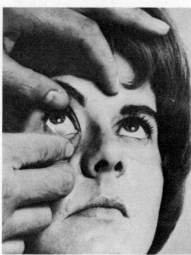

On the sclera only: Here the lens can remain with relative safety until experienced help is available; other white areas of the eye to the side or above the cornea might also be used. If the lens is to be removed, however, slide it to a position directly over the cornea.

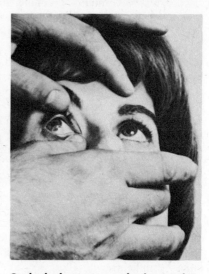

On both the cornea and sclera: A lens in this position—or a similar one anywhere around the periphery of the cornea—should be moved as soon as possible. If the lens is to be removed, slide it to a position directly over the cornea; if the lens cannot be removed immediately, slide it onto the sclera.

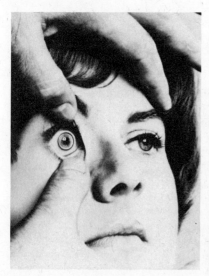

After the eyelids have been separated and the corneal contact lens has been correctly positioned over the cornea, you widen the eyelid margins beyond the top and bottom edges of lens (as shown).

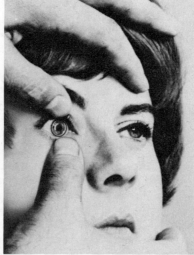

After the lower eyelid margin has been moved near the bottom lens edge and then the upper eyelid margin has been moved near the top lens edge, you are ready (as shown) to move under the bottom edge of the lens by pressing slightly harder on the lower eyelid while moving it upward.

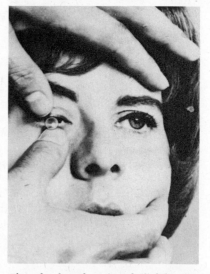

After the lens has tipped slightly, you move the eyelids toward one another and thereby cause the lens to slide out between the eyelids (as shown).

Fig. 21-6. How to remove contact lenses. (From Contact Lens Emergency Care Information & Instruction Packet. Published by American Optometric Association Committee on Contact Lenses.)

since eye irritation may result. It is recommended that any adverse reaction to their use be reported to the prescribing physician immediately.

The nurse should determine whether or not her patient is wearing contact lenses. There may be times when she may be required to remove them if a patient cannot do so. To leave them in place for long periods of time could result in permanent eye damage. This may occur, for example, when the nurse is attending a patient who is unconscious following an accident or sudden illness. Figure 21-6 illustrates and describes how to remove contact lenses when the person is unable to do so himself.

Artificial Eyes

Most patients who wear an artificial eye will prefer to take care of it themselves, and they should be encouraged to do so when possible. However, the nurse should provide the necessary equipment, which usually includes a small basin and solution for rinsing the prosthesis. Normal saline or tap water can be used. Most persons have their own method for cleansing the eye and the area around it. The nurse should ask the patient how he does this and make it possible for him to continue with his usual practice.

If the patient needs assistance, an artificial eye may be removed by putting pressure below the eye until the suction is broken, and then the eye will slip out easily. Another method is to place suction on the artificial eye itself and remove it. A simple method is to use the rubber bulb of an eye dropper. The bulb is compressed to expel the air and placed near the center of the eye. When pressure on the bulb is released, the bulb will cling to the eye and it then can be removed by gentle lifting. The artificial eye is cleansed with normal saline. Care should be taken to avoid scratching an artificial eye. The eye is replaced by pulling down on the lower lid and slipping it in position.

CARE OF THE EARS AND NOSE

Cleaning the Ears

Other than cleaning the outer ears, little more is needed for routine hygiene of the ear. After the ears are washed, they should be dried carefully with a soft towel so that water and wax are removed by capillary action. Forcing the towel into the ear for drying may aid in the formation of wax plugs.

If a wax plug is present in the auditory canal, it is removed by gentle syringing of the ear. Using items such as bobby pins or a hairpin to remove wax is extremely dangerous since the eardrum may be punctured.

Cleansing the Nose

The best way to cleanse the nose is to blow it gently. Irrigations are usually contraindicated because of the possible danger of forcing material into the sinuses. Small objects should be kept away from the nose to prevent aspiration and to prevent injuring the mucous membrane of the nose.

If the external nares are crusted, applying mineral oil aids in softening and removing the crusts. Disposable paper tissues are recommended for nasal secretions.

PERINEAL CARE

An important part of personal hygiene is perineal care. The patient unable to cleanse the perineal area will need the nurse's assistance. To neglect this important part of care may result in physical and psychological discomfort for the patient, a breakdown in the skin, and offensive odors. For patients with indwelling catheters, organisms from the area may reach the bladder, a possibility that increases when microorganisms are numerous in an unclean perineal area.

When practical, the patient is placed on a bedpan. The perineal area is flushed with a warm, mild soap or detergent and water solution. Rinsing well with plain water follows. When flushing is insufficient for cleansing, scrubbing becomes necessary. Using cotton balls or other disposable material for scrubbing is psychologically preferable to using a washcloth. The area is then dried and emollients or powder are used on the skin areas as indicated. If it is not possible to place the patient on a bedpan, the patient is placed on a towel or pad, and the area is cleansed and then wiped free of soap or detergent solution with disposable material.

In the female, the labia are separated carefully and the exposed areas then cleaned. In the uncircumcised male, the foreskin or prepuce is retracted, and the exposed glans penis and prepuce are carefully cleansed. It is important to pull the prepuce back into place over the glans penis to prevent constriction of the penis which may result in serious edema and tissue injury. The penis and scrotum are washed, including the posterior and lateral aspects. The crotch area is cleansed.

The stroke used while cleansing the perineal

area should be long and sufficiently firm to avoid discomfort to the patient. The areas of cleansing should begin at the pubic area and end with the anal area in order to avoid the possibility of carrying organisms from the anal area back over the genitals.

The bidet has long been used for perineal hygiene, especially in Europe and South America. A stream of water is directed over the perineal and anal area as one sits on the bidet. The water leaves the bidet with a flushing-type action or, in the case of the portable bidets, by draining into a toilet or tub. Persons using them report satisfactory results although they are not intended to replace the bath or shower.

THE DECUBITUS ULCER

A *decubitus ulcer* is an area where skin tissue has been destroyed and there is a progressive destruction of the underlying tissue. The terms decubitus ulcer (or simply decubitus), *pressure sore*, and *bedsore* are used interchangeably. The plural of decubitus is *decubiti*.

Causes of Decubitus Ulcers

The earliest forerunner of a decubitus is blanching of the skin. This is followed by reddened, irritated, and tender skin. The skin eventually breaks and a decubitus has formed. The nurse should be especially alert to early signs. She should pay particular attention to those patients most likely to develop pressure areas and to those parts of the body where they are most likely to develop.

Decubiti result from interference with circulation and nutrition in the area. There are several factors that can result in poor circulation and nutrition. Usually, not one factor but a combination of factors is responsible for the development of a decubitus ulcer.

A patient who is debilitated by illness and in a poor nutritional state is less likely to have the same protection from the skin that he has when in good health. Older patients whose skins are wrinkled because of loss of subcutaneous fat are more prone to develop decubiti than the young. The skin forms folds and becomes irritated quickly. Some patients who have lost considerable weight also may have loose, flabby skin with very little turgor. Thin people are more prone than others to develop pressure sores; also they occur more often in men than women. If fever is present or if the function of the cells is altered, destruction of tissues may be relatively easy.

Preventive Measures

Skin that is dry and without its usual amount of resistance is irritated easily by feces, urine, and drainage from wounds. Keeping the patient clean and free from irritation is of extreme importance in the prevention of decubiti. Dressings may need to be changed more frequently and arranged to keep drainage from irritated areas. Patients who are unable to control urinary or bowel excretions require special consideration. As a precautionary measure, an indwelling catheter may be inserted into the patient's urinary bladder if the patient is in constant danger of urinating and seems to be a likely candidate for a decubitus ulcer.

The skin always has microorganisms on it. While the skin manages well with its own flora, the presence of organisms from infected wounds or from feces is potentially dangerous if the skin is irritated. If the skin is moist and warm, and the area dark, conditions become ideal for the growth of transient bacteria. Infection of the skin may occur, and, once the area is broken, the problem of healing it complicates the patient's plan of care and his illness. Patients who are in danger of developing decubiti should be washed locally following each bowel evacuation.

Patients who must lie for long periods of time on sheets over rubber or protective materials perspire, and evaporation of the moisture is prevented. The constant presence of the moisture along with continuous pressure predisposes to decubitus formation. Good results have been reported from placing patients especially prone to bedsores on a piece of sheepskin. The wool is cropped. The air spaces in the wool allow air circulation and help keep the patient's skin dry. The wool also eases pressure on the area and helps to distribute weight. However, testing has indicated that sheepskin probably cannot be rendered sterile by machine washing. This would make it unsafe for use by more than one patient. Synthetic sheepskins can be used and then discarded after use or when soiled.

In addition to keeping the skin surfaces clean and dry, light rubbing of the areas which receive a great deal of pressure is helpful. These areas are the heels, the elbows, the coccyx, the scapulae, and the back of the head. The iliac crests are also danger areas if the patient is very thin and must be on the abdomen much of the time. These areas should be examined frequently and massaged with a lotion. The lotion reduces friction to make massaging easier and more comfortable. The massaging stimulates circulation to the area. Lanolin is frequently recommended for dry skin areas.

One of the best protective measures is to prevent pressure against any one area of the body. Pressure constricts vessels and hence impedes blood supply. This can be done by frequently alternating the patient's position. The position in bed that is most likely to cause the greatest amount of pressure to the largest number of areas is the back-lying position. Congestion of blood reduces the activity of the cells, since oxygen and other nutrients are not brought in and waste products are not removed adequately. If this local state is maintained for hours at a time, death of tissue cells occurs, and a decubitus has been produced. To keep patients from having pressure exerted against any one area for long periods of time, nurses frequently provide for the patient to turn or be turned at frequent intervals. The details for such a plan should then be indicated in the patient's plan of care.

Decubiti are apt to develop on the ankles and heels of some patients. Good results have been reported from the use of polystyrene foam blocks to protect these areas from pressure. The blocks, one for each ankle, are cut in half, hollowed to fit the ankle, padded (preferably with sheepskin), and gripped together around the patient's ankles. The device keeps the foot above the mattress level, thus preventing pressure and irritation. Hyperextension of the knees can be eliminated by placing a pillow under them.

While mattresses should be firm to help maintain good alignment of the body, their firmness also may be cause for concern. The alternating pressure mattress pad has been designed to help reduce this constant pressure. The principle on which it operates is that sections of the pad distend with air or fluid while other sections remain flat. Then those that remained flat distend, and the other sections deflate. In this way, no one area of the body is receiving constant pressure. These pads are placed over the regular bed mattress. Caution is necessary with such a pad because puncture by sharp instruments and pins can cause a leak of the fluid or the air.

The alternating pressure pad is not disturbing to the patient. The fact that it does produce occasional tickling sensations which cause muscular contractions is considered to be beneficial. For the most part, however, patients become adjusted to them and do not seem to realize that they are on the pad.

The use of the water bed has caught the consumer's attention in recent years, and many are now used in hotels, motels, and homes. They had been in use for years for patients with decubiti or for those most prone to develop them but on a limited basis.

In recent years, the materials and designs have made them cheaper, lighter in weight by using less water than once was the case, and easier to handle and maintain. As a result, they are becoming more commonplace in health agencies, especially those where there are many patients likely to develop or have decubiti. Their effectiveness in the treatment and prevention of decubiti is based on the following physics principle. *An increase in pressure on an enclosed liquid will be distributed uniformly and undiminished to all parts of the liquid.* Hence, a water-filled mattress distributes pressure evenly over the body surface in contact with it. This results in better delivery of oxygen to those areas of the body where ordinarily, pressure from a firm mattress is sufficient to decrease blood supply. To avoid chilliness when lying on the water mattress, extra bed covering may be necessary. A study situation at the end of this chapter refers the reader to water-filled pads that can be made at home for protecting parts of the body from pressure.

There are sources of irritation to the skin which could predispose to the formation of a decubitus for which the nurse must be alert. They include wrinkled bedclothes which cause pressure, crumbs and other objects in the bed, top linen so applied that it restricts freedom of movement, and pressure and irritation from casts, adhesive, tubing, arm boards, and the like.

A decubitus, while often called a bedsore, is not confined necessarily to those persons who are in bed. Some patients who are able to be out of bed but remain in a chair for a good portion of the day are also likely to develop decubiti if not cared for properly. Old as well as young patients are vulnerable.

The great variety of methods that have been used to treat decubiti suggests that no one way has been found to be entirely effective. A study situation at the end of this chapter describes several methods that reportedly have been helpful in caring for decubiti. Unquestionably, the best treatment is to prevent their formation.

CONCLUSION

Personal hygiene habits differ rather substantially. As the nurse remains loyal to the principle that each individual is a unique being, she will demonstrate respect for those patients with personal hygiene habits that may differ from her own.

If one follows advertising in our communications media, it would seem that we are all either very clean for using the many personal care products available to us, or very dirty for needing so many different products. Certainly, personal cleanliness is an important aspect of health and grooming. It is also an important part of nursing care as nurses assist patients to meet personal hygiene needs. But in addition to meeting personal care needs, the nurse plays an important role as a health teacher in helping to differentiate fads and fallacies from facts while still being supportive of a wide variety of perfectly acceptable personal hygiene habits.

Study Situations

1. As this chapter points out, no single best way has been found to treat a decubitus ulcer. Here are various methods reported in the literature as helpful.
   a. The following reference indicates that patients with decubitus ulcers reacted well to topical hyperbaric oxygen treatments; between treatments with oxygen, the lesions were covered with dressings soaked in a solution of normal saline and glacial acetic acid.
   Torelli, M.: Topical hyperbaric oxygen for decubitus ulcers. **Am. J. Nurs.,** 73:494–496, Mar., 1973.
   b. Decubiti washed with hydrogen peroxide, rinsed with normal saline, dusted with a powder containing an antibiotic, and coated with a collagenolytic agent, showed marked improvement according to the following article:
   Barrett, D., Jr., and Klibanski, A.: Collagenase debridement. **Am. J. Nurs.,** 73:849–851, May, 1973.
   c. Good results were reported with this treatment: After thoroughly cleansing a decubitus, including debridement if it was necessary, the ulcer was packed daily with white granulated sugar and protected with heavy, airtight dressings. The theory on which this care was based is that the irritating effects of the sugar granules caused local injury that initiated wound repair, and the acidity of the sugar solution tended to increase blood supply by vasodilation in the area.
   Sugar sweetens the lot of patients with bedsores. **JAMA,** 233:122, Jan. 8, 1973.
   d. Honey was reported as effective treatment for decubiti in the following reference:
   Blomfield, R.: Honey for decubitus ulcers. **JAMA,** 224:905, May 7, 1973.
   e. The following article describes a device used to float or levitate a patient with decubitus ulcers on air streams in order to relieve pressure and promote healing of tissue:
   Harvin, J. S., and Hargest, T. S.: The air-fluidized bed: a new concept in the treatment of decubitus ulcers. *In* **The Nursing Clinics of North America.**

Philadelphia, W. B. Saunders, 5:181–187, Mar., 1970.
   f. In the following summary of an article dealing with bedsores in the chronically ill, systemic care that included optimal nutrition and vitamin supplements, was recommended:
   Bedsores and tissue vitality. Medical highlights. **Am. J. Nurs.,** 73:334, Feb., 1973.
   g. The following article tells how cushions that can be made from easy-to-obtain materials, were used effectively to help in preventing decubiti:
   Blass, M. A.: Improvised cushions. Ideas that work. **Am. J. Nurs.,** 70:2605, Dec., 1970.
2. In the following article, the author likens a back rub to a conductor of messages:
   Temple, K. D.: The back rub. **Am. J. Nurs.,** 67:2102–2103, Oct., 1967.
   How does the author describe a back rub as being helpful in developing good interpersonal relationships with patients? Describe briefly the four back rub techniques illustrated in the article.
3. In the following article, what reasons did the author offer concerning why a student nurse felt she could not comb the hair of a black patient?
   Giles, S. F.: Hair: the nursing process and the black patient. **Nurs. Forum,** 11:78–88, No. 1, 1972.
   Recall the first principle concerning man's uniqueness as discussed in Chapter 3. Does the author feel this principle was being observed in the child's care she described? Now recall the four subsystems of the nursing process system as they were described in Chapters 6 through 9. In what parts of the nursing process system had the nurse failed when she neglected the patient's grooming?
4. In the Nurse's Notebook section in **Nursing '72,** 2:35, June, 1972, read the description of the towel bath. Describe situations when you believe "Gus's Bath" would be especially indicated? Do you see any disadvantages in using the towel bath?
5. The following booklet is available from the Superintendent of Documents, U. S. Government Printing Office, Washington, D. C. 20402:
   Feet first: a booklet about foot care. 45 p. U. S. Department of Health, Education, and Welfare, Public Health Service, 1970.
   The booklet is intended primarily for older people and people who have diabetes. However, the nurse will find it to be an aid in teaching anyone about foot care.
   After reading the booklet, see if you can write instructional objectives, stated in behavioral terms, and a content outline, similar to the objectives and content shown in Study Situation 1 of Chapter 16, on page 155. If the booklet is not available to you, select any topic discussed in this chapter and write objectives and content for a patient teaching situation. Here is a start on objectives and content for teaching. Objective: Patient will demonstrate bathing his feet in a satisfactory manner without assistance.

Content: Supplies—Warm water (not hot)
     Basin or tub
     Mild soap
  Technique—Wash between toes using
     friction
     Wash all of feet
     Rinse thoroughly
     Dry completely, especially
     between toes

References

1. Allen, L., ed.: The Look You Like. Chicago, American Medical Association, 1971.

2. Brownlowe, M. A., et al.: New washable woolskins. **Am. J. Nurs.,** 70:2368–2370, Nov., 1970.

3. Burnside, I. M.: Accoutrements of aging. *In* **The Nursing Clinics of North America.** Philadelphia, W. B. Saunders, 7:291–301, June, 1972.

4. Contact lenses: care for the injured. *In* **The Nursing Clinics of North America.** Philadelphia, W. B. Saunders, 5: 369–370, June, 1970.

5. Davis, E. D.: Give a bath? **Am. J. Nurs.,** 70:2366–2367, Nov., 1970.

6. Drimmelen, J. V., and Rollins, H. F.: Evaluation of a commonly used oral hygiene agent. **Nurs. Res.,** 18:327–332, July–Aug., 1969.

7. Feminine hygiene sprays may cause irritation. **Am. J. Nurs.,** 70:2638, Dec., 1970.

8. Flores, A. M., and Zohman, L. R.: Energy cost of bedmaking to the cardiac patient and the nurse. **Am. J. Nurs.,** 70:1264–1267, June, 1970.

9. Foot bath boot. **Am. J. Nurs.,** 72:337, Feb., 1972.

10. Gibbs, G. E.: Perineal care of the incapacitated patient. **Am. J. Nurs.,** 69:124–125, Jan., 1969.

11. Gordon, R. H.: Meeting dental needs of the aged. **Am. J. Public Health,** 62:385–388, Mar., 1972.

12. Gosnell, D. J.: An assessment tool to identify pressure sores. **Nurs. Res.,** 22:55–59, Jan.–Feb., 1973.

13. Harvin, J. S., and Hargest, T. S.: The air-fluidized bed: a new concept in the treatment of decubitus ulcers. *In* **The Nursing Clinics of North America.** Philadelphia, W. B. Saunders, 5:181–187, Mar., 1970.

14. Horn, W. E., and Horn, Y.: Building sound teeth for life. **Parents' Magazine and Better Family Living,** 47:56–57; 117; 118; 128, Nov., 1972.

15. McGregor, R. R.: Geriatric foot care. *In* **The Nursing Clinics of North America.** Philadelphia, W. B. Saunders. 3:687–695, Dec., 1968.

16. Martin, E. J., and Smith, J. E. D., Diabetic Foot Care: Knowledge and Practice. pp. 143–149. ANA Clinical Conferences. New York, Appleton-Century-Crofts, 1970.

17. Passos, J. Y., and Brand, L. M.: Effects of agents used for oral hygiene. **Nurs. Res.,** 15:196–202, summer, 1966.

18. Redman, B. K., and Redman, R. S.: Oral care of the critically ill patient. *In* Bergersen, B. S. et al., eds.: Current Concepts in Clinical Nursing. pp. 107–118. St. Louis, C. V. Mosby, 1967.

19. Reitz, M., and Pope, W.: Mouth care. **Am. J. Nurs.,** 73:1728–1730, Oct., 1973.

20. Robertson, C. E.: Gel pillow helps prevent pressure sores. **The Canadian Nurse,** 67:44–46, Oct., 1971.

21. Storz, R. R.: The role of a professional nurse in a health maintenance program. *In* **The Nursing Clinics of North America.** Philadelphia, W. B. Saunders, 7:207–223, June, 1972.

22. Toothpaste. **Consumer Reports,** 37:251–255, Apr., 1972.

23. Williams, A.: A study of factors contributing to skin breakdown. **Nurs. Res.,** 21:238–243, May–June, 1972.

CHAPTER 22

Providing for Exercise and Activity

GLOSSARY · INTRODUCTION · PRINCIPLES OF BODY MECHANICS ·
HELPING THE PATIENT TO MAINTAIN OR ATTAIN AN AMBULATORY STATUS ·
PROVIDING PROTECTIVE MEASURES FOR THE PATIENT CONFINED TO BED ·
LEISURE-TIME ACTIVITIES FOR THE PATIENT ·
CONCLUSION · STUDY SITUATIONS · REFERENCES

GLOSSARY

Active Exercise: Joint movement activated by the person.

Atony: Absence of muscle tone.

Atrophy: Decrease in size of muscle.

Body Mechanics: Efficient use of the body as a machine and as a means for locomotion.

Contracture: Permanent contraction state of a muscle.

Dropfoot: Complication resulting from extended plantar flexion.

Fowler's Position: Semisitting position.

Hernia: Protrusion of contents through a weakness in the muscular wall.

Hypotonia: Decrease in muscle tone.

Passive Exercise: Manual or mechanical means of moving the joints.

Prone. Lying position with face downward.

Resistive Exercise: Active exercise using an external resistive force.

Supine: Back-lying position.

Tonus: Partial steady state of muscle contraction.

INTRODUCTION

Research has demonstrated that an inactive body suffers both physically and psychologically. Therefore, exercise and activity, including leisure time activity, are of concern to the nurse who has physical and psychological well-being as her goal when offering care to her patients. This chapter will focus on exercise and activity as important considerations in high-quality nursing care.

The concept of rehabilitation becomes important when providing exercise and activity for patients. In the past it has usually referred to the restoration of health or function to a handicapped person. This is still true, but the dimension of prevention has been added to the concept. The purpose of rehabilitation is to prevent loss of function as well as to restore as many functions as possible. Both physical and psychological functions are included.

Because the process of rehabilitation is so broad, many specially prepared persons are usually involved, and many special facilities are utilized: phy-

sicians with advanced preparation in physical as well as psychic functioning; physical, occupational, speech, and recreational therapists; mental health workers of many kinds; and vocational workers and employers join nurses in promoting rehabilitation. Teamwork among these persons is important to promote reinforcement of efforts and goal achievement. Facilities such as special units or hospitals; social, educational, and recreational agencies; employment services; residential treatment centers; day care centers; and halfway houses are among the many agencies designed to promote rehabilitation.

There are extensive variations in patients' needs and their potential for rehabilitation. Nurses play important roles in both prevention and restoration of function loss in health agencies and in the homes. They very often work with family members almost as much as with the patient to provide necessary teaching, assistance, and support.

Since a major goal of rehabilitation is prevention of disability, this chapter focuses heavily on preventive measures. There is some discussion of function restoration, but that aspect can be found in greater detail in more advanced texts. Because physical rehabilitation of the patient often involves much physical exertion for the nurse or family members providing the care, measures to protect those responsible for the patient are discussed also.

PRINCIPLES OF BODY MECHANICS

No one would question the relationship of rest to health or of good nutrition to health. Also, there is a direct relationship of body mechanics to the effective functioning of the body. *Body mechanics* has been described as the efficient use of the body as a machine and as a means for locomotion. Good health depends not only on how expertly we choose our foods, but also on how carefully and efficiently we utilize our body parts in relation to internal and external forces. For example, a truck driver may eat adequately nutritious meals; but if he does not understand how to use his body properly to lift a heavy object onto his truck, he may injure himself. Or the homemaker may be well aware of the essentials of proper menu planning, and she may have many modern conveniences to assist her. But improper use of her body in activities performed throughout a good part of her day, such as reaching, bending, stooping, or standing, may tire her.

The importance of understanding body mechanics is universal for everyone, regardless of health-illness status. The basic principles of body mechanics should be in evidence in every activity and even during periods of rest. Because correct use of the body is another phase of prevention of illness and the promotion of health, the nurse has a major teaching responsibility, both directly and indirectly, by example.

To remember to use the correct muscle groups for the correct activity is indeed a chore when one already has developed a life pattern of using muscle groups in another way. However, as with all habits, it takes time to learn a new pattern, especially when the process involves breaking down an established one. In the final analysis, good body mechanics will pay dividends in good health and appearance and body function, which in turn produces happiness and comfort for the person using them. Good body mechanics is not accomplished by following a set procedure; it is achieved through knowledge which guides actions in every activity performed and is a fundamental concept of nursing.

To be able to evaluate the patient's musculo-skeletal needs and to teach by example, the nurse must understand and utilize the principles of body mechanics. Every activity in which she engages will require understanding and use of these principles, from as simple a thing as moving a chair closer to the patient's bedside to lifting a patient out of bed.

Terms and Concepts of Body Mechanics

All that is involved in body mechanics is sometimes referred to as basic *orthopedic principles in nursing care*. Orthopedics means the correction or the prevention of deformities. Since body mechanics is concerned with prevention of injury to or limitation of the musculoskeletal system, these terms could understandably be interchangeable.

Nurses have long recognized that body orthopedic principles are applicable to all areas of nursing and not just to the patient who has a bone fracture or some other skeletal pathologic change. For example, the patient who is on complete bed rest is in danger of losing muscle tonus. Should the bed rest be prolonged there is the danger also of developing contractures if he does not have exercise and joint motion and if provision is not made for maintaining good posture. Functioning of various internal body processes is also influenced by position and movement or their absence.

Tonus, a normal quality of healthy muscle, is a partial, but steady state of contraction present except during sleep. Muscles usually contract by shortening their fibers, but in some types of muscle contraction the length of the muscle fibers remains the same while the tension within the muscle increases.

A *contracture* is a permanent contraction state of a muscle. It usually results from prolonged contraction and is observed in flexor muscles rather than in extensors because generally flexors are stronger. Flexor muscles when they contract decrease the angle of a joint formed by two adjacent bones. Extensors increase the angle. Knee and elbow contractures are common complications when bedridden patients have not had proper preventive exercises.

While the plight of the patient in bed might be easy to comprehend, everyone who is up and about faces problems as well. A person who is hyperactive may very well exhaust himself and become fatigued. Or, on occasions when patients are depressed or for one reason or another become quite inactive, they may have diminished muscle tonus because of inactivity. This is due to the fact that the use of muscles is essential for maintaining muscle tone. Inactivity leads to *hypotonia* or *atony*, decrease or absence of tone, respectively. Continued inactivity also leads to *atrophy*, a decrease in size (and a loss of normal function) in a muscle.

The woman who is going to have a baby, if taught how to adapt to her weight changes, is able to continue her routine activities more easily. If she understands how to use her muscles effectively during pregnancy, she also helps prepare herself for an easier labor and delivery.

The nurse who understands how to help maintain musculoskeletal functioning is able to care for patients in such a way that their recovery may be speeded, their limitation from inactivity reduced to a minimum, and their convalescence shortened.

A first step in understanding body mechanics is to consider posture.

Good posture or good body alignment is that alignment of body parts which permits optimum musculoskeletal balance and operation and promotes good physiologic functioning. Good posture is essential in all positions: standing, sitting, or lying down. M. C. Winters describes the body as being in good functional alignment when:

...the feet are at a right angle to the lower legs and face forward in the same direction as the patellae; the weight-bearing line passes through the center of the knee and in front of the ankle joints; the knees are extended but are not tense or hyperextended; the thighs are extended on the pelvis; the spine is elongated, and the physiologic curves are within normal limits; the chest is upward and forward and the head is erect (35). Figure 22-1 illustrates.

Posture in itself is a key point in body mechanics and should not be considered as merely the simple procedure of holding onself erect. Good standing posture involves maintaining balance, which constitutes an effort even though we are not consciously aware of it. To balance the body and maintain good alignment in the standing position, and to engage in various activities such as lifting, stooping, pushing, and pulling, require more effort on the part of the body than sitting or lying. This everyone knows from experience, but probably few persons stop to analyze the reasons. There are forces which are present constantly and must be overcome. There are laws of physics which, if utilized properly, will help to reduce the effort expended in maintaining good posture and balance, and in lifting and moving.

Concepts most helpful to the understanding of body mechanics are those concerned with the effect of gravity on balance—balance of all objects, not alone that of humans. Figure 22-2 illustrates these.

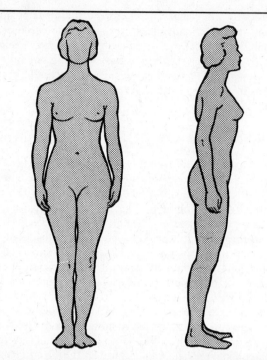

Fig. 22-1. (Left) Anterior view of the body in good alignment. (Right) Lateral view of the body in good alignment.

The *center of gravity* of an object is defined as the point at which its mass is centered. In humans, when standing, the center of gravity is located in the center of the pelvis approximately midway between the umbilicus and the symphysis pubis.

The *line of gravity* is a vertical line which passes through the center of gravity.

To understand further what is involved in the struggle to maintain balance and good posture, it is also necessary to know that there is an accelerating tendency of all bodies toward the center of the earth, referred to as gravity (equal to the earth's attraction minus the centrifugal force arising from the rotation of the earth on its axis; equal to about 32.16 feet per second). This constant pull toward the earth's center is a phenomenon which nurses should understand, since it is a factor in innumerable nursing activities, such as gravity suction, the flow of fluids, drainage of body areas, and the stability of objects.

From the diagrams in Figure 22-2, several basic points can be made—namely, that an object is more stable if its center of gravity is close to its base of support; if the line of gravity goes through the base of support; if it has a wide base of support.

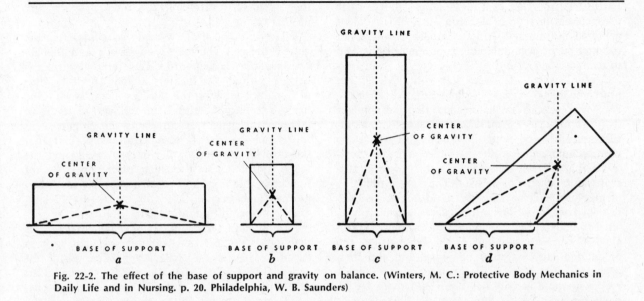

Fig. 22-2. The effect of the base of support and gravity on balance. (Winters, M. C.: Protective Body Mechanics in Daily Life and in Nursing. p. 20. Philadelphia, W. B. Saunders)

While these three points are important facts to be considered with every inanimate object, they are equally important to humans. To demonstrate that these three points have a direct relationship to stability, try standing with the feet close together and then begin to lean forward. As soon as the line of gravity is out of the base of support, you will place one foot forward in order to avoid falling. When standing, a person provides a base of support wide enough so that the line of gravity goes through the base, and he thereby stabilizes himself.

But the act of standing is not merely one of providing a base of support. Synergistic muscle groups contract sufficiently to steady the joints, such as those formed by the head of the femur in the acetabulum of the hip and the knee joint formed by the lower end of the femur and the upper end of the tibia. Usually, muscles work in groups, and synergistic action is smooth coordinated action.

An additional point developed from the three basic ones mentioned is that the stability of an object is also dependent on the height of the center of gravity and the size of the base of support. The wider the base of support and the lower the center of gravity, the greater is the stability of the object. For example, a can of evaporated milk requires little manipulation in order to stabilize it on a table; however, a candle, perhaps, could be made to balance itself, but in order to insure its remaining erect it is necessary to provide a base of support for it.

In humans, as was mentioned, muscular effort is necessary to maintain the erect position. Therefore, the amount of effort required by the muscles is related directly to the height of the center of gravity and the size of the base of support. Again, as an example, the ballet dancer while on her toes is utilizing more effort to maintain herself erect than when she has her feet directly on the floor.

The Need for Body Activity

The values of exercise and good posture have long been recognized. From past experience, we know that sitting in a chair in a class for a period of an hour or more with the shoulders and the head brought forward may cause fatigue and altered breathing. If, in addition, the muscles of the legs have not contracted during that period of time, there may be a certain amount of swelling of the feet. This is because skeletal muscles serve many functions in addition to movement, heat production, and maintenance of posture. When the muscles contract they squeeze veins. This squeezing action helps to move the blood back to the heart. Together with breathing which changes the pressure within the closed chest cavity and the tiny valves located along the inner surface of the veins, venous circulation is maintained even against the pull of gravity. If inactivity eliminates most of this squeezing action and if poor posture prevents normal breathing, then venous circulation is slowed down.

Fatigue will develop as a result of too much waste material accumulating and too little nourishment going to the muscles. Muscle fatigue usually is attributed to the accumulation of too much lactic acid in the muscles.

We have already seen that work load of the heart and blood vessels is influenced by body activity. Many persons are not readily aware of some of its other influences on the body. Because the movement of gases and fluids in the lungs is related to position and activity, the acid-base balance determined partially by the blood's carbon dioxide content, can be altered by activity. The ease or difficulty of ingestion and movement of food in the gastrointestinal tract, as well as intestinal evacuation, are related to body movement. Activity also influences calcium moving into and out of the bone tissue, the production and excretion of urine, and the metabolic activities of cells. If the reader has observed a person whose activity has been limited for an extended period, he is also aware of the influence movement has on the self-concept and psychological functioning. Body activity, then, has a widespread effect on the total well-being of an individual.

Posture while both standing and lying, as well as exercise and maintenance of balance, are only initial phases of body mechanics. While there is concern if the body is not kept in good alignment and active, there is equal concern when the body is put to use. When motion of the body is extended to include activities such as moving and lifting, there are additional aids which should be considered, since efficient use of the muscles will conserve energy and reduce the possibility of strain.

How to Use Muscles Effectively

One of the primary factors in efficient musculoskeletal activity is that the longest and the strongest appropriate muscles should be used to provide the energy needed. When muscles which cannot provide the best strength and support are forced into exertion, strain, injury, and fatigue frequently result.

Origin is the name given to the less movable attachment of a skeletal muscle to a bone. *Insertion* is the name given to the more movable attachment of the muscle to the bone, in other words, the attachment to the bone that is being moved.

In addition to using the longest and the strongest muscles of the arms and legs properly, the muscles in the pelvic area also must be prepared for any vigorous activity. This preparation of the muscles to stabilize the pelvis, to support the abdomen, and to protect the body from strain comprises two activities—namely, putting on the internal girdle and making a long midriff.

The internal girdle is made by contracting the gluteal muscles (buttocks) downward and the abdominal muscles upward. The internal girdle is helped further by making a long midriff. This is done by stretching the muscles in the waist. One has the feeling of standing up tall, and of trying to increase the length of the waistline. Figure 22-3 shows this posture. It is especially important that the muscles involved in the internal girdle and the long midriff assist the long strong muscles of the arms and the legs in activities such as lifting, moving, and carrying heavy objects. Figure 22-4 indicates proper lifting movement.

Another factor in musculoskeletal physiology is that persistent exertion without adequate rest is harmful. Muscles must have alternate periods of rest and work. Therefore, activities should be conducted accordingly, especially if the task is a strenuous one.

Using the combination of the longest and the strongest muscles of the arms and the legs, the in-

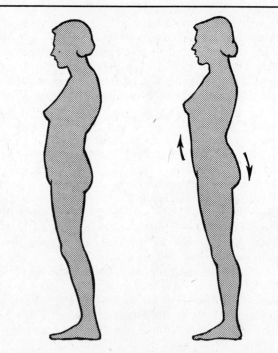

Fig. 22.3. (Left) Slouch position, showing abdominal muscles relaxed and body out of good alignment. (Right) Internal girdle "on." Abdominal muscles contracted, giving feeling of upward pull and gluteal muscles contracted, giving a downward pull.

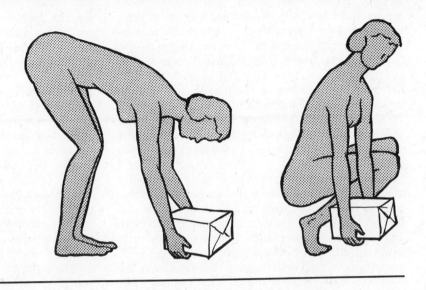

Fig. 22-4. (Left) Poor position for lifting (pull exerted on back). (Right) Good position for lifting (use of long and strong muscles of arms and legs).

ternal girdle and the long midriff in lifting or moving heavy objects is as much a protective measure as it is an efficient use of muscles. Both the back and the abdominal wall are susceptible to injury. It will be recalled that the spinal column is composed of a series of irregularly shaped bones called the vertebrae. These are separated from each other by cushions of cartilage (disks) and held together by strong bands of connective tissue called ligaments. Viewed from the side, the vertebral column looks somewhat like a double S. It has a concave curve at the neck (cervical), and a convex one at the chest (thoracic), another concave curve (lumbar), and then a convex one at the end of the spinal column (sacral). Muscles are attached to the vertebrae and permit flexion and extension as well as a certain amount of lateral movement in certain areas.

When severe strain is placed on the muscles attached to the vertebrae and the force is transmitted to any one of the curves in the spinal column, injury can result. Many low-back (lumbar) injuries are caused by such strain as lifting heavy objects incorrectly. The so-called whiplash injury occurring in the cervical area is a frequent result of an automobile accident in which the car is hit from the rear and the person's head is thrown backward suddenly and forcefully. Even in the course of everyday activities, strain and fatigue can be felt in the thoracic or the cervical regions if we sit with the head flexed forward for periods of time when reading or writing. If our backs were absolutely straight many of these in-

juries would not occur, but then neither could we enjoy the degree of mobility that we have.

While the back is susceptible to injury because of its general structure and muscle groups, the abdominal wall also can be injured by improper use of muscle groups. Weakened musculature of the abdominal wall from decreased tone or from cutting muscle fibers as in surgery can contribute to making the back more susceptible to injury. Because the organs in the abdomen are not protected by any anterior or lateral bony cage, they rely on strong and supportive abdominal muscles. If they are not protected, the organs can cause a protrusion of the abdominal wall which in turn can result in an exaggeration of the lumbar curve (sometimes called swayback). Exaggerated back curves are sufficiently serious that they can cause some individuals to be excluded from occupations where lifting is required. They may also be prevented from engaging in some sports or other activities.

The abdominal wall has its own points of inherent weakness. These are areas subject to hernias (ruptures, in lay terminology). A *hernia* is the protrusion of an abdominal structure through an area of weakness in the musculature. (Technically, the term "herniation" can be used to describe such occurrences elsewhere in the body, but for purposes of this discussion it is concerned with the abdominal wall.) These areas of weakness are at the umbilicus, the inguinal canals which transmit the spermatic cords in the male and the round ligaments in the female, and at the femoral rings which transmit the femoral vessels to the legs. A hernia can occur in any of these areas if a strain imposed on the abdominal muscles exceeds the capability of the muscles at these points. Some persons having had abdominal surgery have suffered incisional hernias because of weak musculature and improper use of the muscles when lifting or moving heavy objects. Those who have hernias often describe the discomfort they experience when sneezing or coughing and their need to protect the area on such occasions by pressing their hands against it.

When practiced consistently, using the longest and the strongest muscles of the extremities and putting on the internal girdle and the long midriff can become almost an automatic act. Many nurses have saved themselves from injury by just such action. It is not an infrequent occurrence in nursing to have a patient or a visitor feel faint and start to slide to the floor or to have a patient almost fall out of bed while reaching for something. The nurse must act instantly and put herself in the best protective position in order to avoid injury to herself as well. It could be disastrous for the nurse to attempt to hold someone up or for that matter to ease him down when in a position that is putting strain on her back or the abdomen.

The nurse will need to teach many patients how activities can be done with greater ease and less fatigue. There is an efficient and safe way or a wrong way of performing such taken-for-granted acts as picking up a baby from a play pen, shoveling snow, raking leaves, skiing, dancing, lifting a turkey out of the oven, or unloading heavy objects from the trunk of a car.

The nurse must be physically fit as well as have good habits of body mechanics also. A regular routine of conditioning exercises will help the nurse strengthen her own muscles. Exercises which develop the knee and hip extensors and the abdominal wall are especially helpful.

Principles of Physics Guiding Body Mechanics

Correct application of some basic laws of physics is essential for good body mechanics.

Essential to the performance of acts of moving, lifting, and carrying which reflects good body mechanics is the correct application of some of the basic laws of physics. If applied effectively, they will conserve energy, reduce the amount of effort exerted, and prevent injury. A few guides based on laws of physics are as follows:

Use the longest and the strongest muscles of the arms and the legs to help provide the power needed in strenuous activities.

Use the internal girdle and a long midriff to stabilize the pelvis and to protect the abdominal viscera when stooping, reaching, lifting, or pulling.

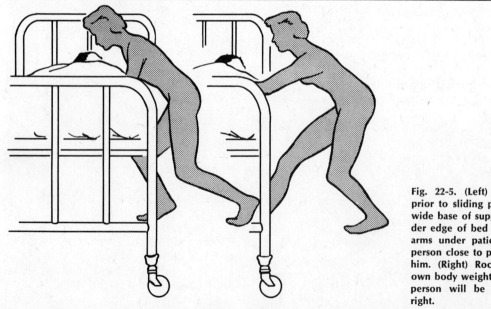

Fig. 22-5. (Left) Shows good position prior to sliding patient to edge of bed; wide base of support with one knee under edge of bed and both knees flexed; arms under patient as far as possible; person close to patient and leaning over him. (Right) Rocking backward to use own body weight to assist in the "pull," person will be in position shown at right.

Work as close as possible to an object which is to be lifted or moved. This brings the center of gravity of the body close to the center of gravity of the object being moved, thereby permitting most of the burden to be borne by the large muscles.

Use the weight of the body as a force for pulling or pushing by rocking on the feet or leaning forward or backward. This reduces the amount of strain placed on the arms and the back.

Slide, roll, push, or pull an object rather than lift it in order to reduce the energy needed to lift the weight against the pull of gravity.

Use the weight of the body both to push an object by falling or rocking forward and to pull an object by falling or rocking backward.

Place the feet apart in order to provide a wide base of support when increased stability of the body is necessary.

Flex the knees, put on the internal girdle, and come down close to an object which is to be lifted.

The nurse can protect herself as well as demonstrate to patients and family members the proper way of using the musculoskeletal system if she consciously develops good habits of movement. The remainder of this chapter discusses additional ways of providing therapeutic activities for patients.

HELPING THE PATIENT TO MAINTAIN OR ATTAIN AN AMBULATORY STATUS

Maintaining an Ambulatory Status

For most patients, fortunately, prolonged periods of bed rest are no longer considered necessary in illness. The benefits of keeping persons up and about as much as possible are evident. A regular exercise routine in health, especially for the elderly whose activities have decreased, is important to maintain body functioning. Activity, even as mild as a stroll around the room, down the hall, from the bedroom to the living room, or out into the yard, is a protective measure for all body systems. It improves circulation and respiration, helps maintain muscle tonus, and aids in elimination from the urinary bladder and intestines. One only has to have a mild case of an upper respiratory infection and rest in bed for a day or two to emerge with "sea legs." Decreased activity because of age or disinterest can result in physiologic as well as mental disfunctions.

Most persons do not wish to be kept in bed and so present no problem. Keeping some persons *in* bed does present a problem many times. Occasionally some persons, especially elderly ones, will decrease their ambulatory activities. Many factors contribute to this, such as arthritis, aches, and stiffness. Some of their problems are in a sense self-induced by lack of exercise of certain joints and muscles over a long period of time. Since these persons are frequently at home, they and family members need to be encouraged to move about, take walks, climb stairs, do toe-heel exercises, and perform any other activity that helps keep them in condition to be on the move.

Patients who have surgery may need some encouragement to take that first walk the day of or following their surgery. Incisional discomfort, a running intravenous infusion, or fear of harming themselves act as deterrents. However, most patients understand that it is to their benefit to do so. Assistance in moving them and supporting them in their first efforts will make the process easier.

Physical Conditioning in Preparation for Ambulation

Patients who are not confined to bed for long periods and have good nights of sleep and possibly short periods of rest during the day may not require special considerations for increased physical activity. However, there are other patients who will have to be prepared for the day when ambulation is resumed. They may need to do conditioning exercises to maintain their muscle tone during extended periods of enforced inactivity, or they may need to strengthen weakened muscles before activity can be resumed. Even if they are active in bed, preparation for walking will have to be a consideration for some persons who have not ambulated for a long period. Certain exercises can be done in bed, at home, or in the health agency, that strengthen the overall efficiency of the musculoskeletal system.

QUADRICEPS DRILLS (SETS): One of the most important muscle groups used in walking is the quadriceps femoris. This muscle group helps to extend the leg on the thigh and flexes the thigh. In addition to walking, it helps lift the legs as in stair climbing. The "sea legs" following even short periods of bed rest result from disuse of these muscles. To help to reduce weakness and make first attempts at walking easier, bed patients should be encouraged to contract this muscle group frequently. It is done by asking the patient to contract the muscles which pull the kneecap up toward the hips, during which the patient has the feeling that he is pushing the knee downward into the mattress and pulling the foot upward. This should be held to the count of four: 1-and-2-and-3-and-4. The exercise should not be done so that fatigue of the muscle group results.

It is a very simple exercise that can be done two or three times hourly.

Push-Ups or Sit-Ups: In preparation for getting out of bed, the muscle strength of the arms and the shoulders also may need to be improved. Exercises improve the strength needed to hold on to or get into a chair and to move about better. They are part of the preparation for all patients who must learn to walk on crutches.

A trapeze attached to the bed of a patient who has limited use of the lower part of his body helps him to move about in bed. However, this does not strengthen the triceps, which is the muscle group necessary for crutch walking or moving from bed to chair. More suitable exercises are sit-ups or push-ups, frequently considered by some physical therapists to be two different types of exercises.

The exercise may be done by having the patient sit up in bed without support and then lift the hips up off the bed by pushing the hands down into the mattress. If the mattress is soft, it may be necessary to use blocks or books under the hands. The other form of the exercise is to have the patient lie face downward on the bed. The arms are brought up so that the patient pushes his head and chest up off the bed by completely extending his elbows. This is repeated several times each time the exercise is done, and the exercise is repeated several times a day. Some patients would find the latter method more difficult to do.

Daily Activities for Purposeful Exercise: In addition to teaching the patient specific exercises, many other activities can be carried out with benefit to the patient. These include such things as placing the bedside stand so that the patient may use shoulder and arm muscles to reach what he needs instead of placing it so as to require little effort to take things from it; placing the signal cord so that the patient must engage in either arm or shoulder action in order to reach it; encouraging the patient to sit up and reach for the overbed table, to pull it close to him, and then to push it back in place; encouraging a patient to try to wash his back; and having him put on his socks while still in bed. There are innumerable ways in which patients can be helped to exercise, and when they understand the purpose, they very often adopt other exercises for themselves.

Preparing for the Patient to Get Out of Bed

In addition to the attention given to the patient's physical state, the nurse is concerned with the necessary items needed, such as a chair or a wheelchair when the patient first gets out of bed. If the patient is going to stand or to walk about, a walker or crutches may be necessary. Positioning of the chair may be important to conserve the patient's energy. If the patient is to move from the bed to the chair without walking, the chair should be positioned parallel to the bed. If the patient is to ambulate, the chair can be positioned an appropriate distance from the bed. The selection of chair varies with the patient, but generally patients who are having difficulty moving find a supportive straight chair easier to get into and out of than a soft upholstered chair.

If the patient is going to walk, it is best for him to wear his shoes or supportive slippers. Having to walk with loose slippers or with shoes that have little support adds to the difficulty of ambulation if there is any physical limitation. This applies to all patients, whether young or old and whether sick for a long or a short time. Patients who are asked to walk immediately following surgery or after long illness are not able to walk as steadily as they would be if their feet were supported properly.

While it is not possible to set the exact manner in which any one patient should be dressed when out of bed, several points should be mentioned. The amount and the type of clothing worn by the patient will depend on the temperature and the air movement in the environment. It is the nurse's responsibility to protect the patient from discomfort due to overdressing and against the danger of having him becoming chilled because he is insufficiently clothed. Changes in the physical state as a result of illness usually make patients more susceptible to environmental factors such as drafts. Patients who may be permitted to sit out in the open on porches or patios may need to be given some sort of head covering. For most patients, it is usually better for their morale if they can be dressed in their usual attire. Agencies for the chronically ill make every effort to reduce the association with illness by having their patients dress in clothing other than that which is worn in bed. The same should be true at home and in hospitals when possible.

Assisting the Patient Out of Bed

If a patient has sufficient strength to stand and to support his own weight, getting him out of bed is a relatively simple matter. However, during the time that the patient is being assisted out of bed, he should be observed for signs of faintness and difficulty in breathing. It is not uncommon for patients to become faint due to an alteration in blood pressure. It is best to assist the patient to the sitting position slowly and to provide a short period of rest between each move. Taking the pulse is a good way to determine the patient's reaction to the activity. If the pulse rate is more rapid than usual, proceed with caution.

If the patient is too weak to walk, the preparation of the chair should precede the preparation of the patient. If a wheelchair is used, the wheels should be locked. If this is not possible, place it against the wall or have it held in place by another person.

The patient is brought to the side of the bed and assisted to the sitting position. The head of the bed should be elevated to help support him in this position. As soon as the patient feels comfortable in this position, the nurse supports his shoulders and legs and pivots him around so that his legs are off to the side of the bed. If the bed is not low enough so that his feet rest on the floor, the feet can be placed on a chair or footstool so that he can support his body and so that pressure against the posterior thigh is reduced. If the feet are not supported, the patient may not feel comfortable, and there is always danger of his sliding off the bed. This position frequently is used preparatory to ambulation and is referred to as *dangling*.

While the patient is sitting on the edge of the bed, it is easy to dress him in his robe and to put on his shoes. A footstool should be provided for stepping down if the patient's feet do not touch the floor.

When helping the patient out of bed, the nurse stands directly in front of the patient. The patient places his hands on the nurse's shoulders. The nurse places her hands in the patient's axillary region with thumbs pointing upward. In this position, she is able to support the patient's shoulders should he begin to fall. If the nurse's hands are held against the chest instead of up in the axillary region as described, she would need to press the patient's chest tightly if he were to fall. This would be extremely uncomfortable for the patient. As the patient pushes himself to a standing position with his legs, the nurse assists by lifting the upper part of his body.

The patient is permitted to stand for a few seconds to make certain that he is not feeling faint. The nurse continues to face the patient and pivots him around so that his back is toward the chair. Then she lowers the patient to the edge of the chair first. While doing this, the nurse should have one foot forward and the knees flexed and again come down

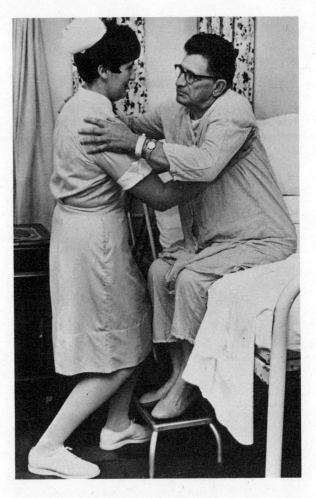

Fig. 22-6. Assisting the patient out of bed. The nurse's hands are in a position to support the patient in the event that he becomes weak and also to assist him to the standing position. (Photo, Warren R. Vroom)

with the patient. She may even wish to brace her knees against the patient's knees for added leverage as she lowers him into the chair. Next she assists the patient to sit well back in the chair and adjusts the footrests if it is a wheelchair.

If a high-low bed is used, the nurse may wish to prepare the patient and permit him to dangle his legs while the bed is in the high position. This creates less strain on her arms, and she is in a better position to support the patient. When the patient is ready to stand, the low position would eliminate the need of a footstool. However, if the patient is very weak, the nurse is in a better position to support him and to use her long and strong arm and leg muscles, if she does not lower the bed and follows the procedure described above.

Assisting the Patient to Walk

Many patients who have been confined to bed for a long period of time find that they must almost learn to walk all over again. An activity which needed no special teaching or encouragement in childhood now becomes a real challenge. Often, it is the nurse who plays a major role in the patient's recovery and mental outlook, his hope and faith, especially when he must stick to a rigid and often difficult schedule of reeducating muscle groups. Physicians have said that a patient able to raise his leg only 1 inch from the bed is considered to possess sufficient power to permit walking.

Where a major problem of muscle reeducation presents itself, the patient will need the assistance of experts in physical medicine. However, nurses are often asked to assist patients out of bed and to help them to walk when the presence of a physical therapist is not possible. There are several aspects to this problem of ambulation with which the nurse should be familiar.

WALKING: The normal pattern of walking is to move alternate arms and legs. For example, the right arm and the left leg move forward, and then the left arm and the right leg move forward. If a patient is able to be supported from the rear at the waist while he practices these movements and has no real limitations to the muscle groups of the hips, the legs, and the feet, he will soon be walking well again. A walking belt with handles for the assistant's hands is often worn by the patient for this purpose.

If the patient is quite weak and is reluctant to try to stand with support only at the waist, it may be necessary to support him under the arm until he feels that he is able to try the other method. A patient who seems to be very weak can be assisted to regain a sense of balance and stability by supporting himself with a walker or the backs of two chairs. Then when the patient walks, if he needs some additional support for a while, the nurse should walk alongside him, keeping her arm which is near the patient under his arm. It is an arm-in-arm position. The advantage of this position is that, if the patient begins to feel faint, the nurse's arm is in a position to slide up into the patient's axilla. The nurse throws one foot out to the side to make a wide base of support and rests the patient on her hip.

To assist patients in the retraining process of walking, there are a number of supportive measures

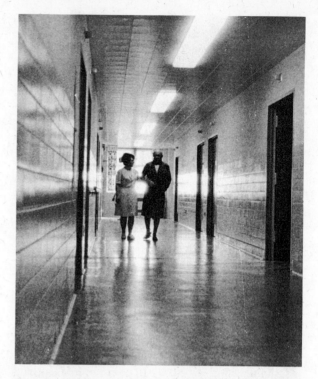

Fig. 22-7. For the patient who has just gotten that invitation, "Let's try a walk down the hall this morning," it may seem more like walking the last mile. All the more reason why bed exercises and quadricep sets are so important. (Courtesy of Muhlenberg Hospital, Plainfield, N. J.)

available. Patients may be given canes, walkers, or crutches, or assisted to use the supportive bars often found on hospital corridor walls.

Crutch Walking

Sometimes, it is necessary for patients to use crutches for a period of time in order to avoid using one leg or to help strengthen one or both legs. This procedure is taught best by a physical therapist; however, there are numerous instances when the nurse is called on to measure patients for crutches and to teach them to use the crutches. Even if a patient is being taught to crutch-walk by a physical therapist, it is necessary for the nurse to understand the patient's progress and the gait he is being taught. The nurse must often guide the patient at home or in the hospital after the initial teaching is completed.

There are several ways by which crutches can be measured, but the two methods described here are considered satisfactory. These are done when the patient is in bed. One way is to measure from the anterior fold of the axilla straight down to the heel and then add 2 inches. The other way is to measure from the anterior fold of the axilla diagonally out to a point 6 inches away from the heel. The patient should be measured in the shoes he will be wearing as he learns to walk. The measurement to the crutches includes the axillary pads and the crutch tips at the bottom. Then the crutches will need to be adjusted for the location of the handgrip according to the height of the patient. This may be done when the patient is in the upright position. The handgrip should be placed so that the elbows are slightly flexed while the patient is using them. The elbows should not be extended and the wrists should be hyperextended.

GAITS: Essentially, there are three gaits: four-point, three-point, and two-point. There is also a swing-through gait which is used by some patients

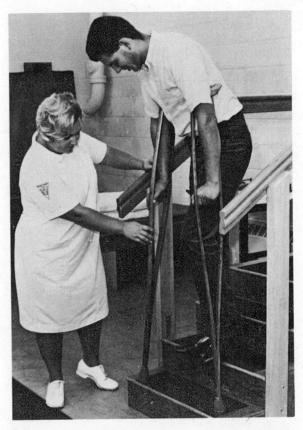

Fig. 22-9. It is important for the nurse to understand which crutch gait the patient is learning from the physical therapist. (Photo, Warren R. Vroom)

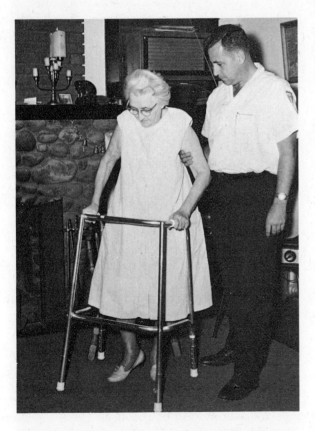

Fig. 22-8. After discharge from the hospital many patients require supervision of other health workers in addition to a visiting nurse. In this instance, the physical therapist is helping the patient in her struggle for more mobility. The nurse will be aware of this as she visits the home, and she too can supervise the patient in her efforts. (Courtesy Good Samaritan Hospital, Phoenix, Arizona)

when they become more accustomed to the crutches and wish to get about quickly and by patients who have had a leg amputated. The swing-through gait, however, does not simulate normal walking and extended use will lead to atrophy of the muscles of the lower extremities.

Four-Point Gait: Weight-bearing is permitted on both feet, and the pattern is as follows: right crutch, left foot, left crutch, right foot. It is the normal reciprocal walking pattern.

Two-Point Gait: Weight-bearing is permitted on both feet and the pattern is a speedup of the four-point gait: right crutch and left foot forward at the same time, left crutch and right foot forward at the same time.

Three-Point Gait: Weight-bearing is permitted on only one foot. The other leg cannot support, but it acts as a balance in the process. It is used also when partial weight-bearing is allowed on the affected extremity. The pattern is as follows: both crutches and the nonsupportive leg go forward, and then the good leg comes through. The crutches are brought forward immediately, and the pattern is repeated.

EXERCISES PREPARATORY TO CRUTCH-WALKING: Before the patient is asked to use the crutches, several exercise drills will help him to be more confident and skillful. The patient must begin by strengthening the arm and the shoulder muscles. The sit-up exercise described earlier is most helpful. The muscles of the hand must also be strengthened. Squeezing a rubber ball 50 times a day by flexing and extending the fingers helps to do this.

The patient should be assisted into a chair which is close to the wall. Then he should be helped to stand against the wall and the crutches placed in his hands. Next, standing slightly away from the wall, he should sway on the crutches from side to side. This accustoms the hands and the arms to weight-bearing.

After this, he should be asked to lean against the wall and pick one crutch up about 6 inches from the floor and then place it down. This should be repeated with the other crutch and the whole exercise done six to eight times. Then, still leaning against the wall, he should be asked to pick up both crutches from the floor and place them down. This too should be repeated several times.

After these exercises, it will be possible to judge the patient's ability to hold and manage the crutches without the added concern for movement. If the patient is judged capable of proceeding into the practice of a gait, if possible begin with the four-point gait.

The patient's posture with the crutches should be guided by the earlier stated physics principles. The line of gravity should go through the base of support, and the base of support should be wide. The crutches should be placed about 4 inches in front and about 4 inches at the sides of the feet for best balance.

Patients using crutches with the axillary support should be cautioned about exerting pressure against the axillae. When patients first begin to use crutches, they should be taught that the support should come primarily from the arms and the hands. The crutches should not be forced into the axillae each time the body is moved forward.

There are crutches available which have no axillary support. A supportive frame extends beyond the handgrip for the lower arm to help guide the crutch. Such crutches are more likely to be used by patients who have permanent limitations and will always need crutch assistance for ambulation.

PROVIDING PROTECTIVE MEASURES FOR THE PATIENT CONFINED TO BED

One of the greatest challenges in nursing is the care of the patient confined to bed. This is particularly true if the person's illness renders him immobile. He is truly dependent upon others to do for him what he cannot do for himself and to help keep him in the best possible physiologic and psychological state. A review of the first part of this chapter would be helpful, because it is essential that persons caring for helpless patients be aware of and use principles of body mechanics to protect themselves as well. One person can generally manage a helpless patient safely and easily if knowledge of body mechanics principles is applied.

General Principles Guiding the Nursing Care of the Bedfast Patient

The body requires alternate periods of rest and activity. Going to bed for the purpose of resting, as for sleep, is truly therapeutic. However, prolonged periods of confinement to bed, whether prescribed or induced by a state of illness, can bring about undesirable results. Close observation of the patient, careful planning for activity within the patient's scope of endurance, and the use of protective measures become an essential part of the patient's nursing care.

The body strives constantly to function coordinately. Optimal functioning of the body, psychologically and physiologically, depends upon all systems being "go." When certain systems are not functioning well, others will be affected. Therefore, when locomotion and movement of the body cease, or are reduced to a minimum, there is urgent need to prevent disruption of other functions.

THE DANGER OF BED REST: As was mentioned in the previous part of this chapter, keeping the patient as active as his physical condition allows is a goal in the treatment of any patient. Obviously, being able to walk about is of great psychological value. Therefore, when a person must be confined to bed it can be expected that this will strongly affect his behavior.

The physiologic damage that can result from

prolonged bed rest is not confined to damage of the musculoskeletal system, such as muscular weakness, difficulty in walking, foot drop, or contractures that limit joint movement. The effects can be far more damaging than the illness the patient had at the onset. For example, circulatory stasis can cause the formation of thrombi (blood clots), or there can be a dilation of blood vessels in the abdomen; respiration can be affected and inadequate exchange of gases will result; lymphatic disturbances can cause edema (swelling due to the accumulation of fluid in the tissues); impaired digestion; constipation; breakdown of tissues, such as bedsores; even chemical imbalance resulting in brittleness of bones. These are but a few of the complications that must be prevented in the bedfast, inactive patient.

Even persons who are not confined to bed for long periods can lose muscle tone and coordination so that simple activities of dressing, bathing, eating, and moving are difficult. While the limitations are temporary, they frequently need not occur if the nurse or family members take adequate precautions. The nurse needs to initiate preventive measures from the beginning of bed confinement.

Nurses need to encourage the patient to engage in routine activities of daily living (sometimes abbreviated A. D. L.) to the extent he is capable. For the bedfast patient, these include such activities as sitting up alone in bed, rolling over from side to side while in bed, brushing the teeth, combing the hair, cutting meat into small pieces, lifting a cupful of liquid, buttoning a shirt button, and the like.

Orders for bed rest can have many different interpretations. It is important that the degree of limitation be clearly understood by the nurse as well as the family. The term bed rest may mean absolute rest, including being fed; or it may mean the patient may feed and bathe himself; or it may mean he is to remain in bed at all times except for elimination when he may use the bathroom. An exact understanding of the patient's activity regimen is needed to plan his nursing care.

Devices for the Safety and the Comfort of the Patient

Resting in bed usually is very comfortable if the body is held or supported in a restful position. Merely being in a horizontal position does not insure rest. It is as important to be in good alignment and posture when lying down as it is when standing or sitting. To sit with the knees crossed may be comfortable for a short while, but it soon becomes uncomfortable and fatiguing. Having the knees crossed

while sitting is not too different from having one leg adducted and rotated inwardly while lying on the side. It is only when the body is supported properly and the position changed frequently enough to rest certain muscle groups and utilize others that rest in bed can serve its best purpose. Modern adjustable beds used in homes and in health agencies make it possible to adjust the patient's position and still provide adequate support. Both electric and manually operated beds facilitate positioning and movement.

There are many devices which help to maintain good body alignment and muscle tonus in bed and to alleviate discomfort or pressure on various parts of the body.

PILLOWS: The primary purposes of pillows are to provide support or to provide elevation of a part. Variety in sizes of pillows increases their usefulness. Pillows intended for the head are usually full- or large-sized pillows. Small pillows are ideal for support or elevation of the extremities, shoulders, or incisional wounds. Specially designed heavy pillows are useful to elevate the upper part of the body when an adjustable bed is not available, as for example, in a home situation.

MATTRESS: For a mattress to be comfortable and supportive, it must be firm but have sufficient "give" to permit good body alignment. Figure 22-10 shows the effect of a supportive and a nonsupportive mattress on body alignment. If a patient were to remain in a bed, such as is depicted at the bottom of the illustration, he might very well complain of backache and other discomforts.

A well-made and well-supported foam-rubber mattress retains a uniform firmness and therefore helps to protect the patient. These mattresses are made of natural or synthetic rubber, or both in combination. A large volume of air is incorporated. The foam-rubber mattress conforms to the contours of the body and supplies support at all points. Its greatest advantage is that it does not form slopes and valleys as the innerspring mattresses are likely to do. Nor does the foam rubber mattress create as much pressure against bony prominences, such as the ankles, the elbows, the scapulae, and the coccyx.

BED BOARD: If the mattress does not provide sufficient support, a bed board may help to keep the patient in better alignment. Bed boards usually are made of plywood or some other firm composition. The size varies with the needs of the situation. If sections of the bed can be raised, such as the head and the foot of a hospital bed, it may be necessary to have the board divided and held together with

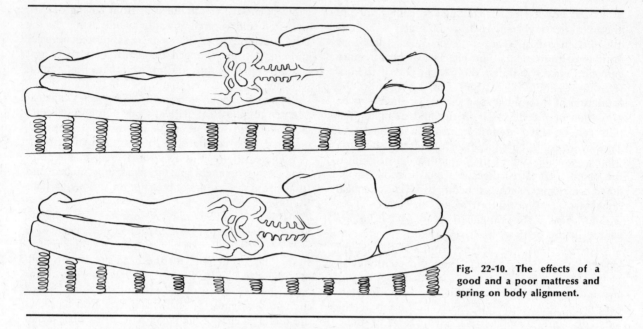

Fig. 22-10. The effects of a good and a poor mattress and spring on body alignment.

hinges. For home use, full bed boards are available commercially or can easily be made at home from available materials.

HIGH-LOW TILT BED: Another useful device is the bed which can have its height as well as total angle adjusted. The value of having an adjustable-height bed has been discussed earlier. These beds also permit the angle to be changed so that the head is higher than the feet, or vice versa. Such beds are extremely helpful for patients forced to lie flat. They have several advantages, one of which is the fact that when the head is up the patient is able to see about him without extreme flexion of the neck. Also, the patient is assisted to a more nearly vertical position without the effort of standing. The shift in the position of the abdominal organs and the alteration in the circulation in the extremities and other body areas help to prevent complications and prepare for the day when weight-bearing and standing will begin.

ROCKING BED: The rocking bed, while used in the care of patients with vascular or respiratory diseases, is also of great value in the care of other immobile patients. This bed is mounted on a frame rather than the usual bedstead. By means of a motor, the bed can be made to rock rhythmically up and down in seesaw fashion. There is a footrest on the bed to help keep the patient from sliding and also to help to keep the feet in good alignment. If the patient is in a moderate sitting position there is little danger of the patient's sliding. The bed is adjusted to rock at the same frequency of the patient's respirations. The rocking aids respiration by shifting the abdominal viscera, which in turn helps to move the diaphragm upward and downward, helping air to be drawn into and forced out of the lungs.

Also, the constant alteration of position aids the flow of blood. The same principle (pull of gravity) is in operation when the tilt bed is used. In some vascular diseases, it is helpful if venous circulation is assisted during the time the patient must be confined to bed.

Other patients, because of their inactive state, also need some measure to assist or improve circulation. It will be recalled that venous blood is assisted in its return to the heart by the contraction of muscle groups in the legs. Pressure against the veins helps to move the blood along its course. If activity is at a minimum, elevation of the extremities is helpful in that the position aids the blood in its return flow.

CHAIR BED: Another type of bed used in the care of patients requiring bed rest is one that can be made into a chair position. These beds were designed primarily for the patient who has a heart ailment. In some instances, they are referred to as the cardiac bed. They permit the patient to be in a semisitting position which may aid the patient's cardiac output.

CIRCULAR BED: The electric circular bed is a 6 or 7 foot metal frame with a diameter support for the patient. The direction of the support can be changed so the patient can be placed in a variety of positions, including supine, prone, and vertical. This bed is especially useful for the patient who will be completely helpless for an extended period of time.

RUBBER AIR RINGS, CUSHION RINGS, AND DOUGHNUTS: Inflated rubber rings, cushion rings, and handmade doughnuts for relieving pressure on bony prominences by lifting them from the mattress surface, have been used extensively in the past. Their disadvantage lies in the fact that, in protecting one area, they create pressure in immediately surrounding areas. This pressure, in turn, impairs circulation to the area of most concern and thus reduces the supply of oxygen and nutrients.

There are more effective means of relieving pressure on bony prominences and protecting the patient from developing pressure sores. A piece of sponge rubber large enough to be supportive placed adjacent to the pressure point so that it fills the space and thus reduces some of the pressure is effective. Small pillows, if available, are also helpful in elevating an area such as the heels, so that the pressure is reduced. Pieces of synthetic sheepskin are useful and protective.

Rubber air rings have some value for patients who are having sitz baths following rectal and perineal surgery. In such instances, they provide comfort for the brief period when the patient must sit in the tub. They are not recommended as a device for the prevention of a bedsore on a patient's coccygeal area.

FOOTBOARDS: A board placed at the foot of the mattress and perpendicular to it is often used to help to keep the top bed covers from pressing on the feet. Footboards are usually made so that they can be wedged between the mattress and the bedframe or so that an extension slides under the mattress. The board should be of sufficient height to hold the bedclothes above the toes when the feet are held in the walking position (dorsal flexion). If the board is too high, it may prevent the top linen from resting on the patient's thighs and legs, thus causing a feeling of chilliness. A footboard may be used to keep the feet in dorsal flexion if the patient is tall enough for his feet to touch the board or if a firm support is used to build up the area from the board to the patient's feet. If the patient is of small stature, a more suitable method for supporting the feet is to use a foot block.

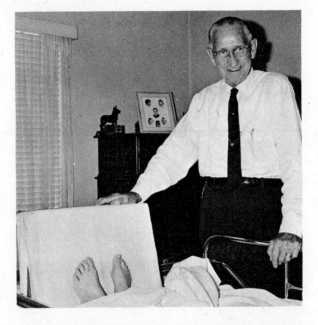

Fig. 22-11. This man prepared a footboard for his wife and is obviously very pleased with the results, since they met with the approval of the visiting nurse. (Courtesy Good Samaritan Hospital, Phoenix, Arizona)

FOOT BLOCKS: A foot block is a firm object placed on the mattress at the foot of the bed so that the patient's feet can rest against it in the correct position, dorsal flexion. A foot block can be made from a sturdy box, a carton, or a wooden block. The block is covered with a pillow case or some other suitable piece of linen before being placed against the feet.

Like other devices, foot blocks must be adjusted to the needs of the patient. If the patient is short, a foot block may need to be of considerable size in order to reach the patient's feet. If the patient is tall, a small foot block is necessary. If a foot block is not readily available or if it is not suitable for the patient, an improvised foot support can be made from a pillow and a large sheet. The pillow is rolled in the sheet, and the ends of the sheet are twisted before being tucked under the mattress. The ends should be tucked under the mattress at an angle toward the head of the bed to help to keep the pillow in place. A pillow foot support does not provide the firmness of a carton, a box, or the foot block, nor does it assist in stimulating proprioceptor senses, muscle contractions, and circulation; but it will suffice for a few hours until a better support can be obtained.

If the patient is in a sitting position while in

bed, the foot block must be placed at an angle. This is to prevent hyperextension of the knees which would result if the feet were kept in dorsiflexion while the trunk was flexed forward.

CRADLE: If pressure of the top bedding is a problem, or if the top bedding must be kept off the patient's lower extremities, a device called a cradle is used. A cradle is usually a metal frame. There are any number of sizes and shapes of cradles. If used, the cradle should be fastened securely to the bed so that it does not slide or fall on the patient.

SANDBAGS: Some patients must have an area of the body held in position by a firm supportive device. For example, the patient may have a tendency to rotate his leg outward. In order to prevent his lying in this position for extended periods of time, the leg can be held in good alignment by placing sandbags alongside the outer surface of the leg from the hip to the knee. Sandbags have numerous uses and their value is enhanced if they are available in various sizes. When properly filled, they are not hard or firmly packed. They should be pliable enough to be shaped to body contours and to give support. They should not create pressure on a bony prominence.

TROCHANTER ROLLS: If sandbags are not available to help prevent a patient's legs from rotating outward, it is possible to improvise a support that will serve the same purpose. Fold a sheet lengthwise and place the narrow dimension under the patient so that it extends from the patient's waist to his knees. A large, bulky piece of linen should not be used because of the discomfort it will cause to the patient's back. Under each end of the sheet, which extends on either side of the patient, place a rolled bath blanket or two bath towels. Roll the sheet around the blanket so that the roll is under. In this way, it cannot unroll itself, and the weight of the patient helps to hold it secure. When the trochanter roll is in place properly, the patient will be lying on a piece of linen which has a large roll on either side of it. Fix these rolls close to the patient and tight against the hip and the thigh so that the femur does not rotate outwardly. If the roll is not sufficiently long, very little support can be expected. Pillows properly placed can also serve as trochanter rolls.

HAND ROLLS: If patients are paralyzed or unconscious, it may be necessary to provide a means for keeping the thumb in the correct position; namely, slightly adducted and in apposition to the fingers. To do this for short periods of time, any number of improvisations can be made. For example, a rubber ball of the appropriate size, sponge rubber, or a folded washcloth may be used. However, if the hands are going to need protective support for many days or weeks, securing a commercial plastic or aluminum splint may be considered. In this way, the thumb is held in place no matter what position the hand is in. Patients who are not moving their fingers should be encouraged to do finger exercises with special attention to having the thumb touch the tips of each finger.

BED SIDERAILS: One of the greatest safety concerns of nursing personnel is to prevent patients from falling out of bed. Hospital accident reports show a high proportion of such events; hence, in many agencies, it is routine to use extra protection on the beds of unconscious and disoriented patients and on the beds of elderly patients. The terms "bedrails" and "siderails" are used synonymously with the term "bed siderails."

There is no question that the presence of siderails often has an unfortunate psychological effect on rational and oriented patients and on their families. Therefore, the use of them requires explanation beyond passing it off as "routine." The patient should be helped to understand how the siderails offer protection if he is weak, or receiving certain drugs and cannot prevent himself from falling, should he roll to the edge of the bed.

Bed siderails, even if they are the full length of the mattress, may not deter some patients from getting out of bed. Many a patient has gone to the foot of the bed and gotten out that way.

The adjustable-height bed seems to be one answer for certain types of patients such as the ambulatory elderly patient. The bed can remain at the lowest point so that when the patient brings his feet over the side of the bed, he is able to place them directly on the floor. He is then safer and more stable. If on the other hand, his feet must dangle from a higher height as from an older hospital bed, he may slide off the edge, lose his balance, and fall to the floor. Many nurses note that the incidence of hospital falls when the bed is lowered to the usual height of the home bed is greatly decreased.

As mentioned in Chapter 18, bed siderails are used for the patient's safety, but they also have value for many weakened patients. For example, siderails make it possible for the patient to roll himself from one side to the other or even to sit up without calling for assistance. This in itself is a very good activity measure to help to retain or regain muscle efficiency.

RESTRAINTS: Restraints are physical devices used to limit bodily movement. They can be used to restrict the movement of an extremity, for example, when an infusion is running. They also are helpful to prevent patients who are not voluntarily able to cooperate from pulling at wound dressings and tubings leading from the body and to prevent patients who are unsteady and in danger of falling when trying to get out of bed or from a chair. There are a variety of types of restraints available commercially. They can also be fashioned from a sufficient length of any sturdy cloth. Figures 18-2 and 18-3 on pages 170 and 171 illustrate restraints.

It is important to remember when using restraints that care should be taken when limiting a patient's movements to prevent impediment of circulation or respirations and irritation to the skin. Confining movement to a safe area may be necessary, but restriction of all movement can have detrimental effects.

It is also important to convey to the patient and his family the reason for the application of the restraint—a protective device for the patient and not a punishment measure. Some patients find it helpful to consider the restraint as a reminder not to move their arms or legs. There are some patients who become so fearful and agitated by the use of restraints that the stress induced by their presence is felt to be more detrimental than the movement. The frightened patient will often relax and become more comfortable if someone stays and calms him. Quiet talking to even the patient who appears to be unaware of his surroundings will generally have a soothing effect. Under no circumstance should the use of restraints be looked upon as alleviating the nurse's responsibility to observe the patient. Frequent observation of the restrained patient is important to insure that the restraints are properly positioned.

Protective Positions for the Patient

Unless medical orders specify restriction of activity, bed patients can be prevented from developing physical limitations by changes in position. The protective side-lying, back-lying, and face-lying positions are intended to help to maintain good body alignment. The semisitting position can provide variety for the patient. To place the patient in any of these positions, it is essential to understand the position of body parts when in good posture. Briefly, these can be recalled: for a person in the standing position the feet perpendicular to the legs (dorsal flexion); the knees in a slight degree of flexion (5° to 10°); the patellae facing forward; the hips straight; the arms alongside the body, the forearms slightly adducted toward the body; the hands pronated; the thumbs adducted into the hands; the fingers in the grasp position; the head held erect on the shoulders so that vision is horizontal with the floor.

THE PROTECTIVE BACK-LYING (SUPINE) POSITION: In the back-lying position, two areas of the body are in need of particular attention. These are the feet and the neck. Of course, if the patient is unable to move at all, then all areas of the body require attention.

The greatest danger to the feet occurs when they are not held in the dorsal flexion position. The toes drop downward, and the feet are in plantar flexion. This position of the feet occurs naturally when the body is at rest. If maintained for extended periods of time, plantar flexion can cause an alteration in the muscles, and the patient may develop a complication referred to as *dropfoot*. In this position, the foot is unable to maintain itself in the perpendicular position, heel-toe gait is impossible, and the patient will experience extreme difficulty in walking. If it is severe enough, the patient will not be able to walk at all. Intensive physical therapy over a long period of time may be required, and, in some instances, surgery has been necessary to help to lengthen the shortened muscle group. The use of a foot support aids in avoiding this complication.

During the time that a patient is in bed, pillows almost always are used to support the head. It will be noted that the patient frequently uses the pillows to tilt the head forward in order to improve his field of vision. This produces flexion of the cervical spine. Often one may see patients who are out of bed continue to walk about with this same flexion of the cervical spine. Since the back-lying position is the one in which the patient often spends the greatest length of time, the thorax, the neck, and the head should be supported properly.

If the patient is active in bed and able to move his arms, use his hands, and roll from side to side, these activities are protective in themselves and reduce the need for some supporting devices. However, if the patient is unable to move, supportive measures are necessary. Preventive measures for keeping the patient in good alignment while on his back are included in the box on page 286. The decision as to whether one, more, or all measures are necessary is dependent on the condition of the patient, his illness limitations, his activity status, and his body build.

THE PROTECTIVE SIDE-LYING POSITION: Lying on the side is a welcome relief from prolonged

THE PROTECTIVE BACK-LYING POSITION

COMPLICATION TO BE PREVENTED	SUGGESTED PREVENTIVE MEASURE
Exaggerated curvatures of the spine and flexion of the hips.	Provide a firm supportive mattress. Use a bed board if necessary.
Flexion contractures of the neck.	Place pillow(s) under the upper shoulder, the neck, and the head so that the head and the neck are held in the correct position.
Internal rotation of the shoulders and extension of the elbows (hunch-shoulders).	Place pillows or arm supports under the forearms so that the upper arms are alongside the body and the forearms are pronated slightly.
Extension of the fingers and abduction of the thumbs (clawhand deformities).	Make hand rolls or use small towels for the hands to grasp. If the patient is paralyzed, use thumb guides to hold the thumbs in the adducted position.
External rotation of the femurs.	Place sandbags or a trochanter roll alongside the hips and the upper half of the thighs.
Hyperextension of the knees.	Place a small soft roll or sponge rubber under the knees, sufficient to fill the popliteal space but not to create pressure and not to exceed 5° of flexion.
Plantar flexion.	Use a foot block or make an improvised firm foot support to hold the feet in dorsal flexion.

THE PROTECTIVE SIDE-LYING POSITION

COMPLICATION TO BE PREVENTED	SUGGESTED PREVENTIVE MEASURE
Lateral flexion of the neck.	Place a pillow under the head and the neck.
Inward rotation of the arm and interference with respiration.	Place a pillow under the upper arm.
Extension of the fingers and abduction of the thumbs.	Provide a hand roll for the fingers and the thumbs.
Internal rotation and adduction of the femur.	Use one or two pillows as needed to support the leg from the groin to the foot.

periods of lying on the back. Patients who have difficulty turning themselves from side to side appreciate a frequent change of position, which is also essential for alternate rest and activity of muscle groups. The side-lying position removes pressure from the prominent areas of the back.

While on the side, the feet are usually in a lesser degree of plantar flexion because the toes are not being pulled downward by gravity. The neck is also held in a more erect position. The primary concern for the patient in this position is the degree of inward rotation of the upper thigh and the upper arm. The pull created by both of these extremities can become very fatiguing. If, in addition, the upper arm pulls the shoulder girdle forward and compresses the thorax, respiration is impaired.

Preventive measures for keeping the patient in good alignment while in the side-lying position are listed in the box on this page. Again, the decision as to whether one, several, or all measures are necessary depends on the condition of the patient, his illness limitations, his activity status, and his body build.

Pillows are arranged to support the patient's extremities, while a heavier pillow is tucked at his back to prevent him from rolling backwards. Figures 22-12, 22-13, and 22-14 show this position.

THE PROTECTIVE FACE-LYING (PRONE) POSITION: Lying on the abdomen, face down, can be a valuable and relaxing position. Unfortunately, many patients are unwilling or unable to be placed in this position.

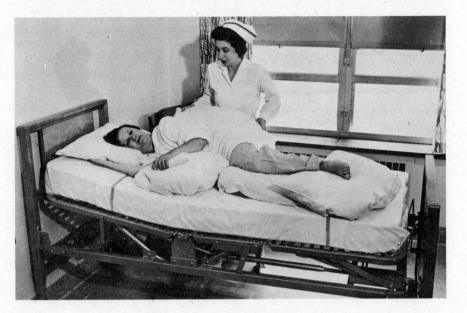

Fig. 22-12. Nurse placing a pillow to keep patient from rolling back.

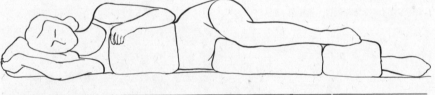

Fig. 22-13. Diagram illustrating anterior view of patient in protective side-lying position.

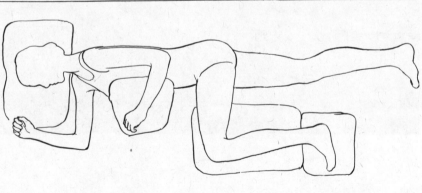

Fig. 22-14. Diagram illustrating side view of patient in protective side-lying position.

From the standpoint of alignment, the prone position offers the fewest sources of concern. If the patient is comfortable in the position and enjoys it, the feet are the only area of real concern. Unless supported or allowed to go over the end of the mattress, they are forced into plantar flexion, and the legs rotate inward or outward. Because the position is helpful, nurses should encourage patients to assume it on their own if they have complete freedom of activity. If the patient needs assistance, the time of the bath is often a good one for placing the patient in the prone position as when washing the back. In some instances, patients are ordered to be placed prone for specified periods of time each day.

THE PROTECTIVE FACE-LYING POSITION

COMPLICATION TO BE PREVENTED	SUGGESTED PREVENTIVE MEASURE
Plantar flexion.	Move the patient down in bed so that his feet are over the mattress; or support his lower legs on a pillow just high enough to keep the toes from touching the bed.
Flexion of the cervical spine.	Place a small pillow under the head.
Hyperextension of the spine. Impaired respiration.	Place some suitable support under the patient between the end of the rib cage and the upper abdomen if this facilitates breathing and there is space there.

The advantages of the face-lying position are as follows: the shoulders, the head, and the neck are placed in the erect position; the arms are held in good alignment with the shoulder girdle; the hips are extended; the knees can be prevented from marked flexion or hyperextension; and the arms can be abducted and flexed. In a sense, it can be said that the body can be "straightened out" when placed in the face-lying position. Preventive measures for maintaining good alignment are discussed in the box on this page. Figures 22-15, 22-16, and 22-17 demonstrate this position.

THE SEMISITTING (FOWLER'S) POSITION: The semisitting position is often used to promote cardiac output, respiratory movement, urinary elimination, and intestinal elimination. It also provides for ease

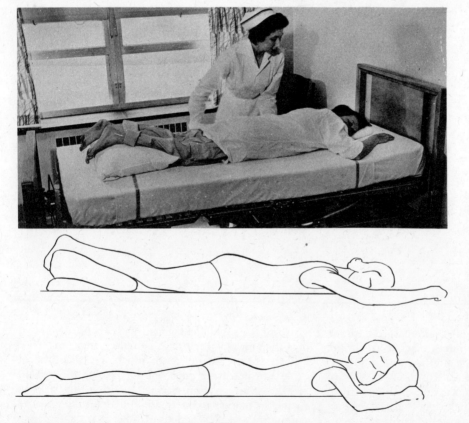

Fig. 22-15. Nurse placing patient in protective prone position.

Fig. 22-16. Diagram illustrating correct protective prone position.

Fig. 22-17. Diagram illustrating incorrect prone position.

THE SEMISITTING POSITION

COMPLICATION TO BE PREVENTED	SUGGESTED PREVENTIVE MEASURE
Flexion contracture of the neck.	Allow the head to rest against the mattress or be supported by a small pillow only.
Exaggerated curvature of the spine.	Use a firm support for back. Position the patient so the angle of elevation starts at the hips.
Dislocation of the shoulder.	Support the forearms on pillows so they are elevated sufficiently so that no pull is exerted on the shoulders.
Flexion contracture of the wrist.	Support the hand on pillows so it is in natural alignment with the forearm.
Edema of the hand.	Support the hand so it is slightly elevated in comparison to the elbow.
Extension of the fingers and abduction of the thumbs.	Provide hand rolls for grasping and thumb supports if necessary.
Impaired lower extremity circulation and knee contracture.	Elevate the knees for only brief periods of time. Avoid pressure on the popliteal vessels.
Plantar flexion.	Support the feet in dorsal flexion.

of eating, conversing, and vision. The completely helpless person should be well-supported. The head of the adjustable bed can be elevated to the desired degree. Usually a 45° to 60° angle is used. A wedge-type, firm support can be used to elevate the patient's body from the hips up if an adjustable bed is not available. The patient should be positioned so the spine is straight and supported.

In this position, the head can be supported with a small pillow if desired. Support of the arms, especially if paralysis exists, is important because the weight of the arms and the force of gravity causes a downward pull on the shoulders and can affect shoulder joint motion in the future. Wrist and finger supports of paralyzed hands also prevent contractures and loss of joint motion. The knees can be slightly elevated with pillows or the bed knee-rest for brief periods, but they should not be in this position for a prolonged period. Impairment of circulation and knee contractures can occur from continued flexion of the knee. Foot supports may be necessary to promote dorsal flexion. Preventive measures for promoting the semisitting position are included in the box on this page.

Protective Exercises and Activities for the Patient

Keeping the patient in good alignment while in bed helps to prevent unequal muscle pulls which may cause limitations of movement. It is often the only activity possible for some patients, such as those who are paralyzed or unconscious. However, when a patient is permitted some exercise, additional measures should be considered to help keep him in good condition.

As little as several days in bed is sufficient time to produce muscular weakness and difficulty in walking. Therefore, efforts to assist patients to maintain good muscle tone must often begin with the first day of confinement to bed. When this is not possible, carefully planned exercises must be started and increased gradually in frequency and endurance on a day-to-day basis. Some patients may require the services of a physical therapist.

The goal of the activities discussed here is to keep the patient in the best possible physical state while bed rest is enforced. This, in turn, should help to prevent physical limitations and to reduce the length of the convalescing period. Nurses and family members can carry out therapeutic regimens. Where the following exercises are not considered as routine nursing measures, the patient's physician must be consulted first.

FULL RANGE OF JOINT MOTION: The framework of the body is the skeleton. The bones of the skeleton are of various sizes and shapes and are held together by ligaments. These points of approximation are the joints. It is by means of the muscles and the joints that body motion is possible. The type of

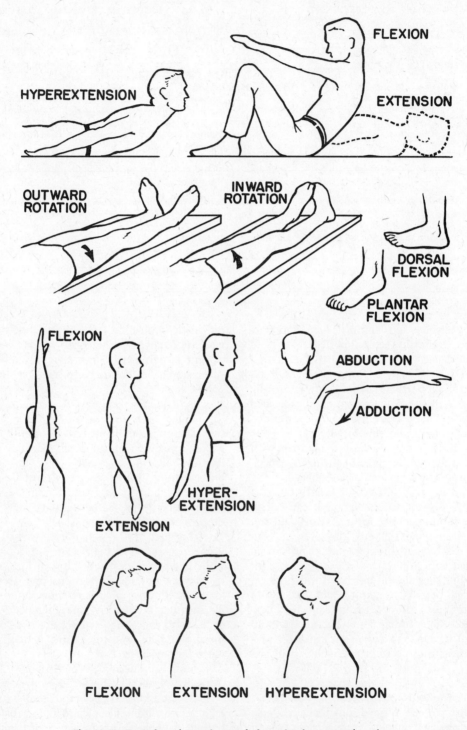

Fig. 22-18. Examples of exercises to help maintain range of motion.

movement possible at the various joints of the body depends on the shape of the terminal portion of the bones and the number of bones forming the joint. It will be recalled that there are six classifications of movable joints: gliding, saddle, hinge, pivot, ball-and-socket, and condyloid. Knowing the classification and the structure of a joint is essential to understanding the type of movement it is capable of performing

As mentioned previously, if muscle groups are altered, as in the formation of a contracture, movement of the joint is altered, and physical limitation occurs. It is essential that the nurse understand the range of motion of the various joints so that preventive measures can be instituted, especially for the patient who is unable to assist in his own care to any great extent. Engaging in routine tasks, such as bathing, eating, dressing, and writing, helps to utilize muscle groups which keep many joints in effective range of motion. When all or some of these activities are impossible for various reasons, attention should be given to the joints not being used, either at all or to their fullest extent.

If a patient is incapable of moving himself, it may be necessary for his joints to be placed through full range of motion several times a day. This can be done during the bath or while changing his position. However, the mere procedure of the bath does not insure that all joints will have been put through range of motion. It is possible to wash the extremities without fully abducting, extending, and flexing the joints. Therefore, purposeful planning for full range of joint motion is necessary. Figure 22-18 shows examples of range of motion exercises. For the helpless patient, this activity is necessary several times a day. In the regimen for some patients who have suffered strokes, full range of motion for specific joints, as the shoulders, the hips, and the thumbs four times a day may be required. The extent to which such exercise is necessary depends on the patient's illness, physical state, and potential for recovery.

Some patients are unable to perform any joint movements themselves. When this is true, another person must move the joints through their range of motion. Manual or mechanical means of moving the joints and related tissues is called *passive exercise*. The patient is a passive recipient of the movement. *Active exercises* are self-activated range of joint movements. The patient is active in the process. *Resistive exercises* are active exercises performed by the patient using an external resistive force. The resis-

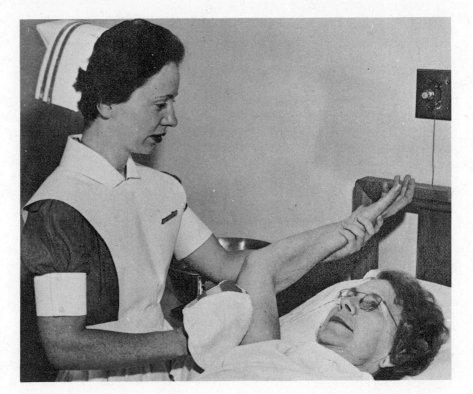

Fig. 22-19. Nurse extending patient's arm during bath as a part of placing shoulder through full range of joint motion.

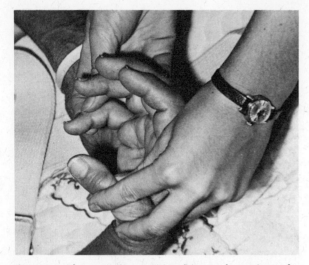

Fig. 22-20. The nurse is exercising fingers of a patient who cannot move his hand. (Good Samaritan Hospital, Phoenix, Arizona)

tive force can be manual exertion applied by another person or by a mechanical device. Passive and active exercises generally can be initiated by nurses. Resistive exercises are most often used by physical therapists.

Occasionally, it is necessary to teach a patient to observe a daily routine of range of motion. In such instances, emphasis may be placed on moving the joints in directions least likely to be used by the patient. The following suggestions could be included:

While sitting up in bed without support:
move the head backward so that the cervical spine is hyperextended.
flex the trunk laterally from side to side.
rotate the trunk.
flex the arms up over the head.
extend the arms to the side of the body and then swing them in circular fashion.

While lying face downward on the bed:
hyperextend the spine by lifting the head and the chest off the bed without the aid of the arms.
hyperextend the arms by lifting them off the bed toward the ceiling.
hyperextend the legs by lifting them up off the bed toward the ceiling.

While lying on the back:
flex the knees by drawing the legs up against the thighs.
rotate the ankles inward and outward.
flex and extend the toes.

While standing and holding onto a chair back:
swing each leg forward and backwards and in a circular fashion.
raise the body on the toes coming down on the heels.

Attention to the thumb is of special importance. If the thumb is abducted permanently so that it cannot be brought into contact with each one of the fingers, the patient will be limited seriously. Without the full use of the thumb, it is difficult to put buttons through a buttonhole, turn a doorknob, and hold various everyday devices securely.

Whenever any of the protective positions, exercises, or devices are used to help to prevent physical limitations or to restore functions, directives should be included on the nursing care plan. It should explain what, how, and when, so that all who care for the patient observe the same routine.

Means by which to Move, Lift, or Carry a Helpless Patient

Frequently, it is necessary to move a helpless patient either in the bed or from the bed to a stretcher or a chair, or vice versa. In addition to keeping him in good alignment while being moved, it is necessary that he be protected from injury.

Protection of the patient's skin from abrasion caused by friction is important because the skin of a helpless patient is usually very fragile and susceptible to injury. Friction burns can occur from pulling a patient across the bed or by pulling his bed linens or a bedpan from underneath him. Reducing friction by using powder or cornstarch sprinkled on the patient's dry skin and/or the linen can be helpful. Rolling, turning, and having adequate assistance are also important. Mechanical devices are usually available in health agencies for moving heavy patients, and many persons have these aids in their homes. Care should be taken to make certain the operator understands how to use the device, that the patient is properly secured, and that he is instructed as to what will occur. The fears of patients who do not understand or are afraid of the devices can result in their refusal to cooperate and possible injuries.

Protection also involves understanding how to support muscles and joints which the patient cannot control voluntarily. When moving a patient, care should be taken to avoid grabbing and holding an extremity by a muscle group. The caution, "avoid grabbing the muscle bellies," is quoted frequently. An extremity should be held at the location of the insertion of the muscle tendons.

When a patient is to be moved or lifted, his

comfort and safety and that of the persons involved should be considered as being equally important. First of all, those who lift patients must be realistic about the effort involved. Two small-statured, 100-pound women must realize immediately that they are physically incapable of lifting a 250-pound patient. He may be pushed, pulled, or slid in bed, but lifting him from one area to another is another matter. Labor laws in some states specify that the maximum a woman can be expected to lift is 35 to 40 pounds. This may act as a guide in some situations, but it is not a specific guide; in certain situations and under some circumstances a woman can safely lift considerably more weight.

By using good body mechanics and the principles of mechanical laws, moving and lifting helpless patients can be made relatively easy. It is essential that the nurse understand such procedures so that she is not entirely dependent on assistance from others. Waiting for assistance which may not be necessary often means that patients cannot be moved as often as or when they would like to be. This is also true of helpless patients in home situations. If the family is taught how to move the patient easily, home care is accepted more readily.

USING TWO PERSONS TO MOVE A HELPLESS PATIENT UP IN BED: Children and light-weight adults are relatively easy to slide toward the head of the bed without the assistance of a second person. Average-weight adults of about 140 to 150 pounds begin to pose a problem. Many nurses have devised ways of moving heavy patients up in bed without assistance, but these methods are usually at great risk to the nurse. When moving a heavy, helpless patient up in bed, two persons should be available.

If the patient is able to push with his feet, the procedure is simple and easy. The wheels of the bed are locked first. One nurse stands on one side of the bed and the other nurse on the other side, near the patient's chest and head. Both nurses face the head of the bed. The patient is asked to flex his knees. Each nurse places the arm nearest the patient under the patient's axilla. One nurse assumes responsibility for supporting the patient's head. The other nurse places the pillow up against the head of the bed so that the patient does not hit the bed frame. Both nurses flex their knees, place one foot forward, come down close to the patient and upon a signal given by one of the nurses, the patient pushes with his feet, and the nurses rock forward, thus moving the patient up in bed.

If a patient is unable to assist by pushing with his feet, the nurses will need to hold him so that the heaviest part of his body is moved by them and not by the patient. The wheels of the bed are locked. It may be easier when the patient's knees are flexed and held in position if necessary by a third person or a pillow. A pillow is placed against the head of the bed. The nurses standing at either side of the bed face each other at a point between the patient's waist and hips. Both nurses give themselves a wide base of support, flex their knees, and lean close to the patient. They join hands under the widest part of the patient's hips and under his shoulders. At a given signal, both rock toward the head of the bed and slide the patient on the bed. The procedure may need to be repeated if he is heavy and is far down in bed. Care should be taken to avoid injury to the patient's neck and head.

USING A DRAW SHEET PULL TO MOVE A HELPLESS PATIENT UP IN BED: While the method described previously may be necessary or convenient, the amount of effort expended by the nurses can be reduced. A draw sheet or a large sheet may be placed under the patient so that it extends from his head to below the buttocks. The sides of the sheet are rolled close to the patient so that they may be grasped easily. The wheels of the bed are locked. The patient's knees are flexed. The nurses stand at opposite sides of the bed at a point near the patient's shoulder and chest and face the foot of the bed. They have a wide base of support with the leg nearest the bed behind them and the other leg in front. Holding the sheet securely at a point near the patient's neck and the lumbar region, they first lean forward and then rock backward. As they rock backward, the weight of their bodies helps to slide the draw sheet and the patient. At the completion of the rocking motion, each nurse usually has the elbow nearest the patient on the mattress.

The procedure can be done with the nurses facing the head of the bed. It seems easier when the backward rock is used. In the forward rock there seems to be a certain amount of upward pull necessary. Figures 22-21 and 22-22 illustrate the draw sheet pull.

MOVING A PATIENT FROM THE BED TO A STRETCHER: Considerable care must be taken, when moving a patient from the bed to a stretcher, or vice versa, to prevent injury to the patient. If he is unconscious or helpless, the extremities and the head must be supported. Mechanical devices are available to move such patients. In the absence of such an aid, the most convenient way to move the patient is to use a sheet underneath him and then carefully pull on the sheet to slide the patient from

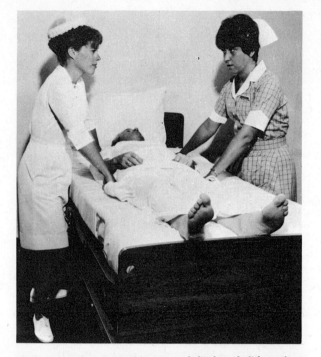

Fig. 22-21. Nurses in position to rock back and slide patient up in bed. Each one has a hand grasping the rolled draw sheet under the patient near his neck in order to support it. When they have a grasp of the sheet close to the patient's body in the hip area, one will give the signal and they will rock back.

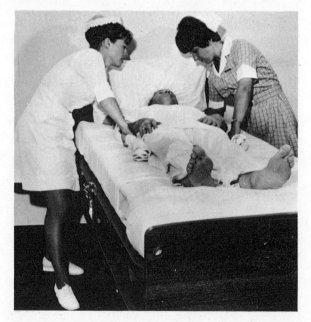

Fig. 22-22. Nurses in position following completion of the draw sheet pull.

one surface to the other. However, there are instances when patients must be lifted and carried. This can be done by means of a three-man lift. If it is done properly, the patient will feel secure, and those lifting will not suffer strain. The three-man lift is detailed in the box on page 296.

When returning the patient to the bed from the stretcher, the same principles are observed. However, the carriers should first move the patient onto the bed, leaving him at the edge. Then, one member of the team supports the patient on the edge of the bed to prevent his falling off while the other two members of the team go around to the opposite side of the bed and place their arms underneath the patient in preparation for sliding him to the center of the bed. Once the two persons on the opposite side of the bed have a good grip on the patient, the third person is able to join them and assist in sliding the patient to the center of the bed. Sliding the patient requires much less effort than attempting to place him directly in the center of the bed. If this is attempted, the group usually is unable to hold the patient, and he is dropped onto the bed.

The three-man lift is used in various other situations, such as lifting a patient who has fallen to the floor and is unable to get up by himself, or lifting a patient out of a chair into the bed. Once the principles of such a lift are mastered, it becomes relatively easy to analyze situations in which it may be used.

For patients who present special problems because of their excessive weight or a cast, the three-man lift may not be sufficient. It may be necessary to have an additional person who is used to help support the heaviest or most cumbersome part of the patient. The persons distribute their arms while carrying so that the heaviest part is well-supported.

Moving a Helpless Patient From Bed to Chair: There are occasions when a patient is permitted to be out of bed but loss of various body functions makes it impossible for him to assist in the process. If the patient is able to help by using his arms for support, the problem is reduced considerably. However, some patients cannot use their arms, and nurses must be prepared to face this problem. In the health agency several persons usually are available to lift the patient from the bed to the chair. Whenever possible, lifting is preferred to prevent friction-induced skin injury. To a great extent the technique is dependent on the size and the weight of the patient and the style of chair that the patient is to use. Chairs often complicate the procedure be-

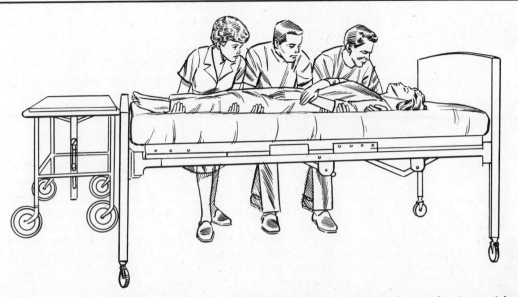

Fig. 22-23. The three-man lift. The patient has been brought to the edge of the bed, the stretcher is at a right angle to the foot of the bed and the three persons preparing to lift the patient have their arms well under the patient with the greatest support being given to the heaviest part of the patient. Each has a wide base of support and each is leaning over close to the patient in preparation for the lift.

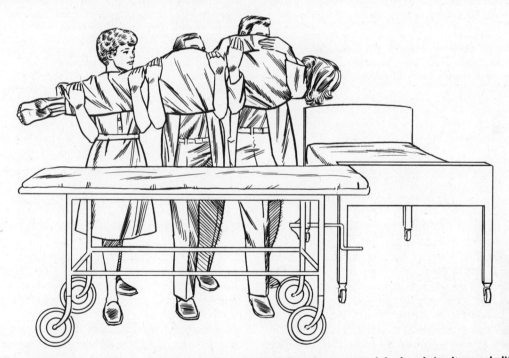

Fig. 22-24. The three-man lift (Continued). On a given signal, the three persons rock back and simultaneously lift the patient and logroll her onto their chests. They then pivot and place the patient on the stretcher. As the patient is being lowered onto the stretcher, all three carriers maintain a wide base of support and flex their knees.

THE THREE-MAN LIFT

The purpose is to move a patient from one place to another while maintaining his horizontal position. (From bed to stretcher is described.)

SUGGESTED ACTION	RELATED BODY MECHANICS FOR THE NURSE
Place the stretcher at a right angle to the foot of the bed so that it will be in position for the carriers after they pivot away from the bed. Lock the wheels of the bed and the wheels of the stretcher.	
Arrange the persons lifting the patient according to height, with the tallest person at the patient's head.	The tallest person usually has the longest arm grasp, making it easier for him to support the patient's head and shoulders.
Stand facing the patient and prepare to slide the arms under him. The person in the middle places the arms directly under the patient's buttocks; the person at the head has one arm under the patient's head, neck, and shoulder area and the other arm directly against the middle person's arm; the person at the patient's feet has one arm also against the middle person's arm and the other arm under the patient's ankles.	The greatest weight is in the area of the buttocks. Having the middle person's armspread smaller than that of the other two persons helps to prevent strain on this person. Having the arms of the first and the third persons touch the arms of the middle person provides additional support in the heaviest area.
Slide the arms under the patient as far as possible and get in a position to slide the patient to the edge of the bed.	Place one leg forward, the thigh resting against the bed and the knees flexed, and put on the internal girdle.
Lean over the patient and on signal simultaneously rock back and slide the patient to the edge of the bed.	Movement is accomplished by rocking backward and attempting to "sit down"; the weight of the nurses and the power of their arms, hips, and knees move the patient.
Place the arms farther underneath the patient. Prepare to "logroll" the patient onto the chests of all three at the same time the patient is being lifted from the bed.	Place one leg forward, flex the knees, and put on the internal girdle. "Logrolling" the patient onto the carriers brings the centers of gravity of all objects closer, thereby increasing the stability of the group and reducing strain on the carriers.
Pivot around to the stretcher and, on signal, lower the patient onto the stretcher.	Flex the knees, have one foot forward, and bring your own body down with the patient, thus letting the large leg and arm muscles do the work of lowering the patient.

cause the backrest and the arms get in the way of the persons lowering the patient.

It is possible for only one person to get a helpless patient into a chair, although two people simplify matters. The single-person technique is a valuable procedure for nurses to know for the home care of invalids and for emergency use. Often, only one family member is available to assist the patient out of bed and to return him to it. More than one person should be available if the bed and chair seat are not the same height. The technique for a single person to move a patient from a bed to a chair and to return him to the bed is included in the boxes on the following page.

Self-help Devices for Patients Having Activity Limitations

While it is recognized that abilities totally lost cannot be recreated, those abilities which remain should be developed to their fullest capacities. Patients who have lost the full use of a muscle group can be helped to learn new ways in which to continue their activities of daily living when they are no longer confined to bed. Of considerable help to such patients are the numerous self-help devices which are being designed and manufactured. Some of these items are available through mail-order houses and department stores. Others are sold by medical supply companies. Items such as walkers, canes, bed

SINGLE PERSON MOVING A HELPLESS PATIENT FROM BED TO CHAIR

The purpose is to move a helpless patient out of bed when his weight makes it impossible for the only available person to lift him.

SUGGESTED ACTION	RELATED BODY MECHANICS FOR THE NURSE
Place the chair facing and against the bed at a point near the patient's buttocks to receive the patient and to use as a brace.	
Slide the upper portion of the patient's body to the edge of the bed. (This makes the patient lie diagonally on the bed.)	Place the arms under the patient's head and shoulders. Place one foot forward and rock backward.
Place the arms well under the patient's axillae from the rear. (The patient's head and shoulders will be resting on the nurse.)	Support the upper portion of the patient's body on yourself to reduce the weight of the patient to be moved.
Move around to the back of the chair, pulling the patient into the chair while so doing.	Lean against the back of the chair to keep it from moving and to brace yourself. Rock back and pull the patient into the chair.
Pull the chair away from the bed until the patient's feet are on the edge of the bed, being careful not to pull the chair out from under the patient.	Flex the knees, grasp the chair near the seat, and rock back.
Support the patient's legs while lowering the feet to the floor.	Flex the knees while lowering the patient's feet to the floor.

SINGLE PERSON MOVING A HELPLESS PATIENT FROM CHAIR TO BED

The purpose is to move a helpless patient from a chair into a bed when his weight makes it impossible for the only available person to lift him.

SUGGESTED ACTION	RELATED BODY MECHANICS FOR THE NURSE
Bring the chair directly alongside the bed with the patient facing the foot of the bed. Place a pillow on the arm of the chair.	Slide the chair rather than lifting one side at a time. If the floor has a polished surface, slide the chair on a small rug or rags.
Lift the patient's legs onto the edge of the bed.	Flex the knees and lower the body and support both the patient's legs when coming to an erect position.
Go behind the chair, grasp the patient under the axillae from the rear and roll him onto the bed.	Face the back of the chair and the bed at an angle. Have a wide base of support and rock to move the patient onto the bed.
Move the chair and help the patient into the desired position.	Slide the chair with your foot and brace yourself against the bed to prevent the patient from falling off.

trapezes, and wheelchairs are all available for home use. Some patients find that braces and prosthetic devices give them added support.

Examples of self-help items used in personal care include elastic shoe laces which eliminate the need for tying laces, long-handled shoehorns which eliminate the need for bending down to put on shoes, handbrushes and toothbrushes which need not be grasped, and a nail clipper which can be worked by a foot pedal.

For the handicapped homemaker there are numerous items which facilitate activities associated with cooking and cleaning, such as a one-handed eggbeater, a safety cutting board which holds food in place while it is being pared or cut, a long-handled dustpan, a one-handed food chopper, an auto-

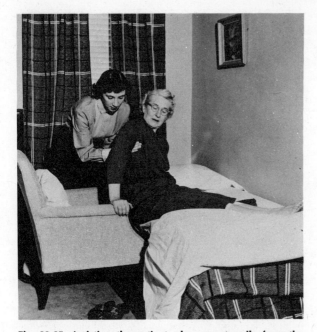

Fig. 22-25. Assisting the patient who cannot walk, from the bed to the chair. The chair is placed facing the bed, and the patient is assisted to the edge of the bed so that she is able to support herself on the arms of the chair. With assistance from a family member, she is guided and supported as she slides into the chair.

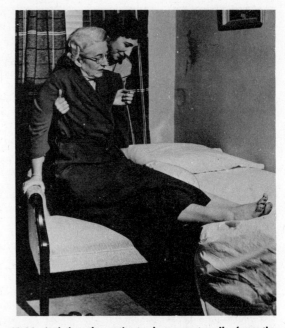

Fig. 22-26. Assisting the patient who cannot walk, from the chair to the bed. The chair is placed next to the bed. A pillow is wedged alongside the arm of the chair nearest the bed, and the patient's feet are brought up on the bed. The family member then assists the patient to lift up in the chair and guides and supports her onto the arm of the chair and the pillow before completing the move into bed.

matic pressure saucepan, mixing bowls with a suction base, and an interchangeable grater, slicer, and shredder held securely on a frame. Many of these items are of value to anyone. They reduce the amount of energy expended and therefore lessen fatigue.

Self-help items for the handicapped are varied in number and complexity. They can range from homemade devices to specially designed automobiles. The purpose of all of them is to promote the independence and individuality of the patient.

LEISURE-TIME ACTIVITIES FOR THE PATIENT

It was stated earlier in this chapter that the concept of rehabilitation involved prevention as well as restoration and physical as well as psychological functioning. Thus far, primarily physical measures have been discussed. While it is true that the physical body cannot truly be separated from the psychosocial, the remainder of the chapter will focus on nonphysical aspects of rehabilitation.

The concept of rehabilitation implies active involvement of the patient. Since the intention, desire, or inner drive must be present in order to be involved, the patient must possess some motivation. Motivation is usually a response to a felt need. One person cannot create or provide motivation for another, but it is possible for an individual to stimulate, support, and foster motivation in someone else. This responsibility is often part of the nurse's role. There are various types of motivational techniques that are described in other texts. The discussion here will be a brief general introduction.

Persons often are or can be motivated to initiate the exercises and activities mentioned earlier for both the well person and the ill person. They can also be motivated to use their leisure time in a meaningful fashion. Leisure time can be planned and desired, or it can be unexpectedly enforced. Diversion or recreation are terms that are frequently associated with leisure-time activities. Activities that fill this time in a meaningful way can be productive to the individual in terms of his self-concept, learning of new ideas and skills, and enjoyment and satisfaction. They can be a means to develop muscles, to

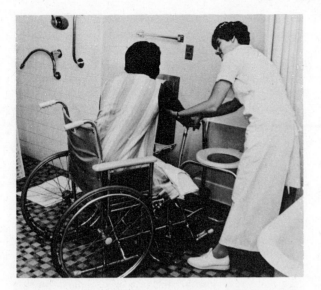

Fig. 22-27. Many hospitals now have continuing care (or interim care) units. Here patients who are not acutely ill but not able to be self-sufficient at home can learn to take care of themselves. In this training unit this patient is receiving some assistance from the nurse. She will be helped onto the shower chair which is secured against the wall. After she is undressed she can be wheeled into the shower which has a low water spigot so that her head does not become wet. There is a disposable mat at the doorway to the shower, and the nurse wears a long plastic apron to protect her uniform and legs. (Photo, Warren R. Vroom)

be involved in therapeutic social interaction, to learn new skills, to retain or gain independence and dignity, or to express emotions. Or, activities can serve to help the time pass more quickly or to provide pleasure. The motivation that a person has toward an activity is dependent on his felt needs.

There are a wide variety of types of leisure-time activities that may be helpful to a patient, but like all other aspects of care, the nurse must consider the individuality of the particular patient in order to be helpful to him. Some patients and families develop their own activities while others need the support and assistance of the nurse.

The nurse has to consider the patient's needs and his strengths, the specific purposes activities are to achieve, the patient's interests and limitations, and available facilities and resources.

Probably the most important single factor in helping a patient with planning diversional activities is his participation in decision making. In order for the activity to have some positive value for him, it must be something he wishes to do. Some patients will want to pursue previous interests. Others can often be assisted to develop interests they did not have previously.

Diversional activities are seen as so important in daily living that extensive investigations of the concept of leisure time and ways it can be used are

Fig. 22-28. The active teen-ager who is convalescing usually needs varied diversional activities to keep him occupied. Here, the young patient looks as if he is enjoying making a successful move against his mother.

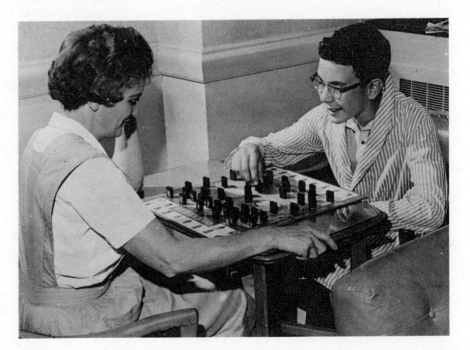

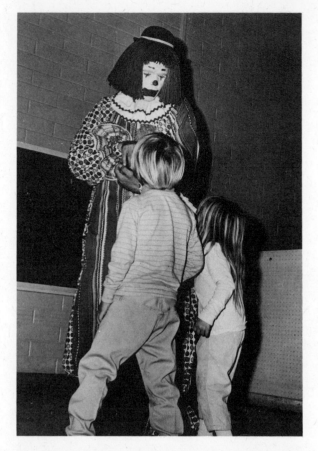

Fig. 22-29. Memories are likely to be pleasant for these young patients who enjoy a visit from Mr. Clown in the health clinic's playroom. (Courtesy Good Samaritan Hospital, Phoenix, Arizona)

being conducted in this country. Many different community and private groups organize efforts to provide leisure-time activities. There are recreational facilities with specially prepared persons who supervise activities that appeal to all age groups and a wide variety of interests and abilities. Health institutions, especially those dealing with the chronically ill patient, often have both recreational therapists and occupational therapists, and extensive programs for both children and adults.

Helping to Select Diversional Activities

Diversional activities can serve a variety of purposes. Very often they are intended primarily to help a person to relax while doing things that are of interest to him. This is especially true of patients who are convalescing after acute illnesses but who can expect to return relatively soon to their usual leisure and work.

It is possible to purchase or to select games or projects on the basis of age, size of group, and degree of difficulty of the activity, in relation to the desired purpose. For example, it is possible to assist quiet and withdrawn individuals to participate comfortably in a group situation or to select a diversion which will help to quiet and relax the more active individual.

When illness or incapacity is prolonged or chronic, recreation that a person enjoyed before his illness may not interest him, or certain activities may no longer be appropriate. Recreation then may be planned to find new and suitable means of spending leisure time. For example, a person with partial permanent paralysis following a cerebrovascular accident may have to give up certain sports and find substitutes. He may lose all interest or become a passive participant.

Recreation is often a good way to keep a child contented in bed and relatively quiet during illness and convalescence. Although activity is restricted, imagination can travel far and wide through toys and games, making confinement seem less bridling. Robert Louis Stevenson's poem, "The Land of Counterpane," illustrates poignantly how toys can help the ill child roam far from his confining bed:

When I was sick and lay a-bed,
I had two pillows at my head,
And all my toys beside me lay
To keep me happy all the day.

And sometimes for an hour or so
I watched my leaden soldiers go
With different uniforms and drills,
Among the bed-clothes, through the hills.

And sometimes sent my ships in fleets
All up and down among the sheets;
Or brought my trees and houses out,
And planted cities all about.

I was the giant great and still
That sits upon the pillow-hill,
And sees before him, dale and plain,
The pleasant land of counterpane.

For older children, group games offer both companionship and challenge for the participants. Play can also promote learning and provide an emotional outlet.

Children's play often serves a useful purpose in aiding to evaluate physical and mental development. The observant nurse can use play as a tool for planning not only a youngster's recreation but many aspects of his care as well.

Diversional activities often are used in occupational therapy. Occupational therapy is a prescribed and supervised rehabilitation procedure involving manual and/or creative activities. For instance, a patient may be referred to the occupational therapy department for an activity which will exercise certain muscle groups in the hand and the arm. There the patient may be required to do something that he never has done before, but in all instances the therapist will try to offer a choice of suitable activities so that the patient may enjoy doing it. Some patients may be referred to the occupational therapy department to learn a new vocation so that they may seek employment after they have recovered. Typical would be an amputee who previously was a bus driver. Or, some patients may be referred to the occupational therapy department to engage in an activity in which they already have some skill. For such a patient the immediate interest in a constructive activity is therapeutic because it gives him self-confidence from the beginning and occupies his time constructively. In still other situations, patients may wish to engage in activities which help merely to pass the time.

The diversional needs of acutely ill patients may be little other than perhaps visits with family and friends and receiving and reading mail. When convalescence is short, patients may require very little assistance in finding diversional activities, since they quickly begin to assume their usual way of life. Their ordinary interests appear, and these are pursued with little effort needed on the part of the nurse.

The person with a long term illness or disability may require assistance. Very often, the diversion is akin to a person's occupation, but it can also be the opposite. For example, it is not uncommon to see a person with excellent manual dexterity, such as a surgeon, paint or sculpt as a diversion, or a highway engineer building a model railroad layout at home. On the other hand, one with a confining occupation, such as a research chemist, may like gardening or golf or other outdoor hobbies. Helping a patient to feel more comfortable while ill very often requires the nurse's display of interest in his usual hobbies or diversions. It may be that he had not thought of them because he was confined. If it is not possible for him to enjoy the identical diversions, close sub-

stitutes perhaps can be found. Any diversion that can be provided which makes the patient more at ease contributes to a therapeutic climate.

Like adults, children are unsatisfied with activities that are of no interest to them. The diversion selected will have to be considered carefully from the standpoint of the child's interest in it, the amount of physical activity involved, and the possible emotional reactions to it.

In certain instances, the patient may prefer group activity to solitary diversion, but here again his condition must be taken into account. Obviously, a patient in a full body cast cannot join in a game of ping pong, but probably he can play cards; a game of solitaire may suffice during times when other persons cannot come to join him in a group game.

Wherever group activities are concerned, like interests are involved. When organizing such events and inviting patients to join them, it should be remembered that recreation for one individual may not be such for another and that points of difference can cause stress and conflict for a patient. For example, if a nurse were to say to a group of patients on a sun porch, "I'll turn the television on so you can all watch the baseball game this afternoon," she may annoy those who have no interest in the game. In other words, the nurse should avoid making patients feel compelled to join in.

For persons confined for long periods of time, group activities usually are enjoyable. Just being in a group may be satisfying in itself. Some agencies have parties on patients' birthdays and on certain holidays, as well as planned events for other special occasions. If given the opportunity, some patients enjoy the challenge of organizing, decorating, and planning for group recreation such as a party, a skit, or a game.

When helping to select diversions, remember that most people need variety. Few care to pursue a single thing all day or day after day. Children and young adults are especially likely to succumb to boredom.

Common Diversions for Patients

READING AND WRITING: Many persons enjoy at least some reading during their leisure time. Books, magazines, and newspapers are usually available in most health agencies. For those unable to visit the library, volunteers in many agencies bring reading materials to the patients.

Some persons also enjoy writing while hospitalized. This is especially true with those who have long-term illness or are not acutely ill. Chronically ill persons often enjoy pen pals. New mothers usually write birth announcements while hospitalized.

The arrival of mail generally is a pleasant experience for confined patients. It is a way to keep in touch with family and friends, and many patients derive great pleasure in displaying the cards that they receive. Very ill patients, or those unable to open their mail, may appreciate help with this. The person bringing the patient his mail should offer to open the envelope and read the card or message to the patient if he so desires. It may be a comforting message from someone who is unable to visit.

TELEVISION AND RADIO: Most health agencies and homes have provisions for patients to use television and radio sets. For those hospitalized patients who are ambulatory, sets often are available in patient lounges and recreation rooms. Many people enjoy watching television or listening to a radio for at least part of every day; and except for the very ill and the very young, this usually is appropriate. It should be remembered that television and radio programs may be a source of annoyance for other persons in a health agency setting; therefore, the volume should be kept at a moderate level.

ARTS AND CRAFTS: Recreation involving any of the arts and the crafts can be especially rewarding in that something is created, and the end-products are useful and decorative. Frequently, arts and crafts are suggested to patients if the activity involved is also beneficial for a specific physical limitation.

TOYS: Toys can be the source of much pleasure for the hospitalized child. They should be carefully selected on the basis of factors discussed earlier in this chapter. In addition, safety must be kept in mind when selecting toys. Those with small removable parts should be avoided because of the danger of swallowing them. Also to be avoided are toys with sharp edges or points. Interesting and inexpensive toys can be made from common objects found in the home. Toys that stimulate the imagination can provide diversion for older children.

EATING AND SOCIALIZING: Eating with others is a symbol of family life and is taken for granted in many cultures. Almost no one likes to eat alone, and efforts to bring a patient to the family table or into a dining area with other patients usually are rewarding. Many of the chronic-illness hospitals have patient dining rooms, and often ambulatory patients may go to the dining room or cafeteria for meals.

Many pediatric services arrange to have children eat together. Often, children eat more willingly when with others, and the handicapped are stimu-

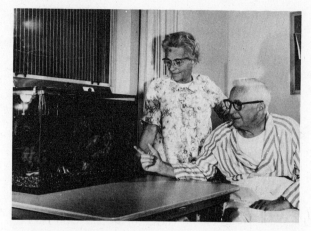

Fig. 22-30. For these patients in a chronic disease unit, a visit to the aquarium and opportunities to socialize with others offer pleasant diversion. (Courtesy Good Samaritan Hospital, Phoenix, Arizona)

lated to do their best to be more like their peers.

Patient lounges are seen commonly in psychiatric hospitals, rehabilitation centers, and chronic-illness hospitals. Here, patients can enjoy games together, meet for chatting, watch television, and so forth. For persons who do not socialize readily, a patients' lounge with opportunities to meet or be near others often can make the difference between loneliness and the satisfaction of being one of a group.

VISITORS: Most patients enjoy visits with family members and friends. At one time most health agencies observed very limited visiting privileges, the reason being that visitors often were thought to upset patients as well as the hospital routines. However, most hospitals have become increasingly lenient in the provision of visiting privileges, as health personnel have observed the therapeutic value for patients. On pediatric services, visiting privileges in the past often were extremely limited. But in agencies where most barriers for visiting have been removed, the children have demonstrated a marked increase in morale, resulting in definite therapeutic benefit.

Visitors in the home as well as the health agency can be therapeutic for the patient. In addition to the pleasure the patient has when a relative or friend visits, some agencies permit the visitor to aid in the patient's care. Examples include assisting the patient with eating, with walking, and with caring for the nails and hair. Under some circumstances, it may even be helpful to the patient if a family member can aid in administering medications or convincing the patient to take them.

Visiting can be overdone, and health personnel generally agree that some limitations still must be observed. For the very ill, a limitation on the length of time visitors may stay or on the number of visitors present at one time may be necessary. While visiting policies are necessary, good judgment still must be used on the basis of the individual situation. In certain instances, because of the danger of infection (such as following organ transplants) no visitors may be allowed for some hospitalized patients.

PATIENTS AS HELPERS: There was a time when patients were expected to help each other and to assist with work in health agencies when such work did not interfere with their recovery. However, using patients as helpers is uncommon today in acute care facilities. In those agencies where this system has been used judiciously, the results have been impressive. For some patients, being able to help is gratifying and gives a feeling of personal accomplishment, besides relieving boredom. A few examples of things that patients can do to help are: acting as interpreter when language barriers occur, reading to patients who are unable to do so, making telephone calls for bedridden patients, writing letters for patients who are incapacitated, making beds, and assisting with landscaping care.

OTHER MISCELLANEOUS DIVERSIONS: Some agencies have facilities for swimming, movies, operating a radio station, canteens, auditoriums for social events, and the like. In general, it seems that as facilities and opportunities for diversion increase, patients' attitudes toward health agencies would improve. Long-term confinement agencies need not be as dreary and impersonal as was often the case in previous years.

Community recreational facilities promote activities such as singing, dancing, group exercises, game playing, and craftwork for patients of all ages. Special activities for the handicapped and chronically ill in their homes or in community centers are available in some areas.

CONCLUSION

Maintenance or restoration of body function is strongly influenced by posture, movement, and activity. Well persons and ill persons and family members frequently need assistance from the nurse in the form of instruction and explanation, demonstration, and support. The nurse can protect herself and promote the most effective learning of others by developing good habits in her own personal life.

Study Situations

1. Assume you are a community health nurse and have just had a patient referred to you who is partially paralyzed below the waist following an auto accident. What information would you want to collect about your patient in regard to posture, exercise, and activity? Make a list of the specific data you would gather and the sources you would use.

2. Gaining independence for the paraplegic requires intense and deliberate practice. The pictures in these two articles show how paralyzed persons can be helped to transfer from their bed to a chair and to a commode and back:
   Kern, F. C., and Poole, L.: Transfer techniques: an illustrated guide. **Nurs. '72,** 2:25–28, July, 1972.
   Jordon, H. S., and Kavchak, M. A.: Transfer techniques. **Nurs. '73,** 3:19–22, Mar., 1973.
   What are the five points the July 1972 article suggests that the nurse remember? How could these suggestions be implemented with nonparalyzed patients?

3. Disabled persons usually prefer to remain in their own homes whenever possible. Read how one state took steps to make it possible for 3,200 dependent persons to stay out of nursing homes and other long-term care institutions.
   Stohl, D. J.: Preserving home life for the disabled. **Am. J. Nurs.,** 72:1645–1650, Sept., 1972.

4. Most persons find group activities enjoyable. This article discusses the approach one hospital used to promote group exercises:
   Griffin, W., et al.: Group exercise for patients with limited motion. **Am. J. Nurs.,** 71:1742–1743, Sept., 1971.
   How do the authors suggest the exercise routines could be carried out in institutions where patients are in four-bed rooms?

5. Many families with young children exist on very limited budgets. What are some of the ways the author of the following article suggests safe and stimulating toys can be prepared inexpensively for young children?
   Alexander, M. M.: Homemade fun for infants. **Am. J. Nurs.,** 70:2557–2560, Dec., 1970.

6. There are various views on the concept of recreation. The author of the following reference reminds us that the word has a Latin origin meaning "to refresh, to restore, or to create anew." Read the chapter to see how she distinguishes between the "experience" of recreation and the "activities" of recreation. What relationship does she see between recreation and self-image development?
   Heinly, J. L.: The patient's need for recreation. In Bergersen, B. S., et al., eds.: Current Concepts in Clinical Nursing. pp. 137–153. St. Louis, C. V. Mosby, 1967.

References

1. Barry, E. M., et al.: Hospital program for cardiac rehabilitation. **Am. J. Nurs.,** 72: 2174–2177, Dec., 1972.

2. Bierbauer, E.: Tips for parents of a neurologically handicapped child. **Am. J. Nurs.,** 72:1872–1874, Oct., 1972.

3. Brooks, M. M.: Why play in the hospital? In **The Nursing Clinics of North America.** Philadelphia, W. B. Saunders, 5:431–441, Sept., 1970.

4. Brower, P., and Hicks, D.: Maintaining muscle function in patients on bed rest. **Am. J. Nurs.,** 72:1250–1253, July, 1972.

5. Campbell, E. B.: Nursing problems associated with prolonged recovery following trauma. In **The Nursing Clinics of North America.** Philadelphia, W. B. Saunders, 5:551–562, Dec., 1970.

6. Carnevali, D., and Brueckner, S.: Immobilization—assessment of a concept. **Am. J. Nurs.,** 70:1502–1507, July, 1970.

7. Carroll, B.: Fingers to toes. **Am. J. Nurs.,** 71:550–551, Mar., 1971.

8. Chazov, E.: Activity breeds relaxation. **World Health,** 14–19, Feb.–Mar., 1972.

9. Courtial, D. C.: The patient with low back pain: bed positioning. **Hosp. Manage.,** 109:66–70, Apr., 1970.

10. Drury, J. H. Jr.: Handbook of range-of-motion exercises. **Nurs. '72,** 2:19–22, Apr., 1972.

11. Foss, G.: Body mechanics: use your head and save your back. **Nurs. '73,** 3:25–32, May, 1973.

12. ————: The 'how to's' of bed positioning. **Nurs. '72,** 2:14–16, Aug., 1972.

13. Germain, C. P.: Exercise makes the heart grow stronger. **Am. J. Nurs.,** 72:2169–2173, Dec., 1972.

14. Goldstrom, D. K.: Cardiac rest: bed or chair? **Am. J. Nurs.,** 72:1812–1816, Oct., 1972.

15. Hagerman, C. W., and Moore, V. B.: Handbook of bed positions and guide to electrically operated beds. **Nurs. '72,** 2:19–26, Mar., 1972.

16. Hahn, J., and Burns, K. R.: Mrs. Richards, a rabbit, and remotivation. **Am. J. Nurs.,** 73:302–304, Feb., 1973.

17. Hott, J.: ℞; play PRN in pediatric nursing. **Nurs. Forum,** 9:288–309, No. 3, 1970.

18. Hrobsky, A.: The patient on a circOlectric bed. **Am. J. Nurs.,** 71:2352–2353, Dec., 1971.

19. Kamenetz, H. L.: Exercises for the elderly. **Am. J. Nurs.,** 72:1401, Aug., 1972.

20. ————: Selecting a wheelchair. **Am. J. Nurs.,** 72:100–101, Jan., 1972.

21. Kelly, M. M.: Exercises for bedfast patients. **Am. J. Nurs.,** 66:2209–2213, Oct., 1966.

22. Kinnaman, P.: The last word. **Nurs. Outlook,** 18:52–53, Feb., 1970.

23. Kottke, F. J., and Blanchard, R. S.: Bedrest begets bedrest. **Nurs. Forum,** 3:56–72, No. 3, 1964.

24. Lavin, M. A.: Bed exercises for acute cardiac patients. **Am. J. Nurs.,** 73:1226–1227, July, 1973.

25. Lowman, E. W., and Klinger, J. L.: Aids to Independent Living: Self-Help for the Handicapped. New York, McGraw-Hill, 1969.

26. Lyon, G. G.: Stimulation through remotivation. **Am. J. Nurs.,** 71:982–986, May, 1971.

27. Merton, P. A.: How we control the contraction of our muscles. **Sci. Am.,** 226:30–37, May, 1972.

28. Millen, H. M.: Physically fit for nursing. **Am. J. Nurs.,** 70:520–523, Mar., 1970.

29. Murphy, D. C.: The therapeutic value of children's literature. **Nurs. Forum,** 11:141–164, No. 2, 1972.

30. Olson, E. V.: The hazards of immobility. **Am. J. Nurs.,** 67:779–797, Apr., 1967.

31. Palmer, E. M., and Griffith, E. W.: Effect of activity during bedmaking on heart rate and blood pressure. **Nurs. Res.,** 20:17–25, Jan.–Feb., 1971.

32. Quigley, J. L., and Walcott, A.: Recreation renews interest in life. **Hospitals, J. Am. Hosp. Assoc.,** 46:53–57, Nov. 1, 1972.

33. Ranalls, J.: Crutches and walkers. **Nurs. '72,** 2:21–24, Dec., 1972.

34. Stop think—then lift. **Nurs. Mirror,** 134:9–11, June 23, 1972.

35. Winters, M. C.: Protective Body Mechanics in Daily Life and in Nursing: A Manual for Nurses and Their Co-Workers. Philadelphia, W. B. Saunders, 1952.

36. Works, R. F.: Hints on lifting and pulling. **Am. J. Nurs.,** 72:260–261, Feb., 1972.

CHAPTER 23

Promoting Comfort, Rest, and Sleep

GLOSSARY • INTRODUCTION • DESCRIPTION AND CHARACTERISTICS
OF PAIN • GENERAL PRINCIPLES IN RELATION TO PAIN •
NURSING MEASURES TO PROMOTE COMFORT • DESCRIPTION
AND CHARACTERISTICS OF SLEEP • SLEEP DEPRIVATION •
COMMON DISORDERS OF SLEEP • GENERAL PRINCIPLES
IN RELATION TO SLEEP • NURSING MEASURES TO PROMOTE
REST AND SLEEP • CONCLUSION •
STUDY SITUATIONS • REFERENCES

GLOSSARY

Delta Sleep: Deep sleep, occurring during Stage III and especially Stage IV in NREM sleep.

Diffuse Pain: Discomfort that covers a large area.

Dull Pain: Discomfort of a gnawing type but less intense and acute than sharp pain.

Enuresis: Involuntary urination.

Insomnia: Difficulty in falling asleep, intermittent sleep and/or early awakening from sleep.

Intermittent Pain: Discomfort that comes and goes.

NREM or Non-REM: Refers to non-rapid eye movement that characterizes four stages of sleep.

Pain: Sensation of physical and/or mental suffering or hurt that usually causes distress or agony to the one experiencing it.

Phantom Pain: The sensation of pain without demonstrable physiologic or pathologic substance.

Referred Pain: Pain in an area removed from that in which stimulation has its origin.

REM: Refers to rapid eye movement that characterizes the dream state of sleep.

Rest: Condition when body is in a decreased state of activity with consequent feeling of being refreshed.

Sharp Pain: Quick, sticking, and intense discomfort.

Shifting Pain: Discomfort that moves from one area to another.

Sleep: A state of relative unconsciousness.

Somnambulism: Sleepwalking.

INTRODUCTION

Chapter 22 pointed out the dangers of bed rest and discussed patients' needs for activity even when confined to bed. Without negating the importance of exercise and diversional activities, provisions for comfort and rest also are essential patient needs. In addition, when patients are comfortable and are meeting needs for rest and sleep, encouraging necessary activity often becomes an easier task, both for the patient and for the nurse. This chapter discusses some basic theory in relation to pain and sleep and measures that help to promote comfort and rest.

DESCRIPTION AND CHARACTERISTICS OF PAIN

Pain has intrigued the curiosity of science and has led to a huge array of pain-relieving techniques since time immemorial. Yet despite its universality and eternal presence among mankind, the nature of pain remains an enigma.

Pain has been defined, and occasionally still is, on a philosophical and religious basis as punishment for wrongdoing. Aristotle defined pain as well as anyone when he wrote that it is the "antithesis of pleasure . . . the epitome of unpleasantness." A typical dictionary definition indicates that *pain* is a sensation of physical and/or mental suffering or hurting that usually causes distress or agony to the one experiencing it. This general definition of pain becomes more precise when stated thus: "Pain is a basically unpleasant sensation referred to the body which represents the suffering induced by the psychic perception of real, threatened, or phantasied injury." (7:45)

There is still another aspect of pain. "Human pain is that condition which occurs when the human being is hurt . . . it is the spirit which is affected. The greatest hurts are the loss of loved ones or the loss of their love, but pain may be felt whenever there is abuse of person . . ." (25:910.)

Another approach to defining pain focuses on the person who experiences the pain. The nurse, along with the physician and other health practitioners, cannot see or feel the pain to which they will attend. They function in this area of care through experiences only the patient senses and describes. Therefore, one can say that pain ". . . is whatever the experiencing person says it is and exists whenever he says it does." (17:8) Recalling the content from Chapter 13, people communicate both verbally and nonverbally. In any definition of pain, therefore, the patient may well describe pain verbally; that is, he may state that he has a throbbing pain in the foot he has injured. Or, he may communicate nonverbally; that is, he may say nothing, but he refuses to walk on the affected foot and is reluctant to let the examiner touch it.

Pain is interpreted as a threat to the organism's integrity. It is an imperative sensation and has a preoccupying characteristic that tends to make us negate other sensations in its presence. Although pain may warn of tissue injury or disease, the degree of pain is not necessarily in direct proportion to the amount of tissue damage, nor is tissue damage always present when pain occurs.

There are two facets to pain—perception and reaction or response. *Perception* is concerned with the sensory processes when a stimulus for pain is present. It is based on previous experiences with pain along with a knowledge of pain and its characteristics. The reaction or response to pain is concerned with the organism's method of coping with the sensation. Although this distinction is made, the reader's attention is called to the fact that not all literature on the subject makes this same differentiation.

Perception of Pain

The threshold of perception is the lowest intensity of a stimulus that causes the subject to recognize pain. This threshold is remarkably similar for everyone. Still, it is theorized by some authorities that a phenomenon of *adaptation* does occur; that is, the threshold for pain can be changed within certain ranges. This phenomenon has been studied, for example, when prisoners of war reported that the pain of repeated torture was not as acute as it would have been under different circumstances. Many factors might well have played a role, but at least some adaptation appeared likely.

Another example of adaptation occurs when a person's hand is immersed in warm water. A sensation of pain eventually occurs as the water is heated. However, the person can tolerate a higher temperature as water is gradually heated to the pain level than he could have, had he plunged his hand into hot water without any preparation. This observation has practical implications, for example, when hot applications are applied to the body over a period of time. Even though tissues are damaged, the patient may not necessarily complain of pain when increasingly hot applications are made as he becomes accustomed to the heat.

Pain sensations are conducted along a pathway which has been rather clearly defined in certain areas, although it is still somewhat questionable in others. There are no specific pain organs or cells in the body. Rather, an interlacing network of undifferentiated nerve endings receive painful stimuli. Sensation is carried to the dorsal gray horn cells of the spinal cord, then to the spinothalamic tract and eventually to the cerebral cortex. Although the autonomic nervous system is an efferent system—that is, it carries impulses *from* the central nervous system —pain sensations from the viscera apparently course along the autonomic system. Through that system, these sensations from deep-lying structures reach the spinal cord by way of the dorsal roots and then continue along the same pathways as sensations from the skin and superficial body structures. Pain impulses are also carried by the cranial nerves to the central nervous system. There is integration (perception as well as reaction) of the sensory impulses of pain along its entire central nervous system route, but the highest level of integration occurs in the cortex.

Stimulants for Pain

When the threshold of perception for pain has been reached and when there is injured tissue, it is believed that the injured tissue releases chemicals that modify pain receptors by increasing their sensitivity. Receptors in the skin and superficial organs, although incapable of responding selectively, are stimulated by mechanical, thermal, chemical, and electrical agents. Friction from bed clothing and pressure from a cast are examples of mechanical stimulants. Sunburn and cold water on a tooth with caries are examples of thermal stimulants. An acid burn is the result of a chemical stimulant. The jolt of a static charge illustrates an electrical stimulant.

Stretching of the hollow viscera, pulling on the omentum, and muscle spasms result in pain. Some investigators believe that at least some of the deep-lying organs have their own individual pain receptors, the uterus being an example. Some organs are insensitive to pain, for example the lungs.

When tissue injury results in pain in an area removed from that in which stimulation has its origin, it is called *referred pain*. Very often, for example, patients with diseases of the gall bladder complain of pain in the upper back or shoulder areas. Several theories have been advanced concerning the phenomenon of referred pain, but none has widespread acceptance.

There are essentially three responses the body makes to pain: voluntary, involuntary, and emotional or psychic.

Voluntary Responses to Pain

Voluntary responses are muscle reactions that trigger efforts to remove the painful stimulus. It is a kind of fight-or-flight reaction that spells protection or defense. One example is removing the hand hurriedly from a hot object. Grimacing and pacing the floor are examples also. Another person reacts by placing the injured part in a position that tends to relieve pain and by keeping the muscles rigid to maintain that position in efforts to avoid further injury. An example is to pull the knees up to the abdomen when abdominal pain is severe. These voluntary responses are protective in nature; also, through cognizance of pain, one remembers its causes and makes voluntary and purposeful attempts to avoid them in the future.

Involuntary Responses to Pain

Involuntary responses, often called autonomic responses, also are protective in nature, in that they increase the body's alertness to pain and promote organic homeostasis. In other words, the body prepares for emergency action. Examples include increases in perspiration, blood pressure, pulse and respiratory rates, pupil dilatation, and an increase in the output of adrenalin. The physiology of these in-

voluntary responses teaches how each one prepares the body for necessary action when a threat to its integrity exists.

Emotional or Psychic Responses to Pain

The emotional or psychic responses to pain have a wide and varying threshold among individuals. A person's previous experience with pain and his racial, cultural, and religious backgrounds all play a part. As one example, in certain cultures weeping, crying loudly, and other overt expressions of distress are part of the pain phenomenon. In other cultures, this behavior may be considered unacceptable. Personality characteristics also influence pain responses. Highstrung, neurotic persons in general have a low threshold of reaction, while stoic individuals appear to have a high threshold.

Preoccupation with other things has been observed to distract from pain. For example, soldiers severely wounded while under fire often indicate that they felt little pain until the excitement of battle subsided. Players injured during the exciting moments in a competitive game may be unaware of injury and pain until the game is completed. Making a loud noise, gripping an object (such as the dentist's chair), clenching the jaws, or experiencing pain elsewhere can alter pain and responses to it.

Pain is almost always accompanied by anxiety and fear, sometimes anger too. These emotional reactions tend to intensify the emotional reactions to pain. Under these conditions, a vicious circle forms that may be difficult to break. Increased irritability, depression, feelings of loneliness, fatigue due to poor resting, and anorexia often add to the problem of relieving pain.

GENERAL PRINCIPLES IN RELATION TO PAIN

From the previous discussions in relation to pain, some general principles can be stated that will guide the nurse when intervention is necessary.

Pain is a subjective and a personal experience, more often unpleasant but occasionally giving rise to ultimate pleasure for some persons, that is influenced by psychological, social, and cultural factors.

One human being cannot accurately assess the type and intensity of pain that another human being is experiencing. The nurse can only observe a patient and, by his verbal and nonverbal behavior, deduce that pain is present. For example, the nurse can presume a patient is in pain when he moans and flexes his legs sharply on his abdomen. But only the patient can describe the experience of pain, its location, and its severity.

While most often pain is unpleasant and is associated with misery and distress, some individuals appear to experience pleasure and use pain to meet certain needs. For example, when pain brings attention to a patient or possibly serves as punishment that relieves feelings of guilt, the ultimate result for the patient is satisfaction.

Cultural influences may teach some persons that to display signs of pain is to display personal weakness. Stoicism and self-control are virtues in such instances. On the other hand, outward behavioral displays when pain is present are accepted in other cultures.

It has been observed that anxiety and stress tend to influence pain. A vicious circle may develop as pain intensifies with increasing anxiety and stress.

Pain is a mixed sensation. To state this principle in another way, pain is not a pure sensation. It is associated with other sensations, as for example, the sensations of stretch, pull, pressure, squeeze, heat, or cold.

Generally speaking, pain correlates with the intensity of stimulation. Usually, the more intense the stimulation, the more likely it will produce pain. For example, there normally is pressure from a cast on the body part where it has been applied. The sensation of the pressure is not painful until it increases to the threshold of pain perception. Generally, it will increase sharply when injury to the tissue due to pressure of the cast occurs. However, it has also been observed that pain may be present without injury and may not be present with injury. Therefore, *tissue injury does not necessarily accompany pain in all instances.* For example, tissue injury is present when the patient experiences pain due to a burn. On the other hand, while physiologic changes occur, tissue injury or destruction is not necessarily present when the patient has a headache due to psychological tension. In addition, *intensity of pain may not accurately relate to the seriousness of a particular condition giving rise to the pain.* For example, the patient may not experience pain until the ravages of a malignancy are beyond control, while the severe pain that usually accompanies a bunion is not generally in keeping with the degree of pathology involved.

Stimulation of sensory receptors and intactness of their nerve supply are neither necessary nor sufficient conditions for pain. It would seem that a receptor for pain and a nerve route that eventually carries the impulse to the brain is necessary when pain is present; yet, it is well known that this is not always necessary. For example, the pain that is often referred to an amputated leg where receptors and nerves are clearly absent is a very real experience for the patient. This type of pain is called *phantom pain* and is without demonstrated physiologic or pathologic substance. As another example, the person who is hypnotized can describe pain when there has been no stimulation to produce pain.

Consciousness and attention are necessary to experience pain. The unconscious patient does not experience pain. Even during a conscious state, however, attention appears to be necessary in order to experience pain. For example, as pointed out earlier, a soldier in battle may not experience pain even when injury is marked until after the combat when he directs attention to the injury. Distraction from pain-producing situations, then, is often an effective method to assist in the relief of pain. This can be observed when a child is given a favorite toy to distract attention from a procedure that may be associated with pain, such as giving the child an injection.

NURSING MEASURES TO PROMOTE COMFORT

Understanding the Patient

Inasmuch as a patient's background is very likely to influence his reaction to pain, it is well to start learning something about the patient who is complaining of pain by using the process of data gathering described in Chapter 6. Here are some typical questions to which the nurse will wish to find answers. What cultural factors may be playing a role in the patient's experience of pain? How much does the patient know about his present illness and of the pain he is experiencing? What types of pain has the patient experienced in the past? How did he react then? What environmental and personality factors may be influencing his reactions to pain? Can the family assist in attempting to understand the patient's reaction to pain? Answers to questions such as these will help the nurse in selecting measures that are likely to promote the patient's comfort.

In addition, the nurse will want to familiarize herself with the patient's medical history, his diagnosis, and the physician's plan of therapy.

Understanding the Nature of the Pain

Observation is an important aspect of data gathering. The nurse should consider the quality, the intensity, and the location of pain. In addition, the nurse will want to know which factors tend to provoke pain and which ones tend to relieve it. What was its mode of onset? What has been its duration? If the patient has had previous experiences with similar pain, what measures tended to relieve pain at that time?

Listed below are some commonly used terms to describe the quality of pain.

Sharp: Quick, sticking, and intense.

Dull: Not so intense or acute as a sharp pain, possibly more annoying than painful.

Diffuse: Covering a large area. Usually, the patient is unable to point to a specific area without moving his hand over a large surface, such as the entire abdomen.

Shifting: Moving from one area to another, such as from the lower abdomen to the epigastric region.

Intermittent: Coming and going. It may or may not be regular.

Removing the Source of Pain and Decreasing Pain Stimuli

Although the source of pain is often illusive, in some situations it can be determined rather readily. Removing the source of pain is ideal and sometimes possible. Here are a few examples: removing or loosening a tight binder if permissible; seeing to it that a distended bladder is emptied; taking steps to relieve constipation and/or flatus; changing the patient's position in bed, and giving him a back rub if muscles have become tense and sore; and changing soiled linen that may be irritating the skin. It is often the nurse who identifies a source of pain that can be remedied with relative ease.

There are factors that may be contributing to discomfort and removing their source often promotes comfort. For example, although the factors given in the previous paragraph are not the actual or only sources of pain for certain patients, they may be contributing to discomfort. Hence, the suggested nursing measures given above apply also in helping to decrease painful stimuli. The hungry or thirsty patient may need a snack or a drink to feel more comfortable. Fatigue tends to increase sensitivity to pain, and promoting rest with measures as discussed later in this chapter is helpful. If the source of pain is an exuding wound, a soiled wet dressing may be the source of trouble and changing it will promote comfort. For the patient uncomfortable

with a cast after the fracture of an extremity, elevating the extremity may relieve pressure sufficiently to promote comfort. The patient in pain usually feels more comfortable when the environment is quiet and restful. Taking steps to eliminate unnecessary noise and glaring lights is helpful. Sometimes the nurse may want to speak with visitors who may be tiring the patient in pain. These measures are also useful when caring for patients in their homes.

These are just a few examples of nursing measures that experience has shown can aid in promoting patient comfort. Almost every chapter in this text offers still more additional suggestions for alleviating discomfort. The ingenious and resourceful nurse who has observed her patient with care is armed with a host of measures that, when used with skill, aid in assisting the patient suffering with pain.

Offering Emotional Support

Experience and research on controlling pain have shown that nursing measures offering emotional support to the patient are essential aids in relieving pain. The reader is encouraged to review Chapters 11 and 12, which offered suggestions in helping patients who are anxious and fearful.

One study found that reduction of a patient's pain occurred following certain nurse/patient interactions. After introductions to initiate the interaction, the process included discussing pain with the patient, suggesting various pain-relieving measures other than medications, and allowing the patient to decide on the method of relief. In the experimental group of adult patients with moderate pain, most of them experienced relief with this type of nursing care. (21)

In another reference at the end of this chapter, the authors describe discussing pain with the patient, remaining with the patient and providing touch as important tools for providing comfort. (18)

Experience has demonstrated that patients who feel confident in health personnel caring for them do not require as much therapy for the relief of pain as those who are less confident. Without confidence, nothing seems to work. With it, often amazing results have been obtained using measures that ordinarily are only modestly effective.

Teaching in Relation to Pain

The well-informed patient is often better able to cope with distressing situations, pain being an example. The nurse should share knowledge with the patient experiencing pain to the extent possible as an aid in promoting comfort. Sometimes assisting the patient to understand the cause for his pain is helpful in reducing it. Or, helping the patient to know that it is usual and acceptable to have pain and to express it may be important. In most situations, teaching in relation to pain will include family members in order that they too may help the patient in pain.

Medically Prescribed Measures

There are times when medically prescribed measures become important. There is available a wide variety of analgesic drugs that certainly play an important role in pain control. When medication is required and is used judiciously, its administration is indeed desirable. However, using drugs as a substitute for good nursing care is an act indefensible for nurses interested in holding to high standards of patient care.

In certain instances, when pain is intractable, the physician may find it necessary to use procedures that obliterate or sever pathways for pain impulses. Even when such are indicated, they do not replace the patient's need for high caliber and individualized care which includes physical as well as emotional support.

The procedure of acupuncture has gained much attention recently and has reportedly been used often with success to control pain. At present, there is no widespread acceptance of a theory to explain the phenomena associated with acupuncture. One area of research deals with a neurological approach and is investigating whether the acupuncture needles block the transmission of pain from peripheral nerves to the central nervous system and/or whether there is a shutting off of pain in the cerebral cortex. The possibility of the patient being in a hypnotic or posthypnotic state also is being investigated as a plausible explanation.

Table 23-1 offers a pain profile that serves well as a summary for this section dealing with pain.

DESCRIPTION AND CHARACTERISTICS OF SLEEP

The word rest has a very broad meaning: refreshing ease or inactivity after exertion; relief from anything that wearies, troubles, or disturbs. In this chapter, *rest* connotes a condition in which the body is in a decreased state of activity with the consequent feeling of being refreshed. For some, rest occurs while leisurely enjoying a break in the day's activities. For others, rest may not come until sleep.

Sleep is a state of relative unconsciousness. The scientist recognizes that sleep, contrary to most laymen's beliefs, is not a quiescent and passive state but rather a progression of repeated cycles, each representing different phases of body and brain activity. These cycles have been studied and analyzed with the help of the electroencephalograph which receives and records electrical currents from the brain. The depth of unconsciousness during sleep is not uniform. Rather, it fluctuates during the different stages of sleep. This is demonstrated when it is observed that varying degrees of stimuli produce wakefulness.

The depth of unconsciousness for the sensory organs also varies. For example, the depth is greatest for the sense of smell, which may explain why home fires gain headway unbeknownst to the sleeping occupants, who do not smell the smoke. The depth is least for pain and for hearing. This explains why ill persons often are wakeful, because pain frequently accompanies illness.

REM Sleep and NREM Sleep

Research illustrates that there are two major states of sleep: rapid eye movement, referred to as *REM* (sometimes also referred to as Stage I-*REM*); and nonrapid eye movement, referred to as *non-REM* or *NREM*.

During the REM state, it has been observed that the eyes tend to dart back and forth, respirations increase, the heartbeat becomes more rapid, and blood pressure increases. If persons are awakened during this state, they almost invariably report that they have been dreaming. In fact, many researchers now state that everyone dreams; those who state they do not simply are unable to recall dreams they had.

When dream deprivation occurs experimentally, that is, when persons are awakened during REM, the subjects become irritable, insecure, and anxious. Inability to concentrate, often leading to poor judgment, usually can be observed with sleep deprivation. Relationships with other people also suffer. Depression is a common mental symptom, and in extreme cases, a person's ethical standards have been known to deteriorate. Symptoms of psychoses have appeared in rational people after prolonged REM sleep deprivation. These same subjects, when allowed to sleep uninterrupted, experience more frequent REM periods, as if the body were trying to make up for losses.

The REM state of sleep is sometimes referred to as paradoxical sleep because it seems as though

TABLE 23-1: Pain profile in relation to source of input*

	Location	Intensity	Temporal aspects	Description	Associated physiologic aspects	Behavior
Superficial Somatic	Surface; well localized	Basically correlated with intensity of stimulation	Correlates with tempo of input and extent of after-discharge	In terms of familiar surface injuries; mainly determined by spatial-temporal intensity dimensions	Intensified by contact; alleviated by gentle stimulation in adjacent areas	Guarding of involved area; application of warmth, cold, soothing agent, counter irritation
Deep Somatic	Segmental; deep; poorly localized; radiates; referred to surface	Basically correlated with intensity of stimulation	Correlates with tempo of input and extent of after-discharge	Vague, aching, sharp, boring, pounding; mainly determined by spatial-temporal intensity dimensions	Intensified by movement, compression, pulsation, (artery); alleviated by inactivity	Avoidance of movement, pressure; awkward movement due to protective spasm
Visceral	Segmental; deep; poorly localized; radiates; referred to surface	Basically correlated with intensity of stimulation	Correlates with tempo of input and extent of after-discharge	Griping, cramping, aching, squeezing, crushing, stabbing, burning; mainly determined by spatial-temporal intensity dimensions	Intensified by motor activity or compression of involved viscus, correlates with secretory or motor rhythms of involved viscus	Trial and error behavior to relieve pain, based on physiologic concomitants, previous experience, psychic factors
Neurogenic	Within neural distribution; surface or deep; radiates	Excessive response to stimulation	No correlation with input	Indescribable; unlike any naturally occurring pain; unusual combination of painful sensations	Provoked by any peripheral stimulation in involved zone; trigger points "spontaneous" paroxysms	Vigilant guarding of involved part—apprehensive concern
Psychogenic	According to body image or appropriate to fantasy; surface or deep; well or poorly localized; may radiate	Variable; correlates with psychic needs for suffering, intensity of guilt, aggression, depression; inconsistent with severity of concurrent organic process	Variable; correlates with individual notions of injury, suffering, or disease	Vivid psychic imagery; correlates with notions of suffering, punishment, torture; variable; inconsistent; elaborated; spatial-temporal intensity dimensions vague or inconsistent with organic processes	Inconsistent or no correlation with physiologic processes	Emphasis on suffering; discrepancy between appearance and intensity of pain reported; distractible; background of violence or aggression; sadistic or masochistic attitudes: guilt. Importance of pain in past or current relationships; prominence of pain in family; pain seen as punishment; response to loss

* From Engel, G. L. Pain. *In* MacBryde, C. M., and Blacklow, R. S., eds.: Signs and Symptoms: Applied Pathologic Physiology and Clinical Interpretation. ed. 5, p. 59. Philadelphia, J. B. Lippincott, 1970

the sleeping person is close to wakefulness. Yet, it is more difficult to arouse a person during REM sleep than during NREM sleep. In normal adults, the REM state consumes 20 to 25 percent of a person's nightly sleep.

NREM sleep consists of four stages, I through IV. *Stages I* and *II*, consuming approximately 5 and 50 percent respectively of a person's sleep, is light sleep and the person can be aroused with relative ease. *Stage III* sleep and *Stage IV* or *delta* sleep are deep sleep states during which time blood pressure, pulse and respiratory rates, and oxygen consumption fall to low average values.

During a person's nightly sleep, it has been demonstrated that he normally goes through the four NREM stages and the REM Stage in a circular order but with some cyclic variations. For example, an individual usually has four or five REM periods, and these periods tend to become longer as morning approaches. Also, ordinarily more sleep occurs in the delta stage in the first half of the night, especially if one is tired or has lost sleep. These findings confirm the old saying that sleep before midnight is the best sleep since proportionately more is spent in deep sleep early in the night than toward morning when more REM sleep occurs.

Stage IV sleep can be said to be the sleep of the weary. If delta sleep is denied, we try to catch up on it, just as deprivation of REM sleep is followed by what appears to be an effort to catch up with it. It is not clearly known what restorative powers delta sleep has, but it is known as being important sleep for everyone.

Figure 23-1 illustrates a normal sleep pattern for young adults, as just described. Variations in the sleep cycle are observed to vary according to age, as Figure 23-2 illustrates and as its caption explains.

It has been theorized that there are possible centers in the central nervous system that suppress and activate wakefulness. It appears as though they may be in a collection of nerve cells in the brain stem. Research also indicates that there is a biochemical process associated with sleep. For example, certain enzymes may be necessary to produce sleep and to arouse one from sleep. The exact nature of these enzymes is still not clearly defined. However, the chemistry of sleep may well be the next frontier for further explorations on the phenomenon of sleep.

For no known reason, eight hours of sleep every night has been the accepted standard, despite obvious variance shown in the general population. Factors such as the person's physiologic metabolism, age, physical condition, type of work, amount and kind of exercise, and the like, can influence patterns of rest. In other words, there is no rigid formula concerning periodicity and duration of sleep. Of importance, however, is that each person follow a pattern of rest that will maintain his well-being.

Despite variations, some generalities can be stated. On the average, infants sleep from 18 to 20 hours each day. Growing children require from 12 to 14 hours of sleep. Adults average seven to nine hours. Those who are able to relax and rest easily, even while awake, often find that less sleep is needed, while others may find that more sleep is required in order to overcome fatigue. The sleep patterns of older persons vary as much as those of younger persons.

A large segment of our society is geared to working during the daytime hours and sleeping during night hours. However, many night workers learn to sleep equally well during daytime hours once they become accustomed to this routine.

Evidence indicates that there are "larks" and "owls" among our population. The "larks" experience their greatest peaks of energy early in the morning and prefer an early bedtime hour. The op-

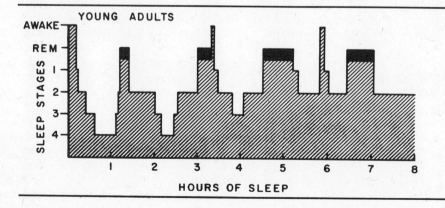

Fig. 23-1. Nocturnal sleep pattern in young adults. Note the absence of Stage IV and the decreased length of NREM periods during the latter part of the night, and the short first REM period. (From Kales, A., ed.: Sleep: Physiology and Pathology. p. 20. Philadelphia, J. B. Lippincott, 1969.)

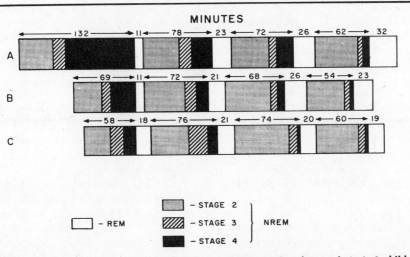

Fig. 23-2. NREM-REM cycles during nocturnal sleep for three age groups (first four cycles). A, 8 children, mean age 8.4 years; B, 15 young adults, mean age 26.6 years; C, 15 normal elderly, mean age 77 years. The figure is arranged so that the onset of the first REM period coincides for the three groups. Differences in amount of Stage IV sleep apparently account for these striking differences in the length of the first NREM period. The decline in Stage IV sleep in the normal elderly may also permit the relatively long first REM period found in this group. In general, age exerts considerable effects on the durations of the sleep cycle components without greatly affecting the number of cycles. (From Kales, A., ed.: Sleep: Physiology and Pathology. p. 45. Philadelphia, J. B. Lippincott, 1969)

posite is true of the "owls." There is no indication that either one of these patterns is better than the other.

Fatigue can be considered a protective mechanism of the body, nature's warning that sleep is necessary. Fatigue is normal; if ignored, it usually results in nervousness, restlessness, and below-par functioning. However, chronic fatigue is abnormal and is often a symptom of illness. A person who complains of chronic fatigue should be advised to see his physician.

SLEEP DEPRIVATION

Symptoms of sleep loss occur in a relatively slow but predictable pattern, mounting as time goes on. As weariness begins, normal performance fades off with lapses in attention and concentration. Unpleasant sensations such as blurred vision, itching eyes, nausea, and headache are common symptoms of fatigue. Hallucinations and illusions eventually become vivid, and mental confusion and inability to determine reality occur. There may be a lack of memory, a decrease in intellectual effort, and an attitude of not caring what happens.

It appears that loss of sleep changes brain function and causes alterations in biochemical processes in the body. It is not known whether irreversible damage to body tissue results from prolonged or chronic sleep deprivation although animal experimentations suggest that there very well might be.

Occasionally, shortchanging one's sleep rarely produces dramatic changes in personality. However, a tired person is often irritable and depressed and may experience some hallucinating such as seeing a fog around a light. Also, a tired person is often observed to perform less well on his job.

The accusation often is made that a hospital is a poor place to rest. It may well be. Many patients already anxious and fearful because of illness suffer with added problems when they are surrounded by complicated and noisy equipment in a monotonous environment, are interrupted frequently with nursing and medical measures, and are bombarded with the noise of loudspeaker systems, talking, and housekeeping chores. Some patients, for example, who have presented symptoms that include hallucinations and illusions following a few days in sophisticated and complex care units where monitoring is often constant, experienced no such symptoms after a night or two of uninterrupted sleep in a private room. Common patient complaints are that they are awakened to take sleeping pills and are aroused at early morning hours to prepare for breakfast long before it is served.

The importance of sleep for physiologic and

psychological well-being is well-known even though possibly not as well-understood. Sleep loss can result in errors and tragedy as judgment fails. Today's living, requiring many split-second decisions, depends to a great extent on the rested person. It behooves the nurse to use measures wherever and whenever possible to promote rest and sleep for her patients. Also, the nurse will wish to observe sensible sleep habits for herself in order that she can function effectively and safely.

COMMON DISORDERS OF SLEEP

Insomnia

Difficulty in falling asleep, intermittent sleep, and/or early awakening from sleep describe *insomnia*. Usually, persons complaining of insomnia have been observed to sleep more than they report. But the condition can lead to such distress as to cause further wakefulness. Although there are some physical conditions that lead to wakefulness, insomnia usually results from overstimulation by anxiety and stress. When a patient complains of being wakeful, the nurse should investigate further and take every step possible to aid in promoting relaxation and sleep. In severe cases, skilled psychological management may be necessary.

Somnambulism

Somnambulism, or sleepwalking, is seen more commonly in children than in adults. Most children outgrow sleepwalking. It has been observed that somnambulism does not occur during REM sleep but during Stages III and IV of NREM sleep. It will be recalled that it is easier to waken a person in deep sleep than one in the dream state of sleep. Therefore, it is generally relatively easy to waken a sleepwalker. The danger for the somnambulist is that he may suffer injury, and measures to provide a safe environment are essential, as for example, using secure locks on doors. In at least some instances, drugs that suppress Stage IV sleep have been found effective in decreasing sleepwalking episodes; one such drug is diazepam (Valium). If a patient with a history of sleepwalking is admitted to an inservice health agency, a record should be made of this, and proper precautions to prevent injury should be taken.

Enuresis

Enuresis is involuntary urination and is often called bed wetting. Since nocturnal enuresis occurs during sleeping hours, it is frequently referred to as a disorder of sleep. The cause is unknown although some physicians now believe that it may possibly not be only of psychological origin as was once thought. Most texts dealing with the care of children describe common measures to assist in preventing bed wetting such as limiting fluid intake for several hours before bedtime and being sure that the bladder is empty prior to bedtime. Certain drugs have been found helpful. Those used seem to increase bladder capacity.

Sleep Talking

From observations, it appears that almost everyone talks in his sleep at some time. It occurs just prior to REM sleep and rarely presents a problem unless the talking interferes with the rest of persons sharing the same room.

Sleep and Disease States

Investigations have demonstrated that sleep correlates with certain disease states. For example, the pain frequently associated with diseases of the coronary arteries is often associated with REM sleep. Normally, gastric secretions are at a low level during the night, but they have been demonstrated to increase considerably during REM sleep in the patient with duodenal ulcers. Some research, especially when children were studied, has demonstrated that asthma attacks appear to occur less frequently during Stage IV sleep, and hence, efforts to increase Stage IV sleep is advisable. One method is to increase exercise of the nature the patient tolerates in order to assist in promoting extended periods of deep sleep.

GENERAL PRINCIPLES IN RELATION TO SLEEP

The body requires periods of decreased activity in order to refresh itself. This principle, which recognizes rest as essential to well-being, becomes the basic guide to nursing practice in relation to rest.

Exactly why prolonged sleeplessness leads to ill health is not known; however, the fact remains that sleep deprivation does produce changes that can markedly alter physical and mental functioning. When in doubt, it is best that the nurse err on the side of safety and employ efforts to promote rest as a need essential to well-being.

Rest and sleep are more likely to occur under conditions of reduced stress. This principle can be stated in another way: stress and anxiety-producing situations tend to interfere with a person's ability to relax and to obtain sufficient rest for well-being.

For example, illness and hospitalization are stress and anxiety-producing situations for nearly everyone. Hence, nursing measures should be directed toward relieving them as much as possible.

Periodicity and duration of rest and sleep vary among individuals. Just as was true with pain, rest and sleep are individual matters. Some people require more than others; there are "good" sleepers and "poor" sleepers; and there are the restless and the quiet sleepers. Habits also apparently play a role in sleep patterns, and rest and sleep are promoted when they can be observed. The sleeping person is just as much a whole and integrated person with a unique personality as is the awake person.

Just as quantity of sleep is important, *the quality of sleep is also important to well-being.* As discussion in relation to the sleep cycle indicated, sleep that disallows for completing the circle of both NREM and REM sleep has been observed to decrease physiologic and psychological well-being. Some sleeping medications influence the length of both the NREM and REM states; therefore, even though the person is asleep, the refreshing effect of the sleep does not occur.

NURSING MEASURES TO PROMOTE REST AND SLEEP

Determining the Patient's History in Relation to Rest

Realizing that there are differences in rest patterns, the nurse can begin by determining the patient's usual routines. It can also be helpful to inquire about the patient's activities that have tended to promote sleep in the past. For the acutely ill, for children, and for the elderly, conferring with family members often is helpful.

By observing a sleeping person carefully, one can determine when REM sleep is in progress by looking for the rapid eye movements. If the nurse finds it necessary to waken a patient for some reason, it is best not to waken him during the dream state if possible, since the importance of REM sleep has been demonstrated clearly.

Promoting Relaxation

To relax means to become less rigid, to slacken in effort, and to decrease tensions. One can relax without sleeping, but sleep rarely occurs until one is relaxed.

Relaxation is an individual matter. For some, purposeful effort may help. For example, a patient can be assisted to relax by having him take several deep breaths; on the last breath, encourage him to try to feel as limp as possible. Then, while the patient is in a comfortable position, instruct him to contract the muscles in his leg and then purposely allow the leg to go limp. Have him repeat this for the other leg, the gluteal muscles, each arm and shoulder, and the face, each time stressing that he must first purposely contract the muscles and then allow them to go limp. Gentle massage helps muscles to relax; therefore, massage of the back is often helpful in producing sleep.

Relieving monotony is in itself frequently relaxing. This is especially helpful to remember when caring for patients undergoing long convalescence. Diversional activities were discussed in Chapter 22. Suggestions made in relation to diversion may assist the nurse in promoting her patient's relaxation.

Some people have a bedtime ritual that tends to aid relaxation and promote sleep. For some, having something to eat is a *must*. A cup of coffee may relax one person despite the presence of caffeine, a central nervous system stimulant. Other persons may prefer milk or tea. Reading, listening to the radio, or watching television are common before-sleep activities. Children display similar idiosyncracies. A favorite stuffed animal or blanket, or bed-rocking, are examples. Readiness for sleep is preceded by a personal hygiene routine for many persons, such as brushing the teeth, washing the hands and face, voiding, or taking a bath or shower.

There are no scientific explanations for bedtime rituals. The important thing is that they work for the persons using them. The wise nurse will be alert to the patient's bedtime rituals and make every effort to observe them as far as possible to aid in promoting relaxation and sleep.

Important for relaxation is a comfortable position in a comfortable bed. The bottom linen should be tight and clean. Upper linen, while secure, should allow freedom of movement and not exert pressure, especially over the legs and feet. Having the body in good alignment, as discussed in Chapter 22, is conducive to relaxation. For patients who must assume unusual positions because of their illness, ingenuity and skill are necessary in order to keep muscle strain and discomfort at a minimum. For example, the patient who must remain in the orthopneic position to aid breathing should be supported in a manner that relieves muscle strain, as with the use of a foot support, an armrest, and possibly some support in the lumbar curve. Although most individuals relax best while lying down, other positions are not contraindicated.

Providing an Environment Conducive to Sleep

A quiet and darkened room, with privacy, is relaxing for nearly everyone. In a strange environment, unfamiliar noises such as people walking or entering and leaving the room, and the closing of elevator doors bring complaints from most hospitalized patients. Although some of these sources are difficult for the nurse to control, every effort should be made toward reducing disturbances to promote relaxation and sleep.

Undue stimulation of the temperature receptors also interferes with rest. The temperature of the room, the amount of ventilation, and the quantity of bed covering are matters of individual choice, and the patient's wishes should be met whenever it is at all possible.

Alleviating Pain, Anxiety, Fear, and Stress

One of the greatest detriments to relaxation and sleep is pain and it is often a realistic complaint when illness is present. Nursing measures to promote relief from pain were discussed earlier.

The emotional reactions of anxiety, fear, and stress, common when illness and hospitalization occur, were discussed in Chapters 11 and 12. The knowledge that these reactions interfere with rest is accepted as fact. Measures to alleviate them are applicable to the discussion here.

Promoting Sleep in Children

The measures just described also apply to children. Approximately the same things interfere with rest in children as in adults. Emotional reactions are somewhat different to handle because most youngsters have not learned how to express fears and anxieties. Rather, they demonstrate these reactions by wakefulness, crying, irritability, and so on.

Picking up children, holding them securely, rocking them, and being readily available are measures that often appear to relieve their reactions to a strange environment and separation from parents. Also, leaving a night light near a frightened child often is helpful. A child's fears are very real to him, and respecting them will aid in helping to promote relaxation and sleep.

Teaching in Relation to Rest and Sleep

The nurse should remember to include content on rest and sleep in her teaching programs. For both the ill and well person, rest and sleep have been found to be equally important to well-being. There have been many jokes and amusing anecdotes told about sleep, and much folklore, mystery, and magic have been associated with it. Helping patients and their families understand the nature of rest and sleep and their importance to high-level wellness through teaching is an important nursing function.

Drugs to Promote Sleep

Although drugs that promote sleep are studied more fully in pharmacology courses, the nurse's role in relation to their administration is worth mentioning at this time. Because no one enjoys restless, interrupted sleep and long periods of wakefulness, most patients accept a medication readily if they are anxious about how well they will sleep. Accepting a drug without a real need often starts patients off on habits that last long after an illness episode. Therefore, the nurse should attempt to promote sleep without the use of drugs whenever possible. If the patient is still unable to sleep, a medication may be offered. When the patient knows he can have a medication if necessary, often he will fall asleep naturally.

As sleep has become a better understood phenomenon, drugs to promote sleep have undergone study. For example, it has been found that most hypnotic drugs suppress REM sleep and when these drugs are withheld after regular use, REM sleep increases in order to make up for the loss. The increased dreaming, often associated with nightmares, can be so distressing that persons are reluctant to give up the drugs once they have become accustomed to their use. Drugs that do not suppress REM sleep are preferred; one example is chloral hydrate, according to research.

CONCLUSION

Among the most common problems patients present are those related to the relief of pain and the promotion of sleep. While certain drug therapy may be indicated at times, the use of drugs in no way eliminates the need for high-quality nursing care, including nursing measures to promote comfort and rest.

The number of over-the-counter remedies for relieving pain and promoting sleep are countless. Many have proven to be ineffective; others have been shown to be dangerous. Using them indiscriminately may delay medical attention the patient needs. Due caution and good judgment are important before using many of these products and the nurse will wish to assist patients when they are observed to be using them without discrimination.

Study Situations

1. The following study looked at different types of nursing approaches to the care of patients complaining of pain:

   Diers, D., et al.: The effect of nursing interaction on patients in pain. **Nurs. Research,** 21:419–428, Sept.–Oct., 1972.

   Note the last paragraph in the article, on page 426, that described the authors' conclusion. What appeared to be the best type of nurse-patient interaction in terms of relieving pain? What effect resulted, according to the authors, when only medications were used to relieve pain?

2. "Thus, nurses need to use their physical nursing care skills, knowledge from sleep and drug research, and knowledge of interpersonal relations and communication to promote good sleep. The panacea for poor sleep may not be the sleeping pill." This quote completed the following article:

   Fass, G.: Sleep, drugs, and dreams. **Am. J. Nurs.,** 71:2316–2320, Dec., 1971.

   What nursing measures does the author describe as helpful in promoting sleep and in preventing overuse of drugs for sleep? What stage of sleep has been found to be suppressed in the chronic alcoholic?

3. The following reference is recommended to increase your knowledge and understanding of the phenomenon of pain:

   McCaffery, M.: Nursing Management of the Patient With Pain. 248 p. Philadelphia, J. B. Lippincott, 1972.

   Consider a patient you are presently caring for who complains of pain. Using the above book to assist you, set up a plan of care for the patient, using the nursing process system as described in this text. For example, what types of information does the author discuss that you should collect in your data-gathering process? How will you assess the patient's pain? Set up a nursing care plan for your patient. What nursing measures should you implement with your patient? How will you evaluate the effectiveness of your care? Use Chapter 7 of the above reference, on pages 219 to 232, as a guide to assist you in setting up a plan of care.

   Prepare a similar plan for caring for a patient who presents problems in relation to rest and sleep.

References

1. Acupuncture. editorial. **JAMA,** 223:77–78, Jan. 1, 1973.

2. Allison, S. E.: The meaning of rest: an exploratory nursing study. pp. 191–205. *In* **ANA Clinical Sessions.** New York, Appleton-Century-Crofts, 1971.

3. Armstrong, M. E.: Acupuncture. **Am. J. Nurs.,** 72: 1582–1588, Sept., 1972.

4. Billars, K. S.: You have pain? I think this will help. **Am. J. Nurs.,** 70:2143–2145, Oct., 1970.

5. Blaylock, J.: The psychological and cultural influences on the reaction to pain: a review of the literature. **Nurs. Forum,** 7:262–274, No. 3, 1968.

6. Cashatt, B.: Pain: a patient's view. **Am. J. Nurs.,** 72:281, Feb., 1972.

7. Engel, G. L.: Pain. Pp. 369–380. *In* MacBryde, C. M., and Blacklow, R. S., eds.: Signs and Symptoms: Applied Pathologic Physiology and Clinical Interpretation. ed. 5. Philadelphia, J. B. Lippincott, 1970.

8. Felton, G., and Patterson, M. G.: Shift rotation is against nature. **Am. J. Nurs.,** 71:760–763, Apr., 1971.

9. Jouvet, M.: Biogenic amines and the states of sleep. **Science,** 163:32–41, Jan. 3, 1969.

10. ————: The states of sleep. **Sci. Am.,** 216:62–72, Feb., 1967.

11. Kales, A., ed.: Sleep: Physiology and Pathology. Philadelphia, J. B. Lippincott, 1969.

12. Kales, A., and Kales, J.: Evaluation, diagnosis, and treatment of clinical conditions related to sleep. **JAMA,** 213:2229–2235, Sept. 28, 1970.

13. Kleitman, N.: Sleep and Wakefulness. Chicago, University of Chicago Press, 1963.

14. Long, B.: Sleep. **Am. J. Nurs.,** 69:1896–1899, Sept., 1969.

15. Luce, G. G., and Segal, J.: Sleep. New York, Coward-McCann, 1966.

16. McBride, M. A. B.: The additive to the analgesic. **Am. J. Nurs.,** 69:974–976, May, 1969.

17. McCaffery, M.: Nursing Management of the Patient With Pain. Philadelphia, J. B. Lippincott, 1972.

18. McCaffery, M., and Moss, F.: Nursing intervention for bodily pain. **Am. J. Nurs.,** 67:1224–1227, June, 1967.

19. McFadden, E. H., and Giblin, E. C.: Sleep deprivation in patients having open-heart surgery. **Nurs. Research,** 20:249–253, May–June, 1971.

20. McKee, K.: Neurotic bodily pain in children. **Am. J. Nurs.,** 70:130–131, Jan., 1970.

21. Moss, F. T., and Meyer, B.: The effects of nursing interaction upon pain relief in patients. **Nurs. Research,** 15:303–306, Fall, 1966.

22. Pain: part 1: basic concepts and assessment: programmed instruction. **Am. J. Nurs.,** 66:1085–1108, May, 1966.

23. Pain: part 2: rationale for intervention: programmed instruction. **Am. J. Nurs.,** 66:1345–1368, June, 1966.

24. Rickels, K., and Hesbacher, P. T.: Over-the-counter daytime sedatives: a controlled study. **JAMA,** 223:29–33, Jan. 1, 1973.

25. Sobel, D.: Love and pain. **Am. J. Nurs.,** 72:910–912, May, 1972.

26. Storlie, F.: Pain: describing it more accurately. **Nurs. '72,** 2:15–16, June, 1972.

27. Webb, C.: Tactics to reduce a child's fear of pain. **Am. J. Nurs.,** 66:2698–2701, Dec., 1966.

28. Williams, D. H.: Sleep and disease. **Am. J. Nurs.,** 71:2321–2324, Dec., 1971.

CHAPTER 24

Maintaining Fluid and Electrolyte Balance

GLOSSARY • INTRODUCTION • DEFINITION OF TERMS • FLUID AND
ELECTROLYTE BALANCE • ACID-BASE BALANCE • FLUID AND
ELECTROLYTE IMBALANCES • ACID-BASE IMBALANCES •
SIGNS OF POTENTIAL FLUID AND ELECTROLYTE DISTURBANCES •
PREVENTION OF FLUID AND ELECTROLYTE DISTURBANCES •
ORAL INTAKE MEASURES TO ASSIST IN CORRECTING FLUID AND
ELECTROLYTE DISTURBANCES • INFUSION MEASURES TO ASSIST IN
CORRECTING FLUID AND ELECTROLYTE DISTURBANCES • GASTRIC
AND DUODENAL SUCTION • INTAKE AND OUTPUT MEASUREMENT •
CONCLUSION • STUDY SITUATIONS • REFERENCES

GLOSSARY

Acidosis: Condition characterized by a proportionate excess of hydrogen ions in the extracellular fluid.

Active Transport: Movement of substances, including electrolytes, against a concentration gradient where energy is required.

Air Embolus: Large quantity of air circulating in the blood.

Alkalosis: Condition characterized by a proportionate lack in the extracellular fluid concentration of hydrogen ions.

Anion: An ion which carries a negative charge.

Blood Donor: Person giving blood.

Blood Typing: Laboratory determination of a person's blood type.

Buffering Action: Taking up or releasing of hydrogen ions by a solution to maintain its pH.

Cation: An ion which carries a positive electrical charge.

Cellular Fluid: Fluid within the cell; also called intracellular fluid.

Crossmatching: Determination of compatability of two blood specimens.

Cubic Centimeter: Unit of measurement, 1/100 of a meter; abbreviated c.c. Approximately equivalent to a milliliter.

Cut-down: Incision into a vein for purpose of infusion.

Dehydration: Decreased extracellular water volume.

Diffusion: Movement of fluid and its nonprotein components from an area of higher concentration to an area of lower concentration until equilibrium is established.

Direct Transfusion: Infusion of blood while it is being collected from donor.

Edema: Excessive fluid stored in body tissue spaces.

Electrolyte: A substance capable of breaking into ions and developing an electrical charge when dissolved in solution.

Embolus: Circulating foreign body in the blood.

Extracellular Fluid: Fluid outside the cells; includes intravascular and interstitial fluid.

Homeostasis: State of balanced internal body environment.

Hydrostatic Pressure: Force exerted by a fluid against the container walls.

Hyperalimentation: Infusion of nutrient solution into the superior vena cava.

Hyperkalemia: Excess amount of potassium in the extracellular fluid.

Hypernatremia: Excess of sodium in the extracellular fluid.

Hypertonic: Having a greater concentration than the solution with which it is being compared.

Hypervolemia: Excess amounts of fluid and electrolytes in extracellular area.

Hypodermoclysis: Infusion of fluid into the subcutaneous tissue.

Hypokalemia: Insufficient amount of potassium in the extracellular fluid.

Hyponatremia: Insufficient amount of sodium in the extracellular fluid.

Hypotonic: Having a lesser concentration than the solution with which it is being compared.

Hypovolemia: Deficiency in amount of water and electrolytes in the extracellular fluid.

Indirect Transfusion: Infusion of blood from container after it has been collected from donor.

Infiltration: Escape of fluid into the subcutaneous tissue.

Infusion: A large quantity of fluid injected intravenously or subcutaneously.

Interstitial Fluid: Fluid between the cells.

Intracellular Fluid: Synonym for cellular fluid.

Intravascular Fluid: Fluid within the vascular system; also referred to as plasma.

Ion: An atom which carries an electrical charge in solution.

Isotonic: Having approximately the same concentration as the solution with which it is being compared.

Lysis: Bursting of cell membrane due to excessive water absorption.

Metabolic Acidosis: Proportionate deficiency of bicarbonate ions in the extracellular fluid.

Milliequivalent: Unit of measurement to describe electrolyte chemical activity; abbreviated mEq.

Milliliter: Unit of measurement, 1/1000 of a liter. Abbreviated ml. Approximately equivalent to a cubic centimeter.

Osmosis: Movement of fluid through a semipermeable membrane from an area of lower concentration to an area of higher concentration until a balance is established.

Osmotic Pressure: Attraction for water exerted by solute particles.

pH: Expression of hydrogen ion concentration and resulting acidity of a substance.

Phlebitis: Inflammation of a vein.

Plasma: Synonym for intravascular fluid.

Preformed Water: Water in food.

Rales: Bubbling respiratory sound.

Recipient: Person receiving blood.

Respiratory Acidosis: Proportionate excess of carbonic acid in the extracellular fluid.

Respiratory Alkalosis: Proportionate deficiency of carbonic acid in the extracellular fluid.

Thrombi: Blood clots.

Transfusion: Infusion of whole blood.

Turgor: Normal tension within a cell.

Venipuncture: Entry into a vein.

INTRODUCTION

In her delightful book, *The Sea Around Us,* Rachel Carson indicated that as organisms came from the waters, they took with them a heritage from the sea that has been passed on to every succeeding generation. Interestingly enough, whatever man's origin, there are striking similarities between man's body fluid and the sea around us.

Within the last three decades or so, remarkable progress has been made in the knowledge of body fluids and their role in health and disease. We know that our very life depends on maintaining the proper amount of body fluid as well as maintaining the fluid's proper constituents and proper placement, each in relationship to the other.

This balanced internal state is called *homeostasis.* The term was first used in this context by the physiologist, Walter B. Cannon, in 1932, in his book *The Wisdom of the Body.* Credit for the original concept, though not the word, is given to the French scientist Claude Bernard. Cannon described homeostasis as a bodily condition produced by coordinated processes which resulted in a relatively constant but not unchanging internal environment. Although this chapter will discuss the concept of homeostasis in relation to body fluids, it can also be applied to other aspects of man's internal functioning, as for example, in relation to body temperature, blood pressure, respiration, and hormone secretions.

Fluid and electrolyte balance is maintained by ongoing physiologic processes. Some circumstances in the healthy person and virtually all illness states threaten that balance. For example, participating in extensive outdoor physical activity on a hot day, going for a long period of time with an inadequate water intake, or eating a poorly balanced diet for an extended period can cause disturbances of fluid and electrolyte balance. Conditions resulting in vomiting, diarrhea, and pyrexia, or illness states such as diabetes mellitus, burns, surgical procedures, and infectious processes frequently create imbalances. Therapeutic regimens also may upset fluid and electrolyte balance. For example, the use of diuretics and of some of the adrenal cortex hormones has been known to upset this balance if not used judiciously. Specific disease entities and their common therapeutic regimens are discussed in other nursing and medical texts and the reader is urged to seek biochemistry and physiology references for more detailed discussions of fluids and electrolytes. In this chapter, fundamental information necessary for administering intelligent nursing care to aid in the maintenance of fluid and electrolyte balance, without regard to specific clinical problems, will be presented.

If the nurse's responsibility in relation to fluid and electrolyte balance had to be spelled out in one word, the most appropriate one would no doubt be *observation.* Therefore, the nurse with a knowledge of fluid and electrolyte balance, of how imbalances occur, and of what symptoms characterize them is in a position to observe and to take action intelligently.

DEFINITION OF TERMS

Fluids are present in two body spaces. There is fluid within each of our millions of body cells. This is referred to as *cellular or intracellular fluid*. All fluid outside of the cells is *extracellular fluid*. The extracellular fluid consists of fluid within the vascular system, called *intravascular fluid* or *plasma*. The fluid in which tissue cells are bathed is called *interstitial fluid*. All body fluid, intracellular and extracellular, contains electrolytes. However, the amount of fluid and the distribution of electrolytes differ considerably between intra- and extracellular fluid.

An *electrolyte* (sometimes called a salt or a mineral) is a substance capable of breaking into ions and developing an electrical charge when dissolved in solution. *Cations* develop positive charges and include such electrolytes as calcium, sodium, potassium, and magnesium. *Anions* develop negative charges and include electrolytes as chloride, bicarbonate, phosphate, sulfate, proteinate, carbonic, and other organic acids. An *ion* is an atom which carries an electrical charge in solution.

Each cell is nourished and gets rid of its wastes through the extracellular fluid. We know that the exchange of waste for nutrients, including fluid and electrolytes, is vital to life itself; but science has as yet to explain the basis for this exchange. However, it is known that the passage of fluid from intracellular to extracellular space, and vice versa, occurs by diffusion, osmosis, and active transport.

Diffusion is the simplest type of fluid movement. Fluid and its nonprotein components move from the area of higher to lower concentration until equilibrium is established.

Each cell is enclosed in a semipermeable membrane which allows easy passage of water back and forth. The membrane is more selective in allowing passage of other substances. *Osmosis* is the passage of fluid through a semipermeable membrane from an area of lower to higher concentration until a balance occurs.

Osmotic pressure is the attraction for water exerted by the solute particles. The greater the concentration of electrolytes, the greater the osmotic pressure. Because of the distribution of electrolytes, normally the osmotic pressure is relatively constant on both sides of the cell membrane and fluid moves freely through the membrane without a net loss or gain. However, if the concentration of electrolytes becomes greater on one side of the membrane, the osmotic pressure and attraction for water will in-

crease, and fluid will move in that direction. When a body cell is placed in an *isotonic* solution, that is, a solution having approximately the same concentration of electrolytes as the cell, the size and shape of the cell do not change because there is no net gain or loss of water in the cell. If placed in a *hypertonic* solution, solution having greater concentration than the intracellular fluid, water moves out of the cell, causing it to shrivel and become smaller. In a *hypotonic* solution, a solution having less concentration than intracellular fluid, the cell absorbs water, swells, and eventually bursts. This is called *lysis*. Knowledge of the osmotic process is important when, for example, the patient receives intravenous fluids. Distilled water is rarely given intravenously for fear of creating hypotonicity of plasma that will cause blood cells to swell and burst.

Osmotic pressure is primarily responsible for any net exchange of water between the intracellular and interstitial fluids. Water exchanges between the intravascular and interstitial fluids are the result of osmotic pressure and hydrostatic pressure. *Hydrostatic pressure* of the blood is the force exerted by the blood against the walls of the vessels. Hydrostatic pressure is sometimes called filtration force. The physics principle that states fluids move from an area of greater to lesser pressure explains that hydrostatic pressure forces fluid out through the semipermeable membranes of the blood vessel wall. However, blood also has osmotic pressure determined by its protein and electrolyte constituents which exert a pulling effect on the fluid. The difference between these two opposing forces will determine whether fluid moves into or out of the intravascular space for a net loss or gain. This pressure relationship has significance in the control of blood pressure, the filtering process of the kidney, and the accumulation of fluid in the tissues, a condition called *edema*.

Active transport is the movement of substances, including electrolytes, against a concentration gradient in which energy is required to accomplish the movement. The process is not completely understood but is used to explain the movement of ions not facilitated by diffusion or osmosis. Movement across a concentration gradient is an "uphill" movement, so to speak. The energy requirement is affected by characteristics of the membrane, specific enzymes, and concentration of the ion. This process provides the explanation for the sodium-pump mechanism which is responsible for moving sodium out of the cell.

The unit of measure commonly used to describe body fluid volume is the *milliliter*, abbreviated ml. Each milliliter is 1/1,000 of a liter. It is roughly equivalent to a cubic centimeter, abbreviated c.c.

The unit of measure used to describe electrolyte chemical activity is a *milliequivalent*, abbreviated mEq. From chemistry one recalls that the atomic weight of an ion does not necessarily describe its chemical power. The unit of chemical power of any ion is equivalent to the chemical power of 1 mg. of hydrogen. For example, one sodium ion carries one positive charge while calcium carries two. In terms of chemical power, a calcium ion can be said to be twice as strong as a sodium ion, weight being no factor. A chloride ion has one negative charge; it takes two chloride ions to combine with one calcium ion to form a molecule, while it takes only one sodium ion to combine with a chloride ion. Almost any cation can unite with any anion to form a molecule, and 1 mEq. of any cation is equivalent chemically to 1 mEq. of any anion. The concept of milliequivalents is used to express chemical activity on an equal basis. It is like the common denominator concept in mathematics. Using milliequivalents as a unit of measure eliminates the need for calculations and conversions when electrolyte therapy is indicated.

Hydrogen is also the basis for pH calculations. The term pH is an expression of hydrogen ion concentration and resulting acidity of a substance. Hydrogen ions with their positive charges are balanced by hydroxyl (OH) with negative charges. Thus, the pH of pure water (H_2O) is 7.0, which is neutral. Because pH is based on a negative logarithm, as the hydrogen ions increase and a solution becomes more acid, the pH becomes less than 7.0. When the concentration of hydrogen ions is exceeded by the hydroxyl ions, the solution is alkaline, and the pH is greater than 7.0. For example, gastric secretions which are strongly acid have an approximate pH of 1.0 to 1.3, while strongly alkaline pancreatic secretions have an approximate pH of 10. Normal blood plasma is only slightly alkaline and has a pH of approximately 7.35 to 7.45. The extracellular fluid range of pH conducive to normal body cellular function is very limited. It is maintained by buffering systems and by respiratory and kidney function. When the normal range is exceeded, the person develops symptoms of illness and if not corrected, death can result. *Acidosis* is the condition when there is a proportionate excess of hydrogen ions in the extracellular fluid and the pH falls below 7.3. *Alkalosis* is the bodily condition in which the extracellular fluid has a proportionate lack in the concentration of hydrogen ions and the pH exceeds 7.4.

FLUID AND ELECTROLYTE BALANCE

This section discusses the following basic principle: *In health, fluid and electrolyte gains and losses are maintained in balance and in harmony with bodily needs.*

Healthy human beings maintain fluid and electrolyte balance automatically. The task is indeed a formidable one. We ingest a wide variety of materials of various quantities, often unmatched with bodily needs, and dispose of wastes and excesses as a result of intricate chemical mechanisms, to maintain a relatively small range of normality. What is normality?

The average total body fluid in adults comprises approximately 60 percent of body weight, a little less in females than males. Approximately one-third is extracellular fluid. About one-quarter of the extracellular fluid is intravascular, and three-fourths is interstitial fluid. Approximately two-thirds of the body fluid is cellular fluid.

In infants, total body fluid comprises about 75 percent of body weight, with approximately three-fifths being intracellular and two-fifths being extracellular. Because infants have a higher basal metabolism rate, a proportionately greater body surface, and a larger percentage of body fluid than the adult, they suffer from fluid deficits more quickly than older persons. Also, infants normally require relatively greater fluid intake in proportion to body weight than do adults.

While it has already been indicated that body fluids move freely between the extracellular and intracellular spaces, the net change in volume in any of the spaces is extremely small in states of health. While the body will attempt to maintain a balance in all of its fluid spaces, if circumstances demand, the intravascular fluid will usually be protected at the expense of interstitial and then intracellular fluids. The nurse's understanding of fluid sources and their losses is essential to providing care which promotes fluid balance.

Water for the body arrives from the ingestion of liquids and food and from metabolic oxidation. While the amount of water available to the body tissues varies with the individual, average daily amounts have been established for the healthy adult. Table 24-1 shows these amounts.

TABLE 24-1: Average daily adult fluid sources

Amount of fluid	Sources of fluid
ml.	
1200–1500	Ingested water
700–1000	Ingested food
200–400	Metabolic oxidation
2100–2900	

As can be observed from the table, oral ingestion of liquids makes up the largest amount of fluid normally taken into the body. Personal habits and circumstances are responsible for the variations.

Water in food, referred to as *preformed water*, makes up the next largest water source. This also varies extensively depending on the dietary items that are eaten. Foods such as melons and citrus fruits have a high water content, while cereals and dried fruits have a relatively low water content.

Water made available through metabolic oxidation is also dependent on the food intake. When food is oxidized during metabolism, water is one of the end products. The amount of water varies with the nutrients. For example, metabolism of 100 Gm. of fat produces 107 Gm. of water while 100 Gm. of carbohydrate will yield 55 Gm. of water, and 100 Gm. of protein will produce 40 Gm. of water. Therefore, a person eating a high-fat meal will have a proportionately greater amount of water resulting from his metabolic process than a person having a high-protein meal.

Thirst is a normal regulatory mechanism related to water balance. Thirst is a subjective experience and an important factor in determining fluid intake. The mechanism responsible for thirst is poorly understood. The hypertonicity of body fluids stimulates the production and release of the antidiuretic hormone which acts upon the kidney to retain water. Psychological as well as some physiologic factors are involved, but it is particularly important to remember that the person who is unable to respond to the thirst stimulus as well as the person who seems to have no stimulus may need professional assistance.

Water is lost from the body normally through the kidneys via the urine, through the intestinal tract via fecal material, and through the skin as perspiration. Water is also lost in insensible or nonperceptible ways. Insensible vaporization from the skin and respiratory tract result in a significant loss of fluid. Like fluid intake amounts, fluid losses vary with the individual and his circumstances, and no absolute standards can be given. Average ranges, however, have been established. Table 24-2 indicates these averages.

TABLE 24-2: Average daily adult fluid losses

Amount of fluid	Exit route
ml.	
1200–1700	Urine
100–250	Feces
100–150	Perspiration, insensible losses
350–400	Skin
350–400	Lungs
2100–2900	

The nurse needs to be aware of factors which influence a patient's fluid losses as well as the volume of his losses. A person may have an increased fluid loss because of an elevated environmental temperature, decreased relative humidity, increased physical activity, or an extended period of mouth breathing. Pyrexia, vomiting, diarrhea, kidney malfunction, blood loss, or wound drainage also all influence fluid loss. The body's own homeostatic mechanisms will attempt to conserve fluid loss from one exit route when the loss is increased from another. Table 24-3 illustrates how a normal adult's fluid losses can vary with changing circumstances.

As indicated, the amount of fluid intake and loss varies extensively with individuals. The body normally attempts to control fluid loss proportionate to intake to maintain a homeostatic state. Authorities indicate a range of 1500 ml. to 3500 ml. per 24 hours is a desirable adult fluid intake and loss. The majority of individuals have a 2000 ml. average intake and loss per day. While the preceding figures

TABLE 24-3: Average daily water losses of healthy adults under varying circumstances*

Exit route	When body temperature is normal	When pyrexia is present	Following prolonged exercise
	ml.	ml.	ml.
Urine	1400	1200	500
Feces	200	200	200
Perspiration, Insensible losses	100	1400	5000
Skin	350	350	350
Lungs	350	250	650
	2400	3400	6700

* Adapted from Shepard, R. S.: Human Physiology. p. 390. Philadelphia, J. B. Lippincott, 1971.

are helpful to establish a standard, the patient's balance between his intake and loss must also be considered when assessing his nursing needs. An individual's fluid intake should normally be approximately balanced by his output or fluid loss. A general rule is that in the adult, the output of urine normally approximates the ingestion of liquids, and the fluid from food and oxidation is balanced by the fluid loss through the feces and skin and the respiratory process. The intake should of course be within the desirable range. The intake-output balance may not always exist in a single 24 hour period but should normally be achieved within two to three days.

KIDNEYS: The kidneys are the chief means by which water balance of the body is maintained. The relationship between the kidneys and the endocrine system is involved in this complex process. The antidiuretic hormone, usually referred to as ADH, is released by the posterior pituitary and acts primarily on the kidney tubules to regulate the amount of water reabsorption. When the amount of ADH is increased, the permeability of the collecting ducts of the kidneys is increased which promotes greater water reabsorption and thus, less urine formation. When ADH is decreased, the collecting ducts reabsorb less water and thus, the urine output is increased. The stimulus for ADH release is generally thought to be the osmotic pressure of the extracellular fluid which is determined by its electrolyte and water relationship. Thus, we see that the composition of extracellular fluid itself influences water balance throughout the body.

ELECTROLYTES: A number of electrolytes in varying amounts are found in the intravascular (plasma), interstitial, and intracellular fluids, as shown in Figure 24-1. The normal electrolyte composition of body secretions also varies. The major electrolytes—sodium, potassium, chloride, calcium, and bicarbonate—will be discussed briefly here.

Sodium is the chief cation of the extracellular fluid. It is also found in smaller quantities within

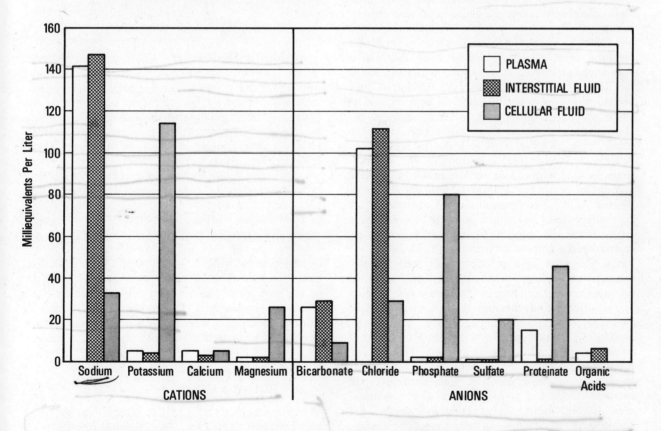

Fig. 24-1. Electrolyte composition of normal body fluids. (From Snively, W. D., Jr., and Beshear, D. R.: Textbook of Pathophysiology, p. 136. Philadelphia, J. B. Lippincott Company, 1972.)

the cell. Since it moves easily between the vascular and interstitial spaces, it is primarily responsible for regulating the osmotic pressure of the extracellular fluid and therefore, also controls water distribution. The old adage, "where goes sodium also goes the water," is essentially true. Sodium also plays a role in acid-base balance and is instrumental in many chemical reactions, particularly within nervous and muscle tissue cells. Sodium excesses are eliminated primarily by the kidney, although small amounts are normally lost in the feces and perspiration also. The kidneys are very effective in conserving sodium through reabsorption stimulated by aldosterone, and hence, the body fluid levels are relatively easy to maintain. The extracellular fluid level of sodium is 135 to 145 mEq./1 in the average adult. Sodium is found normally in many foods such as milk, meat, eggs, and some vegetables and in water in some areas of the country. Sodium is also ingested by most persons in the form of sodium chloride (salt) added to foods. The average American diet includes 3 to 7 Gm. of sodium daily, an amount which more than adequately meets the daily minimum requirements.

Potassium is the major cation of the intracellular fluid. The importance of its main function is comparable to the task of sodium in the extracellular fluid. It is the chief regulator of intracellular electrolyte balance. It also plays an integral part in many physiological processes, as for example, in the transmission of electrical impulses particularly in nerve tissue and the heart and also in skeletal, intestinal, and lung tissues; in protein and carbohydrate metabolism; and in cellular building. A small amount of potassium is normally also found outside of the cells. The gastrointestinal secretions are normally rich in potassium; some is also found in perspiration and saliva. Potassium is primarily excreted by the kidneys in urine. Unlike sodium, the kidney does not have an effective method for conserving potassium; therefore, if the excreted amounts are not replaced, a deficiency will develop readily. Because of the high potassium content of gastrointestinal secretions, large losses of these secretions will quickly cause a deficit. Normal adult values of intracellular potassium are 115 to 160 mEq./1, while extracellular potassium is in the 3.5 to 5 mEq./1 range normally. Potassium is found in many foods and is included in a well-balanced diet. Certain fruits, leafy vegetables, meats, and whole grains are all high in potassium. The average daily dietary intake contains 2 to 4 Gm. of potassium which is adequate to replace losses.

Chloride is the chief extracellular anion. It plays an important role in maintaining the normal plasma pH. The highest concentration of chloride is found in gastric secretions. Chloride is excreted primarily by the kidneys in combination with sodium, and like sodium, the major part of chloride is conserved and reabsorbed. A healthy adult's plasma normally contains 95 to 105 mEq./1 of chloride. It is taken into the body primarily in foods to which sodium chloride has been added.

Calcium is the most abundant electrolyte in the body. It is mainly found in bones and teeth in a non-ion form. A small ionized amount is normally found both in the extracellular fluid and in the intracellular fluid. Calcium is necessary for nerve impulse transmission, blood clotting, and muscle contraction, and it acts also as a catalyst for many chemical activities of cells. The normal adult extracellular fluid has approximately 5 mEq./1 of calcium. Dairy products are the most prevalent natural source of calcium.

ACID-BASE BALANCE

Acidity or alkalinity of a solution is determined by its concentration of hydrogen (H^+) ions and hydroxyl (OH^-) ions. The chemical processes of tissue cells produce large volumes of acids, but most body fluids are normally slightly alkaline. The narrow range of normal pH is achieved by the body's buffer system, carbon dioxide excretion by the lungs, and the selectivity of ion secretion of the kidneys.

Buffering action is the ability of a solution to take up or discharge hydrogen ions to maintain its pH. Some buffer solutions are weakly ionized acids in combination with a salt. Proteins (cellular, plasmatic, and hemoglobinic) also have buffering action. One portion of the protein molecule can accept hydrogen ions, while another portion can give up hydrogen ions. The capacity of a buffer is limited by the number of anions it has available to trap the positive hydrogen ions. The carbonic acid—sodium chloride buffering system is the most important one in the human body. For example, if an acid is added to an alkaline fluid, the body's buffering system would cause the following response:

$$HCl + Na\, HCO_3 \rightarrow NaCl + H_2CO_3$$

When hydrochloric acid (HCl) is added to sodium bicarbonate ($NaHCO_3$), the chemical results are sodium chloride (NaCl) and carbonic acid (H_2CO_3) as indicated in the above formula. This process occurs frequently and very rapidly in the body. Normal extracellular fluid has a ratio of 20 parts bicarbonate to one part carbonic acid. This buffering system carries a major responsibility in maintaining the plasma pH in a 7.35 to 7.45 normal range. 7.4 ph

The lungs are the primary controller of the body's carbonic acid supply. Carbon dioxide (CO_2) is constantly produced by cellular metabolism and enters the extracellular fluid. As it does, the carbon dioxide and water are acted upon by the enzyme, carbonic anhydrase, to produce carbonic acid (H_2CO_3), as shown below:

$$CO_2 + H_2O \xrightarrow{\text{Carbonic anhydrase}} H_2CO_3$$

Since they are reversible reactions, the carbonic anhydrase can also later break down the carbonic acid into carbon dioxide and water as follows:

$$H_2CO_3 \xrightarrow{\text{Carbonic anhydrase}} H_2O + CO_2$$

The carbon dioxide of the above reaction can be excreted by exhalation. As the amount of carbon dioxide in the blood increases, the sensitive respiratory center of the medulla is stimulated to increase the rate and depth of respirations in order to eliminate more carbon dioxide. When the blood level of carbon dioxide is below normal, the center will decrease the rate and depth of the respirations to retain the carbon dioxide so carbonic acid can be formed and the delicate balance maintained. This total respiratory process also occurs frequently and nearly as rapidly as the buffering action described previously.

The concentration of bicarbonate (HCO_3) in the plasma is regulated by the kidneys through the excretion of hydrogen ions and by forming additional bicarbonate as needed. When the pH of the plasma reaches the lower range of normal, hydrogen ions are eliminated, and bicarbonate is formed and retained. When plasma pH is elevated or above normal, hydrogen ions are retained and bicarbonate excesses are excreted. The kidneys regulate hydrogen and bicarbonate ions in three ways: reabsorbing bicarbonate, forming ammonium salts, and forming phosphate salts. Sodium (Na) is exchanged for a hydrogen ion in the tubule cells, after which it combines with bicarbonate (HCO_3) to form sodium bicarbonate ($NaHCO_3$) which is reabsorbed by the plasma, thus conserving the bicarbonate ion, as this formula illustrates:

$$Na^+ + HCO_3^- \rightarrow NaHCO_3$$

As a result of amino acid metabolism, ammonia (NH_3) is formed in the kidney tubule cells and is secreted into the tubule where it unites with hydrogen to form an ammonium ion (NH_4). Ammonium further unites with chloride (Cl) to form ammonium chloride (NH_4Cl) and is excreted, thus:

$$NH_3 + H \rightarrow NH_4 + Cl \rightarrow NH_4Cl$$

Phosphate salts are formed by exchanging a sodium ion for a hydrogen ion in the conversion of alkaline sodium phosphate ($NaHPO_4$) to acid sodium phosphate (NaH_2PO_4). The acid sodium phosphate is then excreted thus:

$$Na_2HPO_4 + H \rightarrow NaH_2PO_4 + Na$$

Acid-base regulation by the kidney is a vast combination of chemical processes, and it occurs more slowly than buffering or respiratory regulation. It may take several days for fluid pH to be restored by the kidneys. The pH of urine varies depending upon the ions which are being excreted, but generally, it is in the 5.5 to 6.5 range for the healthy adult. 6.0 ph

The following principle underlies the importance of the acid-base balance maintenance in the body:

Satisfactory functioning of the body's buffering system, kidneys, and lungs is essential to the maintenance of the acid-base balance present in health and ultimately essential to life itself.

FLUID AND ELECTROLYTE IMBAL-ANCES

As discussed earlier, fluid and electrolyte and acid-base balances are essential to health. In some circumstances, the body's compensatory mechanisms are not able to maintain the homeostatic state, and imbalance occurs. Imbalances can relate to either volume or distribution disturbances of the fluid or electrolytes. While in actual situations, the imbalances frequently occur in combination, for purposes of clarity, the major ones will be discussed here individually. Table 24-4 lists the major disturbances with examples of common symptoms and causes of the disturbances.

The body has a desirable balance for fluids and electrolytes in all three spaces—intravascular, interstitial, and intracellular. Constant extracellular and intracellular exchanges mean that extracellular disturbances have implications for intracellular functioning. This fact plus the relative availability for study of the extracellular fluid results in fluid

TABLE 24-4: Various fluid and electrolyte disturbances, common symptoms, and problems likely to produce them*

Clinical entity	Common symptoms	Examples of problems likely to lead to disturbance
Extracellular fluid volume deficit	Dry skin and mucous membranes Scanty urine Weight loss Lassitude Longitudinal tongue furrows Elevated red blood count, hemoglobin, and hematocrit	Insufficient water intake Vomiting Diarrhea Pyrexia
Extracellular fluid volume excess	Puffy eyelids Shortness of breath Dyspnea Moist rales Edema Weight gain Bounding pulse Decreased red cell count, hemoglobin, and hematocrit	Excessive ingestion or injection of fluids with sodium chloride or sodium bicarbonate Renal malfunction Congestive heart failure disease
Plasma to interstitial fluid shift	Fast, weak pulse Pallor Cold extremities Hypotension Apprehension Unconsciousness Elevated red cell count, hemoglobin, and hematocrit	Burns Massive crushing injuries Perforated peptic ulcer
Interstitial fluid to plasma shift	Early—hypertension Late—hypotension Air hunger Moist rales Bounding pulse Engorged peripheral veins Pallor Weakness Decreased red cell count, hemoglobin, and hematocrit	Excessive infusion of hypertonic solutions Compensation following hemorrhage Recovery phase of plasma to interstitial fluid shift
Metabolic acidosis (base bicarbonate deficit)	Disorientation-stupor Deep rapid breathing Unconsciousness when severe Plasma pH below 7.35 Plasma bicarbonate below 25 mEq./1 Urine pH below 6	Decreased food intake Systemic infections Renal insufficiency Diabetic acidosis Ketogenic diet
Metabolic alkalosis (base bicarbonate excess)	Depressed shallow respirations Hypertonic musculature Tetany Plasma pH above 7.45 Plasma bicarbonate above 29 mEq./1 Urine pH above 7	Vomiting Excessive ingestion of alkalies Gastric suction Adrenal cortex hormone administration
Respiratory acidosis (carbonic acid excess)	Disorientation Respiratory embarrassment Coma Weakness Plasma pH below 7.35 Plasma bicarbonate below 25 mEq./1 Urine pH below 6	Pneumonia Emphysema Respiratory suppression Asthma Respiratory obstruction
Respiratory alkalosis (carbonic acid deficit)	Unconsciousness Tetany	Deep rapid breathing Deliberate over-breathing

* Adapted from Snively, W. D. Jr., and Beshear, D. R.: *Textbook of Pathophysiology.* pp. 133–160. Philadelphia, J. B. Lippincott, 1972.

TABLE 24-4: Various fluid and electrolyte disturbances, common symptoms, and problems likely to produce them

Clinical entity	Common symptoms	Examples of problems likely to lead to disturbance
Respiratory alkalosis (carbonic acid deficit)	Convulsion Slow, shallow respirations Plasma pH above 7.45 Plasma bicarbonate below 25 mEq./1 Urine pH above 7.45	Oxygen lack Pyrexia Extreme emotion Salicylate intoxication
Sodium deficit	Apprehension Abdominal cramps Rapid weak pulse Hypotension Convulsions Scanty urine Plasma sodium below 135 mEq./1	Excessive perspiration and drinking water Gastrointestinal suction and drinking water Repeated use of water enemas Infusions without sodium chloride Diuretic administration
Sodium excess	Dry, sticky mucous membrane Thirst Firm tissue turgor Pyrexia Plasma sodium above 145 mEq./1	Inadequate water intake and excessive sodium chloride intake Diarrhea Pyrexia with rapid breathing
Potassium deficit	Weak and faint pulse Falling blood pressure Malaise Anorexia; vomiting Distention Soft, flabby musculature Plasma potassium below 3.5 mEq./1	Diarrhea Intestinal disease Emotional, physical stress Burns Diuretic administration
Potassium excess	Nausea Irritability General weakness Scanty to no urine Intestinal colic Diarrhea Irregular pulse Plasma potassium above 5.6 mEq./1	Burns Crushing injuries Kidney disease Excessive infusion of potassium
Calcium deficit	Tingling of fingers Abdominal muscle cramps Tetany Convulsions Carpopedal spasm Plasma calcium below 4.5 mEq./1	Sprue Excessive infusion of citrated blood Subcutaneous infections—massive Peritonitis Removal of parathyroid glands
Calcium excess	Relaxed musculature Flank pains Kidney stones Deep bone pains, as "shin splints" Plasma calcium above 5.8 mEq./1	Prolonged bed rest Tumor-parathyroid gland Excessive Vitamin D intake Overactivity of parathyroid glands Excessive milk or hard water intake
Protein deficit	Mental depression Fatigue Pallor Weight loss Loss of muscle tone Edema	Hemorrhage Draining wounds or ulcers Burns Inadequate protein intake
Magnesium deficit	Disorientation-hallucinations Hypertension Tremors Hyperactive deep reflexes Convulsions Rapid pulse rate Plasma magnesium below 1.4 mEq./1	Chronic alcoholism Vomiting Diarrhea Impaired intestinal absorption Enterostomy drainage

imbalances being diagnosed and treated in relation to extracellular levels.

Extracellular fluid deficit is a deficiency in the amount of both water and electrolytes in the extracellular fluid. The fluid and electrolyte proportions remain near normal. The state is commonly known as *hypovolemia*. Dehydration is sometimes used as a synonym for hypovolemia, but strictly speaking, this is an inaccuracy. *Dehydration* refers only to a decreased volume of water. Excessive fluid loss or inadequate intake or a combination of the two are common causes of fluid deficit. Both osmotic pressure and hydrostatic pressure changes force the interstitial fluid into the intravascular space. As the interstitial space becomes depleted, it will become hypertonic and cellular fluid will be drawn into the interstitial space, leaving the cells poorly hydrated. Excessively dehydrated cells are unable to carry on their normal functions.

Fluid deficit occurs in persons with excessive body excretion or secretion losses when they are not replaced. It also occurs in persons who are too ill to help themselves to an adequate fluid intake or do not have a sufficient volume of fluids available. The very young and the elderly and those fatigued or weakened by illness are particularly susceptible. A weight loss in excess of 5 percent for adults and 10 percent for infants can occur rapidly. Evidences of dry skin and mucous membranes with thickened secretions are common. The person's tongue develops characteristic longitudinal wrinkles or furrows, and usually he is lethargic and may even become unresponsive. Laboratory examination of the blood reveals an increased concentration of the solid portions; thus, the red blood cell count, hemoglobin, and hematocrit (volume of red cells per circulating unit) are all elevated.

Extracellular fluid excess is a surplus of fluid and electrolyte amounts while maintaining near normal proportions. It is referred to as *hypervolemia*. Overhydration is commonly used as a synonym for hypervolemia, but strictly speaking, this is an inaccuracy. *Overhydration* refers only to an increase in water. Malfunction of the kidneys causing an inability to excrete the excesses is the most common cause. However, cardiac and liver disturbances can also be influential. Since the kidneys are responsible for sodium excretion also, when water is retained in excessive amounts, so is sodium.

Because of the increased extracellular osmotic pressure from the retained sodium, fluid is pulled from the cells to equalize the tonicity. By the time the intracellular and extracellular spaces are isotonic to each other, an excess of both water and sodium are in the extracellular fluid while the cells are nearly depleted. The increase in intravascular fluid volume may cause an increase in blood pressure, a bounding pulse, and engorged peripheral veins. Fluid can also collect in the lungs and cause respiratory changes such as labored breathing; shallow, rapid respirations; and productive coughing. It also usually causes characteristic bubbling respiratory sounds referred to as *rales*. The excessive extracellular fluid may be stored in tissue spaces and is known as *edema*. Edema frequently can be seen around the eyes, the fingers, ankles, and the sacral area. It may result in a weight gain in excess of 5 percent. When the excess fluid remains in the intravascular space, the concentration of solids in the blood is decreased. Therefore, laboratory examinations will show a decreased red cell count, hemoglobin, and hematocrit.

Plasma-to-interstitial shift describes the occasional movement of fluid and electrolytes from the blood to the spaces between the cells. It occurs most often following major tissue damage, as for example, when there has been a crushing or tearing injury or extensive second or third degree burns. The person develops symptoms of decreased intravascular fluid with decreased blood pressure; rapid, weak pulse; generalized weakness; and coolness of the extremities. Since the blood solids remain behind and therefore are in greater concentration, the laboratory examination of the blood will show an increase in the red blood count, hemoglobin, and hematocrit.

Interstitial-to-plasma shift is the movement of fluid and electrolytes from the space surrounding the cells to the blood. This shift is a compensatory response to volume or osmotic pressure changes of the intravascular fluid. This may occur when a replacement is needed for blood lost in hemorrhage or when excessive hypertonic solutions are administered intravenously. Intravascular increases will be demonstrated by venous engorgement, and blood pressure, cardiac, and pulse changes. The increased intravascular volume will cause laboratory examinations to show a decrease in the red cell count, hemoglobin, and hematocrit.

Sodium deficit is an insufficient amount of sodium in the extracellular fluid. This condition is referred to as *hyponatremia*. It can be caused either by an excessive sodium loss or an inadequate intake. An inadequate intake is usually the result of a poorly managed sodium-limited diet or merely an inadequate food intake. Excessive perspiration with associated drinking of a great deal of water, extensive loss of gastrointestinal secretions, kidney reabsorption malfunctions, adrenal cortex disturbance, and administration of diuretics or nonelectrolyte infusions are all fairly common causes of excessive sodium loss. An increase in aldosterone will stimulate the kidneys to reabsorb available sodium, and along with it chloride and water, so the urinary output is decreased. Osmotic pressure changes of the fluid will result in extracellular fluid moving into the cells. This extracellular fluid loss can also cause vascular changes, as a decrease in blood pressure and a weak pulse. The vascular changes may induce disturbances of concentration and thinking. Examination of the blood reveals a plasma level of less than 135 mEq./1.

Sodium excess is a surplus of sodium in the extracellular fluid. This state is also called hypernatremia. The excess of sodium can be the result of either an increased intake or decreased elimination of the electrolyte. It can also occur as the result of a decreased intake or an increased loss of water. An excessive intake can be either by intravenous or oral routes. Kidney and adrenal cortex malfunctions were mentioned earlier as a cause of sodium retention and resulting extracellular fluid excess. Extreme water losses, such as may occur when hyperpnea or diarrhea are present, can cause a proportionate sodium excess. Because of the increased extracellular osmotic pressure, fluids move from the cells, leaving them in a poorly hydrated state. The person with an increase in extracellular sodium usually develops extreme thirst, dry mucous membranes, an elevated temperature, and very firm body tissues. Examination of the blood reveals a plasma sodium level in excess of 145 mEq./1.

Potassium deficit is an insufficient amount of potassium in the extracellular fluid. This state is known as hypokalemia. It can be caused by a decrease in potassium intake, intestinal absorption, or an increased loss. Since potassium is available in so many foods and malabsorption disorders of the intestine are generally treated effectively, excess loss is by far the most common cause of potassium deficiency. Kidney disturbances resulting in tubular malfunction or excessive aldosterone stimulation will cause increased potassium losses. Diuretics promote fluid and potassium excretion. Gastrointestinal secretion losses from vomiting, diarrhea, or mechanical removal by suctioning can be the cause of a deficiency. Tissue trauma resulting in cellular damage also causes potassium losses. When the extracellular potassium level falls, potassium moves out from the cell creating an intracellular potassium deficiency. Sodium and hydrogen ions are retained by the cells to maintain an ionic balance. These shifts not only influence normal cellular function-

ing but also influence the pH of the extracellular fluid. Muscle tissues are generally the first to demonstrate a potassium deficiency. Symptoms include weakness of skeletal muscles, smooth muscle disturbances resulting in a decrease in peristaltic activity, and cardiac muscle changes producing a rapid weak pulse, decreased cardiac output, and an abnormal EKG. In deficiency, laboratory examination of the blood shows a potassium plasma level of less than 3.5 mEq./1.

Potassium excess, also known as hyperkalemia, is an excess of potassium in the extracellular fluid. An excess of potassium can be the result of excessive administration or decreased excretion or a combination of the two. A decrease in urine output for any reason will minimize potassium excretion. Adrenal cortex malfunctions can cause the reabsorption of excessive potassium. Extensive tissue damage causes the movement of intracellular potassium to the extracellular space. Excessive administration of either oral or intravenous potassium, especially in the presence of kidney dysfunction, can cause an extracellular increase. Neurologic disturbances, including numbness and tingling of the extremities, abdominal cramping, cardiac arrhythmias, and muscle irritability, are common symptoms. Mental confusion, gastrointestinal disturbances, and respiratory difficulties can also occur. Laboratory examination of the blood reveals a plasma potassium level in excess of 5.6 mEq./1.

ACID-BASE IMBALANCES

Acid-base imbalances occur when the carbonic acid or bicarbonate levels become disproportionate. Two kinds of disturbances upset the balance. A metabolic disturbance alters the bicarbonate proportion. A respiratory disturbance alters the carbonic acid proportion. When there is a single primary cause, these disturbances are known as metabolic acidosis or alkalosis and respiratory acidosis or alkalosis. Measurements of the blood bicarbonate level are used to determine these acid-base imbalances. The most common laboratory measurements are the carbon dioxide content dissolved in the blood, carbon dioxide combining power, and the carbon dioxide pressure. In each of the tests the bicarbonate is treated to release the carbon dioxide which is then measured.

Metabolic acidosis is a proportionate deficit of bicarbonate in the extracellular fluid. The deficit can occur as the result of an increase in acid components or an excessive loss of bicarbonate. Increased fat metabolism with resultant acidic ketone wastes, ingestion of large amounts of acidic salicylates, or kidney malfunctions which result in reabsorption disturbances are examples of potential causes of metabolic acidosis. The lungs attempt to increase the carbon dioxide excretion by increasing the rate and depth of the respirations. The kidneys attempt to compensate by retaining bicarbonate and excreting more hydrogen; thus, the urine becomes acidic. If the body is unable to maintain the normal balance, the person may lose consciousness as metabolic acidosis occurs. The blood and urine characteristically both have a lowered pH.

Metabolic alkalosis is a proportionate excess of bicarbonate in the extracellular fluid. This may be the result of excessive acid losses or increased base ingestion or retention. Loss of gastric secretions through vomiting or gastrointestinal suctioning decreases the body's acid component extensively. Drinking large amounts of plain water while a patient is undergoing gastric suctioning has the effect of "washing out" the stomach electrolytes along with the water, and thus, predisposes him to alkalosis. Large ingestions of sodium bicarbonate or other absorbable alkaline substances can disturb the balance. The body will attempt to compensate by retaining carbon dioxide. The respirations will become slow and shallow and apnea may even occur. The kidneys will attempt to excrete potassium and sodium with the excessive bicarbonate and will retain hydrogen in carbonic acid. If these mechanisms are unsuccessful and metabolic alkalosis occurs, the pulse usually becomes irregular, the patient's muscles become hypertonic, and disorientation and delirium occur. The blood plasma has an elevated pH along with an increase in the bicarbonate. The urine pH is also increased.

Respiratory acidosis is a proportionate excess of carbonic acid in the extracellular fluid. Any deficiency in respiratory ventilation can cause respiratory acidosis. As the plasma carbonic acid content increases, the lungs are stimulated to "blow off" more carbon dioxide through an increased rate and depth of respirations. The kidneys will attempt to retain more bicarbonate and increase their ammonium excretion. If these compensatory mechanisms are unable to prevent respiratory acidosis, the person usually develops a rapid pulse, mental disorientation, loss of consciousness, and more labored breathing. The urine and plasma pH are lowered and the plasma bicarbonate volume increases.

Respiratory alkalosis is a proportionate deficit of carbonic acid in the extracellular fluid. It is the result of increased alveolar ventilation and, as a result, a decrease in carbon dioxide. An increase in respiratory rate and depth causes the carbon dioxide loss. Since the carbon dioxide is excreted faster than normal, the carbon dioxide combining power is lowered. Hysteria and anxiety may be causative factors. Pyrexia, anoxia (especially at higher altitudes), and some central nervous system diseases may also cause this excessive carbon dioxide loss. Because of the deficit of carbon dioxide which is a chemical respiratory stimulant, depression or cessation of respirations will eventually occur. The kidneys attempt to alleviate the imbalance by increasing the bicarbonate excretion and retaining more hydrogen. When respiratory alkalosis is present, the plasma and urine pH will increase and the plasma bicarbonate level will decrease.

As indicated earlier, imbalances frequently occur in combination. Table 24-5 shows common imbalances resulting from body fluid losses.

TABLE 24-5: Imbalances resulting from fluid loss of specific body fluid *

Fluid being lost	Imbalances likely to occur
Gastric juice	Extracellular fluid volume deficit Metabolic alkalosis Sodium deficit Potassium deficit Tetany (if metabolic alkalosis is present) Ketosis of starvation Magnesium deficit
Intestinal juice	Extracellular fluid volume deficit Metabolic acidosis Sodium deficit Potassium deficit
Bile	Sodium deficit Metabolic acidosis
Pancreatic juice	Metabolic acidosis Sodium deficit Calcium deficit Extracellular fluid volume deficit
Sensible perspiration	Extracellular fluid volume deficit Sodium deficit
Insensible water loss	Water deficit (dehydration) Sodium excess
Wound exudate	Protein deficit Sodium deficit Extracellular fluid volume deficit
Ascites	Protein deficit Sodium deficit Plasma-to-interstitial fluid shift Extracellular fluid volume deficit

* From Snively, W. D. Jr., and Beshear, D. R: Water and electrolytes in health and disease. In Kintzel, K. C., ed.: Advanced Concepts In Clinical Nursing. p. 264. Philadelphia, J. B. Lippincott, 1971.

SIGNS OF POTENTIAL FLUID AND ELECTROLYTE DISTURBANCES

The importance of observation in gathering the data that the nurse uses as her basis for maintaining or restoring fluid and electrolyte balance cannot be overstressed. As indicated in Chapter 6, knowing when and what type of information should be collected is essential. In other words, the nurse must be alert to situations in which the potential for fluid and electrolyte disturbances is increased, and then she needs to know what information is pertinent. Many specific examples of disturbances and symptoms have been given in the previous discussion. They are included here as a summary.

The nurse will want to be familiar with the patient's health state, the history of any present illness, and the medical plan for therapy. Any one, or any combination, of these factors may predispose the patient to fluid and electrolyte imbalance. Because balance is maintained normally when compatibility exists between the intake of fluids and electrolytes on one hand and their output on the other, anything that upsets the scale on either side acts as a warning. For example, typical questions for which the nurse seeks answers are: Has the patient's normal food and fluid intake changed? If so, for how long has it differed? Have there been restrictions for any reason on what he could eat and drink? Has there been any abnormal loss of body fluids? What particular body fluid is involved? What is the patient's intake and output of fluids?

Any situation in which the person has lost excessive fluids and electrolytes is a potential hazard. Examples include situations when there is extreme perspiration with or without pyrexia, vomiting or diarrhea, wound or body secretion drainage, or blood loss. Inadequate fluid and electrolyte intake can result from nausea, a poorly balanced diet, or the unavailability of food or fluids. Excessive ingestion or injection of either electrolytes or fluids can also be a problem. Because the young and the elderly have less effective physiologic compensatory mechanisms at their disposal, they will tend to develop imbalances faster than adults and therefore are higher risks.

No single symptom is in itself necessarily indicative of fluid and electrolyte imbalance. All must be reviewed in relation to the patient's health state. Combinations of symptoms should be reviewed with possible disturbances in mind. Probably more important than any particular sign is how the symptom compares with the person's normal or usual

characteristic. In assessing the data items, then, the selection of standards pertinent to the individual's situation is extremely important. Data considered significant to fluid and electrolyte imbalances and to which the nurse needs to be alert are grouped here as tissue characteristics, behavioral manifestations, and measurements.

Tissue Characteristics

Tissue characteristics pertinent to the determination of fluid deficiency include dryness of the skin and mucous membranes. The mucosa of the mouth and lips may be covered with a whitish coating and/or may be cracked. Generally, the mucous secretions are increased in viscosity. The texture of the tissues can be very significant. A depletion of tissue fluids will cause a characteristic sunken appearance of the eyes, because the supportive fat pads for the eyeballs have been dehydrated. The tissue cells will lose some of their elasticity when interstitial fluid decreases; thus, the cells have decreased turgor. *Turgor* is defined as the normal tension within a cell. When the skin is pinched up between the fingers, normally it resumes its original shape immediately upon release. In poor hydration states, it remains in folds or returns slowly to its normal posture. An excess of fluids in the tissues will cause increased tension and a characteristic firmness and/or swelling. The swelling is often seen initially around the eyes, in the fingers, at the ankles, and in the sacral area. Changes in muscle tissue are particularly prevalent with electrolyte imbalance. Because the neurologic stimuli and/or the ability to respond may be disturbed, the muscle tissues may appear flaccid or limp, or they may be tense and actually twitch or cramp involuntarily.

Behavioral Manifestations

Behavioral manifestations of fluid and electrolyte disturbances vary extensively. They can range from lethargy and coma to disorientation, hallucinations, and hyperactivity. Extreme personality changes can occur. For example, the normally quiet, reserved person can become very talkative and physically active, or the person who normally participates in mental and physical activities shows no interest and becomes withdrawn. A change in the normal behavior of the individual is the most significant factor. Speech changes can occur from a simple slurring to an actual voice change or hoarseness. In situations where thirst is a factor, a person's behavior can be grossly affected. The patient can become so conscious of the thirst sensation that his actions are motivated by it alone.

Measurements

Measurements of various types have already been mentioned. Changes in the vital signs can be significant. An increase in body temperature usually accompanies fluid deficiencies. Respiratory rate and depth are directly affected by carbonic acid blood levels. Fluid disturbances can also influence the pulse rate and blood pressure. Pulse rate and changes in pulse quality are also influenced by potassium disturbances. Weight changes, either a loss or increase, can result when there are fluid and/or sodium disturbances. Usually, the change must exceed 5 percent in a short period of time before it is considered to be fluid balance related. Peripheral veins normally empty or fill in three to five seconds when the hands are moved from a dependent to an elevated position or lowered from an elevated position to a dependent one. With an increased fluid volume, the time for hand vein emptying is usually increased. Measurements which show a disproportion between the fluid intake and output can be indicative of imbalances. Another type of measurement useful for determining fluid and electrolyte imbalances is laboratory analysis of body fluids. Blood and urine test results, which indicate the quantity of their constituents, specific gravity, pH, and other factors, provide important data.

PREVENTION OF FLUID AND ELECTROLYTE DISTURBANCES

Once predisposing factors are known and high-risk persons are identified, the next step concerns prevention of fluid and electrolyte imbalance. Every measure, nursing as well as medical, is ordinarily taken to aid in maintaining balance in the first place. For example, drugs are ordered to handle many infectious processes that predispose to imbalance, before trouble begins. Every effort is made to encourage patients to take adequate nourishment when lack of appetite or vomiting is a problem. Nursing measures are discussed in Chapter 25. Fluid intake should be encouraged or guarded, depending on the circumstances. Efforts are taken, as described in Chapter 21, to avoid the development of decubitus ulcers, which, if allowed to occur, can result in exuding ulcers that may upset balance. The inactivity of bed rest often accompanying illness may result in such disturbances as an increased excretion of nitrogen. Hence, high protein diets often are prescribed for patients requiring prolonged bed rest. Calcium is mobilized from the matrix of bones dur-

ing long periods in bed and excreted through the kidneys. Hence, nursing measures, such as were discussed in Chapter 22, are used to promote activity to the greatest extent possible. Additional measures are discussed in Chapter 26 in relation to elimination and in Chapter 29 in relation to infection and pyrexia.

Because successful prevention of fluid and electrolyte imbalances must actively involve the patient, helping him to understand the significance of disturbances, their symptoms, and preventive measures is extremely important. The nurse may find that an extensive teaching program for the patient and his family may result in prevention of a serious illness for the patient and the conservation of her time in the long run.

The nurse's vigilance is extremely important in detecting the first signs of impending imbalance so that preventive measures can be intensified. The frequency of observation of high-risk patients should be increased because the signs of impending imbalances are often insidious. Once imbalance occurs, the nurse will observe common symptoms as described earlier. The reader's attention is called in particular to deviations in the vital signs, given in Table 24-4. Personnel other than nurses often assist in obtaining vital signs. When fluid and electrolyte balance is in jeopardy, the nurse is encouraged to make her own observations.

ORAL INTAKE MEASURES TO ASSIST IN CORRECTING FLUID AND ELECTROLYTE DISTURBANCES

When fluid and electrolyte imbalances are present, action must be taken to correct them. The degree of imbalance and the body's compensatory mechanisms will determine the type and intensity of the therapy involved. Planning and implementing the nursing care must therefore be based on the individual patient's situation. Because his active participation is highly desirable, whenever possible, the patient should be involved in determining the nursing care objectives and in selecting the actions to achieve the goals. Patient and family teaching is nearly always a key component of this care.

Increasing Ingestion of Fluids and Electrolytes

Some fluid and electrolyte deficiencies can be corrected by increasing the ingestion of the needed substance. For example, bananas and most fish are high in potassium and their inclusion in the diet might help overcome a potassium deficit. A sodium deficiency might be corrected by adding more salt to foods. Supplementary forms of electrolytes are also commonly used to correct deficits.

Mild fluid deficiencies can be corrected by increasing the ingestion of fluids. The reader will recall that the average adult daily fluid intake is 2100 ml. to 2900 ml., but a person with a water deficit may need to take in more than this to correct the disturbance. Or, if his intake has been considerably less than this, a proportionate increase will be an improvement. Recalling that some foods contain more water than others, an increase in foods with high water content may be helpful. Since both food and fluids cause gastric expansion and a sensation of fullness, some persons can ingest larger volumes of liquids if they are spaced between meals. Whenever the patient's situation permits, encouraging as wide a variety of liquids as possible can help to prevent boredom and may make a larger volume more palatable.

Having a specific fluid intake goal is a very helpful aid for many patients, their families, and nursing personnel. It is very difficult to maintain strong motivation and initiate action when the goal is simply "increase fluid intake." For some patients, the setting of short-term or interim goals is most helpful. For example, "a glass every hour," or "by the time your TV program is finished," or "a pitcher of water by lunchtime," can be useful objectives.

If the reader has ever tried to increase his fluid intake when he did not feel thirsty, he realizes how important are the encouragement and support of others. These boosters can come from the nurse or the patient's family. Because normally during the night, fluid intake is limited or nil, the patient is usually able to consume a proportionately greater amount during the early hours of his waking day. Avoiding a large intake of fluid just before retiring is also usually wise to prevent sleep disturbances caused by having to void.

Having fluid available for the person whose goal is an increased intake is so obvious that it seems unnecessary to mention it. However, it is amazing how many persons in homes and hospitals who are unable to secure their own fluids are left with an unfilled water pitcher, an empty glass and a full pitcher out of reach, or with a pitcher that is too heavy to lift.

The person who is unable to help himself often will be able to take only small quantities of fluids at a time. Therefore, the frequent offering of sips and single swallows is essential. Such simple measures as making sure certain fluids are the temperature the patient prefers are also important. If the patient wants and is permitted iced liquids, they should not be at room temperature. If he wants his coffee, tea, or just water piping hot, then it should be steaming. Attractive, clean, and easily handled cups and glasses can also be an encouragement.

Some persons find that the use of a drinking tube requires less effort, while others may have to have the fluids spoon fed. Increasing the fluid intake of patients is probably the single most common nursing care objective. Often, creativity and considerable patience on the part of the nurse are necessary to reach desired goals.

Limiting Ingestion of Fluids and Electrolytes

Decreasing the oral intake of fluid and electrolytes may be necessary to correct imbalances. The foods that are high in excess electrolytes may need to be limited or eliminated; for example, the restriction of sodium is a particularly common practice for persons with cardiovascular or renal diseases. The degree of restriction will vary depending on the patient's condition. Severe sodium limitations will require the use of distilled water in some parts of the country where the natural content is high. Potassium and calcium restrictions are also necessary for some persons.

Oral fluid limitations are less common, but are necessary for some people with cardiac or renal diseases. Securing the patient's understanding and cooperation is important, especially if the restrictions are severe, because it is nearly impossible to prevent a person who is up and about from securing fluids if he is motivated to do so. Examples of patients drinking bath water, water from flower containers, and even urine indicate how strong the desire can be. Spacing of the allowable fluids should be planned with the patient whenever possible. Since food will also provide relief through gastric distention, it is generally preferable to plan the time of maximum fluid intake for periods between meals. Setting short-term goals for hourly or two-hourly intervals may also be helpful.

Because these persons usually experience intense thirst, measures to minimize it are important. Rinsing the mouth with fluid or holding water in the mouth will moisten the mucous membranes and provide short-term relief. (The effect does not ordinarily exceed 15 minutes, however.) Providing oral hygiene at regular intervals can be helpful; various methods were discussed in Chapter 21. Dry and salty foods should be avoided by the patient whose fluid intake is restricted, because they will tend to increase thirst. Hard candy and gum, often thought to relieve thirst by stimulating saliva, may provide temporary relief. However, their use is generally not encouraged because the high sugar content increases the oral cavity tonicity and temporarily draws fluid to the mucous membrane. After a period of 15 to 30 minutes, the mucous membranes are even more dry than before. Diverting the person's attention by involving him in other activities to the degree he is able is often helpful to decrease discomfort. Such measures as the use of small glasses and serving of ice which when melted is approximately one-half of its apparent volume may also be helpful. Since limiting intake for the person who is experiencing extreme thirst is very uncomfortable, the nurse needs to provide understanding and support of his feelings and encouragement for his efforts.

INFUSION MEASURES TO ASSIST IN CORRECTING FLUID AND ELECTROLYTE DISTURBANCES

Intravenous Infusion

A relatively common form of therapy for handling fluid and electrolyte disturbances is the use of various solutions injected intravenously or subcutaneously. An *intravenous infusion* is the injection of relatively large quantities of solution into a vein. A *hypodermoclysis*, to be discussed later in this chapter, is the injection of relatively large quantities of solution into subcutaneous tissues. Although the physician is responsible for ordering the proper kind of solution and the amount to be used, the nurse is usually responsible for initiating and monitoring the therapy. Hence she is in a better position if she familiarizes herself with the solutions commonly used in the agency in which she is studying or working.

The variety of solutions on the market is almost without limit. There are maintenance solutions containing electrolytes in the proportion normally found in the body. There are replacement solutions with electrolyte content similar to fluids being lost. There are solutions containing amino acids, glucose, and vitamins as well as electrolytes. There is whole blood, as well as blood derivatives and replacements. There are isotonic, hypertonic, and hypotonic solutions. In some agencies, solutions are tailor-made to meet a particular patient's requirements. Should the nurse have questions concerning the selection of

a particular solution, two good sources usually are readily available. The physician in charge of the therapy generally is glad to explain his selection. The pharmaceutical companies preparing the solution have excellent literature explaining the nature and common indications of each. Selection of the fluid is based on the patient's needs. Laboratory analysis of the patient's body fluids and clinical symptoms provide the guide for determining the appropriate solution.

There are several ways in which the amount of fluid to be infused is calculated. Although age and weight are important, either one in itself rarely gives sufficient knowledge to calculate amount. It is easy to see that a 40-year-old man weighing 200 pounds requires quite different amounts from a 40-year-old woman weighing 120 pounds. A combination of weight and age is often used as a guide.

Using the patient's weight to estimate his body surface area in square meters also is common. Charts that list estimates of surface area in relation to weight are available, although calculations still are necessary when the patient's body build deviates considerably from the average for his age.

Regardless of the method used—and the nurse will want to be familiar with it—another factor influences the physician's decision always, and that is the patient's clinical picture. A patient suffering from severe depletion or excess of fluids and/or electrolytes has needs different from one with moderate or mild imbalance. The amount is still different from that needed by a patient with no indication of imbalance, who is placed on maintenance dosages because a condition exists that without care may lead to disturbances.

Patients' needs for infusion solutions are usually calculated and ordered on a 24-hour basis. In some health agencies, student physicians, specially prepared nurses, or technicians initiate infusions. In other situations, nurses caring for the patient start the infusions.

SELECTION OF A VEIN FOR INTRAVENOUS THERAPY: Suitability of veins for intravenous infusions vary with individual situations. Selection should be determined after considering several factors: accessibility and condition of veins, type of fluid to be infused, and anticipated duration of the infusion.

Accessibility of a vein is partially determined by the condition of the patient. For example, a person with severe burns of both forearms will not have vessels in these areas available. Veins in a surgical area should not be used, nor usually even those adjacent to the area. For example, infusions in the arm should not occur on the same side as recent extensive breast surgery because of vascular disturbances in the area.

The most accessible veins are not necessarily the most desirable for infusion. For example, the antecubital veins located at the inner aspect of the elbow are among the most accessible. However, often they are not a good choice for infusion because of the need to limit the patient's arm flexion for an extended period of time. Since there is danger of dislocation of the needle and vein trauma even with slight movement, damage to these vessels may limit later use of the lower arms and hand veins that are

distal to it. (Distal means farthest from the center.) These vessels are quite satisfactory for blood withdrawal or for small amounts of intravenous medication administration.

The lower cephalic vein, accessory cephalic vein, and the basilic vein are good sites for infusion. The superficial veins on the dorsal aspect of the hand can also be used successfully for some persons. The metacarpal veins, basilic veins, and cephalic veins are recommended good sites. Figures 24-2 and 24-3 illustrate these locations.

Veins of the legs are generally not recommended for infusions, unless other sites are not accessible, because of the danger of stagnation of peripheral circulation and possible serious complications. Scalp veins are often used, especially for infants, because

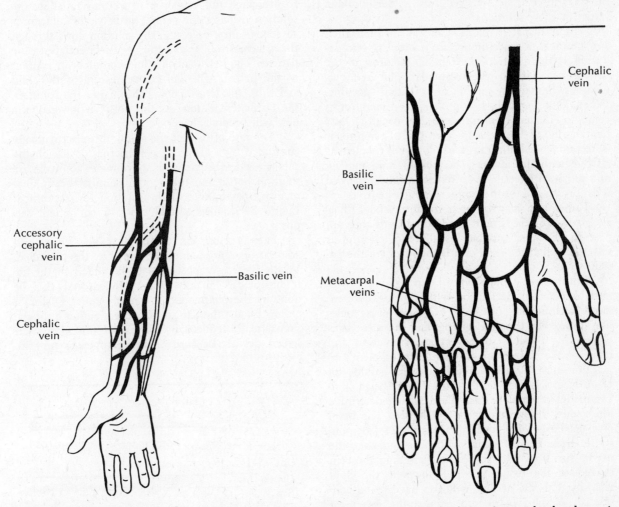

Fig. 24-2. Recommended infusion sites on the ventral aspect of the lower arm.

Fig. 24-3. Recommended infusion sites on the dorsal aspect of the hand.

of their accessibility and relative ease of preventing dislocation of the needle.

Vein condition is an important consideration because it may determine the ease or difficulty of successive entry into the vein. Thin-walled and scarred veins, especially in some elderly patients, make continued infusion a problem. Experience will help the nurse acquire skill in palpating veins to determine their general condition.

The type of fluid to be administered is influential in vein selection because the solution should be compatible with the vein size. Hypertonic solutions, those containing irritating medications, those administered at a rapid rate, and those with a high viscosity should be given in a large vein to minimize vessel trauma and facilitate the flow rate. Generally, the forearm veins are preferred over the dorsum hand veins for these solutions.

The anticipated duration of the infusion therapy becomes a more important factor in vein selection as the duration is extended. Comfort of the patient is facilitated when any restriction in movement is limited to the greatest extent possible. When joint immobility is prolonged, discomfort is common. Trauma from infusions does occur, at least temporarily, at the venipuncture site. Therefore, it is recommended that sites be changed frequently, starting with sites as distal as possible and moving in a proximal direction on alternate arms. (Proximal is defined as nearest the center of attachment.)

Either arm may be used for intravenous therapy. If the patient is right-handed and both arms appear to be equally usable, usually the left arm is selected so that the right arm is then free for the patient's use.

EQUIPMENT COMMONLY USED FOR INTRAVENOUS INFUSIONS: Because a vein is being entered, sterile technique is observed. Most health agencies use disposable infusion tubing and needles, thus eliminating possible sources of contamination and reducing the cost of the aftercare of equipment.

For most intravenous infusions for adults, an 18-, 20-, or 22-gauge needle with a short bevel, 1 to 1½ inches in length is used. Needle gauge determine the size of the inner diameter or lumen. The bevel of a needle is the sloped edge. Figure 24-4 demonstrates these characteristics. Whenever possible, the needle size should be appreciably less than the vein to reduce the tissue trauma. However, the fluid viscosity and rate of flow will also have to be considered. A short bevel also reduces the extent of vein damage. Butterfly needles, which are short-beveled, thin-walled needles with plastic flaps, are also used extensively because of the ease in handling and stabilizing them.

If an infusion is to run for an extended time, an intravenous catheter may be used. Catheters are specially prepared plastic tubes which have been mounted on a needle or are threaded through a needle for insertion. Because of the incidence of serious complications from this type of equipment, only experienced practitioners should attempt to use it.

Normally, the pressure in the patient's vein is higher than atmospheric. Gravity is used to increase the pressure differential between the needle and the solution container. The solution is placed at a level approximately 18 to 24 inches above the level of the vein or at a height where gravity is sufficient to overcome the venous pressure and to allow the solution to enter the vein. The bottle of solution is suspended on a pole, and the solution flows through the attached tubing and the needle directly into the patient. The height of the fluid container in relation to the patient will affect the pressure of the fluid and thus, the rate of flow. The higher the solution, the faster it will run. As the bottle is lowered, the flow will become slower.

The rate of flow of the solution is also manually controlled by a clamp or constricting device on the tubing. A device known as a dripmeter connects the solution bottle and tubing and permits the number of drops per minute of the solution to be counted. Figure 24-5 shows several types of equipment setups.

PREPARATION OF SOLUTION: The kind and amount of solution are determined by the physician. When there are substances to be added to the solution, it is generally recommended that this be done by the pharmacist, preferably under a laminar airflow hood. The danger of contamination has been shown to be reduced by the use of this filtered air screen device. Because of the complexity and in-

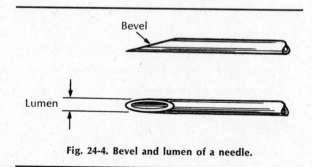

Fig. 24-4. Bevel and lumen of a needle.

compatibility of some additives and the resulting dangers to the patient, having the pharmaceutical personnel prepare the solutions also decreases the likelihood of undesirable combinations being prepared. Any additives should be clearly labeled on the bottle as to type and amount. The precise method of attaching the tubing to the solution varies with the design of the container being used, but sterile technique should always be used to avoid contamination of the ends of the tubing and the solution. After the tubing has been connected to the bottle of solution, the bottle is elevated to allow the air to escape and the fluid to fill the tubing. When all the air is out of the tubing, it is clamped shut. The tip of the tubing can then be attached to the sterile needle.

Before the infusion is started, a final check should be made of the solution to make sure it is clear and contains no particles of any kind. Since some additives create precipitates, this check is es-

pecially important when substances have been added to the solution. In-line filters are commercially available also to filter the solution immediately before it enters the patient's vein.

PREPARATION OF THE PATIENT FOR INTRAVENOUS INFUSION: Since an infusion usually takes several hours to complete, the patient should be made comfortable. If the procedure is unusually long, the patient's position should be changed frequently if he is to remain in bed. If allowed to walk, proper precautions are taken to prevent the needle from slipping out of place.

The arm to be used is abducted slightly from the body and placed on an arm board, if necessary. When the arm is secured to an arm board, attention should be given to keeping it in good position. Very often it is possible to have the forearm pronated and the palm of the hand downward and in the grasping position over the edge of the arm board. This position more nearly resembles the normal position of

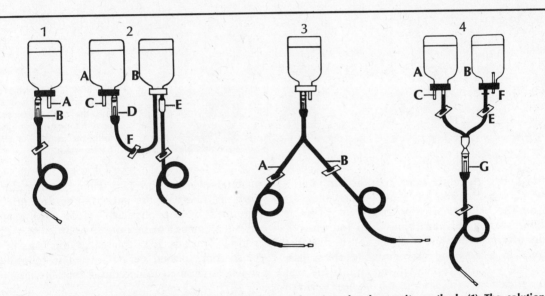

Fig. 24-5. Various means by which intravenous substances can be given by the gravity method. (1) The solution flows through the drip-meter B (which also may be a filter if blood is given) at a rate that can be controlled by a clamp on the tubing. A provides an air inlet so that air may enter the bottle to displace the fluid that leaves. It has a one-way valve which prevents the fluid from running out. (2) This is referred to as a tandem setup. Fluid will leave bottle B if the clamp F is open. As fluid leaves bottle B, an area of lesser pressure is created in bottle B. This lesser pressure exerts its influence on bottle A and draws fluid from it. The system will operate only if C, the air vent, is open and permits air to displace the fluid that leaves bottle A. D is a drip-meter and filter. E is a drip-meter. In this setup, A always will empty before B. If F is clamped off, no fluid will be able to leave bottle B. (3) This Y arrangement is often used for hypodermoclysis. One bottle of solution provides fluid to two injection sites. A and B parts of the tubing each have a clamp to make separate regulation of flow rate possible. (4) Solution may leave either bottle, depending on the regulation of the clamps D and E. In this setup, A is blood and B is normal saline. If D stops the flow of blood from bottle A, the saline will flow from bottle B if clamp E and the clamp below the filter are opened. The reverse also can be made to happen. Therefore, both bottles must have an air inlet, C and F, so that air can enter to displace the fluid as it leaves. In this setup, G is a filter as well as a drip-meter.

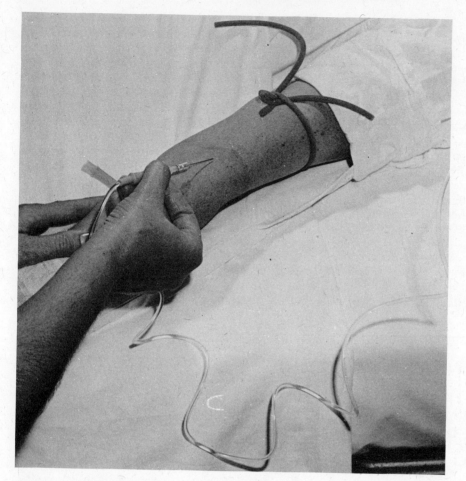

Fig. 24-6. The tourniquet is in place, the vein was located and the area cleansed. With one hand holding the skin taut, the needle is about to be inserted.

the arm and is therefore more comfortable for the patient. Hyperextension of the elbow causes fatigue for the patient, often to the point where it may be impossible for him to move his forearm voluntarily after an infusion is discontinued. It takes assistance in flexing and extending the elbow passively to help regain "feeling" in the arm. If the area is hairy, such as a man's arm, it may be best to shave the area involving the needle site and adhesive.

A tourniquet is applied to aid in distending the vein. The tourniquet is placed under the arm above the selected site and ready to tie. The arm is secured to the board with bandage or ties. Do not obstruct circulation or cause discomfort to the patient, but make it snug enough to hold the arm securely. The skin over the vein where the needle will be introduced is cleansed thoroughly with antiseptic solution.

INFUSION MONITORING: The monitoring of the infusion is the nurse's responsibility and involves maintaining the flow rate while assuring the comfort and safety of the patient. The flow rate is determined by the physician's order. He may indicate the amount to be infused in an 8- or a 24-hour period. The rate is calculated on the basis of drops of solution infused per minute. The following formula can be used to determine the flow rate:

Drops per minute =

$$\frac{\text{Total volume infused} \times \text{drop factor (drops/ml.)}}{\text{Total time of infusion in minutes}}$$

The drop factor, or drops per milliliter, is determined by the size of the opening in the infusion apparatus.

There is no standard size opening; it varies with the commercial company producing the product. Most health agencies use the products of a single company; thus, the nurse should familiarize herself with the products used in her agency. The more

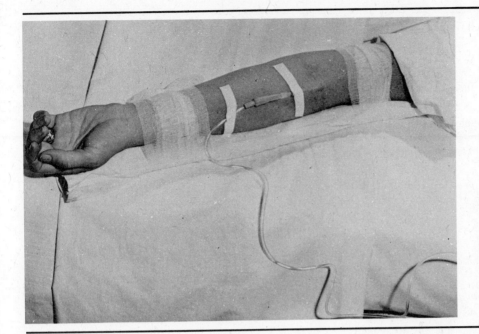

Fig. 24-7. Support under the needle to keep it from touching the wall of the vein depends on the location of the needle and the contour of the surrounding tissues. When the patient held her arm with the palm upward, no support was needed under the needle.

Fig. 24-8. The needle had to be supported with cotton if the patient wished to pronate the hand. Since having the hand pronated is normal body alignment, it is less fatiguing.

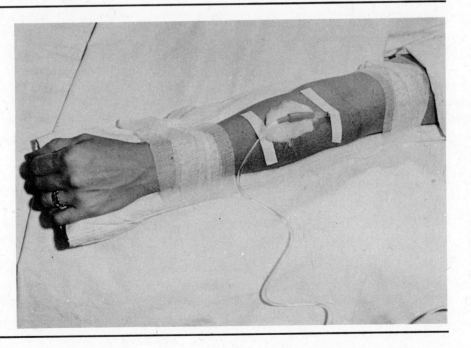

RATIONALE GUIDING ACTION IN PERFORMING AN ARM VENIPUNCTURE

The purpose is to enter a vein to inject a solution.

SUGGESTED ACTION	RATIONALE
Have patient in back-lying position and the bed in semi-Fowler's position.	The back-lying position when venipuncture is performed permits either arm to be used while in good alignment.
Place arm on board with tourniquet under arm, about 1½ inch above intended site of entry. Secure arm to board with bandage or arm board tapes. Fix only snug enough to hold arm securely.	Arm motion will move vein, causing change in position of needle. Circulation of blood can be impaired by constricting objects.
Apply tourniquet to obstruct venous blood flow; direct tourniquet ends away from site of entry.	Interrupting blood flow back to heart causes veins to distend. Interruption of arterial flow would impede venous filling. Distended veins are easy to see, palpate, and enter. Ends of tourniquet could contaminate the area of injection.
Ask patient to open and close his fist. Observe and palpate for suitable vein.	Contraction of muscles of lower arm forces blood along in veins, thereby distending them further.
Using friction, cleanse skin thoroughly at and around site of entry.	Pathogens present on the skin can be introduced into the tissues or the blood with the needle.
Use thumb to retract down on vein and soft tissue about 2 inches below intended site of injection.	Pressure on the vein and the surrounding tissues aids in preventing movement of the vein as needle is being introduced.
Hold needle at a 45° angle usually with bevel up, in line with the vein at a point about ½ inch away from intended site of entry.	Pressure needed to pierce the skin can be sufficient to force the needle into vein at improper angle and possibly through opposite wall.
When needle is through the skin, lower angle of needle until nearly parallel with skin, following same course as vein, and insert into vein.	Following the course of the vein prevents needle from leaving vein at another site.
When blood comes back through needle into tubing, insert needle farther into vein ¾ to 1 inch. Pull back on plunger, if syringe is used, until blood enters syringe.	Pressure of the patient's blood is usually greater than pressure in tubing causing automatic backflow. Pulling back on syringe plunger establishes negative pressure drawing blood into syringe. Having needle placed well into vein helps to prevent easy dislodgment of needle. "Riding" needle into vein while it is distended helps to prevent pushing it through the wall.
Release tourniquet.	Occluded vessel prevents solution from entering circulation.
Start flow of solution by releasing clamp or pushing forward on plunger.	Blood can clot readily in needle if no fluid flow is present.
Support needle with small wipe or cotton ball if necessary to keep in proper position in vein.	Pressure of the wall of the vein against the bevel of the needle will interrupt the rate of flow of solution. The wall of the vein can be punctured easily by the needle.
Anchor the tubing with tape to prevent pull on the needle.	Smooth structure of vein does not offer resistance to movement of needle. Weight of tubing is sufficient to pull needle out of vein.
Adjust rate of solution flow according to patient's situation.	Addition of substances to venous system affect general body circulation in an individualized way.
Apply pressure to venipuncture site when needle is removed.	Pressure promotes blood clotting.

common drop factors are 15 drops/ml., 20 drops/ml., and 60 drops/ml. The small opening required for 60 drops/ml. is used most frequently when small fluid volumes are important, as in infants and small children. There are also adapters available which make it possible to reduce the drop size. If 3000 ml. are to be infused over a period of 24 hours, and the drop factor is 20 drops/ml., the flow rate would be determined as follows:

$$\frac{3000ml. \times 20}{60 \times 24} = \frac{60000}{1440}$$
$$= 42 \text{ drops per minute}$$

It is also relatively simple to determine the desired hourly infusion amount rate. The following formula can be used:

$$\frac{\text{Total infusion volume}}{\text{Total number of hours}} = \text{ml. per hour}$$

In the above example, the hourly rate would be calculated as follows:

$$\frac{3000ml.}{24 \text{ hours}} = 125 \text{ ml. per hour}$$

Many factors can alter the rate of flow of an intravenous infusion. For example, the height of the container in relation to the patient, the patient's blood pressure, and the patient's position are influential. The nurse needs to know the desired rate and then adjust the infusion as necessary to achieve the rate. Her task can be facilitated by calculating the hourly flow rates and by marking them on the bottle. She then regulates the drop per minute rate by timing the flow. As she periodically checks on the infusion, she can determine quickly by glancing at her marking if the solution is being infused at the proper hourly rate. If it is not, she again regulates the flow. Because the patient's movements, disturbances of the regulation mechanism, or change in the height of the infusion bottle or bed can alter the flow rate, even after it is regulated, the nurse needs to continue to check on the infusion at regular intervals. It has been reported that standard intravenous administration sets lose up to ½ of their initial flow rate during the first hour of infusion because of tubing flexibility, and therefore the rate needs adjustment.

Maintenance of the flow rate is important because of the implications relative to the patient's fluid and electrolyte balance. Too slow a flow may result in either the occurrence of deficits because the input is not balancing the loss, or in delaying the restoration of the balance. Infusing intravenous fluid too rapidly can overtax the body's capacities to adjust to the increase in the fluid volume or the electrolytes it contains. Nurses who allow infusions to get behind schedule and increase the rate to catch up may be seriously insulting the patient's compensatory mechanisms and jeopardizing the patient's well-being. Devices which limit the amount of fluid which can be infused at any one time are available on the market. There are also battery-operated rate meters which quickly calculate the milliliter per hour flow rate of a solution as it is infusing. Some agencies use infusion pumps which regulate the flow rate at preset limits and notify the nurse by an alarm system when the solution level of the bottle is getting low.

Possible Complications: After the initial tissue penetration, most intravenous infusions should not create discomfort for the patient. If the patient is uncomfortable, the nurse should check to see that the infusion is entering the vein as intended, that the flow rate is not too rapid, and that the patient's position is satisfactory. Anxiety over the implications of an infusion can also cause discomfort for the patient.

Dislodging the needle or penetration of the vessel wall can cause the fluid to pass into the subcutaneous tissue and result in swelling, pallor, coldness, or pain at the site. This escape of fluid into the subcutaneous tissue is known as *infiltration*. The frequently used method of lowering the solution bottle below the infusion site so the vein pressure is higher than the pressure in the tubing, and then looking for blood to enter the tubing, is not a foolproof way of determining if the needle is in the vein. Blood can return in the tubing when the needle has penetrated only partially through the vessel wall. A backflow of blood in the tubing can then occur even though fluid is passing into the tissue. The needle bevel can be lodged against the vessel wall, and therefore no blood backflow will occur when the bottle is lowered even though the needle is in the vessel. Swelling and discomfort at the infusion site or continued flow of the infusion while a tourniquet occludes the veins are the best indications of infiltration. The needle should be removed when infiltration occurs.

Phlebitis is an inflammation of the vein. It is another potential hazard of intravenous infusions. Mechanical trauma or chemical irritation causes a painful inflammation along the vein. The applica-

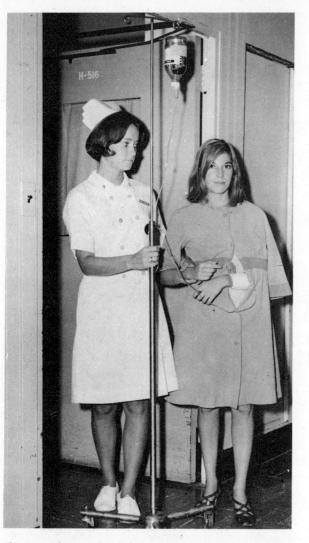

Fig. 24-9. The patient's infusion solution is hung on a pole that is easily pushed ahead of the nurse as she supports the patient.

a solution bottle was allowed to become empty, and when blood was administered under pressure. The quantity of air which would be fatal to humans is not known, but animal experimentation indicates that it is much larger than usually depicted in murder mysteries. Estimates vary from 35 ml. to 350 ml. of intravenous air as being necessary to cause the death of a person. The average infusion tubing holds about 5 ml. of air. Patients, however, are often frightened when they see air in the infusion tubing, and every effort should be made to avoid this happening.

If more than one bottle of solution is ordered for the patient, the nurse attaches the additional bottles. The method by which this is done will depend on the procedure of the agency. Some intravenous equipment is designed to simplify the procedure by making it possible to attach additional bottles with a tandemlike arrangement, as Figure 24-5 illustrates. Because infusions often are continued after the responsibility for a patient's care changes from one nurse to another, it is a good practice to agree on one common method for managing infusions. Without such uniformity, serious errors can occur, or valuable time is lost in checking and rechecking.

DISCONTINUING THE INFUSION: When the amount of solution the physician has ordered has been absorbed, the nurse assumes responsibility for discontinuing the infusion. The adhesive strips are removed, the needle is removed quickly, in line with the vein, and pressure is applied immediately to the site. If the patient is able to do so, he may be asked to hold the pressure dressing for a minute or more.

If the patient's arm or leg has been immobilized for several hours or longer, the nurse should manipulate it carefully in an attempt to put the joint through range of motion and passively move the muscles of the area.

RECORDING THE ADMINISTRATION OF AN INTRAVENOUS INFUSION: The following information is recorded: the date and the time the infusion was started and completed, the kind and the amount of solution infused, the name and the amount of any drugs added, and the name of the person starting the infusion.

Symptoms of reaction are recorded as well as any treatment which the physician may prescribe for it. Symptoms of desired effects are also recorded.

The method just described is the most common one for administering an intravenous infusion. Another method for entering a vein in order to infuse a solution is called a *cut-down*. A cut-down is an in-

tion of moist heat will usually relieve the condition. Further use of the vein should be avoided.

Blood clots, called *thrombi*, can form at the end of the needle or catheter from tissue trauma. When the thrombus is dislodged and circulates in the blood, it is called an *embolus*. Both can do serious damage if vital vessels are obstructed and tissues are deprived of blood.

Air can also circulate in the blood, and when in large quantities, it is referred to as an *air embolism*. While normally well-handled infusions do not permit air to enter the vein, it has occurred in situations when the patient's blood pressure was very low, when cision into a vein for the purpose of administering a solution. It may be a necessary procedure when the superficial veins are not readily accessible. An incision is made by the physician into the skin over a vein. This procedure of entering a vein is carried out under surgical asepsis since it constitutes minor surgery. The physician wears sterile gloves, and many agencies specify that the physician and the nurse wear masks. Plastic tubing (radiopaque) is threaded through the needle and placed into the vein. It is held in place with a suture. The infusion is conducted as described previously. When the plastic tubing is removed, a stitch or two is placed in the skin at the site of incision.

Hyperalimentation

Infusing nutrient solutions into the superior vena cava is called *hyperalimentation*. It is sometimes referred to as central venous hyperalimentation or parenteral hyperalimentation. It is a means of providing amino acids along with glucose, vitamins, and electrolytes for persons who cannot ingest nutrients normally for an extended period of time and for whom standard infusions are not adequate. The method is used generally for seriously ill patients and is discussed in more detail in advanced clinical texts. The hypertonic solution is infused into the superior vena cava through a special tubing threaded through the subclavian or internal jugular vein. The superior vena cava, with its large volume of blood, is needed for the rapid dilution of the hypertonic solution. Various chemical and volume tests are used frequently to adjust the solution components and flow rate to meet the patient's needs.

Hypodermoclysis

Hypodermoclysis is used less frequently since the intravenous method has been perfected. It can be used to administer electrolyte-containing solutions when the oral and the intravenous routes are unsatisfactory. The fluid is injected slowly into subcutaneous tissue where absorption occurs via the blood capillaries. The solution usually used is isotonic or occasionally hypotonic. Hypertonic solutions may cause water and salt depletion and damage to the subcutaneous tissue.

To hasten the rate of absorption, the enzyme (or enzyme complex) hyaluronidase or similar product is used. This drug dissolves cellular protective substances and thus makes it possible for the solution to enter the circulatory system more rapidly. It is effective for this procedure as well as for speeding the absorption of hematomas and certain drugs that ordinarily are absorbed slowly from the tissues.

NECESSARY EQUIPMENT FOR HYPODERMOCLYSIS: Hypodermoclysis usually is administered to adults by the gravity method. For children, the amount of fluid is less and usually is injected slowly at one time, using the syringe method. It is difficult and undesirable to restrain acutely ill children for a prolonged period of time.

Because subcutaneous tissue is being entered, sterile technique is employed for preparing equipment and administering a hypodermoclysis.

The tubing contains a Y connector which makes it possible for the solution to flow in two directions simultaneously. Each of the pieces of tubing to which the needles will be attached has a clamping device. These should be clamped before the tubing is attached to the container of fluid. Figure 24-5 shows this equipment. As it is with intravenous infusions, fluid is permitted to flow through the tubing slowly to force out the air. One tube at a time should be released. The tubes are clamped again, and the tips are protected until the needles are attached, to prevent their becoming contaminated. Safest practice is not to attach the needles until the infusion is to be initiated.

For the adult patient the most common sites of injection are the anterior thighs. However, for the adult female, the area directly below the breasts can be used. A 19-gauge needle, 2½ or 3 inches long, is usually used in these areas. The needles are inserted below the skin into subcutaneous tissue and then moved along horizontally in the tissue.

For children, the sites directly over the scapulae are used. An intramuscular needle of 20- or 22-gauge, 1½ inches long, is usually satisfactory for a child.

To minimize the immediate effect of the needle penetrating the skin, an application of a local anesthetic to numb the area may be used.

PREPARATION OF THE PATIENT: The patient should be made as comfortable as possible and protected from exposure. His position will depend on the area of the body to be entered. If the thighs are used, it will be necessary to divide the top bedclothes so that the tubing is not disturbed. This necessitates adjusting the bed linen to provide appropriate covering considering the patient's age, physical condition, and room temperature. Freedom of movement for the patient is also a consideration. A loin cloth will protect the patient's perineum from exposure.

Since in the gravity hypodermoclysis the solution is absorbed slowly and the procedure continues over a period of several hours, the patient should be turned or at least have his position altered somewhat, every half hour. Patients frequently are reluctant to move for fear of dislodging the needles or of creating discomfort for themselves.

INITIATING THE GRAVITY HYPODERMOCLYSIS: After the patient is in the appropriate position for the procedure, the skin is prepared with an antiseptic. Shave the area if necessary. The needles are inserted at approximately a 30° angle with a quick motion. No backflow of blood into the tubing should be present. Backflow means a vessel has been entered and the needle should be relocated. The needles are secured with supports and tape as necessary. Usual practice is to inject the hyaluronidase as soon as the solution begins to flow. A 2-c.c. syringe and a 25-gauge needle are used to inject the prescribed amount into the rubber inserts in the tubing directly above the needle attachments.

Solutions given by hypodermoclysis must be given slowly enough to allow for absorption. Allowing the solution to enter the subcutaneous tissue too rapidly may damage tissues. The nurse is responsible for adjusting the rate according to the speed of absorption. If administration is too rapid, the fluid accumulates in the tissue, the area of injection becomes swollen, and the skin over the area becomes taut. Should this occur, gentle massage over the area helps to speed the absorption of fluid. In addition to keeping check on the rate of flow and the rate of absorption, the nurse observes the patient for signs that indicate the desired effect of the hypodermoclysis. These signs depend to a large extent on the amount and the kind of solution administered. Reactions rarely occur when solutions are given by hypodermoclysis.

If more than one bottle of solution is ordered for the patient, the nurse adds the additional bottles as necessary.

DISCONTINUING A HYPODERMOCLYSIS: When the amount of solution that the physician has ordered has been absorbed, the nurse assumes responsibility for discontinuing the hypodermoclysis. The adhesive strips are removed, and the needles are removed quickly. Some of the solution tends to escape from the subcutaneous tissue where the needles have been inserted. To prevent this from occurring, a small sterile dressing may be applied snugly.

Blood Transfusion

A blood transfusion is the infusion of whole blood from a healthy person into a patient's vein. Whole blood is usually given when the person's total blood volume has been decreased. Blood components are also sometimes infused when a selective need exists.

The person giving the blood is referred to as the *donor* while the person receiving the blood is called the *recipient*. Blood may be given by either the direct or the indirect method. In the *indirect method* blood is infused after it has been collected from a donor and is the most commonly used method. The technique is similar to that for giving an intravenous infusion. In the *direct method* the blood is infused as it is being collected. This method is rarely used except in emergency situations.

SELECTING BLOOD DONORS: The selection of blood donors must be done with care. It is also important to determine whether or not the donor is free of diseases such as infectious or serum hepatitis. Persons who have allergies usually are not used; nor those with a history of a chronic disease, such as tuberculosis. As a further precaution, some blood banks will not accept blood from a donor who has been immunized recently.

Also, the donor is examined carefully at the time of donation and is permitted to give blood only if his heart and chest sounds, blood count, temperature, pulse and respiratory rate, and blood pressure are within normal ranges.

BLOOD GROUPINGS: Before blood may be given to a patient, it must be determined that the blood of the donor and that of the recipient are compatible. Research in this area indicates that an individual's blood is as unique as his fingerprints. Blood is categorized into four major groups: O,A,B, and AB. In addition to the four groups, there are many hundreds of other factors which differentiate one blood from another. The laboratory examination to determine a person's blood type is called *typing*. The process of determining compatibility between blood specimens is known as *crossmatching*.

All patients should be typed and crossmatched before a transfusion. Blood incompatibility can cause serious and even fatal reactions.

PREPARATION FOR INDIRECT BLOOD TRANSFUSION: Because a vein is being entered, sterile technique is employed. The equipment necessary for the procedure is similar to that used for an intravenous infusion by the gravity method. The drip chamber in a transfusion set contains a filter. A slightly larger needle, usually an 18-gauge, is used because of the viscosity of the blood. If the patient is sensitive to the pain of the larger needle as it pierces the skin, a small amount of local anesthetic intradermally at the site of the injection or a volatile anesthetic spray for numbing the pain receptors may be used.

The blood is dispensed in bottles or in plastic containers by a blood bank or a laboratory and is ready for use. The container is the one used for obtaining the blood from the donor and contains a solution to prevent clotting.

The safe storage of whole blood has been limited to 21 days. It is felt that after this time too large a proportion of the red cells have deteriorated. A new technique of freezing blood has extended the storage life to as long as three years. This process also seems to have the effect of reducing blood reactions.

Blood should not be secured from the laboratory or blood bank until the transfusion is to begin. The desirable temperature range to prevent blood cell deterioration is small. Therefore, storage areas are equipped with precise temperature controls. Nursing unit refrigeration normally does not provide these controls and for this reason, blood which has been dispensed from the laboratory is generally not permitted to be returned.

Blood is normally not warmed before administration in order to prevent cell damage. The blood is warmed sufficiently by the time it passes through the length of the tubing and enters the vein. Exceptions to this are occasionally made in emergency situations when large amounts of blood are transfused rapidly. In order to reduce the adjustment of the patient's body to an extreme volume of low temperature blood, special heat exchange coil units are used to warm the blood. Hot water should not be used to warm blood.

Occasionally, when small amounts are being given, as for children, the syringe method is used. The necessary equipment is the same as that used for intravenous injections.

In the management of blood for transfusion, every precaution should be taken. *Check and double check the labels, the numbers, the Rh factors, and compatibility.* After identifying information on the patient's record is checked, identification of the patient should be reaffirmed at the bedside.

TRANSFUSING THE BLOOD: Gentle inversion of the blood container will resuspend the red cells before the transfusion. Initiating a blood transfusion is similar to a solution infusion. Isotonic saline solution with a Y connection between it and the blood container is frequently used to start the transfusion. Figure 24-5 demonstrates this arrangement. The saline solution makes the blood backflow into the tubing upon vein entry easy to determine; if blood is already present in the tubing, it is extremely difficult to detect the patient's blood backflow. Glucose solution should not be used with blood because the

hypertonicity of the solution causes red cell hemolysis.

After the transfusion has been started, it is the nurse's responsibility to see that the blood is regulated at the rate of flow specified by the physician. During the time blood is flowing, the nurse should check the rate carefully. Changing the height of the bed and elevating or lowering the patient's head can alter the rate of flow. Repositioning the extremity in which the needle is located may also halt or change the rate of flow. The blood container may need to be gently agitated occasionally when the red cells settle to the bottom.

OBSERVING THE PATIENT FOR SIGNS OF A REACTION: Reactions to transfusion even occur when every precaution has been observed in selecting the blood and in sterilizing and preparing the equipment. The nurse should be prepared to recognize the signs and the symptoms of untoward effects of a transfusion. No untoward effects or discomfort should accompany a blood transfusion if all factors of safety and matching of blood have been observed carefully. Incompatibility reactions generally occur after the first 100 ml. to 200 ml. of blood have infused. Any sign of discomfort or any change in the patient's appearance or behavior should be taken into careful consideration if a blood transfusion is being administered or has been recently administered.

The most serious and quickest complication to occur is the hemolytic reaction when incompatible bloods have been mixed. If the patient begins to have symptoms of discomfort, such as headache, sensations of tingling, difficulty in breathing, or pain in the lumbar region, stop the transfusion and notify the physician immediately.

Other reactions may occur after the transfusion has been running for a short time, or perhaps many hours later. They are caused by protein substances to which the patient is allergic. The patient may complain of feeling itchy, especially in areas where the skin is warm, as the back and the buttocks. If hives (urticaria) appear near the site of the needle or on other parts of the body, the reaction is easy to recognize. However, the picture may be complicated if the patient also complains of difficulty in breathing and has laryngeal edema. For allergic reactions, the blood is also stopped immediately.

Febrile reactions, which may be due to some contaminant in the blood, usually occur late in the course of the transfusion or after it has been completed. The patient has an elevated temperature and shows signs of a systemic infection. Flushing of the skin and general malaise are typical.

Occasionally, the addition of blood to the existing supply produces circulatory overload, which is noted by increased pulse rate and dyspnea. This may result in pulmonary edema which can be recognized by signs of respiratory distress, moist coughing, and possibly expectoration of blood-tinged mucus.

Since blood given by the indirect method contains substances to help prevent clotting, it is not unlikely that some individuals may react to these chemicals. Usually, the reaction is mild and of short duration, but it does produce discomfort for the patient and bears careful watching.

TRANSFUSION OF BLOOD EXTRACTS: Some patients do not need all the constituents of whole blood. For example, one may need red blood cells but not the plasma and its constituents. Red blood cells in concentrated form sometimes are given to these patients. In other situations, only plasma is required. Human serum or plasma is particularly useful in emergencies for immediate restoration of fluids, since serum presents no compatibility problem and time need not be lost matching bloods and seeking donors.

Fractions, such as serum albumin and gamma globulin, have been separated out of plasma and used for the treatment and the prevention of certain diseases.

GASTRIC AND DUODENAL SUCTION

Gastric and duodenal suction provides for the continuous removal of contents from the stomach or duodenum or both by use of a partial vacuum. As indicated earlier in this chapter, the removal of these body secretions results in extensive fluid and electrolyte loss. Therefore, the patient having this type of therapy must be observed for indications of fluid and electrolyte imbalance.

Continuous suction is used when it becomes desirable and necessary to keep the stomach and the duodenum empty and at rest. For example, prior to gastric surgery, the surgeon usually wishes to have the area free of gas and undigested food; following surgery performed on the gastrointestinal tract, he may wish to keep the stomach and the duodenum empty and at rest until healing at the site of the operation has begun. The suctioning is effective for removing secretions and air or gas that often accumulate in the gastrointestinal tract following abdominal surgery. This helps to prevent distention. Continuous suctioning is indicated also when there is a paralysis in the gastrointestinal tract and the normal movement of the products of digestion is interrupted, for example, by a paralysis of the ileus. Suctioning then is used to prevent distention, discomfort, and the dangers associated with the paralysis. Suctioning may also be used when the patient is nauseated and the prevention of vomiting is desired. Whatever the reason for removing the gastrointestinal contents, the potential for fluid and electrolyte disturbances is always high.

A variety of tubes is available for use for suctioning gastric and duodenal contents. If simple decompression of the stomach is desired, a long plain tube, such as the Levin tube, is used. The disposable tubes are very satisfactory, since they seem to be comfortable for the patient, are less objectionable when secured to the face, and eliminate the difficult problem of thorough cleaning.

If suctioning of the duodenum is desired and to be continued over a period of several hours or days, then one of a variety of other tubes is used. These usually have a device at the end which keeps the tip of the tube in the duodenum.

One type of tube has a double lumen. One lumen connects with a small rubber bag. After the tube is past the pylorus, the bag is inflated with fluid or air. Another type of tube is injected with mercury, usually 5 ml. The air, the fluid, and the mercury tips aid in the forward movement of the tube. These tips also act to keep the tube in situ by preventing the tube from moving back into the stomach. These tubes are chilled on ice and passed through one of the nares in the same manner as other gastric tubes.

Insertion of a tube into the stomach was described in Chapter 20. If it is desired that the tube enter the duodenum, peristalsis aids in moving it through the pyloric valve. Usually, it is helpful to have the patient lie on his right side so that gravity will aid the tube in dropping into the duodenum. As a rule every 20 or 30 minutes, a few more inches of the tube are passed until the desired length has entered the gastrointestinal tract. Suctioning either is started as soon as the tube has reached the stomach or is delayed until the tube is in the duodenum, depending on the physician's wishes.

Fluids and gases move from an area of greater pressure to one of lesser pressure. To remove liquids and gases from the gastrointestinal tract, it is necessary to decrease the pressure in the collection container and tubing to below atmospheric pressure or create a partial vacuum. Then the greater pressure within the gastrointestinal system will force the contents from the stomach and/or duodenum to move into the tubing and collection container.

The manner in which suction is maintained on

the drainage tube will depend on each agency's equipment. Most agencies have electric pumps which automatically maintain a partial vacuum in the bottle that collects drainage from the patient; others have wall suction which can be connected to the collecting bottle. A syringe attached to the free end of the tube can be used also to create an area of lesser pressure in the tube by partially evacuating the air from the tube.

To remove gastrointestinal contents with a syringe over a long period of time is not convenient or expedient. Therefore, a mechanical device is used to great advantage. The nurse is responsible for seeing that the apparatus is functioning properly at all times. The patient's tube is irrigated at regular intervals, as ordered by the physician. Normal saline or water, usually about 30 ml., is used. When irrigating is done, it is easy to determine whether or not the tube is patent. After the solution has been injected, the suction is started again, and the irrigating fluid should return quickly.

Because the patient often becomes uncomfortable from thirst and from the dryness of his oral mucous membranes, he may be permitted to have ice or liquids in limited quantities. As stated earlier, large amounts of plain water can cause electrolytes to leave the body even faster. Frequent oral hygiene can also increase the patient's comfort.

The nares require special care while the drainage tube is in place. Regular cleansing and the application of a small amount of lubrication help to keep the mucous membrane in good condition.

The nurse is responsible for noting the type and the amount of drainage present. Most agencies provide a routine for measuring, emptying, and cleansing the drainage bottle in every 24-hour period. The amounts of solution used for irrigations and returned, as well as any oral fluids the patient ingested, are also noted. Recording of these amounts are discussed in the next section.

INTAKE AND OUTPUT MEASUREMENT

Measurement of a patient's fluid intake and output is an important part of estimating balance and imbalance states. Intake and output measurements are commonly abbreviated I and O. Securing these measurements is a common part of nursing care. Accuracy of the total intake and output from all sources is important. This means that ingested as well as infused fluids are calculated. Losses include urine, emesis, suction tube drainage, feces (especially if the excrement is liquid), and sometimes wound drainage. Estimates of feces and wound drainage are generally satisfactory, but all of the other liquids are actually measured.

Most health agencies use standard size drinking utensils and have their capacities marked on recording sheets which are kept at the patient's beside. The labels of infusion bottles indicate their volume. Calibrated containers are available for measuring fluid losses.

When the patient at home must maintain an intake and output measurement, the nurse can assist him by determining the capacity of several frequently used drinking containers with a household measuring cup and marking them. A household container of sufficient capacity can also be marked for measuring output.

The patient and his family should be helped to understand the purpose, importance, and technique of intake and output measurement. Their cooperation is important for accuracy. Involving the patient in this aspect of his care is also a means of promoting his independence. Maintaining his own record can be an especially helpful motivating force for the patient whose oral intake is being increased.

Various types of forms are used in health agencies to maintain fluid balance records. In most situations the patient's fluid intake and output are totaled on his record at 8- and 24-hour intervals. Figure 24-10 illustrates an example of such a form. The patient at home can be assisted to adapt this type of form to his needs.

CONCLUSION

The veil of mystery lying over many workings of the body has been lifted with new knowledge established in the science of biochemistry. Science has explained many exceedingly complex processes that, at best, had been left largely to guesswork concerning their nature.

As this chapter has pointed out, the exactness of normal fluid and electrolyte balance and the compensatory mechanisms that maintain relatively little variation in balance have been fairly well-explained. In illness states, when the body needs assistance to maintain fluid and electrolyte balances, the demands for high-quality and exacting care can be seen. Hopefully, this chapter has helped the reader with knowledge that promotes such care and that opens vistas on the marvelous workings of the human body.

INTAKE AND OUTPUT CHART

7:00 A.M. _6/14_ TO 7:00 A.M. _6/15_

GREEN, JOHN
Rm. 316

	INTAKE			OUTPUT					
	ORAL	INTRAVENOUS & MEDICATIONS ADDED	SIGNATURE	Gastric Tube	Urine	Stool	Vomitus	Other	SIGNATURE
7-8	25ml			30ml					
8-9	30			45	250				
9-10		5% D/W; 1000 ml. IV	J. Brown	25		FORMED			
10-11				30					
11-12	25			35	350				
12-1				Discontinued					
1-2	50				150				
2-3	50								
8 HR. TOT.	180			165	750	—	—	—	M. Jones
3-4	50				250				
4-5	75	5% D/W, 1000 ml. I.V.	G. White						
5-6	50								
6-7	100				350				
7-8	75								
8-9	75								
9-10	50				375				
10-11									
8 HR. TOT.	475			—	975	—	—	—	G. White
11-12									
12-1									
1-2									
2-3	75				150				
3-4									
4-5									
5-6									
6-7	50				150				
8 HR. TOT.	125			—	300	—	—	—	
24 HR. TOT.	780 ml.	2000 ml.		165	2025	—	—	—	J. Doe
	TOTAL INTAKE	2780 ml.		TOTAL OUTPUT	2190 ml.				

05-0037

INTAKE AND OUTPUT CHART

Fig. 24-10. Fluid intake and output form.

Study Situations

1. In the following article, the author poses four questions for consideration when making a nursing assessment of the preoperative patient.

   Kee, J.: Fluid and electrolyte imbalances. **Nurs. '72,** 2:22–23, Jan., 1972.

   What sources would you use to collect appropriate data about a patient? Identify standards you would use to judge the data and to arrive at nursing assessments.

2. Ware, A. M., and Chelgren, M. N.: When "Holding On" Brought Change. *In* **The Nursing Clinics of North America.** Philadelphia, W. B. Saunders, 6:125–134, Mar., 1971.

   The above article discusses behavioral changes that were part of the symptoms of Mrs. Blane's electrolyte imbalance. What supportive nursing actions might you have used to respond to her "holding on."

3. The author of the following article indicates that each of us has fluid intake patterns:

   Fenton, M.: What to do about thirst. **Am. J. Nurs.,** 69:1014–1017, May, 1969.

   Do you know what your thirst pattern is? How could the knowledge about a patient's thirst pattern help in planning nursing care when his intake is limited?

4. The author of the following article gives some guides for infusion flow rates on pages 79 and 80. Using these guides and the formulas in this chapter, how many drops per minute should a 150 pound man receive of an isotonic solution? How many drops per minute should this same man receive of a hypertonic solution?

   Abbey, J. C.: Nursing observations of fluid imbalances. *In* **The Nursing Clinics of North America.** Philadelphia, W. B. Saunders, 3:77–86, Mar., 1968.

References

1. Betson, C.: Blood gases. **Am. J. Nurs.,** 68:1010–1012, May, 1968.
2. Buchanan-Davidson, D. J.: A drop of blood. **Am. J. Nurs.,** 65:103–107, July, 1965.
3. Burgess, R. E.: Fluids and electrolytes. **Am. J. Nurs.,** 65:90–95, Oct., 1965.
4. Cannon, W. B.: The Wisdom of the Body. pp. 23–25. New York, W. W. Norton, 1939.
5. Child, J., *et al.:* Blood transfusions. **Am. J. Nurs.,** 72:1602–1605, Sept., 1972.
6. Dickens, M. L.: Fluid and Electrolyte Balance: A Programmed Text. Ed. 2. Philadelphia, F. A. Davis, 1970.
7. Donn, R.: Intravenous admixture incompatibility. **Am. J. Nurs.,** 71:325, Feb., 1971.
8. Drummond, E. E., and Anderson, M. L.: Gastrointestinal suction. **Am. J. Nurs.,** 63:109–113, Dec., 1963.
9. Dudrick, S. J., and Rhoades, J. E.: Total intravenous feeding. **Sci. Am.,** 226:73–80, May, 1972.
10. Duma, R. J., *et al.:* Septicemia from intravenous infusions. **New Engl. J. Med.,** 284:257–260, Feb. 4, 1971.
11. Dutcher, I. E., and Fielo, S. B.: Water and Electrolytes: Implications for Nursing Practice. New York, Macmillan, 1967.
12. Fox, C. F.: The structure of cell membranes. **Sci. Am.,** 226:31–38, Feb., 1972.
13. Grant, J. N.: Patient care in parenteral hyperalimentation. *In* **The Nursing Clinics of North America.** Philadelphia, W. B. Saunders, 8:165–181, Mar., 1973.
14. Heath, J. K.: A conceptual basis for assessing body water status. *In* **The Nursing Clinics of North America.** Philadelphia, W. B. Saunders, 6:189–198, Mar., 1971.
15. Johnson, N. E.: Coping with complications of intravenous therapy. **Nurs. '72,** 2:5–9, Feb., 1972.
16. Kee, J. L.: Fluids and Electrolytes With Clinical Applications: A Programmed Approach. New York, John Wiley and Sons, 1971.
17. Lapides, J., *et al.:* Clinical signs of dehydration and extracellular fluid loss. **JAMA,** 191:413–415, Feb. 1, 1965.
18. Mazzara, J. T., and Ayres, S. M.: Fluid, electrolyte, and acid-base disturbances in the coronary care unit. *In* **The Nursing Clinics of North America.** Philadelphia, W. B. Saunders, 7:549–562, Sept., 1972.
19. Moore, V. B.: I.V. Fluids: Product Survey, **Nurs. '73,** 3:32–38, June, 1973.
20. Parsa, M. H., *et al.:* Central venous alimentation. **Am. J. Nurs.,** 72:2042–2047, Nov., 1972.
21. Payne, J. E., and Kaplan, H. M.: Alternative techniques for venipuncture. **Am. J. Nurs.,** 72:702–703, Apr., 1972.
22. Pederson, B. M.: A solution for post-infusion thrombophlebitis. **Am. J. Nurs.,** 70:325, Feb., 1970.
23. Plumer, A. L.: Principles and Practice of Intravenous Therapy. Boston, Little, Brown and Company, 1970.
24. Potassium imbalance: programmed instruction. **Am. J. Nurs.,** 67:343–366, Feb., 1967.
25. Reed, G. M., and Sheppard, V. F.: Regulation of Fluid and Electrolyte Balance: A Programmed Instruction in Physiology for Nurses. Philadelphia, W. B. Saunders, 1971.
26. Shepard, R. S.: Human Physiology. p. 390. Philadelphia, J. B. Lippincott, 1971.
27. Snively, W. D. Jr., and Beshear, D. R.: Textbook of Pathophysiology. pp. 133–160. Philadelphia, J. B. Lippincott, 1972.
28. ———: Water and electrolytes in health and disease. pp. 246–276. *In* Kintzel, K. C., ed.: Advanced Concepts in Clinical Nursing. Philadelphia, J. B. Lippincott, 1971.
29. Voda, A. M.: Body water dynamics: A clinical application. **Am. J. Nurs.,** 70:2594–2601, Dec., 1970.
30. Wilmore, D. W.: The future of intravenous therapy. **Am. J. Nurs.,** 71:2334–2338, Dec., 1971.

CHAPTER 25

Maintaining Nutrition

GLOSSARY

Anorexia: Loss of appetite or a lack of desire for food.

Antiemetic: Drug used to allay vomiting.

Appetite: The pleasant anticipation of food.

Basal Metabolism Rate: Heat production of the body at its lowest level of cell chemistry and of body activity.

Calorie: Amount of heat necessary to raise the temperature of 1 kilogram of water 1° C.

Emesis: The act of vomiting.

Eructation: Discharge of gas from the stomach through the mouth.

Food Additives: Ingredients added to food to improve color, flavor, consistency, and stability.

Food Supplements: Preparations added to the diet that add nourishment to what is eaten.

Gastric Gavage: Introduction of nourishment into the stomach by mechanical means.

Nausea: Feeling of sickness with a desire to vomit.

Nutrition: Process whereby the body uses food to achieve and maintain health.

Pernicious Vomiting: Persistent and intractable vomiting.

Projectile Vomiting: Expulsion of vomitus with great force.

Regurgitation: Bringing stomach contents to the throat and mouth without vomiting efforts.

Retching: Unproductive muscle movements that ordinarily produce vomiting.

Satiety: Feeling of having had enough to eat.

Vomit: The forceful expulsion of gastric contents through the mouth.

Vomitus: Vomited matter.

INTRODUCTION

Food and its effects on the body have interested mankind for thousands of years. Only during the early decades of the twentieth century did nutrition become a science. Biochemistry and microchemical analysis have become useful tools in the study of food, its digestion and absorption, and metabolism.

Problems in relation to nutrition vary widely and usually have interrelated causes. Insufficient caloric and protein intake are major problems in many parts of the world and usually, anyplace where poverty exists. In areas where people have the wherewithal to consume too many calories, as is true in many places in the United States for example, the problem is one of maintaining a balanced diet. Having too much food in itself is a problem for many people. Eating has many psychosocial implications also. To look only at an individual's diet without regard to his environment and his whole person and personality results in a distorted picture.

MAN'S NUTRITIONAL NEEDS

Nutrition is the process whereby the body uses food to achieve and maintain health. It is concerned with the process by which food is utilized to maintain biological structure through the growth and repair of tissues. The food we eat supplies the energy and cellular materials we need to live.

Nutritional needs have been fairly well-defined. We need a certain number of calories to meet energy requirements. We need specific constituents found in food to maintain health: water, protein, carbohydrates, fats, vitamins, and minerals. Of these needs water is the most urgent. We should also consider needs in relation to palatability, availability, and the cost of food when trying to meet dietary requirements. For example, a person may be observed to need a higher protein intake than he has been getting. There is little benefit in suggesting that he eat more meat if he cannot afford to buy it or if meat is not readily available where he lives.

The constituents described below are necessary in a well-balanced diet. This can usually be accomplished with relative ease when the daily diet consists of two to four or more servings of food selected from each of the four major food groups: milk and milk products; meat, including fish, poultry, eggs, and cheese; vegetables and fruits; and bread and cereals.

Calories

Heat is produced by the oxidation of food. It is a form of energy. Other forms of energy (mechanical, chemical, electrical) can also be expressed in terms of heat. If we measure the body's heat production, we can then ascertain the amount of food needed to produce that amount of heat or energy. Hence, food energy can be expressed in terms of heat.

The measurement for heat is called a calorie. A *calorie* is the amount of heat necessary to raise the temperature of 1 kilogram of water 1° C. We speak of food as having certain caloric value, meaning the

food is capable of furnishing a specific amount of heat or energy to the body.

The heat production of an individual at the lowest level of cell chemistry and of body activity is referred to as the *basal metabolism rate*. For an average adult male, the required calories to cover a basal metabolism rate is roughly 1700; for a female, about 1400. For many hours in every individual's day, metabolism does not go on at a basal or minimum rate because of normal activities in everyday living. Hence, intake of calories must be greater than basal to produce sufficient energy to carry out these activities. Examples of factors that influence an individual's caloric needs beyond basal are age, sex, environmental temperature, and activity. During pregnancy and lactation, a woman needs more calories also.

Protein Requirements

Protein has great practical importance because it is generally the most expensive nutrient, except for legumes such as peas and beans. Protein is observed to be in shortest supply in most instances when malnutrition is present. Not only is protein important for its calories but it is also essential for the structural protein of body tissues and the several nitrogenous materials synthesized in the body. Protein is found in both animal and vegetable foods. The presence of nitrogen, sulfur, and usually phosphorus in the chemical structure of proteins distinguishes them from carbohydrates and fats.

Fat Requirements

Fats are generally more expensive than foods high in carbohydrate content but cheaper than foods high in protein content. Fat is an important food requirement as a source of essential fatty acids, as a vehicle for fat-soluble vitamins and as an important contributor to the palatability of the diet. It provides a more concentrated form of energy than proteins or carbohydrates. Its high caloric content is a disadvantage for persons wishing to lose weight.

Carbohydrate Requirements

Foods rich in carbohydrate content are the main source of calories in most diets and the least expensive source of food for most people. Contrary to what many think, carbohydrates are important for other reasons than calories. For example, cellulose, which makes up much of the stems, leaves, and woody portion of plants, provides necessary bulk that aids digestion. Most plants are primarily carbohydrates. Granulated sugar is pure carbohydrate. Extra carbohydrate in the diet can be stored and used when the body needs it. The liver stores excess in the form of glycogen; if there is still more excess, it can be changed into body fat.

Minerals

In general, minerals are normally present in food in sufficient quantities; thus, a well-balanced, normal diet is rarely deficient of minerals. However, some create problems in certain circumstances. For example, salt may need to be limited when there is water imbalance. Calcium is necessary to build and maintain the skeletal system, especially during childhood, pregnancy, and lactation. When the body is short of calcium, the skeletal system will give up this mineral when required by other tissues. For example, the mother's skeletal system will give up calcium for fetal development and milk production if her diet is deficient in calcium during pregnancy and lactation.

Iron deficiency can be serious because iron is essential for the formation of hemoglobin. Important trace minerals in the diet include phosphorus and iodine. When iodine is in short supply in the diet, the use of iodized salt is recommended.

Vitamins

Vitamins are essential accessory food substances. They do not provide calories in any significant amount, but they play an indispensable role in a number of different processes necessary for health. They are organic in nature; they cannot be manufactured by the body; and they are important in maintaining normal tissue functioning.

Vitamins are either fat-soluble—A, D, E, and K, for example—or they are water-soluble—C and the B-complex vitamins. The number of identifiable vitamins continues to grow as research becomes more sophisticated.

The exact daily requirement for some vitamins is not known. However, certain diseases that occur when vitamin intake is inadequate are well-described. Also, it is known that some disorders result from consuming too large quantities; for example, too much intake of Vitamin D has been observed to be toxic to the body.

Within recent years, there has been much interest in the assertion that daily doses of Vitamin C in much larger than the adult daily requirement of 60 mg. will help to prevent colds and strengthen arteries. Although some well-known scientists have supported the claims, proof following rigorous scientific investigation is lacking. Also, the safety of taking large doses of Vitamin C over a prolonged period of time has not been established.

Water

From 75 to 80 percent of animal tissue is water. The water content of the body must be maintained at a fairly constant level in order to preserve health. It is important for the absorption of nutrients in the body and is the chief ingredient of extracellular fluids. It is an important constituent of body secretions and excretions.

THE REGULATION OF FOOD INTAKE

The mechanism which makes one eat the amount and kind of food required by the body is not clearly understood. Certain factors are known to play a part in the regulation of food intake, but there may possibly be many more than the three usually identified: hunger, thirst, and satiety. *Satiety* is the feeling of having had enough to eat. Certainly, the influence of these factors varies too among individuals. For example, the young and the active feel hungry often while the sedentary may rarely feel hunger pangs. It has been observed that any one or any combination of these three factors may be influenced by illness.

It is theorized that there are centers in the hypothalamus that regulate food intake. Experiments have shown that injury to one part of the hypothalamus results in overeating while injury to another part results in undereating.

A common problem in societies with a high standard of living is obesity. It has been demonstrated rather conclusively that obesity plays an important part in premature death. In addition, it is undesirable from the point of view of comfort and appearance. A variety of reasons have been shown to cause obesity—endocrine imbalance and genetic and psychological factors being included. While these reasons as well as others undoubtedly play a part, in the final analysis, obesity is the result of taking in food in excess of the body's caloric requirements. The excess is stored as fat.

A great variety of diets to lose weight are described in the literature. Many are eccentric and nutritionally unsound. Weight loss after crash dieting is very often temporary since the person usually returns to the same eating habits that brought about obesity in the first place. There are no diet or slimming foods but only different caloric contents in various foods. For many people, the problem of obesity might well be mostly a problem of arithmetic and lack of knowledge concerning the body's caloric needs.

Obesity is no simple matter for most overweight persons. The nurse counseling the obese patient must begin by demonstrating acceptance of the patient and by recognizing that excess caloric intake can rarely be controlled without consideration of psychological as well as physical factors that contribute to the condition. For many people, the will power to follow a reducing diet appears to be strengthened when people work together toward weight loss in groups. For the underweight patient, who is trying to gain weight which may be important to him for the sake of his appearance if for no other reason, the problem may be as irritating and difficult as the problem of losing weight for the obese.

The most efficient and safest way to control obesity is through dietary discretion, exercise, and the change of eating habits. The diet should be well-balanced but limited in the amounts of calories eaten.

Alcohol is a fairly common dietary item and when its intake cannot be regulated, drinking excessive amounts leads to many health problems. In wine-producing countries, it has been estimated that up to 10 percent of the total caloric supply comes from wine. Most of the alcohol is oxidized by the body although some is lost via the respiratory and urinary tract. Because of the caloric content of alcohol, the heavy drinker tends to gain or maintain his weight while eating less. Usually, vitamin and protein intake is insufficient in the diet of heavy drinkers. This in turn leads to some of the common problems of chronic alcoholism.

PSYCHOSOCIAL AND CULTURAL ASPECTS OF EATING

The rituals associated with eating are deeply ingrained in patterns of social behavior and are learned from early childhood. Food is often associated with solemn occasions such as weddings, funerals, and certain religious ceremonies. Eating fads sometimes carry strong emotional overtones. Here are some examples of psychosocial and cultural factors related to food and eating.

• Religious practices often dictate eating patterns. For example, the Buddhist eats no meat and Moslems and many Jews avoid pork. Fasting plays a role in some religions, and bread and wine are used in the sacraments of communion.

• Cultural factors influence eating habits. In western countries, plates, knives, forks, and spoons are used for eating. Arabs use bread and fingers to obtain food from common serving dishes. In the Orient, chopsticks are favored eating utensils. It is customary in the United States, for example, to have coffee, fruit, bacon, and eggs for breakfast while the English often serve meat or fish such as kidneys and kippers.

• Certain foods are associated with certain nationalities. Americans favor hamburgers, hot dogs, and apple pie. The Armenians prefer shish kebab while the Italians favor spaghetti.

• Eating is a time for family and friends to gather in most cultures. It is the rare hostess who does not offer her guests food during their visit.

• For the tense person, food often appears to relieve anxieties.

• Food is used to show love, candy being a typical example. The denial of food is often used to punish: for example, the child who is sent to bed without dinner or the prisoner who is served bread and water.

Many more examples could be cited. The observant nurse will wish to consider psychosocial and cultural factors associated with eating in order to be of the most assistance in helping patients meet nutritional needs.

FOOD ADDITIVES AND SUPPLEMENTS

Americans seem especially obsessed with what, when, and how to eat. While there are those who have inadequate amounts of food to eat in this country, a large majority eat too much and the wrong kind of food. In one way, food may be considered inexpensive since less of the American's disposable dollar is spent on food than in many other countries. However, cost in terms of human life is another matter since it is generally agreed that dietary habits account for many illnesses and premature deaths in this country.

A relatively recent surge in writing on diet and nutrition sometimes appears to threaten the pleasures of eating. Food additives and supplements appear to be at war with the so-called natural or organic foods. Unfortunately, a good deal of myth often shrouds the facts. For example, contrary to some claims, there has been no good evidence to illustrate that organically grown foods are any more nutritious than food grown in the conventional manner.

Food supplements are defined as preparations containing vitamins, minerals, or proteins, or combinations of these and other nutrients. Their purpose is to add nutrition to the diet. For example, vitamins are a commonly used dietary supplement. The extent of their use can be gauged by the fact that Americans spent approximately $500 million on vitamins in 1972.

Certain foods such as cereals and breads may be nutritionally enriched or fortified by adding supplements to replace or restore vitamins and minerals removed by food processing. An example of a commonly fortified product is milk to which Vitamin D has been added. Another example is salt to which iodine has been added. These ingredients are food supplements.

Food additives are ingredients added to food to improve the color, flavor, consistency, and stability of the food. Use of additives is not new. Man has used salt for many centuries, for example, as a food additive to preserve foods. If additives were not used, much of the food we buy today would be uncolored and bland and would have a short shelf life. Rather than this, manufacturers have used additives as a trade-off.

Here are a few examples of types of additives commonly used in food processing today.

• Preservatives to prevent spoilage, for example, in butter, margarine, soft drinks, and beer.
• Antioxidants to retard rancidity, for example, in butter, cream, shortening, and processed meats.
• Surfactants to produce stable mixtures of liquids that would otherwise separate, such as ice cream, peanut butter, and gelatin.
• Thickeners, for example, in cheese, ice cream, jellies, and jams.
• Coloring agents, for example, in ice cream, gelatin, and cake mixes.
• Artificial sweeteners, for example, in soft drinks, cakes, jellies, and jams.
• Bleaches, for example, in bread and cake.

Some of the food additives came under scrutiny when it was demonstrated that they were capable of producing pathology in animals. It had been believed that the additives, ingested more sparingly by man than by experimental animals, were harmless. However, it has been shown that many may be stored in the body and eventually may build up to dangerous levels. Natural or organic foods became popular as the additive scare gained momentum.

The Federal Drug Administration is the agency responsible for enforcing laws in relation to food processing. The *Delaney clause* in the Food Additive Amendment of 1958 prohibits the use of food additives of any that "...is found after tests which are appropriate...to induce cancer in man or animals." The burden of proof is with the manufacturer. While the Delaney clause seems sufficiently clear, the problems are complex since the variety and number of additives are numerous and many have been in use for many, many years without ever having been submitted to rigorous testing. Examples include the commonly used spices and numerous food flavorings.

Final or definitive answers are not known concerning the controversy surrounding food additives and supplements. Most authorities believe that there is a safe middle ground. While the numerous problems become resolved, the best advice for the average consumer is to be alert to news as it develops in this field. Also, due caution is advised in judging assertions that are made by persons holding to excessive claims on either side of the controversy.

The most recent research reported (as this text was being prepared) is concerned with changing the molecular structure of food additives. It is known that food is absorbed when the molecules are sufficiently small after the digestive process to pass through the intestinal wall. Food additives are small molecules that are absorbed almost immediately, just as digested food. The body is programmed to use the products of digestion, but food additives are strangers in the body with no particular place to go. They tend to accumulate in various organs where they may eventually cause problems. The research under way is attempting to increase the size of the additive molecule with polymers so that they cannot be absorbed. Should the research prove successful, many problems believed to be associated with additives will have been solved.

SEPARATING FADS FROM FACTS

As a health teacher, the nurse has a responsibility to assist patients to separate fads from facts in relation to nutrition. The list of claims and facts on the next page was prepared by the Food and Drug Administration, U.S. Department of Health, Education, and Welfare, Public Health Service, in 1971.

Following this list are suggestions offered by the Federal Drug Administration to help protect the public from nutritional fads. These suggestions were also published in 1971 by the Department of Health, Education, and Welfare.

Claim	Fact
1. You are what you eat.	In one sense, yes. You are also what heredity and environment have contributed.
2. Our soil has lost its vitamins and minerals; our food crops have little nutritional value.	In the commercial production of food crops fertilizers are applied in order to produce satisfactory yields. The nutrients which promote good plant growth are added to the soil in these fertilizers, and the food crops produced contain the expected nutritional value.
3. Chemical fertilizers are poisoning our soil.	Chemical fertilizers are not poisoning our soil. Modern fertilizers are needed to produce enough food for our population. Our increasing population further increases the need for these fertilizers.
4. Natural, organic fertilizers are not only safer than chemical fertilizers, but produce healthier crops.	Organic fertilizers cannot be absorbed, as such, by plants. They must be broken down by bacteria in the soil until they finally become the same chemical elements—potassium, phosphorus and nitrogen—that are supplied directly and more quickly by modern chemical fertilizers. Their use may also contribute to the spread of certain infectious diseases.
5. Pesticides are poisoning our nation.	When pesticides on food crops leave a residue, FDA and the Environmental Protection Agency (EPA) make sure the amount will be safe for consumers. The amount allowed, if any, is set at the lowest level that will accomplish the desired purpose, even though a larger amount might still be safe.
6. Modern processing removes most of the vitamins and minerals in foods.	This is not true. While any type of processing, including simple cooking, tends to reduce to some extent the nutrient content or quality of foods, modern processing methods are designed to keep such losses as low as possible. In many instances, nutrients are restored by enrichment after processing.
7. Aluminum cooking utensils are dangerous to health.	Aluminum is the second most abundant mineral element in the soil, and it, therefore, occurs naturally in many foods. Cooking in aluminum utensils is harmless.
8. Cooking with Teflon-coated utensils is dangerous.	Careful testing of this commercial product has proved that there is no danger from normal kitchen use, or the overheating which might occur in the kitchen.
9. If you have an ache or pain, or are just feeling tired, you are probably suffering from a subclinical deficiency.	Feeling poorly, lacking pep, or experiencing an ache or pain occurs in most persons at some time or another. These are symptoms which may be caused by overwork, emotional stress, disease, lack of sleep as well as by poor nutrition. If such symptoms persist, a person should see his physician. It is extremely difficult for the average person to accurately diagnose the cause of these symptoms.
10. You have to eat special foods if you want to correct overweight.	Your physician should prescribe any special diet you may need. Personal experimenting and fad diets can be highly dangerous to your health. Successful weight control depends primarily on self-control of one's total food intake while maintaining a reasonable level of physical activity.
11. Synthetic vitamins are dead and ineffective; vitamins from natural sources are much better.	Vitamins are specific chemical compounds, and the human body can use them equally well whether they are synthesized by a chemist or by nature.
12. Everyone should take vitamins, just to be sure.	Very few of us eat exactly the same foods as our neighbors eat. There is some variation that makes our diet different from everyone else's. It is variety that helps to assure adequate nutrition for most of us. Most healthy individuals whose diet regularly includes even modest amounts of meat and eggs, milk products, fruits and vegetables, bread, and other cereal products need not resort to dietary supplements. Some persons under a doctor's care or in institutions need dietary supplements because of special conditions which greatly restrict their ability to eat a well-balanced diet. Modest supplementation with certain vitamins is generally recommended during infancy, pregnancy, and while breast feeding.

• Don't buy a product or alter your eating habits on impulse or from fear. Take enough time to ask yourself the following questions:

Does the promoter belittle normal foods? This is the first sign of nutritional quackery.

Does the product, or the person, promise or imply a quick correction for a condition you think you may have?

Is the product sold in homes by people who tell you they are interested only in helping people in need. They will agree with any ailment you may say you have, and they have a product to treat your condition. They are not doctors—they are not experts on nutrition—they are salesmen.

• When you see a testimonial, remember that legitimate practitioners do not use them. Testimonials are commonly bought and sold; some are sincere—but essentially worthless, due to the individual's lack of nutritional and medical knowledge.

• Ask known, competent authorities for all information concerning your health. You will receive honest, dependable facts.

GENERAL PRINCIPLES OF NUTRITION

From the previous discussion, several principles of nutrition can be stated.

All body cells require adequate nutrition. Food is basic to life, and there are food substances essential to health. In other words, probably we could eat only what we like and remain alive, but if these foods did not contain the variety of nutrients needed by the cells of the body, physiologic functioning would be impaired.

The nutrients essential to health are carbohydrates, proteins, fats, vitamins, and minerals. Water is essential to maintain fluid balance in the body. All of these are required to build and repair tissue, to furnish energy and to make essential substances, such as enzymes and hormones. They are made available to the body by the process of digestion. The digestive process breaks them down mechanically (chewing and intestinal movements) and chemically (oral and gastrointestinal secretions) so that they can be absorbed into the blood and the lymph.

Food requirements vary among individuals. From birth to old age nutritional requirements continually vary. They are dependent on the demands of the body for growth and tissue repair and also are affected by such factors as activity, climate, emotional status, pregnancy, illness, and so forth. Requirements differ, too, among individuals who would seem to have the same nutritional needs. There are differences in the way their foods are digested, assimilated, and used by the body.

Psychosocial and cultural factors influence the selection of food and patterns of behavior associated with eating. In addition to comments already made in this chapter in relation to this principle, the reader is referred to Chapters 14 and 15 for further discussion concerning influences on food selection and eating.

Hunger, thirst, and satiety are nature's first defenses against malnutrition. Hunger is a sensation that tells us our body needs nutrition. Thirst helps to assure that the body obtains sufficient water to maintain balance. Satiety is important in the control of over- and undereating.

SERVING FOOD IN HEALTH AGENCIES AND TO SHUT-INS AT HOME

Nurses employed in health agencies that serve food will need to acquaint themselves with the details of nursing responsibilities such as forms to use to order diets, time limits for ordering, and ways of changing diets or canceling diets.

Patients on regular or relatively minor restrictive diets often are given menus from which they may select the foods they prefer for the next day's meals. While the type of tray, tray cover, dishes, and silver used are not within the nurse's realm of control, the general appearance of the tray should be the best possible when it is served. Some agencies increase the attractiveness of the tray by using name cards and holiday favors. In the home care of patients, the nurse can do much to please the patient, such as adding a flower, using different colored cloths and napkins, serving one course at a time, and adding treats like cookies or candy if the patient is permitted to have them.

Some health agencies having self-care units permit the patients to be served in a cafeteria or dining room. A dietitian may be present to help patients on special diets to make a selection from the foods available. Even if dining rooms are not available, provisions for groups of patients to eat together, as in a solarium, is a thoughtful gesture. This is true especially for Sundays, holidays, and special occasions. It is the rare person who prefers eating alone.

Some health agencies provide special menus for children and teen-agers. The agencies attempt to offer foods these young folks like and in forms commonly served at home. Youngsters may not care for many vegetables, for example, but may relish vegetable soup. Providing youth-oriented food, these agencies report, has solved at least some dietary problems among the young.

Eligible senior citizens, unable to pick up allotments of donated foods because of poor health or no transportation, can have foods home-delivered through local volunteer efforts in parts of this country. The U.S. Department of Agriculture has developed this program, called the "Drive To Serve Program." Vendors have also begun providing home-delivered meals to shut-ins at home. This service is often called "Meals on Wheels" and the community health nurse should be aware of such programs for home-bound patients without family members who might ordinarily assist with the preparation and serving of meals.

Whenever it seems that some modification in the usual dietary routine or the diet itself would make the patient feel better, the nurse should consider how this might be accomplished. For example, if it is noted that an elderly patient leaves the meat untouched, investigation might show that he has loose-fitting dentures and cannot chew meat. He may be served ground meat instead. Or when cultural patterns affect food preferences to the extent that the patient is not getting an adequate diet, it may be necessary to consult with a dietitian so that substitutes can be made.

Some hospitalized patients find the time span between meals unsatisfactory. Three meals served within an eight- to nine-hour period and then a 15-hour wait for the next meal is not usual routine at home. They may want a snack at bedtime. Some agencies provide this, but many do not. Having the patient save some item, as a piece of cake or fruit, from one of his trays may be an answer. Hunger is distressing, and anything to avoid this should be considered.

Occasionally, hospitalized patients wish to substitute something served on the trays, and this often can be managed through the kitchen on the unit. For example, the patient may have a jar of powdered coffee and he needs only the hot water. Or, he may have a favorite canned item, and all that is required is that it be opened and served.

Size of the food portions may also be a source of discomfort to some patients. For those who eat little and leave a part of the food served, there is no problem. But patients who are accustomed to eating larger portions will feel dissatisfied with the meal. Extra portions can be arranged with the dietary department of the health agency.

Sometimes, patients' wishes cannot be granted because of agency policies or because it would mean doing for one what cannot be done for all. For example, there are patients who would like meals brought from home. Some of the implications can be readily imagined: family members coming in at times other than visiting hours to leave the food; requests being made to heat foods; dishes being left in rooms until family members take them home; food stored in bedside stands; and conflicts with the patient's regular diet. However, an occasional item of food which can be eaten immediately or shortly afterward, such

as a sandwich, a piece of homemade pie or cake, or a jar of cooked fruit might please the patient very much. If hospital policy does not permit the admission of any food, then the nurse is obliged to comply.

Not all likes and dislikes can be acted upon, but when a patient shows obvious distress, some effort should be made in his behalf.

HELPING TO MAINTAIN OR IMPROVE THE PATIENT'S APPETITE

For most people eating is a pleasure. When we recall how much a part of our life and leisure time is associated with food, we can readily see why this is so. Family celebrations, holiday meals, parties, picnics, coffee breaks, informal visits, and watching sports events, movies, and television usually include food in one form or another. We even tend to associate certain foods with particular events, such as hot dogs at baseball games, champagne at weddings, and the like.

Appetite is the pleasant anticipation of food. It is affected by many factors. Disturbances of appetite can interfere with gastrointestinal secretions and hence, digestion. Persons who have been upset while eating or directly afterward have been known to vomit completely undigested food hours later. Not only may his physical condition affect his appetite, but what the patient can see, hear, smell, or taste may influence it as well.

Below are some suggestions nurses will want to consider in relation to maintaining and/or stimulating the patient's appetite.

• See that the patient is in a comfortable position for eating.

• Be sure that the patient is clean and free from damp or soiled garments. Help him wash his hands if necessary.

• Alleviate pain or discomfort, as far as possible.

• Correct such annoyances as a loose or a tight dressing.

• Give the patient an opportunity to void if he desires.

• Avoid treatments such as enemas, dressings, and injections immediately before or directly after mealtimes if possible.

• See that the room is comfortable from the standpoint of temperature and ventilation.

• See that the patient is dressed adequately and comfortably.

• Remove or keep out of sight objects which would be unpleasant to look at while eating, such as urinals, bedpans, dressing trays or carts, drainage containers, suction machines, and the like.

• Screen patients who may be very ill, in pain, or receiving therapy (such as a transfusion or gastric suction) and will not be served a meal. Many patients receiving infusions or transfusions are served meals and should not be screened.

• Make certain that the immediate environment itself is in order, such as removing soiled linen, treatment trays that have been used, dead flowers, and that the furniture is orderly. Many persons who must remain in bed prefer not to have their baths before breakfast if it means having the bed disarranged and bathing items left about the unit.

• Make certain that the person serving the meal is pleasant and courteous and that care has been taken to avoid spilling liquids or disarranging dishes.

• Cooperate with dietary personnel in health agencies so that the meals can be served as quickly as possible. This helps to keep hot foods hot, and cold foods do not melt or become wilted.

ASSISTING PATIENTS TO EAT

Some patients will need assistance with eating and drinking. Physical limitations and the need to conserve strength are some of the reasons. For some patients, such as those in casts or in traction or those with some loss of hand or arm strength, it may be a matter of preparing foods and placing them conveniently. It would include such things as opening the shell of a cooked egg, buttering bread, cutting meat, and preparing other foods so they can be eaten easily.

If it is difficult for a patient to drink from a cup or glass, a drinking tube should be used. Disposable drinking tubes are preferred to glass or plastic because considerable care is needed to keep the nondisposable tubes clean. Accumulated food particles in a drinking tube at room temperature make a good growth medium for microorganisms.

Some patients are unable or not permitted to feed themselves and must be fed by someone else. The patients should be positioned and supported adequately to facilitate ease of swallowing. For those permitted, having the patient in as near an upright position as possible is desirable. Great care must be taken when feeding patients who are in a prone or near prone position. Having liquids and food enter the trachea rather than the esophagus can happen to anyone, but the reclining person is particularly susceptible.

When feeding a patient, a nurse or an assistant should be relaxed and in a comfortable position, so that the patient does not feel rushed. The person feeding should inquire if the patient is accustomed to saying grace. If so, permit him to do so and join by remaining respectfully silent. A comment on his nursing care plan which indicates that the patient says grace would help to individualize his care.

Ask the patient which foods he would like to eat first and other preferences he might have. For example, he might like his coffee with his meal or after it, a piece of bread after each piece of meat or some potato and meat together. Serve the food at the rate the patient wishes it.

If the patient is permitted some slight activity and has some hand and arm functioning, permit him to hold a piece of toast or a roll or to hold the drinking tube in the beverage while he sips it. If there is a beverage that he would like at the end of a meal and it can be placed so that he need only hold the drinking tube, consider doing this. It will prolong the pleasure of the meal and give him some feeling of independence. Avoid having to leave a patient after starting to feed him. If you must, use diplomacy so that he does not feel abandoned.

If a patient being fed is blind or if his eyes are bandaged, it is best to use some method of signaling when the next mouthful of food is ready or when it is wanted. Touching the patient's arm when the

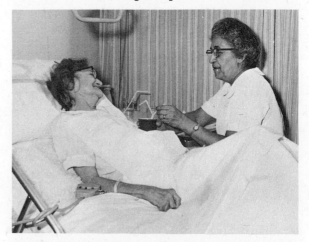

Fig. 25-1. This photo illustrates the various suggestions made in this chapter in relation to assisting a patient with eating. In addition to assisting the patient, the nurse can use the opportunity to learn to know her patient better, to help in establishing a therapeutic nurse-patient relationship, and to teach the patient as indicated. (Courtesy Good Samaritan Hospital, Phoenix, Arizona)

food is ready or having the patient move his hand when he wants more can make the situation much easier for both.

TEACHING IN RELATION TO NUTRITION

Because the nurse is often the central person in relation to teaching patients needing help with nutritional problems, it behooves her to observe general nutrition principles when teaching and to keep abreast of knowledge in the nutritional sciences. In problem areas, a dietitian will gladly assist the nurse, and she should be consulted freely.

Below are a few examples of problems nurses may encounter with suggestions in relation to teaching patients.

An earlier section in this chapter dealt with food fads and facts. Frequently the nurse is in a position to help patients separate fad from fact. Some persons will want and need supportive evidence in order to give up erroneous concepts.

Very often, patients who are on modified diets claim to have lost their appetites; what they are permitted to eat does not give them any pleasure. It is difficult to be denied foods and seasonings we like, and more difficult still for a person to deny himself these pleasures when he no longer feels ill. To have an appetite for foods and to keep reminding yourself that you cannot have them takes considerable self-control. That is why many patients do not adhere to their diets after discharge from the hospital. The nurse has a responsibility to try to help make the special diet as appealing to the patient as possible. If a patient is to be on a special diet, arrangements should be made to teach and to plan with him. This teaching and planning should also include family members as indicated. When possible, having a dietitian meet with the patient can often also do much to help.

Having to eat foods for which you have no appetite can lead to some desperate action. Patients on low sodium or calculated carbohydrate and fat diets have had salt, sugar, or candy brought to them by family or friends. Patients on restricted calorie diets have been known to hide candy and sneak bites secretly.

It is important to support patients by at least indicating an awareness and an understanding of their feelings when special diets do not appeal to them. Reprimanding is not nursing. The patient needs help and support from all—his family, the physician, the dietitian, and the nursing personnel. Nursing care plans for such patients should provide a consistent approach which could help them.

Persons who live alone may have a problem with adequate nutrition. This is particularly true with the older age group. Often they do not wish to cook for one person since they find it no fun to eat alone and maintain that they have no appetite anyway. Meals with friends and relatives are possible suggestions. As mentioned earlier, in some areas food service to the home has been instituted for the ill, the handicapped, or the incapacitated.

The affluent society notwithstanding, an abundant food supply is not available to all in this country. It is disheartening to know that many children and adults are chronically hungry and suffering from severe malnutrition. Sometimes teaching better food selection and using nutritious but inexpensive foods is helpful. In other situations, social agencies may need to be called upon to assist.

ANOREXIA, NAUSEA, AND VOMITING

Anorexia

Anorexia is a loss of appetite or a lack of desire for food. Causes include those having a physiologic basis such as a gastric irritation, or a psychic basis such as any factor that makes eating distasteful, or both. There does not appear to be a physiologic mechanism in the body for anorexia, as is the case, for example, for vomiting. In some instances, persistence of the symptom may require attention to supplying necessary bodily nutrients by ways other than normal eating and drinking.

Anorexia is commonly associated with nausea and vomiting. One has only to recall a personal experience or two with nausea and vomiting to remember the accompanying distress of anorexia.

Nausea

Nausea is a feeling of sickness with a desire to vomit. "Nausea" is a noun. "Nauseous" is an adjective, and to describe a patient as being nauseous is to say that he is sickening or disgusting. The proper wording is to say that a patient has nausea, the patient is nauseated, or nausea is present.

Nausea is felt in the back of the throat, the pit of the stomach, or both. Nausea is accompanied by vasomotor and autonomic disturbances that result in feelings of faintness and weakness, salivation, pallor, perspiration, and tachycardia. Anorexia, dizziness, and headache commonly are associated with nausea. *Retching*, which is the unproductive movements of muscles that ordinarily produce vomiting, also is often present.

It is believed that increased tension, stretching, and pressure on the walls of the stomach and duodenum are responsible for the sensation of nausea. Also, distention of the lower portion of the esophagus produces nausea. If for any reason the stomach descends, tension on this general area of the gastrointestinal tract is present and nausea follows. This last phenomenon is believed responsible when such things as offensive odors and rapid changes in the speed of an elevator bring on waves of nausea. The nausea associated with motion sickness seems to result from semicircular canal stimulation. Some drugs and severe pain also may cause nausea.

Vomiting

*V*omiting is the forceful expulsion of gastric contents through the mouth. It is also referred to as *emesis*. Vomiting is a common and complex symptom associated with numerous clinical entities. It is a reflex act that relieves the upper gastrointestinal tract of its contents. The contents are referred to as *vomitus*. Vomiting is a protective mechanism that enables the body to rid itself of irritating contents.

Projectile vomiting refers to the expulsion of vomitus with great force, often without the presence of nausea. Persistent and intractable vomiting is called *pernicious vomiting*. Bringing stomach contents to the throat and mouth without vomiting effort is *regurgitation*. It occurs commonly among infants when, it is believed, the infant spits up excess food. *Eructation* or *belching* is a discharge of gas from the stomach through the mouth.

The part of the gastrointestinal tract most sensitive to stimulants producing vomiting is the first part of the duodenum. However, sufficient stimulus in almost any section of the tract can produce vomiting. For example, mechanical irritation of the pharynx and fauces produces vomiting in most people. The irritation of an obstruction anywhere along the intestinal tract often produces violent vomiting. When abnormal stimulation of other organs in the body exists, vomiting is often present also. This can be observed when injury or disease affects the uterus, kidneys, heart, semicircular canals, or the brain. Cranial pressure generally produces violent vomiting, projectile in nature. It is a significant sign of deterioration and the physician should be notified when it occurs.

Psychic stimuli for vomiting include nauseating odors, sights, tastes, thoughts, and the like.

It has been demonstrated that a vomiting center is located in the medulla oblongata. Near the center is a trigger zone that apparently collects impulses of chemical irritants, drugs being an example, that in turn produce the vomiting. Other impulses eventually reach the center from the cortex and from other areas in the body, the exact pathways being largely undetermined. Some authorities believe that the vomiting center is not stimulated directly except by chemical irritants. Efferent pathways from the central nervous system carry impulses that influence the mechanical act of vomiting.

The mechanism of vomiting usually begins with a few deep inspirations. The glottis is closed and the nasopharynx is isolated by elevation of the soft palate. Abdominal and diaphragmatic muscular contractions begin and aid in forcing food from the tract. Breathing ceases temporarily and the glottis closes, both mechanisms helping to prevent the aspiration of vomitus into the respiratory tract. In the unconscious patient, the glottis does not close, thus adding to the vomiting problem the danger of respiratory aspiration of vomitus.

NURSING IMPLICATIONS WHEN ANOREXIA, NAUSEA, AND VOMITING ARE PRESENT

Attention has been called to the basic principles that indicate every person's need for an adequate intake of food and fluids. When nausea, vomiting, and anorexia are present, nursing measures are directed toward eliminating them as much as possible, so as to avoid placing the body in jeopardy from lack of food and fluids.

When the cause can be identified and removed, the problem may be largely solved. For example, when a patient is experiencing nausea and vomiting from unsightly odors and sights, removing them may be an easy solution. When the cause has a physiologic basis, nausea and vomiting may be present until therapy begins to make amends. For example, when cranial pressure is relieved, vomiting usually ceases. When gastritis is relieved, so also is nausea.

In some instances, drugs called *antiemetics*, which act to allay vomiting, may be prescribed by the physician. There are drugs too that aid in reducing the nausea and vomiting associated with motion sickness. Some of them have been used effectively with other conditions as well, the nausea and vomiting of early pregnancy being an example. In some cases, certain preparations also assist in stimulating the appetite and help in overcoming anorexia.

The patient who is vomiting needs protection and comfort. The danger of aspirating vomitus is often present and is a serious hazard, especially with the semiconscious and unconscious patient, or with infants and small children. Suctioning may become necessary for these patients to clear the upper gastrointestinal and respiratory tracts. Turning the patient's head to one side helps to rid the mouth of its contents. Gravity helps if the patient's head can safely be lowered slightly. Marked Trendelenburg positions are to be avoided as gravity may then be strong enough to produce more vomiting.

For patients with abdominal wounds, supporting the area with binders, a pillow splint, or with the nurse's hand is helpful. These procedures offer comfort to the patient and help to prevent opening of a wound, although this is an uncommon complication.

Comforting the patient includes special mouth care. This should be instituted as soon as possible after vomiting ceases, because the taste and odor of vomitus often is sufficient to produce more. Soiled linen and clothes are changed and emesis basins are emptied promptly.

The tension often associated with vomiting may be relieved by giving the patient a back rub. A clean, quiet, and comfortable environment also helps.

Additional measures that assist the patient with nausea and vomiting include these: limit the patient's activities as much as possible, especially if motion has brought on the symptoms; assist the patient to assume a comfortable position; take steps to alleviate pain if present; limit the patient's intake until the symptoms subside. Then offer fluids and food separately; offer bland and nonfatty foods; assist infants to bring up air bubbles by burping them; be prepared to offer emotional support when emotional components are present.

Notations are made on the patient's record when vomiting is present—the time it occurred, the nature of the emesis and vomitus, and the amount. An unusual odor such as fecal material or alcohol is also noted. When indicated, a specimen is taken and sent to a laboratory for analysis.

GASTRIC GAVAGE

When the patient is unable to take food and fluids by mouth, other methods to give nourishment are used. The patient may be given nourishment intravenously, as discussed in Chapter 24. Another alternative is to use gastric gavage. A gavage is used most frequently when there is pathology present in the mouth, throat, or esophagus.

Gastric gavage is the introduction of nourishment into the stomach by mechanical means. A gavage usually is indicated when the patient is unable to take nourishment orally but when no stomach or duodenal pathologic changes are present to interfere with normal digestive processes. The procedure is used often when a patient has an obstruction or a stricture in the esophagus or the throat. A tumor may be the cause of an obstruction. A stricture may be congenital or may be caused by scar tissue that has developed following injury to the esophagus.

Gastric gavages are used also for patients who are too weak to take nourishment by mouth. For example, gavages frequently are used for feeding premature infants for whom the physical effort of sucking is too great. They are also used occasionally for patients who are unconscious.

Chapter 20 discussed the introduction of a tube into the stomach when it is done to obtain a specimen. The procedure for introducing a gavage tube is similar, and the reader is referred to Chapter 20 for review purposes.

The nourishment given by gavage is prepared in liquid form, usually with a blender. Drugs that ordinarily are administered orally may be added to the nourishment. When a large amount of nourishment is given at regular intervals, the food is warmed to room temperature so that the patient does not become chilled. Food which is given continuously is not warmed, since it will approximate room temperature while it passes through the tubing to the patient's stomach. In addition, warmed milk and cream will sour more quickly during the period of time it takes for a container of nourishment to enter the patient's stomach.

After the feeding is instilled, a small amount of water should be introduced into the tube. This washes the feeding remaining in the tube into the stomach. It also prevents adhered feeding from souring.

The tube is clamped off after the food is instilled. This prevents it from draining back.

CONCLUSION

This chapter illustrates how the three broad principles discussed in Chapter 3 can be used effectively to guide nursing care. Food selection and eating patterns are usually very individualistic matters and the nurse will wish to consider this as she assists

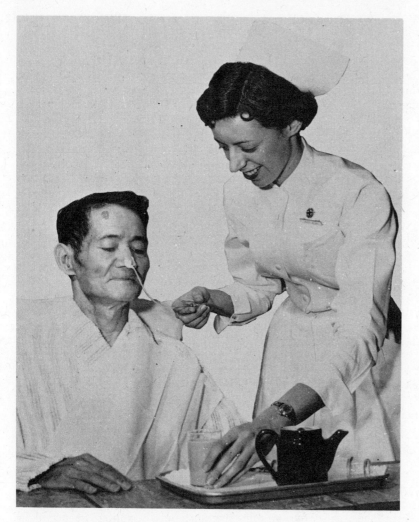

Fig. 25-2. If the patient must be fed by tube, the feeding should be served in an attractive and appetizing manner, so that it is obviously food and not a medication.

patients to maintain adequate nutrition. Also, man functions as a whole, and well-being is attained when both physiologic and psychological needs are being met satisfactorily. Health practitioners sometimes forget the psychological needs as they concern themselves with the patient's physiologic needs. Food and eating have many psychological implications for most people, as this chapter points out, and the nurse will wish to take them into consideration when planning care. Factors in the environment also have been discussed in this chapter as having important influences on nutrition.

Unit 2 described the nursing process system. A study situation in the next section of this chapter directs the reader to a reference which illustrates well how the system can be used as the nurse plans and implements nursing care in relation to meeting the patient's nutritional needs.

Study Situations

1. Obesity and overeating are considered problems of major concern in our affluent society. The following article describes societal stigmas the obese person often faces.

   Kalisch, B. J.: The stigma of obesity. **Am. J. Nurs.,** 72:1124–1127, June, 1972.

   What suggestions does the author give to help combat these stigmas? Note that the first suggestion, on page 1126, indicates that the nurse will wish to explore her own feelings about obesity. Are you aware of prejudices you may have? What suggestion does the author give as the "key" to helping patients who are obese?

2. The consumer has a right to expect that food processors show concern for his health, according to the following article.

Benarde, M. A., and Jerome, N. W.: Food quality and the consumer: A decalog. **Am. J. Public Health,** 62:1199–1201, Sept., 1972.

Note the decalog or ten commandments proposed by the authors for food processors. Can you make any additions? Consider commandment number 10 which is concerned with keeping the consumer informed. Cite examples illustrating that properly informed people generally act pretty sensibly.

3. Food patterns start taking shape early in life and become rather firmly fixed habits. However, patterns of food consumption change, as the following article indicates.

Henderson, L. M.: Nutritional problems growing out of new patterns of food consumption. **Am. J. Public Health,** 62:1194–1198, Sept., 1972.

On page 1194, the author illustrates that vegetable fat consumption increased more than threefold while animal fat consumption declined more than 50 percent in the United States in the last five decades or so. Can you offer reasons that might account for this change in consumption?

On page 1198, the author offers conclusions drawn from national food consumption surveys. List these conclusions and describe what implications they have for nursing care. For example, what implications do you see for nursing when the author indicates that a serious problem in relation to nutrition in this country today is the consumption of too many calories?

4. The reference given below will assist you in putting the nursing process system to work.

Birum, L. H.: Food for thought. *In* Auld, M. E., and Birum, L. H.: The Challenge of Nursing: A Book of Readings. pp. 140–149. St. Louis, C. V. Mosby, 1973.

Using a patient you are presently caring for, plan care in relation to helping the patient meet nutritional needs. To assist you with data gathering, use the diet history on page 145, or develop a similar one of your own. For assessment purposes, describe several standards you will use. The table on page 141, illustrating the required daily servings of the major food groups in a well-balanced diet, is an example of one you may wish to use. When planning nursing care for your patient, you will find helpful ideas on pages 145 and 146. For example, if the patient's diet history told you that the patient has a bedtime snack at home, indicate in your nursing care plan how you will use this information.

Describe how you will implement your nursing care plan. For example, how will you teach your patient of the importance of eating a well-balanced diet if your data gathering tells you that the patient's diet is inadequate in certain areas? If your patient lacks financial resources to purchase an adequate diet, what nursing intervention measures will you take?

References

1. A common sense look at health foods. **Changing Times: The Kiplinger Magazine,** 26:25–28, June, 1972.

2. Afek, L. B., and Hickey, J.: Health classes for migrant workers' families. **Am. J. Nurs.,** 72:1296–1298, July, 1972.

3. Alexander, T.: The hysteria about food additives. **Fortune,** 85:62–65; 138–141, Mar., 1972.

4. Birch, H. G.: Malnutrition, learning, and intelligence. **Am. J. Public Health,** 62:773–784, June, 1972.

5. Bishop, J. E.: Avoiding a hazard: Alza seeks way to make food additives, sugar that won't be absorbed into body. **The Wall Street Journal,** 88:26, June 18, 1973.

6. Chappelle, M. L.: The language of food. **Am. J. Nurs.,** 72:1294–1295, July, 1972.

7. Cox, M., and Wear, R. F., Jr.: Campbell soup's program to prevent atherosclerosis. **Am. J. Nurs.,** 72:253–259, Feb., 1972.

8. Crim, S. R.: Nutritional problems of the poor. **Nurs. Outlook,** 17:65–67, Sept., 1969.

9. Davenport, H. W.: Why the stomach does not digest itself. **Sci. Am.,** 226:86–93, Jan., 1972.

10. Erlander, D.: Dietetics—a look at the profession. **Am. J. Nurs.,** 70:2402–2405, Nov., 1970.

11. FDA fact sheet. Rockville, Md. U. S. Department of Health, Education, and Welfare, Public Health Service, Food and Drug Administration, July, 1971.

12. Gabler, M., and Oh, W.: Nomogram for calculating caloric intake. **Am. J. Nurs.,** 70:816–817, Apr., 1970.

13. Kermode, G. O.: Food additives. **Sci. Am.,** 226:15–21, Mar., 1972.

14. McGuigan, J. E.: Anorexia, nausea, and vomiting. pp. 369–380. *In* MacBryde, C. M., and Blacklow, R. S., eds.: Signs and Symptoms: Applied Pathologic Physiology and Clinical Interpretations. Ed. 5. Philadelphia, J. B. Lippincott, 1970.

15. Nelson, A. H.: Self-recorded diet histories. **Am. J. Nurs.,** 72:1601, Sept., 1972.

16. Pasquali, E. A.: Learning about a poverty budget. **Am. J. Nurs.,** 72:1419, Aug., 1972.

17. Rubin, R.: Food and feeding: a matrix of relationships. **Nurs. Forum,** 6:195–205, No. 2, 1967.

18. Shumway, S., and Powers, M.: The group way to weight loss. **Am. J. Nurs.,** 73:268–272, Feb., 1973.

19. Weiner, L.: The child who refuses to eat. **Bedside Nurse,** 5:28–30, Aug., 1972.

20. Young, V. R., and Scrimshaw, N. S.: The physiology of starvation. **Sci. Am.,** 225:14–21, Oct., 1971.

CHAPTER 26

Promoting Urinary and Intestinal Elimination

GLOSSARY

Albuminuria: Albumen in the urine.

Alimentary Glycosuria: Sugar in the urine due to an unusually large intake of sugar or due to emotional stress.

Anal Incontinence: Inability of the anal sphincter to control the discharge of fecal and gaseous material.

Anuria: Suppression or lack of production of urine.

Atonic Constipation: Dry, hardened fecal material due to sluggishness of the colon.

Bowel Movement: Synonym for defecation.

Cathartic: Drug used to induce emptying of the intestinal tract. Synonym is laxative.

Catheter: Tube used for injecting or removing fluids.

Constipation: Difficult defecation with occasional passage of dry, hard fecal material.

Defecation: Evacuation of the intestinal tract. Synonym for bowel movement.

Diarrhea: Passage of excessively liquid and unformed feces.

Diuresis: Excessive production and elimination or urine. Synonym is polyuria.

Dysuria: Difficult or painful urination.

Enema: Introduction of solution into the lower intestinal tract.

Fecal Impaction: Hardened mass of feces in the rectum.

Flatulence: Excessive gas in the gastrointestinal tract.

Flatus: Intestinal gas.

Frequency: Urinating at frequent intervals.

Glycosuria: Sugar in the urine.

Hematuria: Blood in the urine.

Hemorrhoids: Distended varicose rectal veins.

Hypertonic Constipation: Dry, hardened fecal material due to intestinal spasms. Synonym is spastic constipation.

Intestinal Distention: Accumulation of excessive gas in intestinal tract. Synonym is tympanites.

Laxative: Synonym of cathartic.

Micturition: Process of emptying the urinary bladder. Synonyms include voiding and urination.

Nocturia: Excessive urination during the night.

Oliguria: Scanty production of urine.

Orthostatic: An erect position.

Overflow Incontinence: Involuntary escape of some urine from bladder due to increased volume pressure. Synonym is paradoxical incontinence.

Paradoxical Incontinence: Synonym for overflow incontinence.

Peristalsis: Wormlike contractions of the gastrointestinal tract which propels its contents.

Polyuria: Synonym for diuresis.

Pyuria: Pus in the urine.

Residual Urine: Urine retained in the bladder after voiding.

Retention: Excessive storage of urine in the bladder.

Spastic Constipation: Synonym for hypertonic constipation.

Suppository: Oval or conical substance that is solid at room temperature but melts at body temperature.

Total Incontinence: Inability of bladder to store any urine.

Tympanites: Synonym for intestinal distention.

Urinalysis: Laboratory examination of urine.

Urinary Catheterization: Introduction of a catheter through the urethra into the urinary bladder to remove urine.

Urination: Synonym for micturition and voiding.

INTRODUCTION

Elimination from the urinary and intestinal tracts is essential to rid the body of wastes and materials in excess of bodily needs. Elimination processes are necessary to maintain high-level wellness and even life itself.

Because in our society it is not considered generally acceptable to discuss body elimination freely, intestinal and bladder functions sometimes tend to be neglected in nursing care. The nurse needs to realize these processes are essential to body functioning and handle them in a direct but objective manner. Most persons usually take elimination for granted unless something goes wrong. However, preventive measures may be important in promoting normal patterns of elimination. In some situations, nursing intervention is also necessary to facilitate elimination when malfunction occurs.

Some general principles relating to elimination are followed by brief reviews of the anatomy and physiology of the urinary and intestinal tracts. Nursing actions to promote normal eliminations are then discussed, followed by measures that are used to combat common problems of elimination.

GENERAL PRINCIPLES IN RELATION TO URINARY AND INTESTINAL ELIMINATION

Efficient physiologic functioning requires that waste substances be eliminated from the body. Elimination is essential to life itself. Mechanisms of elimination include not only bowel and bladder, but other organs, namely the lungs and the sweat glands.

Patterns of elimination from the large intestine and the urinary bladder vary among individuals. Despite individual differences, as long as the intestines and the urinary bladder are eliminating wastes efficiently, there is no great need for concern.

Stress-producing situations and illness may interfere with normal habits of elimination. Persons under stress often encounter problems in elimination. For example, a patient confined to bed may find it so difficult to use a bedpan or a urinal that he may be unable to have a bowel movement or to urinate normally. Or, a person experiencing emotional stress may have difficulty maintaining normal intestinal elimination.

In addition to stress, normal elimination, especially from the large intestine, often is affected by change in diet, certain medications, therapeutic and diagnostic measures, and reduction in the patient's normal activities.

Patterns of elimination from the urinary bladder do not vary among individuals so markedly as bowel habits. Most people urinate just before bedtime, upon arising, and several times during the day, depending on their diet, fluid intake, activity, and the like.

ELIMINATION FROM THE URINARY TRACT

The efficiency of the urinary system is vital for the maintenance of good physiologic functioning. Especially during illness, considerable emphasis is placed on the patient's ability to excrete urine normally. Close observation is essential if deviations are to be detected early.

The urinary tract is one of the routes by which wastes are excreted. Certain inorganic salts, nitrogenous waste products, and water are removed from the bloodstream, accumulated, and excreted through the proper functioning of the urinary tract.

Kidneys and Ureters

The kidneys are located on either side of the vertebral column behind the peritoneum and in the posterior portion of the abdominal cavity. They carry a major responsibility for maintaining the composition and the volume of body fluids. The kidneys function in a selective manner; that is, they single out constituents of the blood for excretion for which the body has no need. It is estimated that total blood volume passes through the kidneys for waste removal approximately every half hour. Despite varying kinds and amounts of food and fluids ingested, body fluids remain relatively stable if there is proper kidney function. The waste solution containing organic and inorganic wastes which the kidneys produce is called *urine*.

The nephron is the unit of kidney structure. There are approximately one million nephrons in each kidney. Urine from the nephrons empties into the pelvis of each kidney. From each kidney, urine is transported by rhythmic peristalsis through the ureter to the urinary bladder. The ureters enter the bladder obliquely, and a fold of membrane in the bladder closes the entrance to the ureters so that urine is not forced up the ureters to the kidneys when pressure exists in the bladder.

Urinary Bladder

This is a smooth muscle sac which serves as a

reservoir for varying amounts of urine. There are three layers of muscular tissue in the bladder—the inner longitudinal, the middle circular, and the outer longitudinal. The three layers are called the detrusor muscle. At the base of the bladder, the middle circular layer of muscle tissue forms the internal or involuntary sphincter. This sphincter guards the opening between the urinary bladder and the urethra. The urethra conveys urine from the bladder to the exterior of the body.

Urinary bladder muscle is innervated by the autonomic nervous system. The sympathetic system carries inhibitory impulses to the bladder and motor impulses to the internal sphincter. These impulses result in relaxation of the detrusor muscle and constriction of the internal sphincter, causing urine to be retained in the bladder. The parasympathetic system carries motor impulses to the bladder and inhibitory impulses to the internal sphincter. These impulses result in contraction of the detrusor muscle and relaxation of the sphincter.

The bladder normally contains urine under very little pressure, and, as volume of urine increases, the pressure increases only slightly. This adaptability of the bladder wall to pressure is believed to be due to the characteristics of muscle tissue in the bladder and makes it possible for urine to continue to enter the bladder from the ureters against low pressure. When the pressure becomes sufficient to stimulate stretch receptors located in the bladder wall, the desire to empty the bladder becomes apparent.

Urethra

The urethra differs in men and women. In men, the urethra is common to both the excretory system and the reproductive system. It is approximately 5½ to 6½ inches in length and consists of three parts—the prostatic, the membranous, and the cavernous portions. The external urethral sphincter consists of striated muscle and is located just beyond the prostatic portion of the urethra. The external sphincter is under voluntary control.

The female urethra is 1½ to 2½ inches in length. Its function is to convey urine from the bladder to the exterior. The external or voluntary sphincter is located approximately midurethra. No portion of the female urethra is external to the body as is true in the male. Most literature refers to muscle at the meatus in the female as the external sphincter.

The Act of Micturition

The process of emptying the urinary bladder is known as *micturition;* the terms *voiding* or *urination*

are used also. Nerve centers for micturition are situated in the brain and the spinal cord. Voiding is largely an involuntary reflex act, but its control can be learned.

Following stimulation of the stretch receptors in the bladder, as the urine collects, the desire to void is experienced. Usually this occurs when about 100 ml. to 200 ml. for the child and 200 ml. to 300 ml. for the adult has collected. If the process of micturition is initiated, the detrusor muscle contracts, the internal sphincter relaxes, and urine enters the posterior urethra. The muscles of the perineum and the external sphincter relax, and micturition occurs. The act consists of relaxation of the internal sphincter, contraction of the detrusor muscle, slight contraction of the muscle of the abdominal wall, and a lowering of the diaphragm. The act of micturition is normally painless. During micturition, the pressure within the bladder is many times greater than it is during the time the bladder is filling. The voluntary control of voiding is limited to initiating, restraining, and interrupting the act.

Restraint of voiding is believed to be subconscious when the volume of urine in the bladder is small. But when voiding is delayed, the bladder continues to fill. Discomfort may then be felt when undue distention occurs and the urgency to void becomes paramount.

Increased abdominal pressure, as occurs for example with coughing and sneezing, sometimes forces the escape of urine involuntarily, especially in the female since the urethra is shorter. Strong psychic factors, such as marked fear, may also result in involuntary urination. Under certain conditions, it may be difficult to relax the restraining muscles sufficiently to void, as when a urine specimen is requested from a shy or embarrassed person.

When the higher nerve centers develop after infancy, the voluntary control of micturition develops also. Until that time, voiding is purely reflex in nature. Persons whose bladders are isolated from control of the brain because of either injury or disease also void by reflex only.

Normal Urine

Healthy adults excrete approximately 1200 ml. to 1700 ml. of urine in each 24-hour period. However, this amount may vary, depending on several factors. If large amounts of fluids are being excreted by the skin, the lungs, or the intestine, the amount excreted by the kidneys will decrease. The amount of urine will depend on the amount of fluid ingested: the greater the fluid intake, the larger will be the amount of urine produced and vice versa. Diet influences the amount of urine. Persons on high protein diets will produce more urine than those on a regular diet. Children and infants excrete more urine in proportion to their weight than adults do.

The word *diuresis* is used most often to mean an excessive production and the elimination of urine. *Polyuria* is a synonym. Certain fluids act as diuretics and will cause an increase in the production of urine. Examples are coffee, tea, and cocoa. Certain drugs also produce diuresis.

The color of normal urine is golden yellow or amber. If the urine is scant in amount and concentrated, the color will be darker; if it is dilute, the color will be lighter. Urine has a characteristic odor. Some foods and drugs will alter the odor.

Normal urine is clear. On standing and cooling, cloudiness and a sediment may occur which are due to the presence of urates and phosphates that precipitate as the reaction of urine changes from acidity to alkalinity. Normal urine will clear again rapidly if acid is added and the urine is heated to body temperature.

Laboratory examination reveals that the specific gravity of normal urine varies on the average between approximately 1.015 and 1.025, but it has been observed to vary between 1.002 and 1.040 in healthy persons. The inorganic constituents of normal urine include ammonia, sodium chloride, and traces of iron; and phosphorus, sulfur, sodium, potassium, calcium, and magnesium in combination with oxygen. Organic constituents include urea, uric acid, creatinine, hippuric acid, indican, urine pigments, and undetermined nitrogen. Traces of urobilin, sugar, fatty acids, carbonates, mucin, and cystine may be present.

The urine of persons on a normal diet is slightly acid. Vegetarians excrete a slightly alkaline urine. Normally, the urinary tract is sterile; therefore, urine is free of bacteria. Bacteria are found at the end of the urethra, and if they are washed into a urine specimen, usually they will be identified by laboratory examination. Normal urine values were shown in Table 20-2 in Chapter 20.

Frequency of Urination

The frequency of voiding depends on the amount of urine being produced. The more urine that is being produced, the more often voiding is necessary and vice versa. Normally, from two-thirds to three-fourths of the urine output is voided by ambulatory persons during the daytime hours. Unless the fluid intake is very large, most healthy persons do not void during their normal sleeping hours. The first voided urine of the day is usually more concentrated than urine excreted during the remainder of the day.

Some persons normally void small amounts at frequent intervals because they habitually respond to the first early urge to void. This habit is insignificant and is not necessarily an indication of disease.

NURSING RESPONSIBILITIES IN RELATION TO URINARY ELIMINATION

Nursing personnel are responsible for observing the patient's urine when this is essential to his health problem. The color, odor, amount, appearance, and the frequency with which voiding occurs are noted. Anything unusual is reported to the physician. Difficulty or pain associated with the act of micturition also is reported promptly.

Adequate fluid intake is a prime factor in maintaining urinary elimination. The patient should be encouraged to drink plenty of fluids if his intake is not restricted. Question the patient about his fluid intake if there are signs of concentrated urine.

Some patients find it difficult to void while in bed. Even the sitting bed position is not helpful. They may need to have their legs over the side of the bed while sitting on the bedpan. Some male patients on bed rest may need permission from the physician to be able to stand to use the urinal.

Providing the Bedpan and Urinal

Men patients confined to bed use the urinal for voiding and the bedpan for defecation; women use the bedpan for both. When a woman patient is unable to sit up in bed—for example, when she is in a body cast—a female urinal may be used. Having to use the bedpan and the urinal is considered embarrassing by most patients. In addition, the bedpan is often difficult to use. It "fits" no one. Privacy is important to almost all patients when they use either a bedpan or urinal.

Many bedpans are made of metal. This is important to remember when the room is cold. The bedpan may be warmed by running warm water inside it and then rotating the water around the sides of the pan.

Bedpans of nylon resin are also available. They feel warm to touch and can be asepticized by conventional methods. Also, these bedpans eliminate the problem of noise associated with handling of metal bedpans.

Unless contraindicated, the head of the bed should be raised slightly before placing the patient on the bedpan. This makes it easier for the patient to lift himself onto the pan. If an overhead trapeze is permitted, the patient can also often move himself with less strain. If he is flat in bed, it is necessary for him to hyperextend his back in order to lift himself up onto the bedpan.

After providing privacy, fold a corner of the top bed linen over onto the patient so that it is easy to slip the bedpan under him. It is not necessary to expose a patient for this procedure. When the patient is on correctly, leave the toilet tissue within easy reach, check to see that the signal bell is convenient, and leave the patient alone if physical condition warrants. The patient should be instructed to signal when finished.

If the patient is very weak, it may be necessary for the nurse to place one hand under his buttocks and assist him to raise himself. If the patient cannot help to lift himself, raise the head of the bed slightly, turn the patient over on one side, place the bedpan against his buttocks, and hold it in place while the patient is rolled back onto the bedpan.

Care should be taken to avoid injuring the skin from friction by pushing the bedpan under the patient or pulling it out. If the patient is unable to assist and rolling him is not possible, sufficient assistance should be secured to lift the patient.

Before emptying the bedpan, the contents should be noted carefully. The excretory products are a vital clue to the patient's physiologic state. Any abnormalities in the nature of the urine or in the act of elimination should be reported promptly and recorded on the patient's chart.

After a patient has used the bedpan, offer a basin of water or a wash cloth which has been moistened with water and soap, and a towel for cleansing the hands and/or perineal area.

Commodes can be used for patients allowed out of bed but unable to use the bathroom toilet. Commodes are chairs (straight back or wheel chairs) with open seats and a shelf or a holder under the seat on which a bedpan is placed.

If the patient is able to use the bathroom toilet, the nurse still is responsible for noting any abnormalities of elimination. Patients may need to be taught in some instances to report abnormalities to the nurse and instructed not to flush the toilet until the nurse has seen the urine. In other situations, the patient may go to the bathroom for voiding, but if the urine volume is to be calculated, he may need to urinate in a bedpan or some other receptacle placed on the toilet so the urine can be measured before it is discarded.

A weak patient should be assisted to the bathroom. Someone should remain in attendance if there is any danger of the patient's falling. Bathrooms should not be locked, and, especially in hospitals, a signal bell should be within easy reach of the patient so that help can be summoned easily if the patient feels weak and in need of assistance.

Many a dangerous situation has been created in the absence of a signal bell or bedpan. Patients confined to bed have gotten out to go to the bathroom to void. Some had to climb over or around bed siderails, and others removed oxygen masks or drainage or infusion tubings. For example, an elderly woman was admitted to the hospital in a comatose state. The physician ordered her on *absolute* rest and oxygen as well as other medications. Several hours later when a nurse went in for one of the frequent checks on the patient, the latter was nowhere in sight. She was found in the bathroom. Asked how she got out of bed she said she had crawled around the bottom of the bed siderails. As to why she did it, she said simply, "I had to go." It was recognized that this patient was beginning to have lucid moments; henceforth, she was offered a bedpan frequently.

Offering a bedpan or urinal frequently can save many a patient from a fractured hip or a dislodged infusion. If a patient appears very ill or is sedated, he may not think to ask in time. Family members of patients at home may have to be made aware of this. Remember, the nurse is responsible for the patient's safety at all times.

Securing Urine Specimens

Nurses are frequently responsible for securing urine specimens from patients for laboratory analysis. This urine examination is called *urinalysis*. Urination into a clean receptacle is considered adequate in many routine situations. Other situations may require a "clean catch" specimen. This is especially true if a urinary tract infection is suspected and a urine culture is desired. Culture media are inoculated with the urine to allow any organisms present to grow so that they can be examined.

In the "clean catch" technique, the external meatus area is cleansed thoroughly with soap and water or an antiseptic solution such as aqueous Zephiran. In the uncircumcised male, the foreskin or prepuce should be retracted to expose the glans penis before cleaning. In the female, the labia are well separated before cleansing and kept apart until the specimen is collected. In many agencies, it is recommended that a sterile glove be worn during the cleansing and collection. The patient voids into a sterile container.

Some agencies catch the specimen "midstream." It is expected that any additional organisms harbored at the meatus will have been flushed out by the urine stream. The specimen collected after urination has been initiated will be as near the constituency of the bladder urine as possible. A patient who can be adequately instructed and expected to carry out the aseptic precautions may collect his own "clean catch" or "midstream" specimens and often prefers to do so. Following the specimen collection the foreskin of the male patient should be returned to its reduced position.

Twenty-four hour specimens are required for some types of laboratory studies. Instruction of the patient regarding the importance of collecting *all* urine for a period of 24 hours is important. The collection is initiated at a specified time by having the patient empty his bladder. This specimen is discarded. All urine for the next 24 hours is saved. Depending on the type of examination, the urine from each voiding may be kept in a separately marked container, indicating the time of urination, or all voidings may be put into a common receptacle. The specimens should be refrigerated and sometimes a preservative is added to retard decomposition.

Children who are too young to cooperate in urine specimen collection often require use of special techniques and apparatus. They are described in detail in texts dealing with the care of children.

COMMON NURSING MEASURES FOR DEALING WITH URINARY ELIMINATION PROBLEMS

Before describing common nursing measures to deal with elimination problems, it is necessary to define terms associated with urine and voiding with which the nurse will wish to be familiar. *Anuria* refers to suppression of urine. When total anuria occurs, the kidneys produce no urine; therefore, the bladder remains empty. When the kidneys produce only scanty amounts of urine, the term *oliguria* is used. Anuria and oliguria are usually serious signs. *Polyuria* refers to an excessive output of urine. The term *diuresis* also describes excessive urine production.

At times urine is produced by the kidneys and enters the bladder but is not eliminated. Excessive storage of urine in the bladder is called *retention*. The inability to retain urine voluntarily is called *incontinence*.

Hematuria refers to urine that contains blood. If present in large enough quantities, the urine becomes reddish brown in color. Pus in the urine is called *pyuria*. The urine appears cloudy. Pyuria should not be confused with the cloudiness which may occur when normal urine stands and cools. Albumin in the urine is called *albuminuria*. Albumin is sometimes present in urine that is voided following periods of standing, walking, and running. This is called *orthostatic albuminuria* and is a phenomenon of the circulatory system and not necessarily a symptom of kidney disorders. *Glycosuria* refers to the presence of sugar in the urine. If glycosuria is due to an unusually large intake of sugar or to marked emotional disturbances and is temporary in nature, there is little cause for alarm. This condition is called *alimentary glycosuria*.

Dysuria refers to difficulty in voiding. It may or may not be associated with pain. A feeling of warm local irritation occurring during voiding is called *burning*. *Frequency* refers to voiding at very frequent intervals. Excessive voiding during the night especially when not associated with large fluid intake is called *nycturia* or *nocturia*.

Urinary Incontinence

Incontinence may be partial or complete. If the bladder is unable to store any urine and urine dribbles almost constantly, the condition is called *total incontinence*. If the bladder cannot be emptied normally, urine continues to accumulate, and, when there is sufficient pressure in the bladder, small amounts of urine may be forced out. The dribble of urine ends when the pressure has been reduced somewhat, but the bladder is not empty. This is called *overflow* or *paradoxical incontinence*. This type sometimes accompanies retention. Incontinence may be either permanent or temporary in nature, depending on the cause. It is a problem faced by many elderly persons. Because it is so common, family members often need to be helped to deal with it in the home.

Nursing Measures for Incontinence: As soon as a medical evaluation of the patient's problem has been made, nursing measures should be directed toward helping to restore normal function if there is a possibility of success. As with fecal incontinence, urinary incontinence should not be a situation to which everyone becomes resigned. The psychological value to the patient of knowing that effort is being made to help him cannot be underestimated. For example, suggesting a routine for taking fluids followed by periods of time to try voiding can be successful with some patients. They may not understand the relationship of fluid intake to voiding. Also voluntary efforts either to control or to induce voiding may be sufficiently stimulating to help restore function. For some patients, especially the elderly chronically ill, it may be as simple as taking them to the bathroom or offering a bedpan every two to three hours. For other persons, perineal exercises may be helpful to increase the muscle tone.

A quick course of action is to have an indwelling catheter inserted. An indwelling catheter is a tube into the bladder which provides for constant urine drainage. The cost in terms of physical discomfort to the patient may be exceedingly high. Infection from indwelling catheters is very common. For some patients it will require months after the catheter is removed before the infection is cured.

In addition to efforts to help the patient to regain control of this function, other measures also must be considered, such as keeping the patient dry, clean, and comfortable. Often, great skill and ingenuity are required to prevent odors and discomfort from wet clothing and linens. The ammonia of the urine and lying on wet linen can quickly irritate the skin and predispose the patient to ammonia dermatitis and decubiti.

Various types of external urinary collection appliances are available for male patients. The devices fit directly over the penis and are secured by adhesives or straps. A collection bag is usually attached to the patient's leg to permit ambulation. These devices must be applied carefully to prevent skin irritation and skin breakdown, cleansed regularly to avoid odor, and emptied at appropriate intervals to prevent accidental spillage. Since a man's trousers can cover the entire appliance, his independence and activity can be readily maintained with no embarrassment. Unfortunately, because of the anatomical structure of the female, no such device is available for women.

Patients with incontinence usually are embarrassed and insecure. The nurse can be of assistance by demonstrating tact and understanding while carrying out her nursing responsibilities. Offering emotional support, allowing the patient to talk of his problem, and allowing him to assist with decision making about his care also are helpful. Whenever possible, it is preferable from a psychological standpoint to consult with him about measures to collect

and absorb urine such as absorbent pads, urinary appliances, and waterproof undergarments. Persons who are incontinent or fear incontinence often limit their fluid intake in order to minimize their accidents. They need to be helped to understand the relationship of an adequate fluid intake to their total body functioning.

Obstructions of the urinary tract may require some patients to have surgical diversions of the urinary flow. They may have an abdominal opening for urinary excretion such as the ileal conduit, a connection of the ureter to the ileum with abdominal wall exit for urine. More detailed discussion for care of these patients can be found in advanced clinical texts.

In certain disease conditions, voluntary control of voiding may be impaired, but the reflex act of micturition is intact. These patients may be helped with bladder training. Drugs also are used to assist these patients.

BLADDER TRAINING: Bladder training should be instituted with the consent of the physician, since a complete evaluation of the patient's physical condition is essential. To start a patient on such a program when there is little or no possibility of his achieving results would be psychologically disastrous for him. Even if a patient is considered eligible for bladder training, he must be helped to understand that it will be a slow process and that the gains may be slight and very gradual. As in any situation, it is poor policy to permit a patient to set unrealistic goals for himself.

A primary factor in bladder training is the management of the patient's fluid intake. In addition to liquids such as milk, tea, broth, water, and soup, foods of high liquid content also must be considered. Because of the time relationship between drinking and the occurrence of urine in the bladder, it is best to plan a drinking schedule that will permit convenient occasions for attempting to empty the bladder. For example, most persons urinate shortly after awakening, and this is usually the first and the best time for the patient to attempt to empty the bladder. Having some water immediately on waking is helpful. Other fluids can be spaced throughout the day according to the patient's wishes. Fluids should be limited in the late evening hours, thus limiting the risk of being incontinent during the night.

Position of the Patient: When the patient attempts to start bladder training, it is essential that conditions conducive to the process be provided. For example, the patient should be comfortable and relaxed, and adjustments should be made so that a good sitting position may be maintained. If the patient is not able to get out of bed and is going to use the bedpan, the head of the bed should be raised and the patient well supported by pillows. It is also best if the patient's knees are flexed during the period of time that an attempt to void is being made.

The position found to be most helpful is the normal sitting position. This position can be simulated by some patients if they are permitted to have their feet over the edge of the bed while sitting on a bedpan. In addition, they should have a foot support and a chair or overbed table on which to lean. A toilet or a commode is best if the patient is able to be out of bed.

Time: A regular schedule is also essential for helping the patient to establish a pattern. If there has been any regularity to the patient's incontinence of urine, these times should be considered in the scheduling. For example, if the patient notes that a frequent "wetting time" is 10:30 A.M., then provision for attempting to void should be made at 10:00 A.M.

The times selected for attempting to empty the bladder need not be spaced regularly, such as every four hours. However, they should be at the same time each day. The intervals between each voiding will be dependent on the patient's fluid intake and his bladder capacity.

The Stimulus or Call: Any sensation which precedes the act of micturition is referred to as the *stimulus* or *call.* The patient should be informed that this may not be the usual kind of stimulus produced by a full bladder, but it may include other reactions, such as sensations in the abdomen, chilliness, sweating, muscular twitching, restlessness, and the like. It is important that the patient understand these signs to become sensitive to the clues of a need to empty the bladder.

Methods for Assisting the Process: While the patient is in the sitting position, it is helpful if he bends forward in a slow, rhythmic fashion. This creates pressure on the bladder. It also helps if the patient applies light pressure with the hands over the bladder. The pressure should be directed toward the urethra.

Other measures, such as those which are used to help patients void, also should be used if necessary. These include drinking fluids to the extent allowed or listening to running water.

It is possible for the patient to void during the attempt without any knowledge of it or without any specific stimulus or control. This is still considered as involuntary voiding. Not until the patient is able to use a specific method to stimulate and empty the bladder is the bladder training program considered successful.

For those patients with severe neuromuscular involvement, the best method for inducing the stimulus and emptying the bladder may require considerable exploration; 15 to 20 minutes for each attempt is sufficient. Unsuccessful attempts are discouraging, and the patient should be helped to maintain a positive and hopeful attitude toward the process.

As a means of gauging the success of the attempts, examination for residual urine may be included as a part of the process. Percussion directly over the symphysis is one method. In some programs of rehabilitation, tests for residual urine are made by inserting a catheter. As the amount of residual urine diminishes and the success of emptying the entire bladder increases, the frequency of examination is reduced.

Urinary Retention

Retention occurs when urine is being produced normally but is not being excreted from the bladder. The bladder continues to fill and may distend until it reaches the level of the umbilicus. The abdomen swells as the bladder rises above the level of the symphysis pubis. The height of the bladder can be determined by palpating with light pressure on the abdomen.

Retention is often temporary in nature. It is common following surgery, especially if ambulation is delayed or fluid intake is minimal. Any mechanical obstruction—for example, swelling at the meatus, which often occurs following childbirth—may cause retention. The cause also may be psychic in nature or be due to certain disease conditions.

While urine that is retained in the bladder can be removed by introducing a catheter, every effort should be made to help the patient void. Medical literature abounds in caution against using the catheter too freely. Since urinary catheter-induced infections are the most common nosocomial infections and it is generally conceded that infections of the bladder can occur following even one insertion of a catheter despite the most careful procedure, natural urination should be encouraged by all possible means.

Nursing measures should be instituted as soon as a patient feels that he cannot void even if the interval since the last voiding was only a few hours. This is particularly true if the patient has been having a normal fluid intake. Urine retained in the bladder increases the likelihood of urinary tract infection.

There are several measures that often aid in initiating normal micturition if there is no mechanical obstruction or disease condition causing retention. Placing the patient in the normal position for voiding—that is, in the sitting position—is usually helpful if sitting is not contraindicated. Sometimes, voiding will begin if the patient sits at the edge of the bed on a bedpan and supports his feet on a chair. If the patient is allowed out of bed, the patient can sit on a bedpan placed on a chair, or a commode can be used. The male patient often can induce voiding if permitted to stand. A toilet is best if the patient can walk or be moved to one. The back-lying position has been found to be least successful in helping to initiate voiding. If the patient's condition permits, he should be provided privacy while he attempts to void. In many instances the patient may need to wait several minutes for the urge to void to appear or reappear.

Additional measures which often assist in the voiding process include offering the patient fluids, especially warm drinks; warming the bedpan before use; allowing water to run from a tap within hearing distance of the patient; or placing the patient's hands in warm water or pouring warm water over the perineum (if no specimen is desired).

Retention is painful. The patient often becomes anxious and tense, which usually further interferes with normal voiding.

Occasionally, a patient will void but the quantity is insufficient by comparison with the fluid intake. Or, the patient may say that he feels as though he still needs to void. Urine retained in the bladder after voiding is called *residual urine*. Normally, all but approximately 1 ml. to 3 ml. of urine is excreted from the bladder in voiding.

Catheterization

Catheterization of the urinary bladder is the introduction of a catheter through the urethra into the bladder for the purpose of withdrawing urine. A catheter is a tube for injecting or removing fluids. In recent years, the value of catheterization, formerly unquestioned, has become increasingly dubious in view of the hazards involved.

Several physiologic facts should be recalled. The bladder is normally a sterile cavity. The external opening to the urethra can never be sterilized. The bladder has defense mechanisms, namely, the emptying of urine and intravesical antibacterial activity. These help to maintain a sterile bladder under normal circumstances and also aid in clearing an infection if it occurs. Infections introduced into the bladder can ascend the ureters and lead to kidney infection. A normal bladder is not so susceptible to infection as a damaged one. A patient's lowered resistance, present in many disease entities and stress situations, predisposes him to urinary infection. Therefore, patients should only be catheterized when absolutely necessary because of the danger of acquiring an infection.

The hazards of introducing an instrument or a catheter into the bladder are sepsis and trauma; the possibility of the latter to the male urethra, because of its length, is obvious. An object forced through a stricture or irregularity from the wrong angle can cause serious damage to the urethra. While the urethra in the female is shorter, it also is susceptible to damage if a catheter is forced through it. Bacteria can enter the bladder by being pushed in as the catheter is being inserted. In situations when the catheter is left in place, the organisms may also move up the catheter lumen or the space between the catheter and the urethral wall.

PURPOSES OF CATHETERIZATION: It was formerly considered essential to catheterize for a routine specimen free of contamination, but this practice has been abandoned in most situations. The "clean catch" technique has been substituted. Catheterization may be used before surgery to empty the patient's bladder completely since tension and preoperative sedatives can result in incomplete emptying of the bladder. When this is necessary, it is recommended the catheterization be performed in the aseptic conditions of the operating room. Catheterization is used postoperatively to prevent bladder distention and when patients are unable to urinate after all nursing measures to induce voiding have failed. It is used before and after delivery for the same reasons. Catheterization is also used in some situations when the patient is incontinent.

Catheterization also may be used to remove urine from a greatly distended bladder. It generally is agreed by urologists that gradual decompression of the distended bladder is a safer procedure than rapid removal of all urine. Rapid emptying of the bladder has resulted in damage to the organ with severe systemic reactions, such as chills, fever, and shock. Gradual decompression aids in preventing engorgement in the vessels as well as helping to improve the tone of the bladder wall by adjusting the intravesical pressure in stages.

For patients who have severe retention, for example, if as much as 2000 ml. is suspected, a special apparatus may be used to decompress the bladder over a period of 24 hours or more. However, there are instances when the nurse will need to exercise judgment as to the amount of urine to withdraw at a single catheterization. Safe procedure for catheterization is that no more than 750 ml. of urine be withdrawn from a patient at any one time. If more urine is present in the bladder, it should be removed at a later time.

EQUIPMENT: Commonly used catheters are made of rubber or plastic material. For male patients, there also are silk woven catheters that are firm, yet flexible, and follow the contour of the urethra with ease.

Catheters, like rectal tubes, are graded on the French scale according to the size of the lumen. For the female patient, sizes No. 14 and No. 16, Fr., catheters usually are used. Smaller catheters are not necessary, and the size of the lumen is so small that it increases the length of time necessary for emptying the bladder. Larger catheters distend the urethra and tend to increase the discomfort of the procedure. For the male patient, sizes No. 18 and No. 20, Fr., catheters usually are used, but if this appears to be too large, a smaller caliber should be tried. Sizes No. 8 and No. 10, Fr., commonly are used for children.

In addition to the catheter, a receptacle for collecting urine and materials to cleanse the meatus and area around it and sterile gloves are necessary.

All of the equipment used during a catheterization should be sterile and handled while using strict aseptic technique. Sterilization with steam under pressure is usually recommended.

Disposable catheterization sets are frequently used and are desirable. They are sterile when purchased and are used only once, thereby decreasing the possibility of introducing infection. These sets are easy to use and economical as well. When catheterization must be done in a home, a disposable set is first choice inasmuch as it eliminates sterilization problems.

PREPARATION OF THE PATIENT: It is assumed that the patient will have an adequate explanation of the procedure and the reason for it beforehand. Some patients who have a long-term need for a catheter have been taught to catheterize themselves. A catheter being inserted produces a sensation of pressure in the area rather than one of pain. This should be explained to the patient. In addition, the patient should be assured that every measure to avoid exposure and embarrassment will be taken. The more relaxed the patient can be, the easier it will be to insert the catheter.

The most frequent position for the patient is the dorsal recumbent, and preferably on a solid surface such as a firm mattress or a treatment table. Catheterization in the bed with a soft mattress, especially for the female patient, is not as satisfactory because the patient's pelvic surfaces are not supported firmly, and visualization of the meatus is difficult. Also, sinking into the bed may cause the patient's bladder to be lower than the outlet of the catheter. If the patient is in bed, supporting the buttocks on a firm cushion is helpful.

The Sim's or lateral position can be an alternate for the female patient. It may provide better visualization for the nurse if her stature is short, and it may be more comfortable for the patient, especially one who finds hip and knee movements difficult. Reduced area of exposure also can result in less psychic discomfort for the patient. The patient may lie on either side depending on which position is easiest for the nurse and best in terms of the patient's comfort. The patient's buttocks are placed near the edge of the bed with her shoulders at the opposite edge and her knees drawn toward her chest. The nurse lifts the upper buttock and labia to expose the urinary meatus.

For the female patient, good positioning and lighting are especially essential to locating the meatus quickly and easily. Artificial light is almost always necessary for this procedure. The patient should be protected adequately from unnecessary exposure of the perineal area and from drafts by proper and adequate draping. Figure 26-1 illustrates alternate positions of the female patient for catheterization.

Positioning of the patient should always allow sufficient space for the nurse to prepare and maintain a sterile area adjacent to the perineal area to place the necessary equipment. If the dorsal recumbent position is used, the sterile area is generally between the patient's legs near the perineum. If the lateral position is used, the sterile area is immediately adjacent to the lower buttock. In addition, sterile drapes are usually used to extend the work area beyond the immediate perineal area.

PROCEDURE FOR CATHETERIZATION OF THE PATIENT: As indicated earlier, bacteria can be introduced into the urinary bladder by passing a catheter through the external meatus and the urethra into the bladder. The area around the meatus should be made as clean as possible in order to minimize contamination of the catheter.

It would seem that the best preparation of the glans penis or the labia and the introitus prior to introducing a catheter is to wash the area thoroughly with soap and warm water. Some agencies specify a thorough washing of the local area immediately

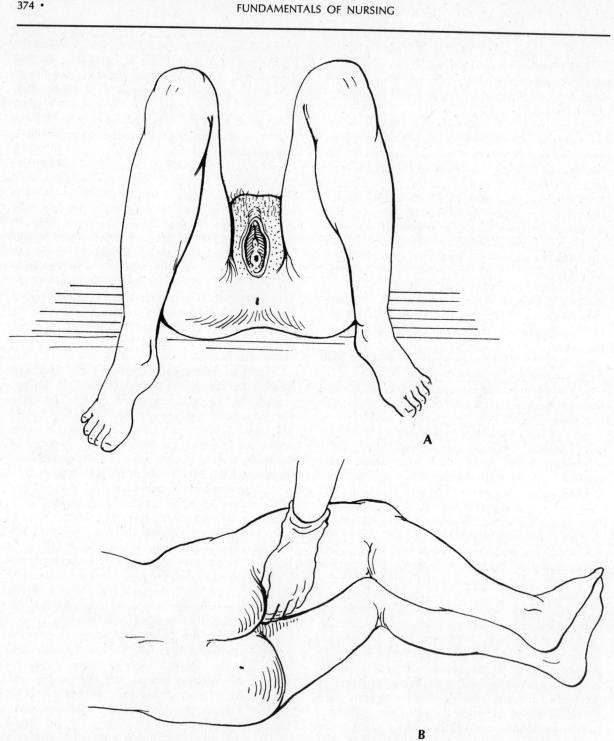

Fig. 26-1. Alternate positions for female urinary catheterization. A shows the patient in the dorsal recumbent position and B shows the patient in the lateral position. Drapes are omitted in the sketches to more clearly show positioning of the patient.

before the procedure, and then cleansing with an antiseptic solution on cotton balls prior to the insertion of the catheter. If soap is used to wash the area, antiseptics should not be used until all of the soap has been rinsed away. Soap destroys the action of some antiseptic agents. The nurse will be guided by local procedure also.

Most authorities recommend the use of sterile gloves for catheterization for the female as well as for the male patient. Most catheterization equipment setups are issued with disposable gloves. The technique for putting on sterile gloves is shown in Figure 26-2. If gloves are not worn, sterile equipment must be handled with sterile forceps. In instances when edema or pathologic changes of the perineum of the female distort the area, sterile gloves facilitate the procedure and make it more comfortable for the patient. If gloves are not worn, the nurse must wash her hands thoroughly under running water im-

mediately before starting the procedure. When a sink is in the patient's unit, it is recommended that the hand wash be done after the patient has been draped, if possible. While this means that the patient must keep the knees flexed if the dorsal recumbent position is used, it also eliminates the possibility of the nurse touching contaminated linens and other objects immediately before handling the catheter. When gloves are worn, the patient is positioned and draped before the gloves are put on.

To catheterize the female patient, good visualization of the meatus facilitates the procedure and reduces the chance of contaminating the tip of the catheter. When the patient is in the dorsal recument position, this can be accomplished by inserting the thumb and the first or second finger well into the labia minora, spreading it apart and then pulling upward toward the symphysis pubis, as Figure 26-3 illustrates. Stretching the tissue in either position "irons

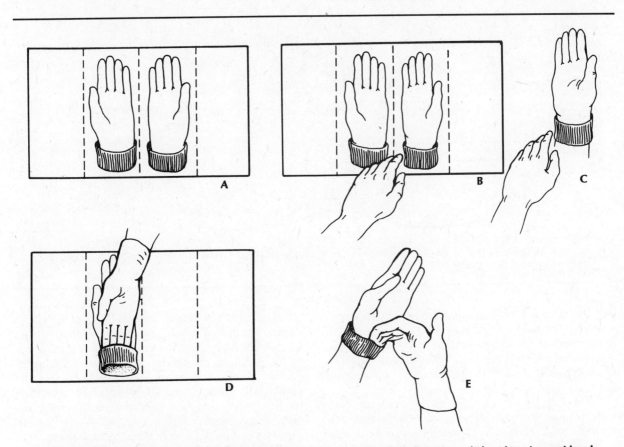

Fig. 26-2. Correct method of putting on sterile gloves. Note that the shaded portion of the glove is considered contaminated and is the only part touched by the skin as the gloves are applied.

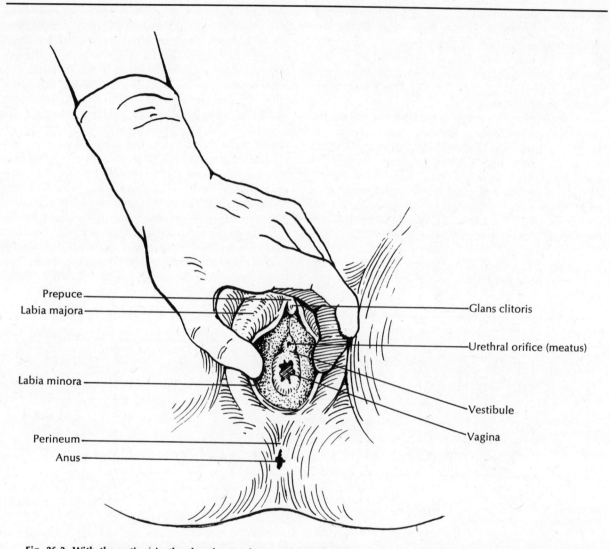

Prepuce
Labia majora
Labia minora
Perineum
Anus

Glans clitoris
Urethral orifice (meatus)
Vestibule
Vagina

Fig. 26-3. With the patient in the dorsal recumbent position, the labia minora are separated in order to cleanse the area and to insert the catheter.

out" the area and makes the meatus visible. In many women, it is rather difficult to find the meatus and it may appear as a small dimple in the area. Once the meatus has been cleansed, do not allow the labia to close over it. This risks the chance of contaminating it.

The foreskin of the penis in the uncircumcised male is retracted for cleansing and the catheter is then inserted. The urethral meatus should be visible at the tip of the penis. The penis should be held upward or near perpendicular to the body to straighten the long urethra and facilitate catheter insertion. Figure 26-4 demonstrates the catheter insertion.

The catheter should be well lubricated with a sterile, water-soluble jelly to minimize friction and to ease insertion. Slight resistance will often be met as the catheter encounters the external sphincter. Pausing briefly and asking the patient to breathe deeply will generally result in sufficient relaxation for the catheter to be passed readily. Rotating the catheter gently may also be helpful. Under no circumstance should force be used. The catheter will need to be inserted approximately 2 to 3 inches in the female patient and 7 to 9 inches in the male. As the bladder is entered, urine will escape through the catheter. Following catheterization, the foreskin

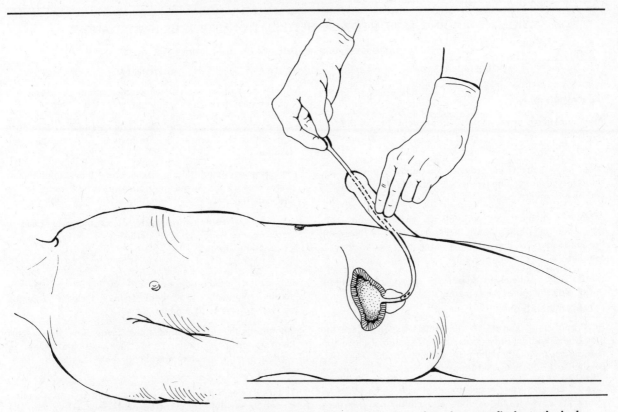

Fig. 26-4. The insertion of a catheter into the male bladder. The penis is elevated nearly perpendicular to the body in order to straighten the urethra.

of the male patient should be replaced over the glans penis. Leaving the foreskin in a retracted position can cause edema and inability to void.

The insertion of the catheter normally does not produce severe pain. If the patient seems to be experiencing unusual discomfort, discontinue the procedure and notify the physician. Some patients have strictures in the urethra, in which case it is best for the physician to introduce the catheter.

Immediately following the insertion of the catheter, some patients react by tightening the muscles in the area, and the flow of urine may be delayed for a few seconds until the patient is able to relax. If the nurse will merely wait a brief time after she believes the bladder has been entered, she may save herself and the patient the necessity of repeating the procedure.

Following catheterization, there are observations which are made and recorded. These include the color and the transparency of the urine and the amount obtained. Occasionally, urine has an unusual odor, and this should be recorded. Any unusual dis-

comfort experienced by the patient should also be noted. A specimen, if desired, is handled according to agency policy.

Indwelling Catheters

If a catheter is to remain in place for continued drainage, an indwelling or retention catheter is used. The catheter used is so designed that it does not slip out of the bladder. Such catheters are used for gradual decompression of an overly distended bladder, for intermittent bladder drainage and irrigation, or for continuous drainage of the bladder.

An indwelling catheter has a portion which can be inflated after the catheter is inserted into the bladder. Because the balloon is larger than the opening to the urethra, it is impossible for the catheter to slip out. There are several types of indwelling catheters available, but the principle on which they operate is similar. The catheter has a double lumen. One lumen is connected directly with the balloon which may be distended with either solution or air, and the other is the portion through which the urine

RATIONALE GUIDING ACTION FOR CATHETERIZATION OF THE URINARY BLADDER

The purpose is to remove urine from the bladder.

SUGGESTED ACTION	RATIONALE
Collect and prepare all necessary equipment before entering the patient's room.	Preparation of equipment where the patient can observe it may be disturbing and frightening.
After providing privacy place the patient in the desired position.	Good visualization of the meatus is essential to introduce the catheter. Comfort of the patient will facilitate relaxation.
Drape the patient to provide minimum exposure. Use sufficient covering, depending on patient's age, condition, and environmental factors.	Embarrassment and chilliness can cause the patient to become tense. Tension can interfere with easy introduction of the catheter.
Arrange equipment for convenience and to avoid contamination of sterile items. Place materials for cleansing the perineum so that reaching over the sterile field is avoided.	Placement of equipment in order of use increases speed of performance. Reaching over sterile items increases the risk of contamination.
Lubricate the catheter for about 1½ inches, being careful not to plug the eye of the catheter.	Lubrication reduces friction and facilitates catheter insertion. Minimizing movements following cleansing of the patient reduces contamination danger.
After putting on gloves, for the female patient, place the thumb and one finger between the labia minora and maintain the separation. For the male patient, lift the penis perpendicular to the body and retract the foreskin as necessary.	Smoothing the area immediately surrounding the meatus helps to make it visible. Lifting the penis straightens the urethra. Microorganisms may be harbored under the foreskin.
Cleanse the area using as many cotton balls as necessary to assure absolute cleanliness. Use one cotton ball for each stroke, moving it from above the meatus downward toward the rectum for the female and in a proximal direction for the male. Keep the labia separated in the female and the penis elevated for the male.	Thorough cleansing of the meatus and the area surrounding it reduces possible introduction of microorganisms into the bladder. Contamination from rectal area can result by stroking from this area toward the meatus. Permitting the labia to close over the meatus or lowering the penis may contaminate the area just cleaned.
Pick up the catheter, taking care not to contaminate it.	The bladder is normally a sterile cavity.
Insert the catheter into the meatus until urine begins to flow. This is usually 2 to 3 inches for the female and 6 to 7 inches for the male.	The female urethra is approximately 1½ to 2½ inches long. The male urethra is approximately 5½ to 6½ inches in length.
Hold the catheter securely in place and prevent pulling and pushing the catheter in the urethra.	Withdrawing the catheter and then pushing it back into the urethra increases the possibility of contaminating the urethra.
When the flow of urine begins to diminish, withdraw the catheter slowly, about ½ inch at a time until urine barely drips.	The tip of the catheter passes through urine remaining in the bladder.
Cleanse all equipment thoroughly immediately after use, if not disposable.	Secretions, lubricant, and other substances are removed more easily when they are not coagulated.

drains. When the balloon is distended, the sidepiece through which the solution or air was introduced is clamped. There are also catheters which are self-sealing. Equipment for inflating the balloon is needed when a retention catheter is inserted. The equipment is included in some disposable setups.

The basic procedure is the same as for catheterization. As soon as the bladder has been emptied of urine, the balloon of the indwelling catheter is distended with air or solution, usually sterile normal saline or sterile water. The balloons are designed to hold from 5 ml. to 30 ml. Each catheter indicates the amount to be injected into the balloon. The means of injecting varies with the make of catheter. Some balloons must be distended by means of a syringe with an adaptor, and then the inlet is clamped off. Other balloons are distended with a syringe and a No. 20 needle because the inlet is self-sealing. If the patient complains of pain or discomfort while the balloon is being filled, empty the balloon and insert the catheter farther, for it may be that the balloon is in the urethra.

After the balloon has been distended, it is best to test the catheter to see that it is secure. Slight tension on it will indicate whether or not it is secure in the bladder. For patients with pathologic changes of the bladder and/or the urethra, it may be necessary to irrigate the catheter after the balloon is distended. This will help to determine whether the catheter is inserted properly.

DRAINAGE WITH THE INDWELLING CATHETER: It is general practice for an indwelling catheter to be attached to a collection receptacle by tubing so that drainage occurs by gravity. This arrangement is also known as straight drainage. The drainage tubing should be of sufficient length to reach the collecting container and still give the patient freedom to move about. If the drainage tubing is too long, urine pools in the tubing, and it may interrupt the drainage from the bladder. If it is too short, movement will be restricted.

When the tubing is attached to the catheter, a glass or plastic connecting rod is used. This makes it possible to examine drainage from the catheter. The drainage tubing should then be secured by some means which permits movement of tubing and prevents tension and pull on the catheter. The catheter is generally taped to the patient's leg and in addition, the tubing may be secured to his clothing or the bed. It is essential that the tubing be placed so that it cannot be compressed by the weight of the patient's buttocks or thigh.

To place the drainage tubing over the patient's thigh has a disadvantage in that urine may pool in the bladder until there is a sufficient amount of pressure to force it up the tubing. Drainage will not occur until the urine forces its way over the thigh, and then gravity will empty the bladder. The distance between the bladder and the container will determine the rate of drainage.

If constant drainage is to be in effect, the drainage tube should be so arranged that accumulation of urine in the bladder or back flow into the bladder will not occur.

The drainage container should be placed so that suction on the bladder is minimized in the event that occasional siphonage should occur. Placement should also be such that the collection container is lower than the catheter's entry into the bladder to prevent urine from re-entering the bladder. This is especially important when the patient ambulates. Attaching it to the bed frame is common practice when the patient is in bed. Figure 26-5 shows the position of the collection container. In addition, it should be inconspicuous to avoid embarrassment to the patient, yet easy to examine. Calibrated drainage containers have several advantages. Amounts of drainage can be determined readily, and measuring when emptying the container is eliminated.

The closed drainage system has been shown to be superior in preventing urinary tract infections. In the closed system, a continuous sterile passageway leads from the bladder to the drainage receptacle. A special air filter permits air to escape from the collection container without bacteria entrance. The catheter, tubing, and receptacle are never disconnected from each other to prevent the introduction of microorganisms. Various types of commercial closed drainage systems are available.

The open system, in which catheter, tubing, and collection container may be disconnected from each other and the receptacle may even have an open top, are still occasionally used in home situations. While the risk is still great, economy and elimination of cross-infection from other patients may be felt by some persons to be ample justification for its use in homes.

Chronically ill patients at home may have indwelling catheters that are cared for by the patient or family members. If nondisposable equipment is used, the nurse may need to teach the patient and/or family how to care for it. It is recommended that the collection receptacle and tubing be washed daily with soap and water and soaked in a vinegar solution. The tubing should be boiled approximately twice a week.

Indwelling catheters have increased the comfort of the ambulatory patient with bladder disturbances, whether he is in a health agency or at home. There are rubber or plastic urinals available, so designed that the catheter fits into the top. The urinal is then attached to the leg and held in place by small, soft straps. These urinals make it possible for the patient to be completely dressed without any evidence of the attachment. However, the patient should be taught that pressure on the container could force urine back into the bladder and should be avoided because of the danger of infection. Some patients

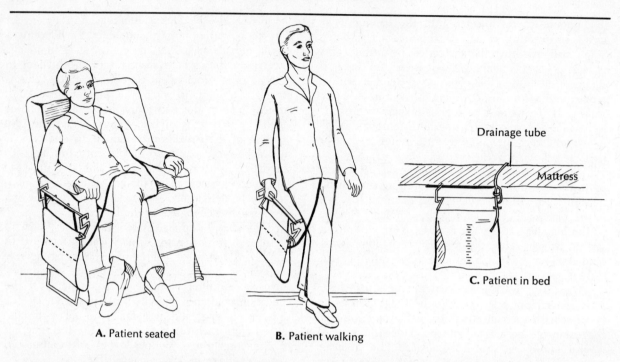

A. Patient seated   **B.** Patient walking

Drainage tube

Mattress

C. Patient in bed

Fig. 26-5. Urine collection receptacle for an indwelling catheter. Note that whether the patient is seated, ambulatory, or in bed, the tube is free of kinks and pressure, and lower than the bladder.

are taught to use a clamp on the catheter and to release it to empty the bladder at specified intervals, such as every two or three hours. This practice makes the use of a collecting container unnecessary.

IRRIGATION OF THE INDWELLING CATHETER: To irrigate a catheter is to flush it with solution to maintain its patency. The physician occasionally orders an irrigation in situations when blood clots or other debris threaten to block the catheter. The procedure was done routinely for almost all indwelling catheters in the past, but because this is another means of introducing pathogens, the current recommendation is that an irrigation should be done only in situations when there is a demonstrated need. "Natural" irrigation of the catheter through an increased fluid intake by the patient is felt to be preferable.

When irrigation is done, strict aseptic technique must be followed. Sterile equipment consisting of a bulb syringe, a basin and solution, and a clean collecting basin is necessary. A catheter with a three-way stopcock is preferred if irrigation is to be done. Otherwise, the catheter should be separated from the drainage tubing so that the solution is injected directly into the catheter. The ends of both the catheter and the tubing must be handled carefully

to prevent contamination. Sterile drainage tube protectors and catheter plugs are commercially available. When it is necessary to use these items, they should be discarded after each use. It is recommended that when catheter irrigations are done at home using nondisposable equipment, the syringe should be boiled for 10 minutes before it is used.

Varying amounts of sterile solution may be specified for irrigation, but 30 ml. per instillation, repeated three or four times, usually is sufficient. The solution should be instilled and allowed to return by gravity. "Milking" the tubing may be necessary if it is obstructed. Suction should not be used routinely because the mucous membrane lining of the bladder can be injured.

NURSING IMPLICATIONS: Great care must be taken by the nurse to prevent introducing a urinary tract infection to the patient with an indwelling catheter. Studies have demonstrated that the hands of nursing personnel are one of the primary modes of transmission of such infections. Careful handwashing between care of patients cannot be emphasized too strongly. Careful body hygiene is urged for all patients with indwelling catheters as still another effort to reduce the possibility of infection. Complete and at least daily cleansing of the area around the meatus is recommended for both female and male patients, because organisms allowed to accumulate in this area can ascend and cause infection. Provisions and reminders for patients to wash their hands, especially following intestinal elimination, are also important, because urinary infections from the intestinal tract can easily be acquired.

The importance of using strict aseptic technique when dealing with any of the urinary drainage equipment has been indicated. If there is any doubt that any piece of equipment is sterile, it should be replaced.

Patients who have indwelling catheters should have the benefit of full explanation on how the system functions and on how they can assist. Teaching points include keeping the tubing free from kinks, maintaining constant downward flow of the urine, maintaining an adequate fluid intake, keeping a record of the output, and preventing contamination.

When an indwelling catheter is in place, note any comments that the patient may make about it, such as irritation, burning sensations, or annoyances with it. Also note the volume and character of the drainage. Any signs of infection should be reported. After an indwelling catheter has been removed, it should be noted on the patient's nursing care plan. There is still need for observation. Frequency, burning on voiding, interference with the urinary stream, such as inability to start it, and cloudy urine may be some of the aftermath of an indwelling catheter. Too often, patients endure the discomfort because they believe that it is to be expected.

While indwelling catheters are sometimes necessary, every effort should be made by the nurse to avoid their use or to minimize the length of time they are used. Studies have shown the incidence of urinary tract infections increases in direct proportion to the length of time the catheter is in place.

ELIMINATION FROM THE INTESTINAL TRACT

Food is ingested and digested by the alimentary canal. The products of digestion which the tissue cells of the body assimilate are absorbed through the mucous membrane of the alimentary canal. Part of the residue that the body does not select for utilization becomes waste products and is excreted by the intestines. This process of excretion of wastes is essential for life and must continue during illness as in health.

Large Intestine

The large intestine is the lower or distal part of the alimentary canal. It extends from the ileocecal valve to the anus. Waste products of digestion are received by the large intestine from the small intestine.

The length of the large intestine in adults is approximately 50 to 60 inches, but variations have been observed in normal persons. The width of the colon varies in different parts. At the narrowest point, the colon is approximately 1 inch wide; at the widest point, about 3 inches. Its diameter decreases from the cecum to the anus.

The barrier between the large intestine and the ileum of the small intestine is the *ileocecal* or *ileocolic* valve. This valve normally prevents contents from entering the large intestine prematurely and prevents fecal matter from returning to the small intestine.

The waste contents pass through the ileocecal valve and enter the cecum, which is the first part of the large intestine. It is situated on the right side of the body, and to it is attached the *vermiform process* or *appendix*. When waste products enter the large intestine, the contents are liquid or watery in nature. While they pass through the large intestine, water is absorbed. Approximately 800 ml. to 1000 ml. of liquid is absorbed daily by the intestinal tract. This absorption of water accounts for the formed, semisolid consistency of the normal stool. When absorption does not occur properly, as when the fecal matter passes through the large intestine at a very rapid rate, the stool is soft and watery. If too much water is absorbed, the stool becomes dry and hardened.

From the cecum, the contents enter the colon, which is divided into several parts. The *ascending colon* extends from the cecum up toward the liver, where it turns to cross the abdomen. This turn is referred to as the *hepatic flexure*. The *transverse colon* crosses the abdomen from right to left. The turn from the transverse colon to form the descending colon is referred to as the *splenic flexure*. The *descending colon* passes down the left side of the body from the splenic flexure to the *sigmoid* or *pelvic colon*. When the waste products reach the distal end of the colon they are referred to as *feces*, and, when excreted, the feces are usually called the *stool*.

The sigmoid colon contains feces ready for excretion and empties into the *rectum*, which is the last part of the large intestine. The rectum is approximately 4 to 6 inches long, 1 to 2 inches being the anal canal. Normally, transverse folds of tissue, usually three, are present in the rectum.

The three transverse folds may help to hold the fecal material in the rectum temporarily. In addition, there are vertical folds. Each vertical fold contains an artery and a vein. Distended veins are called *hemorrhoids*. If hemorrhoids are present, caution must be exercised when a rectal thermometer or tube is inserted. Objects introduced into the anus or rectum should always be lubricated to reduce friction. If force is applied, injury to the mucous membrane may occur. The rectum is usually empty except during and immediately prior to defecation. Waste products are excreted from the rectum through the anal canal and the anus, which is about 1 to 1½ inches long.

The muscular layer of the large intestine plays an important part in excretion. The internal circular muscles are thicker than they are in other parts of the gastrointestinal tract. The outer longitudinal fibers are also thicker and are arranged in three mus-

cle bands called *taeniae coli*. When muscles of the large intestine contract, they are capable of producing strong peristaltic action to propel fecal matter forward. Peristalsis is a kind of wormlike contraction of the musculature.

The contents of the large intestine act as the chief stimulant for the contraction of intestinal musculature. The pressure of the contents against the walls of the colon causes muscle stretch. This in turn causes stimulation of the nerve receptors, which in turn is followed by contraction of the walls of the colon, peristalsis, and haustral churning.

Stimulation occurs by both mechanical and chemical means. The bulk of the contents acts as a mechanical stimulant; as bulk increases, the pressure in the intestine increases, causing the muscles of the large intestine to contract. Bacterial action in the intestinal tract is responsible for chemical stimulation. Certain bacteria act on carbohydrates, causing fermentation, while other bacteria are responsible for the putrefaction of proteins. The end products of fermentation and putrefaction are organic acids, amines and ammonia, which stimulate muscular contraction chemically. Various gases formed by bac-

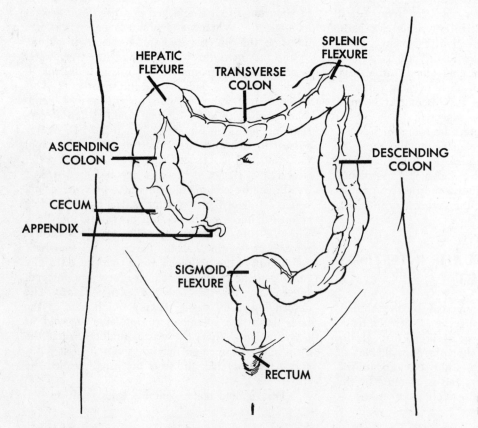

Fig. 26-6. Diagram of the large intestine.

terial action also stimulate muscle contraction by increasing pressure within the colon. Emotional disturbances also have been observed to produce muscle contraction in the large intestine. Such contraction occurs by reflex action.

Waste products in the large intestine are propelled by mass peristaltic sweeps one to four times each 24-hour period in most individuals. The fecal mass is moved during these sweeps. This movement is unlike the frequent peristaltic rushes that occur in the small intestine. Mass peristalsis often occurs after food has been ingested. This accounts for the urge to defecate that frequently is observed following meals. One-third to one-half of ingested food waste products is normally excreted in the stool within 24 hours and the remainder within the next 24 to 48 hours.

Anal Canal and Anus

The internal sphincter in the anal canal and the external sphincter at the anus control the discharge of feces and intestinal gas, or *flatus*.

The internal sphincter consists of smooth muscle tissue and is involuntary. The innervation of the internal sphincter occurs through the autonomic nervous system. Motor impulses are carried by the sympathetic system (thoracolumbar) and inhibitory impulses by the parasympathetic system (craniosacral). It will be recalled that these two divisions of the autonomic nervous system function antagonistically to each other in a dynamic equilibrium.

The external sphincter at the anus has striated muscle tissue and is therefore under voluntary control. The levator ani reinforces the action of the external sphincter and also is controlled voluntarily. Interference with the normal functioning of elimination from the intestines can occur in health as it can during illness. It can be affected by amount and quality of fluid or food intake, degree of activity, and emotional states.

The Act of Defecation

Defecation is an evacuation of the intestines and is often referred to as a bowel movement. There are two centers governing the reflex to defecate. One is situated in the medulla, and a subsidiary one is in the spinal cord. When parasympathetic stimulation occurs, the internal anal sphincter relaxes, and the colon contracts. The defecation reflex is stimulated chiefly by the fecal mass in the rectum. When the rectum is distended, the intrarectal pressure rises, the defecation reflex is stimulated by the mus-

cle stretch, and the desire to evacuate results. The external anal sphincter, controlled voluntarily, is constricted or relaxed according to will. If the desire to defecate is ignored, defecation can often be delayed voluntarily.

During the act of defecation, several additional muscles aid the process. Voluntary contraction of the muscles of the abdominal wall, fixing of the diaphragm, and closing of the glottis aid in increasing intra-abdominal pressure up to four or five times normal pressure that aids in expelling the feces. Simultaneously, the muscles on the pelvic floor contract and aid in drawing the anus over the fecal mass.

Normal Defecation

Normally, the act of defecation is painless. *Normality is associated with the regularity and type of stool.* If the bowels move at regular intervals and the stools are normal, functional problems of frequency of elimination occur infrequently. However, nurses find that many persons show concern if they do not have a daily bowel movement. The normal frequency of bowel movements cannot be stated arbitrarily. Although most adults pass one stool each day, healthy persons have been observed to have more frequent or less frequent bowel movements. Some persons have a bowel movement two or three times a week; others as often as two or three times a day.

Normally, the stool consists principally of food residues as cellulose which is not digested and other foodstuffs which the body has not utilized completely, microorganisms of various kinds, secretions from intestinal glands, biliary pigments, water, and body cells. Unless the diet is high in roughage content, little of the total amount of feces is food residue. The normal stool is a semisolid mass. The amount of stool varies and depends to a large extent on the amount and the kind of food ingested. The color of the normal stool is brown, due chiefly to urobilin, which is a result of the reduction of bile pigments in the small intestine. A change in color is significant, since it frequently indicates impaired physiologic functioning. The stool has a characteristic odor due chiefly to skatole and indole produced by bacterial action on tryptophan. The diet may influence odor, as will certain drugs.

Normally, the stool assumes the shape of the rectum. Change in the shape of the stool is significant if such change persists. For example, pencil-like stools frequently indicate a change in the lumen of the colon and may be due to a growth.

NURSING RESPONSIBILITIES IN RE-LATION TO INTESTINAL ELIMINATION

Nursing personnel are frequently responsible for observing the patient's stool or teaching him or a family member what to observe for. Color, odor, consistency, shape, and amount are noted, and anything unusual such as the presence of blood, pus, parasites, and mucus, should be reported promptly.

It is important for the nurse to know the patient's normal patterns of elimination in order to recognize any abnormality. The frequency with which stools are passed should be noted. It will be recalled that frequency normally varies with individuals, and this should be taken into account when making judgments concerning the frequency of bowel movements.

Passing little or no gas or unusual amounts of flatus are often important symptoms. Difficulty with passing a stool or pain during defecation also should be reported.

The nurse should understand that the establishment of bowel habits begins in childhood. Bowel habits have many psychological implications, depending on accepted practices in various cultural groups. These practices are concerned with consideration for privacy, cleanliness, frequency, and other factors. Having a bowel movement is usually easier when the person is relaxed both physically and mentally. Stress or being away from his usual environment and routine may disturb defecation habits. Individual patterns of living will guide the selection of a convenient time. The urge to defecate often occurs following a meal; after breakfast is a common time for persons who are awake during the usual daylight hours. Responding to the urge to defecate is important in establishing and maintaining an elimination pattern. Sometimes patients are not aware of the implications of not taking the time to have a bowel movement promptly when they experience the stimuli. The nurse may need to consider all of these factors when assisting a patient to establish a satisfactory defecation routine.

A person's food and fluid intakes are probably the largest influential factor in intestinal elimination. Balanced food content with varied bulk is important to the production of feces and its movement along the intestinal tract. The residue after food is absorbed provides bulk which stimulates peristalsis. The food residue must therefore provide this necessary bulk. Some persons find certain foods are acted upon by their intestinal tract bacteria to cause sufficient flatus formation to result in discomfort or distress. Since the offending foods vary with individuals, eliminating their intake becomes a selective personal matter.

Fluid intake has a relationship to stool consistency. Making sure that an adequate amount of liquid is taken in daily to provide for the body's physiological needs and to maintain a soft consistency to the stool is frequently a factor that busy and older persons do not always consider. Some persons find hot liquids on arising or prune juice helpful to stimulate defecation. Teaching and providing for the availability of fluids may be the nurse's responsibility.

Activity influences intestinal elimination by promoting the development of muscle tone as well as by stimulating appetite and peristalsis. The person who has minimal daily activity will generally find his intestinal elimination patterns will be irregular. Encouraging daily activity may be an important role of the nurse.

Positioning during a bowel movement influences ease of emptying the rectum. The nurse may need to assist patients or instruct family members in relation to the best position. The normal physiological semisquatting position permits the most usage of the abdominal muscles for evacuation. This means a person should be in as near a sitting position as possible with the feet resting on a solid surface. A person of small stature may need a footstool or box as he sits on the toilet. Whenever possible, a person who must remain in bed will find positioning the bedpan so his legs can hang over the edge with his feet resting on the floor or a chair will make defecation easier. A person who cannot be helped to the edge of the bed will find it easier to use the bedpan if the head of the bed and his knees are elevated as much as possible.

Securing Stool Specimens

Stool specimens are sometimes analyzed for diagnostic purposes. For example, the fecal material may be examined for blood, bile, urobilin, parasites, and ova. The nurse usually either instructs the patient in the collection of the specimen or she carries out the technique.

Whenever possible, it is preferable if the fecal specimen is uncontaminated with urine or other body excretions. A clean or sterile bedpan can be used for intestinal elimination. The specimen can then be transferred to the appropriate laboratory container by two clean or sterile tongue depressors or a similar disposable instrument. Care should be taken that the outside of the container remains uncontaminated.

Accurate labeling of the container is important. Depending on the examination to be performed, the specimen may be refrigerated or must be kept warm. Ova and parasites cannot sustain life if the environmental temperature varies much below body temperature. The laboratory's directives should be followed closely.

COMMON NURSING MEASURES FOR DEALING WITH INTESTINAL ELIMINATION PROBLEMS

Constipation

Constipation is defined as the passage of unduly dry, hard stools. This definition, it will be noted, makes no mention of frequency. Some persons may be constipated and yet have a daily bowel movement, while others who regularly defecate no more than three times a week are not constipated. The habits of elimination vary exceedingly among healthy persons. Therefore, defining constipation on the basis of frequency of evacuation is meaningless until careful comparisons are made with the person's usual habits.

Constipation is among the commonest and oldest of all medical complaints. It is found in all cultural, economic, and age groups. There are references to laxatives in the Bible and anthropologic investigations suggest the use of enemas even before recorded time. Interestingly enough, many ancient methods for treating constipation are very similar to those used today.

COMMON CAUSES OF CONSTIPATION: Certain organic diseases cause constipation. Other factors causing it require attention once the physician has ruled out organic disease.

When no pathologic changes are involved, a common cause of constipation is the result of poor elimination habits. If the desire for defecation is ignored repeatedly, the feces become hard and dry because of increased water absorption. In addition, the colon becomes insensitive to normal chemical and mechanical stimulation, and eventually the stool in the rectum is no longer sufficient to stimulate the defecation reflex. Neglecting to observe the normal desire for defecation may result from carelessness, occupational demands, the stress of modern life, and, in children, the reluctance to interrupt play.

Many patients resort to the use of laxatives and cathartics which, by either chemical or mechanical means, increase stimulation for muscle contraction. In the habitual use of these the body needs ever larger doses before the urge to defecate becomes apparent.

Certain types of diets predispose to constipation. A diet that is low in roughage often leaves so little residue that the fecal mass is small in amount and becomes dry before sufficient quantity is present to stimulate the defecation reflex. When possible, increasing the bulk of the diet with foods such as fresh fruits and vegetables, bran, and the like, is often sufficient for relief. Heavy-residue foods will pass through the large intestine quickly, while low-residue foods such as lean meats, rice, eggs, and sugar are moved more slowly. Since water increases the rate of movement of residue, an increase in fluids is usually helpful to the person who must consume a low-residue diet.

Investigations indicate that the colon in some individuals absorbs an unusually high percentage of water from the feces, and constipation results. For these persons, increased fluid intake often is the answer. If a bland diet is prescribed for medical reasons, the physician may recommend a medication for the patient to counteract constipation. Certain drugs, such as iron preparations, may be constipating for some persons.

Emotions, as tension, may cause the gastrointestinal tract to become spastic, and fecal content is not moved along the large intestine sufficiently well. The importance of relaxation to aid defecation has been mentioned, and relief is often obtained as the person learns to assume a way of life that allows time for relaxation. Constipation due to spasticity usually is referred to as *hypertonic* or *spastic constipation*.

Authorities differ in opinion concerning *atonic constipation* or constipation that is due to an abnormally sluggish and "lazy" colon. Some state that the condition is doubtful, since the colon and the rectum do not become too weak to propel feces. Others believe that the colon does become too weak to function, especially when debilitating chronic illness, emaciation, or prolonged habitual use of laxatives is present.

In addition to the hard, dry stool, the nurse will observe that some persons who are constipated complain of headache, malaise, anorexia, foul breath, furred tongue, and lethargy. It generally is agreed that these symptoms probably are reflex in nature and are due to the increased pressure in the lower colon. Relief is usually rapid following a bowel movement. These symptoms of constipation have also been produced experimentally by packing the rectum with cotton. Therefore, the general belief that the symptoms are the result of poisons being absorbed when constipation is present is unfounded.

When constipation is not due to pathologic changes, the nurse can help the patient to understand some of the ways in which the situation can be corrected, as by establishing habit patterns of elimination, increasing fluid intake, eating high-roughage foods, and increasing physical activity. Also, the nurse can assist by teaching the patient the importance of establishing an evacuation habit. One suggestion is that the patient go to the bathroom regularly, an hour or so after a meal, and remain there for a while until the defecation urge appears. Distractions, such as reading, are helpful during this period to aid in reducing anxiety. It takes time to develop an evacuation habit just as it takes time to overcome the one that was present originally. But success has been observed among patients whose cooperation has been obtained.

Mr. Bartoni is an example of a person with a normal habit that was interrupted by bed rest. He was distressed about his constipation, a problem he said he had never had previously. He was sure that it was because he was in traction and could not get to the bathroom. In talking with him, the nurses learned that he arose every day at 5:30 A.M. and always had a bowel movement immediately after breakfast.

He was also awake every day in the hospital at 5:30. However, there was no breakfast until 8 or 8:15 A.M. In talking about it a bit more they suggested that he try having a glass of water, and possibly some fruit when he awakened. The first morning did not yield results, but his desire to help himself gave him confidence that it would work. In a short time his former habit had been reestablished.

Cathartics and Suppositories

Cathartics or *laxatives* are drugs which induce emptying of the intestinal tract. Some of these drugs act chemically by stimulating peristalsis. Others act by increasing the intestinal bulk which promotes additional mechanical stimulation on the intestine. Still others act on the fecal material itself by softening it.

Nurses are often in a position to help patients understand the appropriate use and dangers of laxatives. Because many cathartics are available as over-the-counter drugs and because modern advertising promotes their use, many persons take laxatives frequently on their own initiative.

Most persons are aware that because laxatives have a chemical action, they should not be taken when there is abdominal pain because of the danger of intestinal pathology and subsequent harm from increased peristalsis. While many individuals take laxatives because they believe they are constipated, most are unaware that habitual use of laxatives is the most common cause of chronic constipation. Often the person is upset or concerned when he does not have a bowel movement, so he takes a cathartic. The drug's action will stimulate peristalsis enough to empty the entire intestinal tract. Since the colon may not fill for several days and no stimulation of the defecation reflex occurs, he often repeats taking his laxative and continues the pattern. The habitual use of cathartics very soon makes it difficult for him to have a normal bowel movement.

Breaking this habit, often from both a physical and psychological viewpoint, is not easy for a person who has come to depend on laxatives. It often requires a great deal of patience, support, and teaching from the nurse. The patient frequently needs to be helped with diet, fluid intake, activity, and regularity of habits.

Laxatives are necessary at times for persons whose activity is limited, or appetite poor. They are also used for evacuating the intestinal tract in preparation for surgical or diagnostic exploration. Their occasional use is generally not harmful for most persons, but all efforts should be taken to prevent the person from becoming dependent on this means of stimulating defecation.

A *suppository* is a conical or oval solid substance shaped for easy insertion into a body cavity and designed to melt at body temperature. Since a certain amount of absorption can take place in the large colon, some medications for systemic effect can be given by a suppository. However, the most frequent use of the suppository is to aid in stimulating peristalsis and defecation. When effective, results are obtained usually within 15 to 30 minutes, but it could be as long as an hour.

A variety of suppositories is available. Some act as fecal softeners, others have direct action on the nerve endings in the mucosa, and some liberate carbon dioxide when moistened.

Fecal softeners are useful when the stool is very hard, while those substances that stimulate the rectum are helpful for persons with weak muscle tone or poor innervation. The carbon dioxide suppositories liberate about 200 ml. of the gas which causes distention, thus producing stimulation and evacuation impulses.

Suppositories are helpful in a program to aid a patient in regaining good evacuation habits. A procedure which has been found to be satisfactory is to insert one or two suppositories one-half hour before a meal. Since the intake of fluids and food usually results in increased peristaltic action, it is more common to have the urge to defecate after meals.

To be most effective, the suppository should be introduced beyond the internal sphincter of the anal canal. To reduce friction, lubricate the suppository before inserting it. A finger cot or a glove is used to protect the finger when inserting the suppository. If the patient breathes through the mouth while the suppository is being inserted, the anal sphincter is usually relaxed.

Some patients are able to insert suppositories for themselves. In other situations, family members can be taught. The nurse should establish whether the patient has an understanding of the correct procedure since incorrect insertion will not produce the desired results.

Enemas

An *enema* is an introduction of solution into the large intestine, generally for the purpose of removing feces. Enemas are given for three common purposes: to relieve constipation; to prevent involuntary escape of fecal material during surgical procedures and during delivery; and to promote visualization of the intestinal tract by x-ray or instrument examination. There may be some variations in the types of solutions used. Those most frequently used are tap water, physiological saline, soap solution, hypertonic solutions, and oil.

Tap water, physiological saline, and soap solutions are usually given in quantities of 500 ml. to 1000 ml. for the average adult patient. The quantity of solution distends the rectum and colon and usually stimulates peristalsis and defecation within 15 minutes of administration.

Tap water and physiological saline appear to have approximately the same degree of effectiveness in causing bowel evacuation. However, because the colon does absorb solution to some degree, their repeated use for some patients can result in fluid and electrolyte imbalances. Tap water must be administered cautiously to infants or to adults who have altered kidney or cardiac reserve. If a large quantity of hypotonic solution is absorbed through repeated enemas, the blood volume may be increased. This reaction is usually called water intoxication, and

symptoms include weakness, sweating, pallor, vomiting, cough, or dizziness. The colon can conserve sodium quite effectively, so persons with abnormal sodium retention, as in congestive heart failure, may absorb sufficient sodium from repeated saline enemas to cause further electrolyte disturbance.

Soap suds solutions stimulate peristalsis by chemical irritation of the mucous membrane, as well as by intestinal distention. Too much or too strong soap can produce hyperirritation or actual colon membrane damage. Concentrated soap solutions designed for enemas are commercially available and should not be used in quantities of more than 5 ml. per 1000 ml. of water.

Soap solutions can be made by dissolving a bland white soap or castile soap in water. However, estimates of the concentration are very difficult to determine. Bar soap that has been used previously is not recommended because it has been found that these bars often harbor organisms. Household detergents are too strong for the delicate mucosa. Many proctologists discourage the use of soap for enemas, particularly for patients having known or suspected rectal pathology or for patients being prepared for rectal examinations because of the effect on the mucosa of the intestine.

Hypertonic solutions are available in commercially prepared, disposable enema units. The amount of solution given is usually 4 ounces, or 120 ml. The action of the solution seems to be a combination of distention and irritation. The hypertonic solution draws fluid from the body into the bowel by osmosis, thus creating fluid bulk in the colon. In addition, the hypertonicity of the solution acts as a mild irritant on the mucosa. The administration of this type of enema is simple, results are obtained readily within 2 to 7 minutes, and evacuation of the colon is generally good. In many agencies, it has become the method of choice for preparation for examination of the rectum with a proctoscope or for x-ray visualization of the rectum by the barium enema. It is less fatiguing and distressing to the patient. Disposable units of hypertonic solution have been very successful for patients unable to retain large quantity enemas.

Oils such as mineral oil, cottonseed oil, or olive oil, are used for enemas. Their primary action is as a lubricant, although they may also help to soften the fecal material somewhat. Usually, 150 ml. to 200 ml. of oil is given slowly and the patient is requested to retain the oil for as long a period as he is able, at least 30 minutes. Oil enemas vary widely in the length of time in which they are effective, since usually they are administered to severely constipated patients. It is not uncommon for an oil enema to be followed by a soap solution, tap water, or saline enema after several hours if an evacuation does not result from the oil anema.

ENEMA EQUIPMENT: The commercially prepared enema is self contained. It is a flexible bottle containing the solution with an attached prelubricated firm tip of approximately 2 to 3 inches in length. Its ease of use makes it particularly convenient for home situations. Patients can readily administer their own in many instances.

For the tap water, saline, or soap solutions, a container for the solution, rubber or plastic tubing with side openings near its distal end, tubing clamp, lubricant, and the solution are necessary. The solution container varies. Metal cans or plastic bags attached to the tubing are most often used. The plastic containers are usually disposable and used for one patient only, while the metal containers are sterilized for reuse. Pitchers as solution containers may be used occasionally with a funnel attached to the tubing for introduction of the solution. While the commercially produced equipment is sterile, and the reusable equipment is sterilized between patients in the health agency, the enema is an aseptic or clean technique, not a sterile one.

The larger the lumen of the rectal tube, the greater the stimulation of the anal sphincters. This is to be desired if the purpose in giving the enema is to aid in emptying the colon. If the purpose is to introduce a solution which is to be retained, a smaller size rectal tube should be used.

If an enema is to be expelled immediately, the most commonly used rectal tubes are between No. 26 and No. 32, Fr., and for enemas to be retained, No. 14 to No. 20, Fr. The size of the tube used for retention enemas depends on the viscosity of the solution to be administered. The larger sized tubes should be used for solutions of high viscosity because of their resistance to flow.

ENEMA PREPARATION: The maximum amount of solution should generally be prepared even though it may not all be used. If the primary purpose in giving the enema is to stimulate the defecation impulse and to aid in emptying the lower colon, and if this goal is achieved with a lesser amount, it may not be necessary to use the total amount. Quantities less than the maximum are sufficient for some persons and for others, the total amount may be necessary.

The temperature of the solution should generally be slightly higher than internal body temperature, that is, 105° to 115° F. (40.5° to 49° C.) Disposable enemas are frequently given at room temperature, but some authorities feel they are more effective and comfortable for the patient if warmed in a basin of water or under the hot water tap. Solutions that are too hot can injure the mucosa, while those that are too cold can cause cramping and difficulty for the patient to retain the enema.

After the solution is prepared and before administering the enema, the solution should be allowed to fill the tubing and displace the air. While introducing air into the colon is not harmful, it may serve to impede the solution inflow if there is no escape and the intestinal pressure is great enough. Running a small amount of solution through the tubing before introducing it into the colon also warms the tubing.

PREPARATION OF THE PATIENT: Since the enema is a common procedure, many patients understand its use and how it is administered. Other patients who have not experienced an enema before will need an explanation of its purpose, what they can expect, and how they can participate. The procedure offers an excellent opportunity for health teaching, since many persons are not familiar with the principles underlying it. Failure to observe one or more of these principles may be responsible for their considering the procedure a disagreeable one.

Most patients believe that solutions introduced into the colon are to be expelled as soon as possible. When a solution is to be retained, care should be taken to have the patient understand this. If the procedure is explained as a small enema, the patient still may believe that it is to be expelled. It is best if the patient is helped to understand that it is an instillation which is to be retained. An additional precaution is to keep the bedpan out of sight.

Traditionally, the enema has been administered with the patient in the left lateral recumbent position. It was thought that the solution would flow into the colon with less resistance if the patient were to lie on his left side. It now appears that the left lateral is no more effective than the right. For some commercially prepared enemas, it is recommended that the patient be in the knee-chest position. This position helps the solution to flow further into the colon and insures the distribution of the small amount of solution over as wide a surface area of the lower colon as possible. In this way, more fluid is drawn into the colon. The knee-chest position is difficult for some patients to assume and impossible for others. In this event, it is best if the patient is as flat as possible. In addition, it is preferable if the patient is kept in a recumbent position for a few minutes following the administration if possible. If the patient is permitted to sit up, the solution may pool in the lower portion of the colon and this would reduce its effectiveness.

A common misunderstanding about enemas is that the solution can be administered effectively while the patient is in the sitting position. The amount of pressure needed to force the solution up into the colon while sitting is far greater than that needed while lying down. In addition, solution will tend to pool and distend the lower colon since it must go against gravity in order to ascend the colon. This will cause the desire to empty the colon sooner than may be desirable for effective results.

Before the enema is administered, plan with the patient where he will evacuate the solution. If possible, most patients prefer to use the bathroom toilet. If this is not feasible, a bedside commode or the bedpan can be used. Arranging the patient's robe and slippers conveniently, making certain the bathroom is vacant or making the bedpan accessible are all important parts of helping the patient to relax.

ADMINISTERING THE ENEMA: The enema tube should be lubricated before insertion to facilitate its entry. The tip is inserted through the anus approximately 2 to 3 inches at an angle pointing toward the umbilicus. Figure 26-7 illustrates.

Possible injury to the rectal wall is increased with further insertion. Occasionally, the tube seems to meet with some resistance as it is being inserted. In such instances, it is best to permit a small amount of solution to enter, withdraw the rectal tube slightly, and then continue to insert. The resistance may be due to spasm of the colon or failure of the internal sphincter to open. The solution will help to reduce the spasms and relax the sphincter, and the tube may be inserted safely to the desired distance.

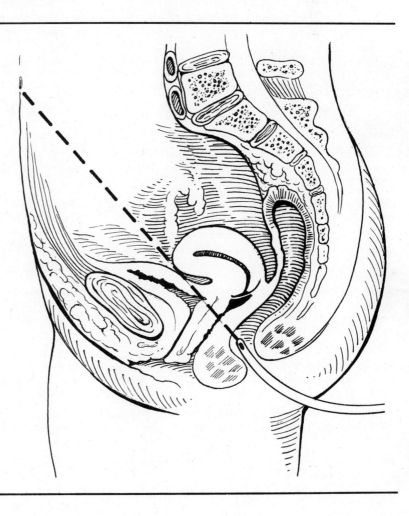

Fig. 26-7. Insertion of the enema tube. The inserted tube should be directed at an angle toward the umbilicus and inserted 2 to 3 inches.

The disposable enema solution is forced into the rectum by applying gentle, steady pressure to the solution container. The large volume enema solution container should be elevated approximately 18 to 20 inches above the anus and the solution introduced slowly, that is, over a 5 to 10 minute period. Faster introduction or greater elevation of the solution container and a higher pressure can result in cramping and difficulty for the patient to retain the solution. Encouraging the patient to mouth breathe during the administration usually results in muscle relaxation and ease of solution retention.

The patient should be encouraged to retain the solution as long as he is able in order to achieve maximum effects. The average time for most patients is 5 to 10 minutes.

Occasionally it is not possible for a patient voluntarily to contract the external sphincter and assist in retaining the solution being given. Such a patient may need to have the rectal tube inserted and then be placed on the bedpan and the solution introduced. The nurse wears a glove to hold the tube in place. The head of the bed should be elevated slightly so that the patient's back is not arched. A pillow support to the lumbar region may be necessary. If the head of the bed is elevated beyond a 30° angle, there is less likelihood of the solution's entering the colon freely. Most of the solution will drain back out, and evacuation of feces in the colon may not be accomplished.

For patients who are unable to retain large quantities of fluid, the commercially prepared hypertonic

RATIONALE GUIDING ACTION WHEN ADMINISTERING AN ENEMA

The purpose is to introduce solution into the colon to aid in stimulating peristalsis and removing feces.

SUGGESTED ACTION	RATIONALE
Secure the commercially prepared enema or prepare the desired enema solution. The temperature of the solution should range from 105° to 110°F. (40.5° to 49°C.)	For maximum stimulation, comfort, and safety, the solution should enter the colon at a slightly higher than internal body temperature. The adult colon is estimated to hold about 750 ml. to 1000 ml.
Lubricate the end of the rectal tube for 2 to 3 inches.	Friction is reduced when a surface is lubricated.
Position the patient in the lateral recumbent, recumbent, or knee-chest (for commercially prepared enema) position, as dictated by the patient's comfort.	Gravity aids the flow of fluids into the colon. The patient's comfort will help him to relax.
Insert the rectal tube for 2 to 3 inches at an angle pointing toward the umbilicus.	The anal canal is approximately 1 to 2 inches in length. The tube should be inserted through the internal anal sphincter, but further insertion may damage the intestinal wall. The suggested angle follows the normal intestinal contour. Slow insertion of a lubricated rectal tube minimizes spasms of the intestinal wall.
Gently and steadily collapse the flexible commercial enema container with hand pressure, or elevate the reservoir to the point where the solution begins to flow *slowly* into the colon. Usually the reservoir is 18 to 20 inches above the anus.	Pressure on the liquid forces the solution into the colon. Force on the container wall or gravity provide the pressure. The amount of pressure exerted on the solution will determine the rate of flow into the colon and the pressure exerted on the colon.
Stop the flow of fluid and remove the rectal tube when the patient has a strong desire to defecate.	Distention and irritation of the intestinal wall, which produce strong peristaltic action, should be sufficient to empty the lower intestinal tract.
Place the patient in a sitting position on the bedpan, or assist him to the bathroom or to a commode if permissible.	Contraction of the abdominal and the perineal muscles which aid in emptying the colon is easier when the patient is in the sitting position.
Wash all equipment thoroughly and sterilize it before reuse, if disposable equipment is not used.	Normally, there is an abundant growth of bacteria in the large intestine.

solution enemas are often more satisfactory. The quantity is small enough so that usually there is no difficulty in retaining that amount.

The results of the enema, character of the evacuation, and the volume and type of solution are recorded on the patient's chart. The nurse also records any unusual effects of the enema experienced by the patient.

Fecal Impaction

A *fecal impaction* is a prolonged retention or an accumulation of fecal material which forms a hardened mass in the rectum. It may be of sufficient size to prevent the passage of normal stools.

The medical literature describes a condition referred to as obstipation which is the accumulation of hardened feces extending well up into the colon and in some instances almost amounting to intestinal obstruction. While it is common for a fecal impaction to prevent the passage of normal stools, the situation may be misleading, because the patient has liquid fecal seepage. Small amounts of fluid present in the colon are able to go around the impacted mass. As a matter of fact, such liquid fecal seepage and no passage of normal feces are almost a confirmation of the existence of an impaction.

Fecal impactions frequently are due to constipation and poor habits of defecation. They may result when parts of a hardened, dry stool become lodged in the folds of the rectum.

Certain conditions predispose to fecal impactions, and the nurse will need to be alert to prevent their development. For example, patients who are required to maintain complete bed rest may find normal defecation difficult, and, unless some action is taken, constipation and fecal impactions may result. This may mean determining if the patient's food and fluid intake can be improved to aid the process. Or, it may mean consulting the physician about the possibility of permitting the patient to use a commode or having a mild laxative daily.

Patients who are required to take constipating drugs over a period of time are also prone to develop fecal impactions; barium enemas for x-ray examinations of the colon are likely to develop fecal impactions if care is not taken to cleanse the colon of barium following examination.

Investigations have shown that some fibrous foods, such as bran and fruit seeds have been known to cause fecal impactions, as have coated pills.

The patient with a fecal impaction may complain of constipation, uncontrolled liquid fecal seepage or both. Usually, he experiences a frequent desire to defecate but is unable to do so. Rectal pain may be present. Very careful observation is needed to prevent fecal impactions. There is no particular time span associated with their formation. Some have been known to occur within 24 hours. There have been reports in the literature of impactions removed by surgical procedures. Prevention is based on observation of the stool as to amount, consistency, and frequency. If the patient is ambulatory, he will need to be instructed to make these observations. If he does not use the bathroom, nursing personnel or family members should assume this responsibility. If the causes are not eliminated, impactions are likely to recur. As with the prevention of constipation, all efforts to help a patient should be entered on the nursing care plan. When fecal impactions are not associated with circumstances beyond the nurse's control, such as antiperistaltic drugs or other therapy, the occurrence of an impaction usually is a sign of less than satisfactory nursing care.

When it has been determined that a fecal impaction is present, an oil retention enema is often used. This is followed by a cleansing enema two or three hours later. This may be followed by enemas twice a day if necessary until normal stools are evacuated. If this procedure fails, often it is necessary to break up the impaction by digital manipulation.

To remove an impaction, the patient should be placed in the Sim's position if possible, the top bedding folded down to the foot of the bed, the patient covered with a bath blanket; use protection for the bedding, such as a disposable pad or plastic sheeting, under the patient. The bedpan should be placed conveniently on the bed so that pieces of removed feces may be deposited in it. Clean gloves should be used. Lubricate the forefinger generously and insert it as gently as possible into the anal sphincter. The presence of the finger added to the mass already present causes considerable discomfort to the patient. By carefully working the finger into the hardened mass, it is possible to remove pieces of it. Use plenty of lubricant in order to avoid irritating the mucous membrane or inducing bleeding. When a severe impaction exists, part of the impaction will need to be removed at one time, possibly more oil instilled, and remaining parts removed at intervals of several hours. This will avoid extreme discomfort and possibly harm to the patient.

Intestinal Distention

Excessive formation of gases in the stomach or the intestines is known as *flatulence*. When the gas is not expelled and accumulates in the intestinal tract, the condition is called intestinal *distention* or *tympanites.*

Any disturbance in the ability of the small intestine to absorb gases or in its ability to propel gas along the intestinal tract usually will result in distention. Irritating foods, such as beans and cabbage, often predispose to flatulence and distention. Constipation is a frequent cause of distention. Certain drugs, morphine sulfate for example, tend to decrease peristaltic action and thus cause distention. Swallowing large amounts of air while eating and drinking can cause distention. Persons who are tense often can be observed to be swallowing large amounts of air, especially when taking fluids. This habit can be overcome by purposely training oneself to eat and drink without swallowing air. Usually, air swallowers will eructate a great deal, and much air escapes in this manner before it reaches the intestines.

Distention can be noted by the presence of a swollen abdomen. Gentle percussion with the fingers produces a drumlike sound. In addition, usually the patient will complain of cramplike pain, and, if distention is sufficient to cause pressure on the diaphragm and the thoracic cavity, shortness of breath and dyspnea may result.

Acting on the cause usually will relieve the distention. Movement in bed or ambulation will often promote escape of the flatus. Temporary relief often can be afforded the patient by inserting a rectal tube.

The sizes of rectal tubes used most frequently for the relief of distention in adults range from No. 22 to No. 32 Fr. Smaller sizes are used for children. The tips of rectal tubes also vary—some have smoothly rounded tips with an opening on the side of the tube near the tip, others have an opening at the tip as well as on the side of the tube. The distinct advantage of the rubber or plastic tube for rectal treatments is that it is flexible, and, with good lubrication and careful insertion, it can be introduced with relative ease beyond the anal canal into the rectum.

After lubricating the rectal tube, it should be carefully inserted for approximately 4 inches. However, since fluids are not being introduced, it is possible to insert it a bit farther if no resistance is encountered and if it is noted that no flatus is being removed.

The rectal tube may be attached to a piece of connecting tubing of sufficient length to reach well into a small collecting container which can be attached to the bed frame. Water then can be put into the collecting container to cover the end of the tubing to determine whether or not the patient is ex-

pelling flatus; air bubbles indicate that gas is being removed.

A rectal tube should be left in place for a short period of time; usually 20 minutes is sufficient. Leaving the tube in place for long periods of time reduces the responsiveness of the sphincters. There is more likelihood of stimulating the sphincters and peristalsis if the rectal tube is reinserted every two to three hours as necessary. If the tube is inserted repeatedly over a period of several hours and no gas is removed, and the patient remains distended, the observation should be reported to the physician.

Medications are also often used to relieve distention.

Diarrhea

Diarrhea is the passage of excessively liquid and unformed stools. Frequent bowel movements do not necessarily mean that diarrhea is present, although patients with diarrhea usually will pass stools at frequent intervals. Diarrhea often is associated with intestinal cramps. Nausea and vomiting may be present, as may be the presence of blood in the stools. Diarrhea is protective in nature when its cause is the presence of irritants in the intestinal tract.

Diarrhea may have a functional basis. The patient may have allergies to ingested food or drugs. The abuse of cathartics, and also certain dietary indiscretions, may cause diarrhea. Some persons know that, for them, certain foods and fluids such as rich pastries, coffee, or alcoholic beverages may produce temporary diarrhea. Avoidance of the factor causing it usually remedies the situation easily.

Diseases in parts of the body other than the intestinal tract may be at the root of the trouble. Examples include uremia and certain cardiac and neurological disorders.

Diarrhea may be caused by certain intrinsic conditions existing in the intestine itself. Examples include these: viral, bacteriologic, fungal, protozoan, or metazoan invasion; alterations in the normal bacterial flora of the intestine; antimicrobial therapy; fistulas; inflammatory conditions such as ulcerative colitis; and tumors in the intestinal tract.

If the cause of diarrhea is psychic in nature, the nurse may be able to play an important part in assisting the patient to understand the cause. Situations in daily living may be disturbing to him. However, diarrhea may be associated with deep-seated emotional problems that require the help of a psychiatrist.

Diarrhea is often an embarrassing and usually a painful disturbance. Local irritation of the anal region and possibly even the perineum and the buttocks from frequent watery stools is not uncommon. To help to prevent irritation the nurse may need to initiate special hygienic measures, such as washing the area after each movement, drying it thoroughly, and possibly using one of the medicated creams or powders. Also, it may be necessary to caution the patient to use only very soft toilet tissue.

When a person has diarrhea it is often impossible to control the urge to defecate for very long, if at all. Therefore, when it is known that a hospitalized patient has diarrhea, a comment to this effect should appear on the nursing care plan. This will alert nursing personnel to watch for his signal light. Or, it may be necessary to place the bedpan within easy reach for the patient, but yet out of sight to prevent embarrassment.

A review of Table 24-4 in Chapter 24 illustrates how very frequently diarrhea leads to or is involved in fluid and electrolyte disturbances. Large amounts of fluids and electrolytes may be lost relatively quickly in the presence of diarrhea. This is especially true with infants; if neglected, such loss may easily place a baby's life in jeopardy. Parenteral fluids may be necessary when diarrhea is present. If oral intake is possible, cold fluids and rich foods, especially sweets, should be avoided.

Anal Incontinence

Anal incontinence is the inability of the anal sphincter to control the discharge of fecal and gaseous material. Usually, the cause of incontinence is an organic disease resulting either in a mechanical condition that hinders the proper functioning of the anal sphincter or in an impairment in the nerve supply to the anal sphincter.

While anal incontinence rarely is a menace to life, incontinent patients suffer embarrassment and may become disturbed emotionally. They require much emotional support and understanding as well as special nursing care to prevent odors, skin irritation, and soiling of the linen and the clothing.

Too often, incontinence is accepted as an inescapable situation. This attitude should not exist until every effort has been made to determine if continence can be achieved. While the situation itself is distressing to the patient, some of the nursing measures may be equally disturbing if not managed with tact, since they are not too different from those used with children before they gain bowel control.

Typical nursing measures follow. Note if there is a time of day when incontinence is more likely to occur, such as after a meal. If so, the patient could be placed on a bedpan at such times. If there is no pattern as to when incontinence occurs, place the patient on a bedpan at frequent intervals, such as every two or three hours. The patient's attempts at trying to use the pan may be successful and may lead to better muscular control. Consult with the physician about the advisability of using suppositories or a daily enema. For some patients, the problem is so severe that moisture-proof undergarments may be necessary in order to limit soiling of the patient and the bed clothing. Disposable bed pads are available and convenient to use. Diapering the patient should be avoided because of its distressing psychological effect.

Anal control is dependent ultimately on proper functioning of the anal sphincter, and nursing or medical therapeutic measures depend on the cause. In certain instances, functioning of impaired anal sphincters can be improved with a planned program of bowel training. For these patients, aid in regaining bowel control becomes an important part of nursing care.

BOWEL TRAINING: The matter of planning a regimen for bowel training is certainly a mutual proposition involving the physician, the patient, his family, and the nurse. As might be expected, it has great psychological implications for the patient, since almost every lucid individual desires normal control of this body function. The physician must first determine the feasibility of initiating such a program. Is there any possibility for success? It would be a disaster to the patient if even partial success were impossible. As a plan is being developed, and once it has been established, it should be a conspicuous part of the patient's nursing care plan, since interruptions may jeopardize the progress being made.

Before beginning bowel training, the patient will need to determine what time of day is best for him to have an evacuation. This can be decided in terms of his past pattern of evacuation and after he has considered his schedule at home and the facilities available. It is also essential that the nurse review the diet, the amount of exercise permitted, and the medications being administered.

Arrangements then should be made so that the patient can try to have an evacuation at the time of day selected. If possible, the patient should be on a toilet or a commode, since in this position gravity and more effective muscular contraction aid defecation.

If the patient is paralyzed, frequently the external sphincter is relaxed, but the training of the internal sphincter is possible. The patient should be encouraged to bear down as is done in normal bowel evacuation. However, straining or persistent bearing down should be discouraged because of the possibility of inducing hemorrhoids.

A time limit for trying should be set, such as 15 to 25 minutes. If the patient had any previous habits that seemed to be associated with bowel evacuation, these should be included. Frequently, patients state that hot coffee or a glass of water upon arising helped. Smoking or reading have some value in the procedure for certain patients. There is merit in taking advantage of any of the patient's suggestions and wishes in relation to his previous bowel habits.

The physician may need to be consulted about using suppositories. Inserting one or two suppositories is often a satisfactory means of helping to create stimulation and subsequent emptying of the rectum. The results from the suppositories may not be obtained until several hours later, so that, during the early training period, the patient may be having results at other than the desired evacuation time.

Because of the many discouraging aspects to such a program, especially the long-time span before any progress is evident, the patient will need much encouragement to continue. He should also receive praise for his efforts.

There is no usual span of time which can be estimated for a bowel-training program. The rapidity with which a satisfactory pattern can be established depends on the patient's condition and often on the perseverance shown by both the patient and the nurse. If the patient becomes discouraged, the nurse may need to modify the procedure from time to time so that the patient has a feeling of some gain.

CONCLUSION

Urinary and intestinal elimination are essential physiologic processes. The nurse assists patients often by observing elimination patterns and by promoting normal elimination. Her functions in regard to elimination frequently involve extensive teaching of the patient and his family. Her goal is to maintain or restore as near normal body elimination as is possible.

Study Situations

1. In the following article, the author reports on a study that used ice successfully to promote micturition.

Bergstrom, N. I.: Ice application to induce voiding. **Am. J. Nurs.,** 69:283–285, Feb., 1969.
What is the technique the author recommended?

2. Try your nursing care planning skills in a fictitious, but common situation. Assume you are caring for a debilitated elderly lady who has frequent urinary incontinence. The nursing care objective is for the patient to develop urinary continence within two weeks so that she remains dry during her waking hours. Identify as many nursing action alternatives as you can that you would consider in formulating your plan of care.

3. Urinary tract infections are a common occurence with indwelling catheters. This article discusses causes and prevention of such infections.

Langford, T. L.: Nursing problems: bacteriuria and the indwelling catheter. **Am. J. Nurs.,** 72:113–115, Jan., 1972.
On page 114, the author indicates that continuous urine flowing down the catheter can impede the ascent of organisms in the catheter and tubing. What flow rate is recommended to prevent the majority of organisms from moving upward? How can the nurse promote this urine flow rate?

4. Enemas are possibly one of the most common nursing techniques provided for hospitalized patients. The authors of the following article discuss some of the hazards of administering enemas.

Tillery, B., and Bates, B.: Enemas. **Am. J. Nurs.,** 66: 534–537, Mar., 1966.
How do the authors indicate intestinal performation may occur? What can be done to avoid this danger?

5. Many persons at home have indwelling catheters. The following reference discusses the care of these patients.

Clark, C. L.: Catheter care in the home. **Am. J. Nurs.,** 72:923–924, May, 1972.
What does the author recommend that the patient and his family be taught about care of the catheter and the drainage system?

6. A frequent nursing problem is met with in persons who suffer from bowel consciousness beyond the point of good reason. Misleading literature and advertisements, especially in relation to frequency of defecation, have caused people to upset habits that were completely normal. For example, some begin taking laxatives rather routinely because they have read in advertisements that bowel "sluggishness" occurs after middle age.
Examine the variety of preparations available the next time you are in the drug department of a store. Read the labels for a description of the kind of action the medication is to induce, where the action occurs, frequency of administration and dosage. Do a count of the varieties available to the public for self-administration. Do not forget to count and examine the labels on those that are refrigerated.

References

1. Birum, L. H., and Zimmerman, D. S.: Catheter plugs as a source of infection. **Am. J. Nurs.,** 71:2150–2152, Nov., 1971.

2. Bortoff, A.: Current concepts: intestinal motility. **New Engl. J. Med.,** 280:1335–1337, June 12, 1969.

3. Cleland, V., *et al.:* Prevention of bacteriuria in female patients with indwelling catheters. **Nurs. Research,** 20:309–318, July–Aug., 1971.

4. Delehanty, L., and Stravino, V.: Achieving bladder control. **Am. J. Nurs.,** 70:312–316, Feb., 1970.

5. Dobbins, J., and Gleit, C.: Experience with the lateral position for catheterization. *In* **The Nursing Clinics of North America.** Philadelphia, W. B. Saunders, 6:373–375, June, 1971.

6. Given, B. A., and Simmons, S. J.: Nursing Care of the Patient With Gastrointestinal disorders. pp. 1–35; 188–192. St. Louis, C. V. Mosby, 1971.

7. Maki, D. G., *et al.:* Prevention of catheter-associated urinary tract infection, an additional measure. **JAMA,** 221:1270–1271, Sept. 11, 1972.

8. Padilla, G. V., and Baker, V. E.: Variables affecting the preparation of the bowel for radiologic examination. **Nurs. Research,** 21:305–312, July–Aug., 1972.

9. Pike, B. F.: Soap colitis. **New Engl. J. Med.,** 285:217–218, July 22, 1971.

10. Rowson, L.: The lateral position in catheterization. *In* **The Nursing Clinics of North America.** Philadelphia, W. B. Saunders, 5:189–190, Mar., 1970.

11. Saxon, J.: Techniques for bowel and bladder training. **Am. J. Nurs.,** 62:69–71, Sept., 1962.

12. Tudor, L. L.: Bladder and bowel retraining. **Am. J. Nurs.,** 70:2391–2393, Nov., 1970.

13. Winter, C. C., and Barker, M. R.: Nursing Care of Patients with Urologic Diseases. pp. 1–223. St. Louis, C. V. Mosby, 1972.

CHAPTER 27

Maintaining Respiratory Functioning

GLOSSARY · INTRODUCTION · GENERAL PRINCIPLES IN RELATION TO
RESPIRATORY CARE · COMMON DIAGNOSTIC MEASURES ·
COMMON NURSING MEASURES TO PROMOTE NORMAL
RESPIRATORY FUNCTIONING · NURSING MEASURES FOR
ASSISTING IMPAIRED RESPIRATORY FUNCTIONING ·
CARDIOPULMONARY RESUSCITATION · CONCLUSION ·
STUDY SITUATIONS · REFERENCES

GLOSSARY

Aerosolization: Suspending medication droplets in a gas.

Anoxia: Oxygen deprivation.

Atomization: Breaking of a drug into comparatively large particles for inhalation.

Biopsy: Removal of a small piece of tissue for examination.

Bronchography: Radiologic examination of the bronchi following injection of a radiopaque dye.

Bronchoscope: Instrument used for visually examining the bronchi.

Bronchoscopy: Visual examination of the bronchi.

Endotracheal Tube: Tube passed into the trachea through upper respiratory passageway.

Expiratory Reserve Volume: Additional amount of air which can be exhaled beyond tidal volume; abbreviated E. R. V.

Inspiratory Reserve Volume: Additional amount of air which can be inspired beyond tidal volume; abbreviated I. R. V.

Intermittent Positive Pressure Breathing: Mechanical means of providing gases or medication under positive pressure for inhalation; abbreviated I. P. P. B.

Intradermal: Between the skin layers.

Laryngoscope: Instrument used for visually examining the larynx.

Laryngoscopy: Visual examination of the larynx.

Nebulization: Breaking of drug into small particles to produce mist or fog for inhalation.

Residual Volume: Air remaining in lungs following maximal exhalation; abbreviated R. V.

Spirometer: Device for measuring respiratory inhalation and exhalation volumes.

Tidal Volume: Amount of air inspired and expired in a normal respiration; abbreviated T. V.

Tracheostomy: Artificial external opening into the trachea through which a tube is passed.

Ultrasonic Nebulization: Use of high frequency sound waves to break a drug into minute particles for inhalation.

Vital Capacity: Maximal amount of air which can be expelled from the lungs following a maximal inspiration; abbreviated V. C.

INTRODUCTION

The mechanism of respiration involves the exchange of gases in which oxygen from the air is delivered to the tissue cells and carbon dioxide is removed. Maintenance of the complex processes involved with this gas exchange is essential to life. Yet, many persons do not consider respiratory maintenance in the total picture of health care. Unless pathology is present, breathing is quiet and auto-matic. It does not command the attention that other bodily activities do such as watching weight, concern about bowel functioning, applying creams or lotion to the skin, or taking tranquilizers to reduce tension.

From time to time we are made aware of respiratory functioning, such as when we "catch" our breath after being forced into a fast walk or run, or when we climb up the stairs; or if hiccoughs (singultus) occur and we hold our breath or blow into a paper bag.

The need for attention to respiratory functioning is as much a part of basic nursing care as any other measure. The increasing incidence of chronic lung diseases and newly developed methods of prevention and treatment have opened another vast area of preventive teaching for the nurse.

Some of the physiologic factors of respiration were discussed in Chapter 20 and will not be repeated here. The problems of respiratory care when specific pathology is present are found in clinical texts containing descriptions of the disease and its treatment. However, some commonly used nursing measures for patients predisposed to or having respiratory difficulties will be discussed in this chapter. Because respiratory arrest constitutes a crisis, cardiopulmonary resuscitation is also included in this chapter.

GENERAL PRINCIPLES IN RELATION TO RESPIRATORY CARE

Respiration is the exchange of gases between the living organism and its environment. Oxygen is inhaled and carbon dioxide discharged, while internal respiration takes place at the cellular level.

All living body cells require oxygen. It follows then that the means by which the body receives this necessity of life should be kept in the best possible state.

The air passageway must remain patent for respiration to occur. The respiratory gases are transported from the nose to the alveoli and returned. Obstruction in any area of the normal passageway will impede respiration. Obstruction can occur from a foreign substance such as a piece of food, a coin, a toy or other small object, or liquids, as is the case for the drowning victim. Obstruction can also arise from tissues or secretions from within the body. For example, excessive or thickened secretions, tumor growths, or edema in the respiratory tract can cause an obstruction.

Muscle movements provide the physical force essential for respiration. The diaphragm and the intercostal muscles are responsible for normal inspiration and expiration. Accessory muscles of the abdomen and back are used to maintain respiratory movements at times when breathing is difficult. The condition of the body musculature can therefore affect the process of respiration.

Incomplete expansion of the lungs can result in atelectasis (collapse or partial collapse of lung tissue). The areas of the lungs affected by atelectasis cannot fulfill the function of respiration.

Adequate hydration is essential to respiratory functioning. Fluid is essential to the production of the watery mucus, which is normally present in the respiratory tract and is being constantly propelled towards the upper respiratory tract by ciliary action. This is an important mechanism because it helps remove foreign particles and "debris" from the lungs. This covering of mucus also protects the underlying tissues from irritation and infection.

Anatomically, the respiratory system consists of the nose, pharynx, larynx, trachea, the bronchial tree (bronchi with its ciliated cells, bronchioles), and the lungs. The lungs contain many alveoli and blood vessels. Gas exchange takes place in the vascular pulmonary tissue. Because all parts are interdependent, it is toward the maintenance of the entire system that nursing measures in this chapter are directed. Other measures, such as exercise, frequent turning and changing of position are related and are discussed in other parts of the text.

Not all lung tissue is active to the same degree with each respiration; that is, ventilation depends upon the extent of perfusion in the area. Blood flow in the lungs is influenced by gravity. Therefore, the amount of blood present in any given area of lung tissue depends partially upon whether the person is sitting up or lying down, prone, supine, or on either side. The use of lung tissue is also dependent upon activity. Greater activity results in increased cellular oxygen need and cardiac output and consequently, increased blood return to the lungs. Like all other body tissues, use of healthy lung alveoli helps to maintain them in optimum condition. The implications for the nursing needs of patients who are bedfast, or sitting in chairs most of the day, should be obvious.

Respiratory maintenance is now considered basic to preventive nursing care. It is not limited to the inactive patient or to the preoperative patient. Other factors also affect respiration, such as drugs, pain, fear, and even sights and odors that seem disagreeable. Pollutants in the air have received attention in recent years because of their influence on breathing. The presence of any of these may indicate a need for preventive nursing measures. In recent years, progress in respiratory care has given rise to another paramedical group, thoracic or respiratory (inhalation) therapists. These practitioners perform diagnostic pulmonary function examinations and instruct patients in breathing and coughing exercises. In addition, they administer varied treatments to patients who have pulmonary pathology. Where such therapists are not available, nurses may help to fill the gap. However, preventive respiratory care is always a part of good nursing.

COMMON DIAGNOSTIC MEASURES

Early detection is one of the prevention measures with which the nurse is often involved. Observations of the breathing rate and respiratory characteristics were described in Chapter 20. The nurse may also assist in diagnostic measures by preparing the patient and by gathering specimens. Results of diagnostic tests found in the patient's record provide her with data basic to nursing care planning and intervention. Many kinds of examinations can be used to determine breathing adequacy and respiratory tract problems. Pulmonary function testing, tissue, blood and secretion examination, skin testing, and radiography are discussed briefly here.

Pulmonary Function Tests

Pulmonary function tests are usually a part of health screening examinations. They are also done on persons with known respiratory diseases for comparative studies of disease progression and effectiveness of treatment. Pulmonary function testing provides information about the status of the respiratory process in the body, but it does not by itself provide definitive diagnostic information. There are numerous complex tests which can be done; the basic ones are described here.

Tidal volume is the amount of air inspired and expired in a normal respiration. It is abbreviated T.V. Volume of air can be measured by having the patient breathe through a mouthpiece connected to a spirometer while wearing a noseclip to prevent air escape. *A spirometer* is a device for measuring inhalation and exhalation volumes.

Inspiratory reserve volume is the additional amount of air that can be inspired beyond tidal volume. It is abbreviated I.R.V.

Expiratory reserve volume is the additional amount of air which can be exhaled beyond tidal volume. It is abbreviated E.R.V.

Vital capacity is the maximum amount of air which can be expelled from the lungs following a maximum inspiration. It is abbreviated V.C.

Residual volume is the air remaining in the lungs following a forced expiration. R.V. is the abbreviation used. The residual air is important to prevent atelectasis. For example, when alveoli are obstructed,

the blood will eventually carry away most of the air and the alveoli will collapse.

The vital capacity and lung volumes vary with individuals according to body size and general health condition. The average amounts for healthy adults are indicated in Figure 27-1. Disease states causing limitation of alveoli tissue functioning, obstruction of the respiratory tract, or decreased respiratory muscle activity will result in lesser lung capacities.

Blood Analysis

Since there is a direct relationship between pulmonary functioning and gas constituents of the blood, examination of blood specimens provides an indirect indication of lung physiology. Arterial and venous blood are both used to determine oxygen and carbon dioxide levels. Examination of blood specimens for these purposes is commonly referred to as a *blood gas analysis*. Examination of arterial blood is used to determine the amount of oxygen and carbon dioxide present as well as to detect the effectiveness of the blood buffer system. Venous blood is more commonly used to determine the blood bicarbonate levels and respiratory acidosis and alkalosis states, as discussed in Chapter 24. Venous blood is also used for analysis of cells, electrolytes, and enzymes.

Respiratory Secretions

Secretions from the respiratory tract are often secured for diagnostic examination. As mentioned in Chapter 20, the nurse may be responsible for securing nasal and throat secretion specimens. Sputum specimens are examined for cells, pus, bacteria, and blood. When collecting a sputum specimen, the nurse will encourage the patient to cough deeply so that secretions are actually raised from the lungs. Early-morning specimens are generally easier to obtain, and usually approximately a teaspoonful is needed for most laboratory tests. Special specimen containers are supplied by the laboratory, and the patient expectorates directly into them. Care should be taken that the outside of the container does not become contaminated. Mechanical suction is sometimes used to secure a sputum specimen from a patient who is unable to raise sputum. Gastric washings are also occasionally used; a tube is inserted into the stomach to secure sputum the patient has swallowed.

Respiratory Tract Tissue

Specimens of respiratory tract tissue are examined generally to determine the presence of a malignancy. Such specimens are obtained by the physician usually with special instruments. A *bronchoscope* is an instrument used for visually examining the bronchi while the *laryngoscope* is used to visualize the larynx. Specimens are obtained at the time of viewing. A visual examination of the bronchi is called a *bronchoscopy*, and of the larynx, a *laryngoscopy*. Securing a piece of tissue for examination is called a *biopsy*.

A bronchoscopy is usually done with the patient in a fasting state, and it is performed in a specially equipped room. The physician will generally order a sedative for the patient prior to the examination. A local anesthetic is also used. Because of this anesthetic, the patient's gag reflex is absent during and following the procedure, until the effects of the anesthetic disappear. To prevent tracheal aspiration, the patient should not be permitted to eat or drink until the gag reflex has returned.

Skin Tests

Skin tests are commonly used to detect the presence of antibodies against organisms commonly causing lung infections. Since the sensitivity of the body is increased following contact with the organism, an antigen-antibody reaction is induced. A small amount of dilute antigen prepared from the organism or its secretions is generally injected *intradermally*, that is, between the skin layers. The patient is observed at specified periods for a reaction which indicates the presence of antibodies resulting from previous contact with the antigen.

Skin testing is commonly part of the diagnostic procedure for tuberculosis, histoplasmosis, and coccidiodomycosis. The technique for intradermal injections is discussed in Chapter 28. If the nurse is responsible for administering the test, she should explain its purpose to the patient and be careful to help him understand that a positive reaction is only an indication of the presence of antibodies, and not necessarily a current infection.

Radiography

X-ray examination of the lungs is another commonly used diagnostic method. The chest x-ray can demonstrate the size and shape of the lungs. Fluoroscopy allows the visualization of lung movement during expansion and contraction. These examinations are most often used to detect space-occupying lesions and infectious processes. No special preparation is necessary for the patient.

Bronchography is the radiologic examination of the bronchi following injection of a radiopaque dye

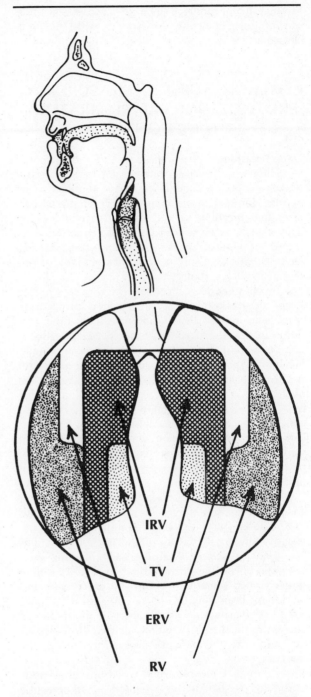

Fig. 27-1. Average lung capacity amounts for the healthy adult. (Figure from Early, M. The gaseous exchange process: nursing implications. In Kintzel, K. C., ed.: Advanced Concepts in Clinical Nursing. p. 208. Philadelphia, J. B. Lippincott, 1971. Numerical data adapted from Shepard, R. S.: Human Physiology. pp. 299–302. Philadelphia, J. B. Lippincott, 1971)

through a bronchoscope. The preparation and after-care of the patient are the same as with the bron-choscopy.

COMMON NURSING MEASURES TO PROMOTE NORMAL RESPIRATORY FUNCTIONING

Deep Breathing

Habits of breathing that are not in the best interests of bodily functioning may develop. Some persons, for one reason or another, develop a pattern of shallow breathing or walk with a "caved-in" chest. The result may be decrease of lung distensibility. A means of combating this is taking deep breaths (hyperinflation). Daily periodic hyperinflation is essential in such instances.

Involuntary deep breathing often occurs during sleep. Persons who snore, although a problem to those who have to listen, may benefit by their condition in that they frequently take deeper breaths.

Positioning for ease of breathing is important. Having the patient assume a position that allows for the free movement of the diaphragm and expansion of the chest wall promotes ease of respiration. Sitting in a slumped position that permits the abdominal contents to push upward on the diaphragm will result in less lung expansion during inspiration. Persons with dyspnea are more comfortable in a sitting position because the accessory muscles can be used more readily.

Because incisional discomfort following chest and abdominal surgery usually results in the person's unconsciously or consciously minimizing his respiratory movements, secondary pulmonary complications can occur. Teaching breathing and coughing exercises and encouraging the patient to practice before surgery, even sometimes before he enters the hospital, have been found to be very helpful in promoting a faster convalescence. Support of the incisional area with the hands, a pillow, or a folded blanket can minimize the patient's discomfort during the exercises.

Although there are some variations in what is considered to be *the* best method for therapeutic deep breathing, physiologic principles guide the actions that are essential. For one, the person should be instructed to inhale slowly and evenly to the greatest chest expansion possible for him. Next, he should hold his breath for at least three seconds. Studies indicate that a longer period does not pro-duce any more benefit than the three second hold. Then the person permits normal recoil of the chest. As to the frequency with which this should be done, the patient's condition is the best possible guide. For some persons two to three times every two or three hours is satisfactory. For patients in danger of pulmonary complications it may need to be as often as every hour.

The person with known lung pathology needs to learn more specific exercises. Persons with chronic pulmonary diseases in particular, profit by developing the auxiliary respiratory muscles through exercises. Several of the references at the end of this chapter and texts dealing with pulmonary diseases describe these exercises in detail.

Coughing

The cough mechanism consists of an initial irritation, a deep inspiration, a quick tight closure of the glottis together with a forceful contraction of the expiratory intercostal muscles, and the upward push of the diaphragm. This causes an explosive movement of air from the lower to the upper respiratory tract. To be effective, a cough should have enough muscle contraction to force air to be expelled and to propel a liquid or a solid on its way out of the respiratory tract. The cough is a cleansing mechanism of the body. It is an effective means of assisting the cilia to keep the airway clear of secretions and other debris. When a cough does not occur as a result of reflex stimulation of the cough-sensitive areas, it can be induced voluntarily.

Patients who are susceptible to airway collections of secretions are frequently taught to cough voluntarily. Coughing is most effective when the patient is in a sitting position and when he is sufficiently well-hydrated so that the viscosity of the secretions permits their movement. Deep inhalation followed by a forceful coughing expiration, using the abdominal and other accessory respiratory muscles, is generally effective.

For the patient who is unable to cough voluntarily, manual stimulation over the trachea and prolonged exhalation can be helpful. If neither of these methods is successful, mechanical endotracheal stimulation with a catheter is sometimes used.

Although the actual teaching of preventive respiratory exercises such as deep breathing and coughing is relatively easy, experience has shown that it is difficult to have the patient follow through and do them. Frequent reminders throughout the day are necessary for most patients. Figures 27-2 through 27-4 illustrate breathing exercises.

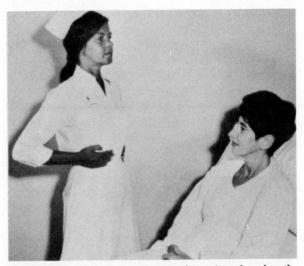

Fig. 27-2. The nurse demonstrates to the patient deep breathing exercises. She is showing her how to take a deep inspiration so that she can feel the pull between the ribs.

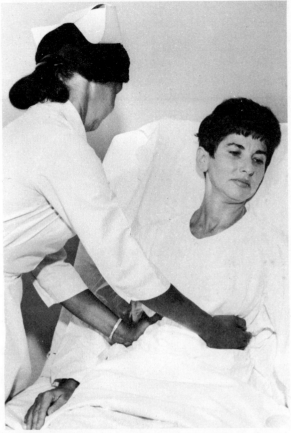

Fig. 27-3. The nurse is showing the patient how she can support the lower chest when doing deep breathing or coughing exercises.

Involuntary coughing is a frequent accompaniment of respiratory tract infections and irritations. As indicated earlier, coughing is a cleansing mechanism of the body and not undesirable unless it is ineffective or becomes so frequent as to cause fatigue. Many persons find a cough annoying and want it suppressed. For this reason, many kinds of cough preparations are available for over-the-counter purchases. Nurses are often asked about them. The nurse may need to help the person understand the useful effects of a cough and explain that it is a symptom of some respiratory irritation which may need medical attention. Frequent nonproductive coughing can, however, be harmful because of its fatiguing effect or because the cough is ineffective in removing the secretions in which case medications may be helpful.

Two of the major types of cough preparations are suppressants and expectorants. Suppressants act upon the cough reflex and depress it. An irritating, nonproductive cough in persons with no evidence of excessive secretions may need to be depressed. Inappropriate suppression of the cough in a person with respiratory tract secretions can result in harmful retention of the substances.

Expectorants reduce the secretion viscosity. Persons with extremely tenacious secretions may need to have secretions liquified in order for the cough to be effective in removing them. Adequate hydration for these persons also is extremely important.

Since cough preparations are so readily available and persons who purchase them are usually eager for relief, they sometimes take more than one type. Understanding the principles of action of the suppressants and expectorants should enable them to make a proper choice.

Postural Drainage

Postural drainage is the promotion of gravity drainage of the lungs by special positioning of the patient. Since the normal movement of pulmonary secretions is in an upward direction propelled by ciliary action, gravity merely assists the normal process by emptying the smaller bronchi toward the main bronchi and trachea so that they can be coughed up and expectorated.

Various positions are used to promote the drainage, depending on the area of the lung where the

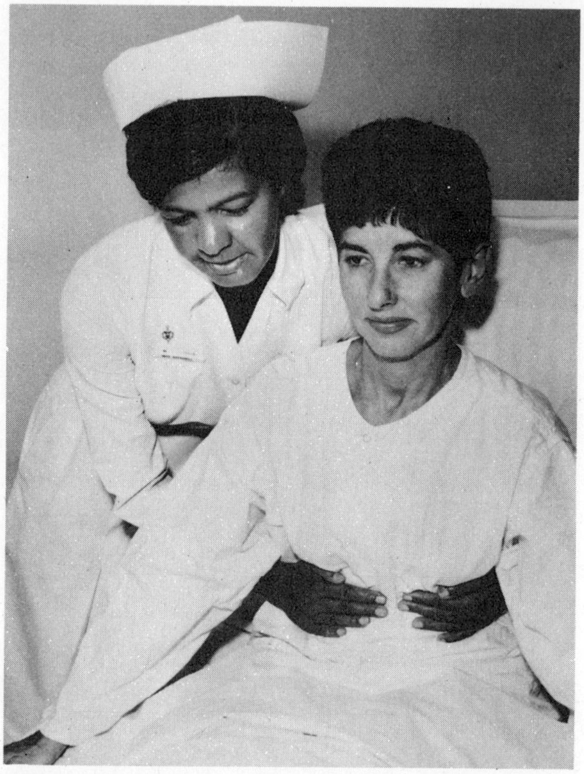

Fig. 27-4. The nurse is assuring the patient that if she has discomfort that there are means for helping her to do deep breathing and coughing exercises. As for example, the nurse will go behind the patient and support her while she does deep breathing and coughing exercises.

secretions have collected. In order to promote drainage, the bronchi segments must be in a near upright position to drain into the main bronchi. Patients can be supported by pillows, a bed, or a chair to maintain the position.

Percussion and vibration of the chest wall are additional methods used to loosen secretions within the bronchi. Several of the references at the end of this chapter contain diagrams and photographs of postural drainage positions and percussion and vibration techniques. Physical therapists and respiratory therapists are responsible for positioning, exercise, and drainage techniques in most health agencies.

Adequate Hydration

In addition to ridding the lungs of accumulated secretions through deep breathing, coughing, and positioning, attention must be given to adequate hydration to minimize the viscosity of secretions. The patient's fluid intake should be within the limits of his regimen. The patient who has an elevated

temperature, is mouthbreathing, or is losing excessive body fluids in other ways, should have special attention focused on his intake. The systemic implications of fluid deficit were discussed in Chapter 24, along with nursing measures to help in increasing fluid intake.

In some circumstances in which the air is dry, that is, the humidity is low, artificial means for humidification may be necessary. The inspiration of dry air further removes the normal moisture in the respiratory passages which is essential to protection from irritation and infection. Room humidifiers may be helpful for some patients. For others, direct humidification of the respiratory tract will be necessary.

NURSING MEASURES FOR ASSIST-ING IMPAIRED RESPIRATORY FUNCTIONING

Oxygen Therapy

Oxygen is essential for life, and the body has no reserve of it. Therefore, when there is insufficient oxygenation of the blood, oxygen must be added to inhaled air in order to sustain life. *Anoxia* is the term for oxygen deprivation, regardless of its cause. Whenever anoxia occurs, it presents an emergency; therefore, it is essential that the nurse fully understand how to manage oxygen equipment and the means for administering therapeutic concentrations. Respiratory therapists are also available in many health agencies to initiate and maintain oxygen therapy.

Numerous conditions result in poor oxygenation of blood when normal air is inhaled. For example, when congestion of the lungs from an infection such as pneumonia is present, the total functional lung surface is reduced. Oxygen is added to the inhaled air so that the blood can be oxygenated more easily. In this example, there is inadequate oxygenation because of an abnormality of the lungs. The need for adding oxygen to inhaled air at high altitudes is an example of aiding oxygenation occurring in normal lungs. When circulation of blood in the lungs is impaired by congestion, as often occurs with certain heart conditions, increasing the intake of oxygen relieves anoxia. Occasionally, when strict rest is essential in a disease condition, oxygen may be given so that the least amount of energy is used by the body in the act of respiration.

Oxygen therapy must sometimes be instituted

with such speed that there is little time for explaining to the patient. However, depending on the situation, some concurrent instruction is generally possible. If there is an emergency, once the patient is out of danger and is breathing easily he should be told about the device and the essentials necessary to serve him effectively. It is a terrifying experience to be unable to breathe, and the patient needs the support and comfort of feeling that all that is possible is being done for him.

Oxygen is delivered to the respiratory tract artificially under pressure. Therefore, excessive drying of the mucous membrane lining the tract occurs unless the oxygen is humidified. Since oxygen is only slightly soluble in water, it can be readily passed through solution with little loss. Regardless of the method of administration, oxygen administered therapeutically should be humidified by water, saline, or a medicated solution before entering the respiratory tract.

There are patients who must become proficient in administering oxygen to themselves. They may have asthma or chronic lung ailments or impaired cardiac functioning and have oxygen at home for self-administration.

Oxygen, which constitutes approximately 20 percent of normal air, is a tasteless, odorless and colorless gas. In addition to its vital importance in sustaining life, it has a chemical characteristic which requires careful consideration. Oxygen supports combustion. Therefore, open flames and sparks must be kept away from the area where oxygen is being administered. This precaution cannot be emphasized enough since periodically tragic accidents occur as a result of this hazard. "No Smoking" signs should be placed in many prominent places in the patient's room and the patient and his visitors taught the necessity of observing this regulation.

All electric devices such as heating pads, stoves, electric bell cords, razors, and radios, should be checked carefully to be certain they are not emitting sparks. The greatest care should be taken also in the management of linens, since many fabrics—including wool, silk, rayon, and nylon—generate static electricity and sparks from such sources are equally dangerous.

In most hospitals, oxygen is piped into each patient unit and is immediately available from an outlet in the wall. This piped-in oxygen is a valuable asset: it increases the patient's safety by eliminating the delay in transporting oxygen in tanks and the constant vigil on the gauge to check on the amount of oxygen remaining in the tank. Some hospitals do not have it in all units, but are providing for it in delivery, operating, and recovery rooms. When oxygen is not available from a wall outlet, it is obtained in portable cylinders. The flow rate of oxygen is measured by liters per minute. The rate will vary depending on the condition of the patient and the administration route being used.

PIPED-IN OXYGEN: The wall outlet source for oxygen can be prepared for use quickly. The oxygen is supplied from a central source through a pipeline, usually at 50 to 60 pounds per square inch of pressure. A specially designed flowmeter is attached to the wall outlet. The flowmeter opens the outlet and a valve makes possible regulation of the oxygen flow. Figure 27-5 shows a flowmeter.

THE TANK OF OXYGEN: Oxygen usually is compressed and dispensed in steel cylinders (tanks). The tank is delivered with a protective cap to prevent accidental force against the cylinder outlet. When a standard, large-size cylinder is full, its contents are under more than 2,000 pounds per square inch of pressure. The force behind an accidentally partially opened outlet could cause the tank to take off like an uncontrolled, jet-propelled monster.

To release the oxygen safely and at a desirable rate, a regulator is used. The regulator valve controls the rate of oxygen output. On the regulator are two

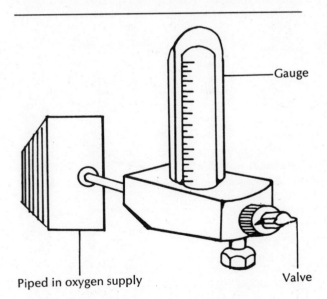

Piped in oxygen supply   Valve

Fig. 27-5. A piped-in oxygen supply with flowmeter. The valve permits regulation of the oxygen flow at the rate indicated on the gauge. The lower connection attaches to the humidifier bottle. The oxygen is supplied from a central source piped into the patient's room.

gauges. The one nearest the tank shows the pressure (hence the amount) of oxygen in the tank. The other indicates the number of liters per minute of oxygen being released. Figure 27-6 shows an oxygen tank with its regulator.

Because of the nature of oxygen, caution must be used in handling the oxygen cylinder and the regulator. The oxygen cylinder should be transported carefully, preferably strapped onto a wheeled carrier to avoid possible falling and breaking of the outlet. Once the cylinder is located, it should be stabilized by securing it in a properly fitting stand. No oil should be used near the gauge or the outlet because of the danger of the oil being ignited.

Because of the possibility of dust or other particles becoming lodged in the outlet of the tank and being forced into the regulator, the tank is "cracked" before a regulator is applied. This calls for slightly turning the handle on the tank which releases the oxygen so that a small amount of oxygen may be released, thus "flushing out" the outlet. The force with which the oxygen is released from this opening causes a loud hissing sound which usually startles anyone who is not aware of what it is. For this reason, it is recommended that oxygen tanks be "cracked" away from the patient's bedside. If this is not possible, the patient should be prepared for the noise by proper explanation. The oxygen can be released slowly and the sound reduced if both hands are placed on the handle. One hand helps control the movement of the other.

NASAL CANNULA: The simplest and the method best tolerated by the patient for administering oxygen is via the nasal cannula. The cannula is a disposable plastic device with two protruding prongs for insertion into the nostrils. It is held in place by an elastic strap around the head.

Before the oxygen is delivered to the cannula, it is bubbled through a humidifier containing distilled water. The patient should be observed for signs of pressure from the positioning or tightness of the cannula. Periodic movement and gauze padding under the cannula may be helpful. This method of administration is generally used by patients who are ambulatory or receiving oxygen at home.

The cannula can comfortably deliver up to 35

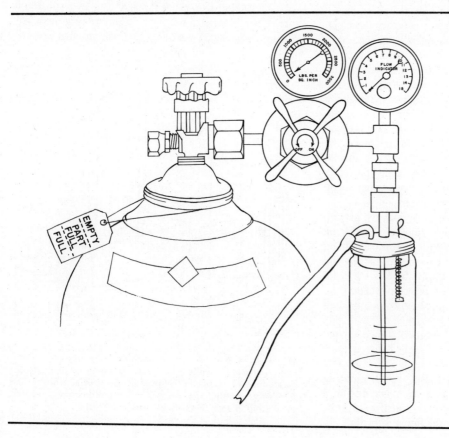

Fig. 27-6. Oxygen tank with regulator. The regulator is fastened to the tank valve and tightened with a wrench. The valve atop the tank admits oxygen to the regulator. When this valve is opened, the left-hand gauge will indicate the tank pressure. The regulator valve (below the tank gauge) then is turned; it releases the oxygen and then is adjusted for the correct rate (shown on the right-hand gauge). A humidifier attached to the apparatus is used when oxygen is administered by all methods except the tent.

percent oxygen concentration at 2 to 4 liters per minute. Higher concentration will cause excessive drying of the mucosa. Figure 27-7 shows a patient receiving oxygen through a nasal cannula.

NASAL CATHETER: A nasal, or oropharyngeal, catheter is a more efficient means for administering oxygen. It is somewhat more uncomfortable for the patient than the cannula but it delivers a higher concentration of oxygen. Moisturization of the oxygen is accomplished through a humidifier bottle attached to the flowmeter. The catheter is inserted into the nostril and passed until it is in full view at the back of the tongue. It should be in the oropharynx. The horizontal distance from the nasal opening to the ear lobe may be used as a guide for determining the length of catheter to be inserted. If the catheter is inserted too far, there is danger of insufflating the gastrointestinal tract; if it is not inserted far enough, much of the oxygen will escape before it is inhaled. Figure 27-8 shows the proper location of the nasal catheter.

Irritation of the mucous membrane by the catheter is minimized when the catheter is lubricated prior to insertion with a water-soluble lubricant. An oily substance used as a lubricant could be harmful if aspirated. Nasal catheters should be removed for cleaning at least once every eight hours. Alternate nostrils should be used whenever possible.

It has been found that, when oxygen is administered at 4 to 6 liters per minute, the patient will inhale a concentration of approximately 42 percent oxygen. A flow of 7 liters per minute yields a 45 to 50 percent concentration. Increasing the flow of oxygen will dry the mucous membrane, and the patient may complain of a sore throat. The box on page 407 outlines the catheter insertion technique.

OXYGEN MASK: Various types of face masks have been devised for administering oxygen. For many patients, a mask is more comfortable than the nasal catheter. The oronasal mask is designed to cover both the nose and the mouth and is necessary if the patient is a mouth breather. It presents problems in eating, drinking, and talking, however. The nasal mask covers the nose and permits the patient's mouth to be exposed. If it is possible for the patient to use it, this mask is more comfortable and convenient.

When a mask is used to administer oxygen, it must be fitted carefully to the patient's face to avoid leakage. If foam rubber is available it is satisfactory. The mask should be comfortably snug but not tight against the patient's face. Frequent care of the face, including washing and powdering, will help to prevent irritation from the mask. In addition, the mask should be kept clean. Frequent washing helps to reduce the odors absorbed by the rubber. Disposable masks are available and eliminate many of the problems of rubber ones.

Lower concentrations of oxygen are administered through masks when the supply tubing connects directly to the mask. Higher concentrations are supplied through masks with a flexible breathing bag to which the oxygen tubing is attached. The masks with breathing bags have values which permit the entrance of room air and exit of carbon dioxide. The bag is distended with oxygen, and during inspiration, oxygen is withdrawn from the bag and air is drawn through valves completing the tidal volume.

A therapeutic concentration by this method usually is determined by rhythmical, easy breathing, during which time the bag almost collapses during inspiration. Depending on the patient's needs, a range of 6 to 8 liters per minute usually produces a therapeutic concentration. However, if a high concentration of oxygen is indicated, the rate of oxygen flow should be increased so that the bag does not collapse during inspiration. Figure 27-9 illustrates one type of mask.

There are masks available that are designed to deliver an exact amount of oxygen. These masks are used for patients having certain conditions such as chronic lung diseases.

Humidity with the oxygen is generally recommended, although the patient's expirations into the mask will provide some humidification.

THE OXYGEN TENT: An oxygen tent is a light,

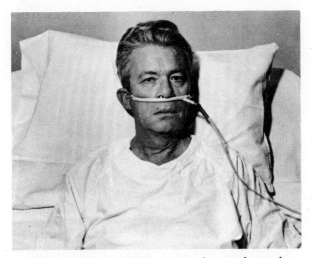

Fig. 27-7. Patient receiving oxygen via a nasal cannula.

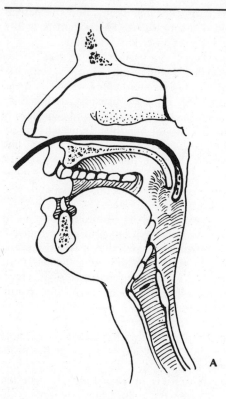

A

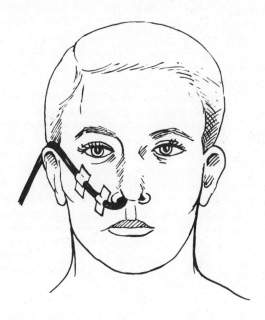

B

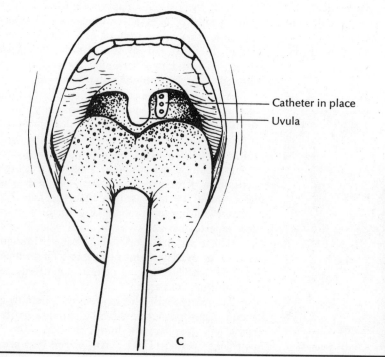

C

Catheter in place
Uvula

Fig. 27-8. (A) Diagram of the correct location of a nasal catheter in the nose and the oropharynx.

(B) To make certain that the catheter is placed properly, it is necessary to ask the patient to open his mouth. The tip of the catheter should be located just below the uvula (see arrow).

(C) The catheter should be taped close to the nares and on the cheek. It can then drape over the ear. This provides freedom of movement of the lips and reduces pull on the catheter.

RATIONALE GUIDING ACTION IN THE ADMINISTRATION OF OXYGEN BY MEANS OF A CATHETER

The purpose is to administer a therapeutic concentration of oxygen to a patient by direct admission of oxygen into the oropharynx.

SUGGESTED ACTION	RATIONALE
Observe precautions to prevent fire, such as checking electrical appliances and posting "No Smoking" signs.	Oxygen supports combustion.
Attach the humidifier bottle to the regulator or flowmeter.	Oxygen forced through a water reservoir is humidified before it is delivered to the patient, preventing dehydration of the mucous membranes.
Attach a nasal catheter, No. 8 to No. 10, Fr., to the connecting tube on the water reservoir.	A small catheter passes through the nose easily and causes minimum discomfort to the patient.
Measure the catheter by holding it in a horizontal line from the tip of the nose to the ear lobe. Mark it with a narrow strip of tape.	The distance from the tip of the nose to the ear lobe usually places the tip of the catheter in the oropharynx when inserted.
Moisten the tip of the catheter with a water-soluble lubricant.	Friction irritates the mucous membrane. The lubricant reduces friction.
Hold the tip of the patient's nose up and insert the tip of the nasal catheter into the nares downward. Move the catheter along the floor of the nose until the marking on the catheter is reached.	Direct connection from the nares to the oropharynx is made most easily by passing the catheter beneath the concha inferior.
Check the position of the tip of the catheter by depressing the tongue carefully with a tongue blade.	If the catheter has been inserted too far, it may stimulate the gag reflex.
Adjust the catheter as necessary so that the tip is visible behind the uvula.	The oxygen stream can be inspired easily at this point.
Adjust the liter flow to the rate specified by the physician, or 4 to 6 liters per minute.	High rates of oxygen flow produce a forceful stream against the mucous membrane which is both irritating and drying.
Secure the catheter with tape to the side of the patient's face.	The weight of the catheter and the moist surface of the mucous membrane will cause the catheter to slip out if not anchored.
Insert a clean catheter in alternate nostrils as often as necessary and at least every 8 hours, to prevent irritation and to keep the nares clean.	Mucous membrane is irritated by continued presence of a foreign object. Prolonged irritation of mucous membrane can cause ulceration.

portable structure made of clear plastic and attached to a motor-driven unit. The motor aids in circulating and cooling the air in the tent. The cooling device functions on the same principles as an electric refrigeration unit. A thermostat in the unit keeps the temperature in the tent at the degree considered most comfortable by the patient. The oxygen tent is used only occasionally today.

An oxygen tent fits over the top part of the bed so that the patient's head and thorax are in the tent. Usually, there is sufficient covering to extend the tent further if necessary. If the tent is well-sealed by tucking the sides under the mattress and by wrapping the front flap into a piece of bed linen, a concentration of 40 to 50 percent of oxygen can be maintained relatively easily. Because oxygen is heavier than air, and thus falls to the bottom, its escape around the tent edges can make maintenance of concentration a problem. The tent should be flooded with oxygen at 15 liters per minute for about two minutes before sealing the tent and after opening it for nursing care. Between floodings, approximately 10 to 12 liters of oxygen per minute usually is given. The technique for administering oxygen by tent is discussed in the boxed material on page 410.

Patients may be frightened by the appearance

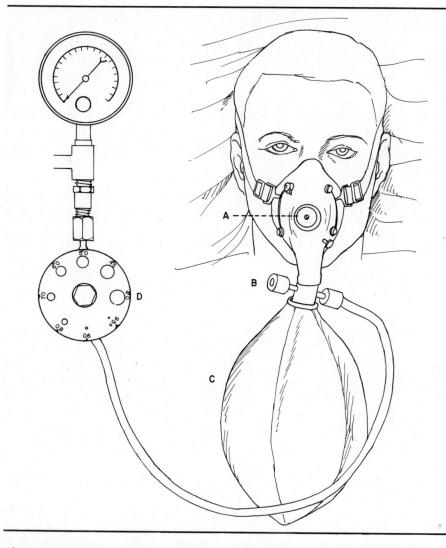

Fig. 27-9. There are many types of face masks. Some provide for an oxygen reservoir, a means for the expired carbon dioxide to be removed, and a means for mixing air with the oxygen, as the one in this sketch. (A) The flutter valve on the oronasal face mask, which provides an outlet for expired air. Pressure of the expired air forces the soft rubber disk away from the mask. (B) A safety valve that provides for an air inlet in the event of an emergency or increased depth of respirations. (C) The reservoir which contains the air and oxygen mixture inhaled by the patient. (D) The meter calibrated from 40 to 95 plus per cent, for adjusting the concentration of oxygen to be delivered to the bag.

of an oxygen tent, since it frequently is associated with critical illness. If the patient is prepared adequately as to its advantages, few object to its use. Many even prefer it to other methods because it is cool, permits movement, and prevents excessive dryness of the mucous membrane.

One of the disadvantages of which the nurse should be aware is the possibility of too great air movement in the tent. Many tents are constructed so that there is a complete exchange of air in the tent every few seconds, in order to prevent an increase in carbon dioxide content. The air movement may create a draft on the patient to the point of real discomfort. The discomfort can be avoided by protecting the patient's head, neck, and shoulders with a combination flannel hood and shawl specially designed for use in a tent, as in Figure 27-10, or an improvised covering made with a towel or other available linen.

The temperature within an oxygen tent can be regulated within a desired range and should be maintained at a level that is comfortable for the patient. The combination of rather rapid air movement and low temperature can make the patient uncomfortably chilly if the temperature within the tent is not watched.

A word of caution is necessary as a reminder that the tent is not soundproof. Usually, the patient is able to hear normal conversation outside the tent. Speak to the patient in normal conversational tones unless he indicates that he cannot hear. It is distressing to the patient to have people outside of the tent shouting at him.

This caution also should be kept in mind when

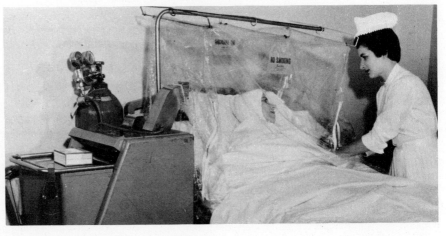

Fig. 27-10. Many nursing activities are carried out easily through the zippered openings provided in the oxygen tent. Because of the air circulation in the tent, protection for the patient's head may be necessary. Care should be taken also to avoid restricting the patient's activity by tucking the draw sheet which helps seal the bottom part of tent too tightly under the mattress.

the patient's condition, progress, or plan of therapy is being discussed in the immediate vicinity of the bedside. Nothing should be discussed within the patient's hearing which may be disturbing to him.

Oxygen tents are so designed that the nurse may slip her arms into the tent at various places in the hood without lifting it up over the patient's head. This convenience facilitates administering medications, foods and fluids, and carrying out other aspects of nursing care. It is essential that there be careful planning and preparation of all needed items in order to reduce oxygen loss through prolonged and unnecessary opening of the tent.

When it becomes necessary to manipulate the hood so that care which involves turning the patient or adjusting the bed linen may be given, the oxygen concentration must be maintained. This may be accomplished best by moving the hood up to the patient's upper chest or neck and tucking the sides securely under the pillow. The oxygen flow should be increased as much as necessary to compensate for leakage from those points where the hood cannot be sealed.

A signal cord that does not have an electric button on it should be used in the tent. If one is not available, a small hand bell, such as a dinner bell, should be provided.

An oxygen tent should be washed thoroughly after use on each patient. While the plastic is easy to clean, the size and the shape of the canopy make it a rather cumbersome chore.

Inhalation Therapy

In addition to oxygen, other gases and certain drugs are administered by inhalation. Most of the absorption occurs on the very vascular surfaces of the alveoli, and, because of the large surface area in the lungs, absorption after inhalation generally is rapid.

Before drugs can be inhaled, they must be vaporized to permit their entry into the body with inspiration. A few drugs are volatile and vaporize when exposed to air. Nonvolatile drugs are added to a vehicle, which, when vaporized, carries the drug into the respiratory tract.

Ammonia is an example of a volatile drug. The gas vaporizes from ammonia water, frequently called smelling salts, and, when inhaled, acts systemically to stimulate the heart and respiration. The ammonia water is poured onto a small piece of absorbent cotton or gauze and held near the nose so that the vapors are inhaled. The gas is very irritating and should be used cautiously for only short periods of time. The patient's eyes should be protected or kept closed.

One way to vaporize a drug so that it may be inhaled is to add it to water which, when heated, produces steam that is laden with the drug to be inhaled. This drug acts locally to soothe irritated, inflamed, and congested mucous membrane and to loosen secretions in the respiratory tract. In addition to the action of the drug, the steam soothes the respiratory membrane. The inhaled air, carrying warm minute droplets of water, carries heat to the area and produces the same results as when heat is applied locally to other parts of the body.

A mistlike spray is another common means of administering nonvolatile drugs for inhalation. A device called a nebulizer is used to separate a drug in solution into minute particles for inhalation. *Atomization* usually refers to the production of rather large droplets, while *nebulization* is the production of a mist or fog. The smallest particles are produced by high frequency sound waves. The procedure is called *ultrasonic nebulization*. Suspending the drop-

RATIONALE GUIDING ACTION IN THE USE OF AN OXYGEN TENT

The purpose is to prepare, place, and manage an oxygen tent so that the patient receives a therapeutic concentration of oxygen.

SUGGESTED ACTION	RATIONALE
Check or remove electrical appliances from the immediate area, including the electric signal bell.	Electric appliances may produce sparks and oxygen supports combustion.
Bring tent unit to bedside, plug in motor, and start unit. Turn on oxygen flow. Check oxygen flow inlet in tent and exhaust outlet. Set temperature control.	Testing the mechanical aspects of the tent reduces the possibility of causing further respiratory distress for the patient in the event of mechanical defect.
Close all openings of the hood. Seal the bottom opening of the hood by bringing the sides together and folding over several times, or by tying, so that the upper half of the hood is flooded with oxygen at 15 liters per minute.	For immediate benefit for the patient, the air in the tent should contain an oxygen content of at least 30 to 40 percent. Oxygen is heavier than air; therefore, flood the area which is to be over the patient's head.
Flood the tent for 2 to 5 minutes while the hood is closed.	A therapeutic concentration usually is established in this length of time.
Move the unit directly into position near the bed before opening the hood.	Having the unit in place prevents oxygen loss when the hood is placed over the patient.
Open bottom of hood and place over patient. Leaving some slack, tuck part at the head of the bed well under the mattress as far as it will go.	Sufficient length of hood is necessary to lower head of bed if desired.
Tuck the sides of the hood well under the mattress as far as they will go.	A tightly closed hood prevents oxygen seepage.
Enclose the part of the hood which goes over the patient's thighs in a piece of linen and arrange so that open spaces between the hood and the bedding are closed. Tuck the ends under the mattress to hold them securely. Avoid binding down the patient's legs.	Oxygen, being heavier than air, will escape through open areas at the edge of the hood. Linen, being more pliable than the hood, facilitates sealing the openings and in addition keeps the edge of the hood in place.
Test inside the tent for drafts by placing the hand in various locations near the patient's head. Protect the patient's head with a hood or other suitable object.	Forced entrance of the oxygen and provision for withdrawal of air in the tent produce air motion in the tent.
Check the oxygen gauge and reduce flow to 10 to 12 liters per minute.	Ten to 12 liters per minute usually maintains a 40 to 60 percent concentration in the tent.
Check the temperature indicator frequently until the temperature in the tent is stabilized. Adjust to the temperature most comfortable for the patient.	A temperature of 68° to 72°F. usually is comfortable for a person who is sufficiently covered and protected from the effects of the air movement.
Empty the drainage spigot near the base of the motor unit as often as recommended, usually once every 24 hours.	Moisture in the air which has been withdrawn from the tent condenses. There is also some condensation from the refrigeration unit.

lets in a gas is called *aerosolization*. The finer the particles, the farther they will travel into the respiratory tract. If the inhalation is intended to produce effects in the nasal passage as well as in the remainder of the respiratory tract, the patient closes his mouth while he breathes and inhales the substance through his nose. Otherwise, the mist is inhaled through the mouth. The vapor produced by this method is often referred to as *cold steam*.

There are several ways in which a spray may be produced. The hand nebulizer uses a bulb attachment which, when compressed, forces air through the container holding the drug in solution. The increased pressure in the unit forces solution into a specially constructed strictured device. The force with which the solution is made to move through this stricture and to leave the container is sufficient to break the large droplets of fluid into a fine mist.

Commercially prepared aerosol containers with medications, such as bronchodilators or mucolytic agents are available. These are helpful for home use since no external source of pressure is necessary.

The nebulization can also be accomplished by using the force of an oxygen stream or compressed air to be passed through the fluid in a nebulizer. This method is valuable for patients who require 10 to 15 minutes of inhalations of a special drug several times a day. The hand nebulizer would prove to be quite fatiguing. The oxygen stream is also useful in the production of vapors when high humidity is needed continuously for long periods of time. One of the most common means of administering oxygen and the nebulized drug is the intermittent positive pressure breathing machine, to be discussed next.

INTERMITTENT POSITIVE PRESSURE BREATHING: Intermittent positive pressure breathing, abbreviated I.P.P.B., is a mechanical means of providing a specific amount of air, air/oxygen, or air/oxygen/ medication under increased pressure to the respiratory tract. The device forces deeper inspiration by positive pressure inhalation and then permits passive exhalation. The amount of pressure varies according to the patient's needs.

The I.P.P.B. apparatus can assist ventilation by being set so that the patient's natural inspiration is the stimulus for the pressure increase. Or, it can control the patient's ventilation by having a preset cycle. Assisted ventilation is used for persons who have respiratory disorders when periods of deeper inhalation would be helpful to further aerate the lungs or to move secretions. Controlled ventilation is used for patients who have no spontaneous respiratory movements, as in brain injuries or respiratory paralysis.

Pressure for the I.P.P.B. is supplied by a compressed air or oxygen source. The air or oxygen is forced through a nebulizer containing distilled water or medication and then is directed to the patient. The patient who is having assisted ventilation inhales the mist through a mouthpiece or a face mask. If a mouthpiece is used, the patient seals his lips tightly around the device and breaths only through his mouth. Noseclips can be used if he has difficulty with mouthbreathing. If the face mask is used, it should fit tightly to avoid air leaks. Controlled ventilation is usually provided through a tube inserted directly into the trachea. This type of therapy is discussed in more advanced texts.

The patient with assisted ventilation needs to be informed that he controls the machine by his breathing and that the machine will turn off automatically when the lungs are filled. He should inhale slowly and deeply and allow his lungs to be filled, then exhale as completely as possible before the next inspiration.

Having the patient in a sitting position for maximum respiratory movement is helpful. Depending on the amount of lung secretions, the I.P.P.B. treatment will usually induce productive coughing following its use. The patient should be encouraged to raise and expectorate as much of the secretions as he is able. Figure 27-11 shows a patient with an I.P.P.B. machine in use.

The physician or the respiratory therapist determines the amount of positive pressure, medications and dosages, and frequency of treatments. Improper pressure or inappropriate medications can cause pulmonary tissue damage. Most often the treatments are done at least upon rising and before bedtime, but they may be done at more frequent intervals for some patients. Treatments should be avoided immediately preceding or following meals because the productive coughing may induce vomiting.

I.P.P.B. treatments are frequently recommended for persons with acute and chronic respiratory tract diseases. Many persons with long-term illnesses have the equipment to continue their treatments at home. They are also used with regularity for patients without specific lung pathology, especially following surgery, as a means of promoting respiratory ventilation and preventing complications. Deep breathing, coughing, and postural drainage are often used in conjunction with intermittent positive pressure breathing.

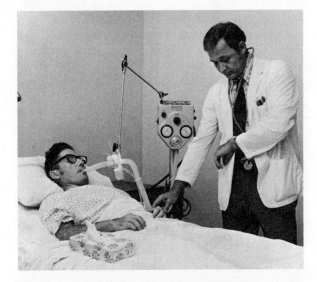

Fig. 27-11. This patient is being given an intermittent positive pressure breathing treatment by the inhalation therapist. (Good Samaritan Hospital, Phoenix, Arizona)

Adequate disinfection of pulmonary ventilation equipment between uses, and especially between patients, is extremely important. Pathogens within the equipment or solution could be forced deep into the lungs by the pressure and cause serious infections.

Like all commercial products, I.P.P.B. machines differ according to the manufacturer. The nurse should take the time to become familiar with the proper use of the I.P.P.B. machines being used for her patients. To assure maximum benefit and safety for the patient, she should be able to detect such conditions as improperly fitting connections, changes in pressure settings, and mechanical malfunctions.

Other Methods for Assisting Ventilation

Other types of respirators are also available for specialized needs of patients having pulmonary ventilation problems. Some of these are available for home as well as health agency use.

Artificial airways are sometimes necessary to provide a patent respiratory tract when obstruction occludes the upper airway. An *endotracheal tube* is a patent tube passed into the trachea through the upper respiratory passageway. A *tracheotomy tube* is one passed through an artificial external opening into the trachea. Both types can be used to supply atmospheric air, oxygen, or other gases. They can also be used to remove tracheal or bronchial secretions by suction.

Respiratory suctioning is the aspiration of secretions from the upper respiratory tract by use of a mechanical device. It is used when the patient is not able to expectorate the secretions for himself. The nasopharyngeal, oropharyngeal, tracheal, and bronchial areas can be suctioned by means of a rubber or plastic catheter attached to a machine providing the necessary suctioning. While mechanical removal of obstructive secretions is necessary for some patients, damage to the delicate respiratory tract mucosa lining, excessive removal of essential oxygen, and the introduction of pathogens are hazards. More advanced nursing texts and respiratory therapy references will provide detailed explanations for the reader who is interested in the more complex ventilation methods.

CARDIOPULMONARY RESUSCITATION

Cessation of breathing may be due to respiratory or cardiac failure. Emergency treatment must be instituted *immediately*. It is the opinion of many medical authorities that as many persons as are capable of learning how to safely administer resuscitation techniques should be taught to do so. In most health agencies there is an on-going program for the teaching and periodic practice of such technique to all health personnel. Such teaching programs extend into the community, over and beyond such groups as police, firemen, and rescue workers.

Recognizing When Resuscitation Is Indicated

Cessation of breathing can be of cardiac or pulmonary origin. If of cardiac origin, breathing usually stops within 30 to 45 seconds. If of respiratory origin, cardiac action may continue, but becomes more and more feeble. Resuscitation *must* begin immediately. No time must be wasted in asking "what happened?", or calling "give him air," or taking blood pressure, and so on. Brain damage may occur quickly from a lack of oxygen. Irreversible damage may occur in about 4 minutes, but for some persons, such as those with vascular disease, damage may occur sooner.

Feel for a carotid or femoral pulse. These areas are considered best. In *cardiac arrest, pulsation in these areas is absent.* Also, the patient lapses into unconsciousness within a matter of seconds (10 to 15). Dilation of the pupils follows. In pulmonary arrest, chest and abdominal wall movements are absent. Dilated pupils occur as a delayed symptom. A distinguishing difference between a person who has "fainted" and a person in cardiac arrest is that the person who has fainted has a pulse—weak, but palpable.

The person recognizing the need for emergency resuscitation should institute action immediately and have someone else get medical aid. In hospital situations there is a plan which calls a team of doctors, nurses, and other therapists into action at any time of the day or night. The person or persons resuscitating the victim continue their efforts until this team arrives. In the community the same holds true. The rescuers continue their efforts until the emergency squad arrives.

Artificial Ventilation

Artificial ventilation is the procedure of forcing exhaled air into the lungs of the victim. It can be done by means of an S tube, mouth-to-mouth, or mouth-to-nose.

The S tube, so named because of its shape, can be inserted into the patient's mouth over the tongue. It has a flange on it so that the patient's mouth can be sealed. Be sure the mouth is clear of any obstructive material. The rescuer then takes a position facing the top of the victim's head, and tilts the head back as far as possible in order to try to open the airway. A small support under the shoulders may be helpful. In some instances this act alone may result in spontaneous breathing as evidenced by movement of the chest and the presence of breath sounds.

Insert the long end of the tube for an adult, and the short end for a child. Use both hands, one on either side of the tube. With thumbs, pinch patient's nose closed and with other fingers hold chin up to hold head back and flange tight over mouth. Take a *deep* breath and blow into the mouthpiece. When the victim's chest rises, take mouth off of tube and allow him to exhale. Take another deep breath and repeat. Do not blow forcefully for a child.

An S tube is usually standard emergency equipment on all units of a health agency. Some agencies have gone so far as to have one in each patient unit. It is a good idea to have one in the home emergency first aid supplies as well. There has been no specific part of this text marked for "home emergencies" or "home first aid," but a point can be made here. No matter where one lives, temporary first aid items should be a part of the environment. This goes beyond emergency treatment of burns and insect bites, and other minor accidents. Instructions for artificial ventilation should also be readily available.

Mouth-to-Mouth Resuscitation

As with the S tube, clear the mouth if necessary, and tilt the patient's head back as far as possible. Again, the rescuer takes a deep breath, pinches the victim's nose closed, and then places his mouth over the victim's mouth, making a tight seal and then exhaling. The volume of air should be sufficient to cause the patient's chest wall to rise. Remove mouth and allow the chest to return to "normal." Repeat once every 5 seconds or at least 12 times a minute.

Mouth-to-Nose Resuscitation

If the rescuer cannot get a good coverage of the mouth so that there is a tight seal, close the patient's mouth and force exhaled air into his nose. The mouth should be open for exhalation because the palate may obstruct, preventing air from leaving through the nose.

Air can be forced into the stomach; therefore, look for signs of bulging of the stomach. If it occurs, press gently but firmly over the epigastric area. It is wise to turn the patient slightly on his side in the event stomach contents are emitted. This facili-

tates clearing the mouth and prevents aspiration of emitted material.

After two deep inflations, check the pulse. The carotid is considered best. Continue to keep the head back while feeling for the pulse. Resume ventilating.

Self-inflating, hand-compressible breathing bags with attached face masks are available in many health agencies for respiratory resuscitation. Their proper use demands familiarity with the equipment.

Artificial Circulation

If no pulse is detected, the person is judged as being in a state of cardiopulmonary arrest. Circulation must be maintained by externally applied compression of the heart. An initial emergency measure is to give the person a sharp, quick blow over the sternum. This may be sufficient to stimulate cardiac action. However, do not waste time doing this repeatedly.

When external cardiac compression is performed it must be accompanied by artificial ventilation.

For external cardiac compression to be effective, the patient should be on a *firm* surface. Place him on the floor if necessary. The rescuer should be at either side of the patient. The point of concentration is the sternum. Place the heel of one hand (part closest to wrist) on the lower part of the sternum, but *not* over the xiphoid process (tip of the sternum) in order to prevent internal injury to the patient. The entire palm of the hand is not used because it covers too large an area and could cause damage to the rib cage. Figure 27-12 shows the correct hand position for cardiac resuscitation. Place the other hand over the first one. For each compression movement the sternum should be depressed 1½ to 2 inches, then relax pressure completely. Do not lose contact with the point of compression over the sternum. The rate of compression should be at least 60 times per minute in adults and 100 times per minute for children.

Palpate for the femoral or carotid pulse at frequent intervals to determine if the compression is being effective. If artificial circulation is being done effectively it can sustain a reasonable cardiac output in most patients.

Artificial ventilation and circulation must be done alternately during the period of emergency. One person can do both. That is, give two to three rapid mouth-to-mouth or mouth-to-nose breaths (this will usually supply the lungs with enough oxygen for about 15 seconds) then do cardiac compression for 15 seconds, doing about one compression per

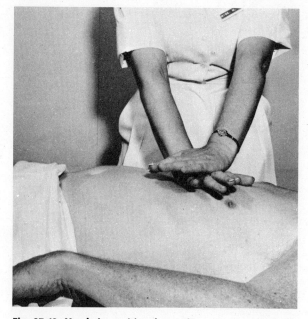

Fig. 27-12. Hands in position for cardiac massage, above the tip of the sternum.

second. If a second person is available, one can concentrate on the artificial ventilation and the other on the artificial circulation. In this case the ratio is one breath to five compressions. Portable mechanical cardiopulmonary resuscitators are available which make resuscitation less exerting for the rescuer and more stabilizing for the patient.

Emergency care continues until the arrival of medical personnel. The physician or specially prepared nurses are then responsible for definitive therapy which includes the use of drugs, such as for stimulating heart action and stabilizing blood pressure or preventing acidosis; the use of oxygen; defibrillating equipment; and so forth. These measures are covered in detail in clinical texts and periodical literature. The implications for nursing care are considerable, not the least of which are: understanding what this episode means to the person, giving emotional support to him and his family, observing for evidence of resulting physiologic disturbances, and maintaining a protective environment.

CONCLUSION

Adequate respiratory functioning is essential for life. The nurse can assist patients by promoting measures that prevent many respiratory problems as well as those that institute therapeutic measures. Because many persons take breathing for granted, preventive respiratory teaching is an important area of need for many individuals. Persons who have difficulty breathing are generally anxious and fearful. The nurse can play a major role in helping to alleviate their psychological distress which is often as significant to improved respirations as specific physical means.

Study Situations

1. The following article applies the nursing process system to a patient with a respiratory problem. Read it while focusing on both the nursing process as well as patient care.

   Griffith, E. W.: Nursing process: a patient with respiratory dysfunction. In **The Nursing Clinics of North America.** Philadelphia, W. B. Saunders, 6:145–154, Mar., 1971.

   Can you parallel the author's nursing process steps with the subsystems described in Unit 2 of this text, even though some of the terms are not the same? Is there other information you would have secured about the patient, for Table 1.? Practice the planning of nursing care by developing another goal, objectives and action, for Table 2.

2. The following article describes a study comparing four different methods for helping patients to breathe deeply and cough effectively. What were the findings of the study? How can you use this information in planning nursing care for postoperative patients?

   Collart, M. E., and Brenneman, J. K.: Preventing postoperative atelectasis. **Am. J. Nurs.,** 71:1982–1987, Oct., 1971.

3. The author of the following article views the human body as an open system.

   Schimpf, K.: The human body as an energy system. **Am. J. Nurs.,** 71:117–120, Jan., 1971.

   How does Mr. M., a patient with a chronic lung disease, demonstrate the characteristics of a system? What does the author mean when she refers to the nurse as a "high energy system"?

4. The articles given below illustrate a variety of pulmonary exercises and postural drainage positions. Ask a friend to practice with you. Can you understand why the patient needs a great deal of support and encouragement from the nurse in order to perform the exercises and postures?

   Wasenius, M.: Physical therapy in the nursing care of respiratory disease patients. In **The Nursing Clinics of North America.** Philadelphia, W. B. Saunders, 3:463–478, Sept., 1968.

   Foss, G.: Postural drainage. **Am. J. Nurs.,** 73:666–669, Apr., 1973.

References

1. Beamont, E.: Portable I.P.P.B. machines. **Nurs. '73,** 3:26–31, Jan., 1973.

2. Betson, C.: Blood gases. **Am. J. Nurs.,** 68:1010–1012, May, 1968.

3. Callard, G. M., and Jude, J. R.: Cardiopulmonary resuscitation in the cardiac care unit. *In* **The Nursing Clinics of North America.** Philadelphia, W. B. Saunders, 7:573–585, Sept., 1972.

4. Collart, M. E., and Brenneman, J. K.: Preventing postoperative atelectasis. **Am. J. Nurs.,** 71:1982–1987, Oct., 1971.

5. Conner, G. H., *et al.*: Tracheostomy. **Am. J. Nurs.,** 72:68–74, Jan., 1972.

6. DeWalt, E. M., and Haines, Sr. A. K.: The effects of specified stressors on healthy oral mucosa. **Nurs. Research,** 18:22–27, Jan.–Feb., 1969.

7. Dyer, E. D., and Peterson, D. E.: Safe care of I.P.P.B. machines. **Am. J. Nurs.,** 71:2163–2166, Nov., 1971.

8. Early, M.: The gaseous exchange process: nursing implications. *In* Kintzel, K. C., ed.: Advanced Concepts in Clinical Nursing. pp. 207–235. Philadelphia, J. B. Lippincott, 1971.

9. Ellis, C. R.: Fundamental breathing exercises. **Nurs. Mirror,** 130:34–35, Feb. 20, 1970.

10. Feeley, E. M.: The new graduate in cardiopulmonary resuscitation. **Am. J. Nurs.,** 70:1304–1307, June, 1970.

11. Finigan, M., and Warm, J.: Ventilatory considerations in cardiac patients. *In* **The Nursing Clinics of North America.** Philadelphia, W. B. Saunders, 7:541–548, Sept., 1972.

12. Flatter, P. A.: Hazards of oxygen therapy. **Am. J. Nurs.,** 68:80–84, Jan., 1968.

13. Foley, M. F.: Pulmonary function testing. **Am. J. Nurs.,** 71:1134–1139, June, 1971.

14. Helming, M. G., Guest ed.: Symposium on nursing in respiratory diseases. *In* **The Nursing Clinics of North America.** Philadelphia, W. B. Saunders, 3:381–487, Sept., 1968.

15. Jacquette, G.: To reduce hazards of tracheal suctioning. **Am. J. Nurs.,** 71:2362–2364, Dec., 1971.

16. Keough, G.: Providing the patient with proper humidification. pp. 206–211. *In* **ANA Clinical Sessions.** New York, Appleton-Century-Crofts, 1971.

17. Kudla, M. S.: The care of the patient with respiratory insufficiency. *In* **The Nursing Clinics of North America.** Philadelphia, W. B. Saunders, 8:183–190, Mar., 1973.

18. Kurihara, M.: Assessment and maintenance of adequate respiration. *In* **The Nursing Clinics of North America.** Philadelphia, W. B. Saunders, 3:65–76, Mar., 1968.

19. Murphy, A. J.: A respiratory screening and surveillance program in a textile industry. **Occup. Health Nurs.,** 20:12–15, Mar., 1972.

20. Nett, L. M., and Petty, T. L.: Why emphysema patients are the way they are. **Am. J. Nurs.,** 70:1251–1253, June, 1970.

21. Olson, E. V., and Thompson, L. F.: Immobility: effects on respiratory function. **Am. J. Nurs.,** 67:783–784, Apr., 1967.

22. Perkins, J. E.: Control of airborne infection in hospitals. **National Tuberculosis and Respiratory Disease Association Bulletin,** 58:10–13, Mar., 1972.

23. Pulmonary care unit. **Am. J. Nurs.,** 70:1254–1255, June, 1970.

24. Roberts, J. E.: Suctioning the newborn. **Am. J. Nurs.,** 73:63–65, Jan., 1973.

25. Rodman, T.: Management of tracheobronchial secretions. **Am. J. Nurs.,** 66:2474–2477, Nov., 1966.

26. Secor, J.: Patient Care In Respiratory Problems. Philadelphia, W. B. Saunders, 1969.

27. Shepard, R. S.: Human Physiology. pp. 291–317. Philadelphia, J. B. Lippincott, 1971.

28. Those critical first minutes. **RN,** 35:46–47, June, 1972.

29. Traver, G. A.: Assessment of thorax and lungs. **Am. J. Nurs.,** 73:466–471, Mar., 1973.

30. Tyler, M. L.: Getting a proper fit with an Ambu Mask. **Nurs. '72,** 2:25, Apr., 1972.

31. ———: Artificial airways: suctioning, tubes and cuffs, weaning and extubation. **Nurs. '73,** 3:21–36, Feb., 1973.

32. Ungvarski, P.: Mechanical stimulation of coughing. **Am. J. Nurs.,** 71:2358–2361, Dec., 1971.

33. Waligora, Sr. B. M.: The effect of nasal and oral breathing upon nasopharyngeal oxygen concentrations. **Nurs. Research,** 19:75–78, Jan.–Feb., 1970.

34. White, H. A.: Tracheostomy: care with a cuffed tuber. **Am. J. Nurs.,** 72:75–77, Jan., 1972.

35. Winter, P. M., and Lowenstein, E.: Acute respiratory failure. **Sci. Am.,** 221:23–29, Nov., 1969.

CHAPTER 28

Administering Medications

GLOSSARY

Hypodermic Injection: Synonym for subcutaneous injection.

Inner Canthus: Medial angle of the eye.

Intra-Arterial Injection: Injection into an artery.

Intracutaneous Injection: Injection under the epidermis.

Intradermal Injection: Synonym for intracutaneous injection.

Intramuscular Injection: Injection into muscle tissue.

Intravenous Injection: Injection into a vein.

Inunction: Rubbing substance into the skin.

Oral: Administer by mouth.

Outer Canthus: Lateral angle of the eye.

Parenteral: Administration route other than oral.

Pharmacist: Person licensed to practice pharmacy.

Pharmacology: Study of actions of drugs on living organisms.

Pharmacy: Profession (or place) of preparing and dispensing drugs.

Prescription: Physician's medication order.

Single order: Directive to be carried out one time.

Standing Order: Directive to be carried out until canceled.

Stat Order: Directive to be carried out immediately.

Subcutaneous Injection: Injection into the subcutaneous tissue.

Topical: Applied directly.

Unit Dose: Separate packing and labeling of an individual drug dose.

INTRODUCTION

A chemical intended to have a therapeutic effect is called a *drug* or a *medication*. Medications can support, improve, or inhibit body functioning. Extensive investigations and experimentation are constantly going on in efforts to discover and perfect substances having a therapeutic effect on the body. The study of the actions of drugs on living organisms is known as *pharmacology*. *Pharmacy* is the profes-

sion (or the place) of preparing and dispensing drugs. A *pharmacist* is a person licensed to practice pharmacy.

Literally thousands of drugs are available on the market today, with new ones being added continuously. It takes efforts from a combination of health practitioners to provide a therapeutic regimen of drugs for patients. In most situations, the physician prescribes the drug, the pharmacist prepares and dispenses it, and the nurse administers it or teaches the patient to administer it to himself. In some health agencies, pharmacists or pharmacy personnel administer as well as teach patients to take their own medications. In some situations, nurses determine some drug prescriptions or at least contribute to the prescription decision. In addition, the biochemist and laboratory technicians may be involved with helping to determine the patient's medication plan. All may be involved in one way or another in observing the person's response to the drug.

Because the nurse generally sees the patient most frequently, whether in the hospital, clinic, office, or his home, she carries a major responsibility for determining whether the desired effect of the medication is occurring or whether an undesirable response has occurred. In order for her to recognize the effect of the drug, she will find the data-gathering process especially helpful. The nurse needs to understand the reason for the drug's use, the action of the drug, its expected effects, and indications of undesirable responses. She may be responsible for teaching these facts to the patient so that he can better understand his health state and treatment and can detect responses induced by the drug.

Drug abuse has become a major health and social problem in this country in recent years. Because of the frequency of her contact with medications and their administration, it is especially important that the nurse learn to respect the effects of drugs and guard against becoming a victim of inappropriate drug use. The nurse must also take precautions not to inadvertently contribute to drug abuse by others. At times she may be responsible for providing care for drug abusers and must therefore understand something of the biochemical as well as psychological complexity of the problem. The reader is encouraged to become familiar with some of the many references that are available on this subject.

Self-medication is the treating of oneself with nonprescription drugs. Occasional treatment of minor problems is a common practice with over-the-counter (OTC) drugs. However, repetitious or long-term, self-medication can be dangerous because of the drug's cumulative action on the body. Also, the use of these drugs may result in the patient's avoiding needed professional health care. The Food and Drug Administration attempts to protect the public by requiring proper labeling and directions on OTC drugs and truthful advertising in relation to the drugs. As an attempt to protect the individual from harm, the Food and Drug Administration has the recommendations listed below.

Information about specific drugs and their actions can be found in pharmacology references. This chapter will discuss techniques for administering drugs by various routes.

GENERAL PRINCIPLES IN THE PREPARATION AND ADMINISTRATION OF THERAPEUTIC DRUG REGIMENS

Physiologic activities of the body can be maintained, improved, or, in some instances, restored by the administration of appropriate therapeutic drugs.

Persons vary in the way they metabolize injected or ingested drugs, or react to medications applied externally.

Appropriate precautionary measures help to avoid errors and accidents in the preparation and the administration of drugs.

Therapeutic measures are those from which the patient benefits. Because every person responds individually, a therapeutic drug regimen must be planned for himself alone.

THE MEDICATION ORDER

Most therapeutic drug plans are developed by the physician. He conveys directives for his plan to

Don't be casual about taking drugs.	Do read and follow directions for use.
Don't take drugs you don't need.	Do be cautious when using a drug for the first time.
Don't overbuy and keep drugs for long periods of time.	Do dispose of old prescription drugs and outdated OTC medications.
Don't combine drugs carelessly.	Do seek professional advice before combining drugs.
Don't continue taking OTC drugs if symptoms persist.	Do seek professional advice when symptoms persist or return.
Don't take prescription drugs not prescribed specifically for you.	Do get medical checkups regularly.

others by a physician's order or a *prescription*. Safe
practice is to follow only a *written* order. A written
order by the physician is least likely to result in error
or misunderstanding. Under certain circumstances,
a verbal order from the physician may be given to
a registered nurse or pharmacist. The legal circumstances of dispensing and administering a drug without a written order vary.

Each health agency has a policy specifying the
manner in which the physician writes his order. In
most cases, orders are written on a form specifically
intended for the physician's orders. This becomes
part of the patient's permanent record or the pharmacy record.

Types of Orders

There are several types of orders that the physician may prescribe. One type is called a *standing
order* and is to be carried out as specified until it
is canceled by another order. Occasionally, the physician writes a standing order and its cancellation
simultaneously—that is, the physician specifies that
a certain order is to be carried out for a stated number of days or times. After that number of days or
times has passed, the order is canceled automatically.
Some health agencies and pharmacies have policies
that specify that standing orders must be reviewed
and rewritten at regular intervals or they will be
canceled. A second type of order is called a *single
order*—that is, the directive is carried out only once,
either at early convenience or at a time specified by
the physician. A *stat order* is also a single order, but
it is one which is to be carried out at once. When a
patient has an operation or when he is transferred
to another clinical service or another health agency,
it is general practice that all orders related to drugs
are discontinued, and new orders are written. To
keep physicians aware of orders in effect, some hospitals specify a day of the week when orders are to
be rewritten or they will be automatically discontinued.

It is usual hospital policy that when a patient is
admitted unless specific orders to the contrary are
written, all drugs which the physician may have
ordered while the patient was at home are discontinued. This sometimes may prove to be a problem
when a patient brings his medications to the hospital. To avoid the possibility of having the patient
continue taking his medications while receiving the
same ones or others under new orders, all medications should be sent home with the family or removed from the patient's unit and placed in safekeeping. Of course, this will require an explanation

to the patient and family of how his drug plan will
be implemented.

In some inpatient facilities, patients keep their
medications at their bedside and learn or continue
to administer them as they would at home. It is
felt this approach helps to promote the independence
of some patients.

Parts of the Drug Order

The drug order consists of seven parts: (1) the
name of the patient; (2) the date when the order
is written; (3) the name of the drug to be administered; (4) the dosage; (5) the route by which it is
to be administered and special directives about its
administration; (6) the time of administration and/
or frequency; and (7) the signature of the person
writing the order. Drug prescriptions to a pharmacist serving an outpatient may also specify whether
or not the name of the drug should be included on
the label and how many times the prescription can
be refilled.

The *patient's full name* is used. The middle
name or initial should be included to avoid confusion with other patients. Some health agencies have
facilities to imprint the patient's name mechanically
on the order form.

The date when the order is written is given.
In some situations, the *time* the order is written may
also be included. Since the nursing staffs in inpatient
facilities change several times during each 24-hour
period, the date and the time help to prevent errors
of oversight as different nurses take charge of a unit.
When an order is to be followed for a specified number of days, the date and the time are important
in order that the discontinuation date and time can
be determined accurately. The period of time that
an order for a narcotic remains valid is determined
by law. Therefore, the date and the time when the
order was written are essential to determine when
the order for a narcotic becomes invalid.

The *name of the drug* is stated in the order
after the physician has indicated the patient for
whom it is intended. Some agencies require that
the physician use generic nomenclature. Certain
trade names are well-known, but the practice of using
the official name is the safest one. If the nurse is
unfamiliar with a drug, she can investigate by referring to certain standard references. In this country,
The United States Pharmacopeia (U.S.P.) and the
National Formulary (N.F.) are official sources. Most
other countries have similar references which describe official therapeutic agents. Many agencies also
provide their own book listing the official drugs

commonly used by the agency. The American Society of Hospital Pharmacists and the American Medical Association's Council on Drugs also publish helpful resources for drug information.

If a patient at home is taking a drug that does not have the name of the medication on the label, the nurse needs to contact the physician or pharmacist to determine the identity of the substance.

The Council on Drugs of the American Medical Association has gone on record as favoring labeling of prescriptions. While it is agreed that at times, for some drugs and for some patients, the drug should be nameless, in most cases labeling is desirable for several reasons. It generally is felt the patient has a right to be informed about his health state and drugs he is taking. With labeling there may be less likelihood of taking incorrect medications, especially when several persons in a home may have prescribed drugs on hand. In case of accident, emergency treatment can be facilitated when the exact content of the drug is known. With the trend in teaching patients concerning their therapy, the patient usually is told what drugs he is receiving.

The *dosage* of a drug can be stated in either the apothecary or the metric system. With planned conversion of this country's measurements to the metric system, apothecary measurements are being used less frequently. Self-administered drugs are frequently labeled in household measurements to facilitate administration. Most agencies post a table of common equivalent dosages for persons who have learned to use one system and find that the agency in which they work uses the other system. Although these tables are convenient and useful, the nurse should be prepared to convert from one system to the other, since such tables are not available in every situation. The nurse should also be familiar with common equivalent measurements when using household equipment such as teaspoons, tablespoons, and the like, since usually the home is not equipped with special measuring devices. Table 28-1 shows some of the common equivalents.

Certain standard abbreviations are used to indicate drug amounts. Before a nurse can administer drugs, she will be required to acquaint herself with these common abbreviations. Table 28-2 indicates some of the most commonly used abbreviations.

TABLE 28-2: Common abbreviations for measures

Abbreviation	Unabbreviated form
c.c.	cubic centimeter
ʒ	dram
gtt.	drop
gr.	grain
Gm.	gram
mg. or mgm.	milligram
ml.	milliliter
m	minim
℥	ounce
tbsp.	tablespoon
tsp.	teaspoon

The nurse also should be aware of common factors that influence dosage calculation; for example, a child's dose for a drug is smaller than an adult's dose. Various formulae have been devised to calculate children's dosage by reducing adult dosages in proportion to the age or the weight of the child. One common formula is Clark's Rule, based on the

TABLE 28-1: Approximate equivalents of fluid and weight measures*

WEIGHTS (approximate)

Metric	Apothecaries'	Metric	Apothecaries'	Metric	Apothecaries'	Metric	Apothecaries'
0.2 mg. = 1/300 grain		3.0 mg. = 1/20 grain		60.0 mg. = 1 grain		1.0 Gm. = 15 grains	
0.3 mg. = 1/200 grain		6.0 mg. = 1/10 grain		0.12 Gm. = 2 grains		4.0 Gm. = 60 grains (1 dram)	
0.4 mg. = 1/150 grain		10.0 mg. = 1/6 grain		0.2 Gm. = 3 grains		6.0 Gm. = 90 grains	
0.5 mg. = 1/120 grain		15.0 mg. = 1/4 grain		0.3 Gm. = 5 grains		10.0 Gm. = 2½ drams	
0.6 mg. = 1/100 grain		25.0 mg. = 3/8 grain		0.5 Gm. = 7½ grains		15.0 Gm. = 4 drams	
1.0 mg. = 1/60 grain		30.0 mg. = 1/2 grain		0.6 Gm. = 10 grains		30.0 Gm. = 1 ounce	

LIQUID MEASURE (approximate)

Metric	Apothecaries'	Household	Metric	Apothecaries'
0.06 c.c./ml.	= 1 minim	= 1 drop	30 c.c./ml.	= 1 fluid ounce
0.5 c.c./ml.	= 8 minims		250 c.c./ml.	= 8+ fluid ounces
1.0 c.c./ml.	= 15 minims		500 c.c./ml.	= 1+ pint
4.0 c.c./ml.	= 1 fluid dram	= 1 teaspoon	1,000 c.c./ml. (1 liter)	= 1+ quart

* Adaptation courtesy of Beacon, Dickinson and Company, Rutherford, New Jersey.

assumption that the average adult weighs 150 pounds:

$$\text{Usual adult dose} \times \frac{\text{weight of child in pounds}}{150} = \text{child's dose.}$$

Weight is a factor in dosage calculation because in general, the heavier the person, the larger the dosage of drugs he can tolerate.

The route of administration influences dosage calculations. Drugs given by mouth are absorbed more slowly and less completely than those given intravenously. Hence, the dosage of a drug given intravenously generally is smaller than when the same drug is given orally.

The general condition of the patient and his drug intolerances are also factors that may influence dosage calculations. Age and the patient's sex may also be significant. Generally, elderly persons and women require smaller dosages than younger adults and men.

The *time* and/or *frequency* with which a drug is to be administered usually are stated in standard abbreviations in the medication order. The most common abbreviations are listed in Table 28-3.

The nursing service department of inpatient facilities usually determines the hours at which routine drugs are given. For example, if certain drugs are to be given every four hours, the nursing service policy indicates the times. Every four hour administration may be at the times of 4 A.M., 8 A.M., 12 A.M. (noon), 4 P.M., 8 P.M., and 12 P.M. (midnight). Another agency may use the hours 5 A.M., 9 A.M., 1 P.M., 5 P.M., 9 P.M., and 1 A.M. If a drug is ordered to be given before or after meals, the time will depend on the hours at which meals are served.

If a drug is to be given only once or twice a day, the decision as to which hours to use will depend on the nature of the drug and the patient's plan of care. Whenever possible, there should be consideration for the patient's choice of time unless there is a need to maintain a constant level of drugs in the blood, such as those controlling cardiac arrhythmia. Not infrequently, patients will ask to have medications left at the bedside. Those patients who have become accustomed to taking prescribed drugs at home may find hospital policy inconvenient or unsatisfactory for personal reasons. When it is possible and safe to make adjustments for the patient, usually it is desirable to do so, and such adaptations should be indicated on the patient's nursing care plan.

The *route* to be used when administering the medication is stated clearly since some drugs can be given in more than one way. If a route is not specified, it is generally understood to be an *oral* medication, that is, it is given by mouth.

As in the case of calculating dosages, there are several factors that influence the choice of route. These include the desired action of the drug, the speed of absorption, the nature of the medication, and the condition of the patient.

The action of drugs can be either systemic or local. A systemic action occurs when the agent is absorbed by the bloodstream and is distributed throughout the tissues and the fluids of the body. For example, an antibiotic given by injection is absorbed by the blood and acts upon certain organisms wherever they may be harboring in body tissues or fluid. Narcotics are given for their systemic effect generally.

A local action occurs when the agent is placed directly in contact with tissue and it is intended to act upon that specific tissue only. An example is applying a drug for athlete's foot where the drug acts directly upon the diseased tissue and the causative organism. Other examples include eye drops containing drugs which can, when instilled, either dilate or contract the pupil, and local anesthetic agents.

Table 28-4 illustrates common routes by which therapeutic agents are administered.

TABLE 28-3: Common abbreviations used in prescribing drugs

Abbreviation	Unabbreviated form	Meaning
a.a.	ana	of each
a.c.	ante cibum	before meals
ad lib	ad libitum	freely
aq.	aqua	water
b.i.d.	bis in die	twice each day
c	cum	with
h.s.	hour of sleep	at bedtime
IM	intramuscular	into muscle
IV	intravenous	into a vein
o.d.	oculus dexter	right eye
o.s.	oculus sinister	left eye
p.c.	post cibum	after meals
PO	per os	by mouth
p.r.n.	pro re nata	according to necessity
q.d.	quaque die	every day
q.h.	quaque hora	every hour
q.i.d.	quater in die	4 times each day
s	sine	without
s.o.s.	si opus sit	if necessary
ss.	semis	a half
stat.	statim	at once
subcu or subq	subcutaneous	into subcutaneous tissue
t.i.d.	ter in die	3 times a day
tinc.	tincture	alcohol base solution

The *signature of the person writing the order* follows the order. The signature is of importance for legal reasons because the authority to prescribe drugs is defined by state laws. Should there be a question concerning the order, the signature indicates who should be contacted.

Questioning the Medication Order

The nurse is responsible for questioning a drug order if in her judgment the order is in error. The suspected error may be in the name of the patient, the medication prescribed, dosage, the time, or the frequency with which it is to be administered, or the route by which it is to be given. The legal implications are serious when there is an error in the medication order and when the nurse involved could be expected, from her knowledge and experience, to have noted the error. On occasion, the nurse may not feel that there is an error in the order, but she may not understand why the medication has been prescribed. In such an instance, the nurse should ask so that she may understand how the order relates to the patient's plan of care.

Occasionally, a nurse may have difficulty reading the order. Guessing is gross carelessness; rechecking with the person who wrote the order is the only safe procedure.

SAFEGUARDING DRUGS

In each health care agency, there is at least one area where drugs are stocked and kept in readiness for dispensing to patients. The cabinet or room is usually locked, and only authorized personnel have access to the key to protect persons from unsafe drug use.

Drugs may be kept in a central area for all patients or they may be kept separately for individual patients. Some inpatient facilities have locked wall cupboards near the entrance to each patient's room for drug storage. Other agencies have locked mobile cupboards which require an individually keyed card for access to each patient's supply.

Unit dose packaging, that is, the separate packaging and labeling of individual drug doses, has become popular in recent years as a means of promoting better drug control, fewer errors, and cleanliness. Pharmacies of some hospitals deliver the single dose of medication, which is ready for administration, to the nurse caring for the patient.

Patients often need to be taught the importance of safeguarding drugs at home. Keeping all medications out of the reach of children is especially important. The number of children who are poisoned from seemingly harmless aspirin and vitamin pills every year is alarmingly high.

Handling of Narcotics

Narcotics are kept in a double-locked drawer, box, or room. This precaution is observed as an additional safety measure. Narcotics may be ordered only by physicians registered under the Harrison Narcotic Act, which is a federal law governing the use of opium and cocoa leaves and their derivatives. According to federal law, a record must be kept for

TABLE 28-4: Routes for administering drugs		
Route	*How drug is administered*	*Term used to describe route*
Given by mouth	Having patient swallow drug	Oral Administration
Given via respiratory tract	Having patient inhale drug	Inhalation
Given by injection	Injecting drug into	Parenteral Administration
	1. Subcutaneous tissue	1. Hypodermic or subcutaneous injection
	2. Muscle tissue	2. Intramuscular injection
	3. Corium (under epidermis)	3. Intracutaneous injection
	4. Vein	4. Intravenous injection
	5. Artery	5. Intra-arterial injection
Given by placing on skin or mucous membrane	Inserting drug into	
	1. Vagina	1. Vaginal administration
	2. Rectum	2. Rectal administration
	Placing drug under tongue	Sublingual administration
	Rubbing drug into skin	Inunction
	Placing drug into direct contact with mucous membrane	Instillation
	Flushing mucous membrane with drug in solution	Irrigation

each narcotic that is administered. Health agencies provide forms for keeping such records, and these forms are kept with the narcotics. Although the forms differ, the following information generally is required: (1) the name of the patient receiving the narcotic; (2) the amount of the narcotic used; (3) the hour the narcotic was given; (4) the name of the physician prescribing the narcotic; and (5) the name of the nurse administering the narcotic. It is common practice to check narcotics daily at specified intervals. For example, in hospitals it is usually with each change of shift. The amount of narcotics on hand is counted, and each used narcotic must be accounted for on the narcotic record. A narcotic count which does not check must be reported immediately. The law requires these special precautions in the use of narcotics in order to aid in the control of narcotic drug addiction. The nurse administering narcotics has a responsibility to see that the federal law is observed.

While in the past it was common practice for nurses to prepare and administer most drugs, today in many inpatient facilities, pharmacy personnel prepare and may administer medications. This practice permits the persons most knowledgeable about drugs to deal with them and provides more time for nurses to spend with patients. Whether nurses actually prepare or administer drugs or not, they still have a responsibility to understand how the medications a patient receives fit into his total regimen of care, to observe their effects, and to teach patients and family members appropriately about the patient's drug therapy. The remainder of the chapter discusses the nurse's role when she prepares and administers the drugs.

PREPARING DRUGS FOR ADMINISTRATION

When the nurse is to give a drug, her first step is to follow the agency's policy specifying the manner in which the medication order is checked. Various systems are used. Some agencies use a card system. Others check with the original written order. Still others use a computer printout sheet. The nurse should be familiar with the system used and implement it correctly to minimize the incidence of errors in administering medications.

Knowledge of the Patient and the Drug
It is essential that the nurse understand the patient's health state and disease process in order to administer drugs intelligently. Understanding the plan of therapy is equally important; otherwise the nurse cannot observe the patient's responses so that they can be used to plan and adjust therapy according to changes in the patient.

The nurse should know the desired action, both local and systemic, of the drugs she administers, their toxic manifestations, and side effects.

Safety Measures in Preparing Drugs
It is important that good lighting be available. Also, while the nurse is preparing drugs, she should work alone. This practice helps prevent distractions and interruptions, which may lead to errors.

Once the nurse begins to prepare drugs for administration, she should not leave them. If interruption is imperative requiring her to leave for a short period of time, the drugs which have been prepared should be placed carefully in a locked area until her return.

The label on the medication container should be read and checked *three times:* (1) when reaching for the container of medication; (2) immediately prior to pouring the medication; and (3) when replacing the container on the shelf. The importance of this checking three times cannot be overemphasized. The safe nurse does not allow automatic habits of preparing drugs to replace *constant thinking, purposeful action*, and *repeated checking* for accuracy.

Safety in Transporting Drugs
Special trays or carts on which to carry medications to the patient are provided. These trays are designed for individual or group use. They usually provide a means by which the identifying information and the medication container can be kept together safely. If a large number of medications are to be given by injection, it is safer as well as convenient to have medication trays or carts which also hold syringes securely. During the time the nurse is administering the medications to the patients, the tray or cart should never be out of her sight. This is to prevent persons from taking medications not intended for them and accidental dislodging of cards or spilling of drugs.

When medications are to be given to more than one patient, it is efficient to arrange the medications in order of administration. This may be according to location of the patients or problems associated with the administration of drugs to certain patients. If a patient requires a great deal of assistance, it seems safer if all other medications are given first and only his medications remain on the tray.

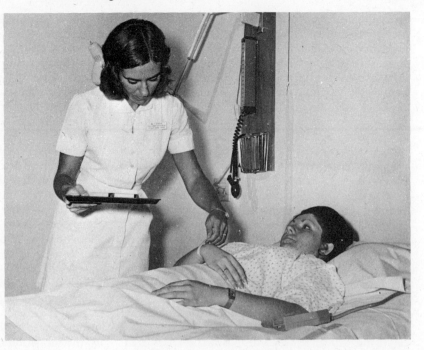

Fig. 28-1. The patient is identified by checking her name on her identification bracelet against the medication card that indicates the drug the patient is to receive.

ADMINISTERING DRUGS

Identifying the Patient

Before the nurse administers the drug, she checks carefully to see that she is giving the drug to the right patient. Patients in inpatient agencies generally wear identification bracelets or have their names posted on their beds. All patients should be called by name. When calling the patient by name, accuracy and clear diction are important so that the nurse can be sure of proper identification. When the patient is unknown to the nurse, he should be asked to state his name. This is particularly important when the patient has a language handicap or is confused.

Administering a Drug

The nurse should remain with the patient while he takes the drug and see that he swallows, injects or applies it before she leaves. If the patient receives several drugs, offer them separately so that if one is refused, or dropped, positive identification can be made and thus recorded or replaced. Leaving medications for the patient to take later, or allowing the patient to give a medication to another, is generally considered unsafe practice. The patient may not take the drug after the nurse leaves. Also, the nurse should not record a drug as given unless the patient has actually received it. If the drug is harmful in large doses and the patient intends to harm himself, he may save a sufficient quantity to do so, as with sleeping pills.

Recording the Administration of Drugs

Every drug administered should be recorded on the patient's permanent record. Most agencies have a special form and a specific policy for such recordings. While there are variations, the drug, its dosage, and route of administration are always included. The location of giving other than oral drugs may be required. For example, policy may require that the nurse record that drops were placed in the right, left, or both ears, or that an injection was given into the left gluteus maximus or right deltoid muscle. Some agencies also require other specific information about the patient. For instance, the pulse rate may be recorded when administering some cardiac drugs or a description of the effects on the patient's pain when administering narcotics.

Omitted or Refused Drugs

Inadvertent omission of a drug should be reported as soon as it is detected to determine whether a dose should be administered at that time. For example, a medication given daily might be given in the afternoon after it was discovered that it had been omitted in the morning. Generally, however, if the omission goes undetected until the following day, a double dose would not be given. A medication administered every six hours would probably be given if its omission was discovered within two to three hours. However, it might be omitted or a partial dose substituted if it was detected four hours later.

Drugs are also omitted for legitimate reasons. The omission and the reason for it are indicated on the patient's chart. For example, if a patient is to have a diagnostic test and is to fast prior to the test, oral drugs usually are omitted or their administration is delayed, depending on the physician's wishes. Another example occurs when a laxative has been ordered for a patient who is constipated; if the patient has a bowel movement and the laxative is no longer needed, the laxative may be omitted. Drugs are also omitted if it is suspected that the patient may be having an allergic reaction to the medication. The symptoms of such reactions vary with the drug. Omitting any drug requires judgment and an understanding of the plan of therapy for the patient.

If the patient refuses a drug which is considered essential to his therapeutic regimen, the nurse will want to report this promptly. In many instances, the nurse can play an important role in determining the reason for the refusal and in helping the patient accept drugs he needs. However, if reasonable efforts fail to accomplish this, it is unwise to continue urging a patient who adamantly refuses a medication. Refusals to take prescribed drugs and the manner in which the situation was managed should be described on the patient's chart.

The Nurse's Role in Case of Error

The conscientious nurse takes reasonable precautions to avoid errors in medication administration. Because human beings are subject to occasional poor judgment, errors do occur. When this happens, the patient's welfare is the first concern. The physician is contacted and remedial measures are begun as necessary. The physician is notified as soon as the error is noted, and the error also is described on the patient's permanent record.

Most agencies require that the nurse responsible for an error fill out a special form for reporting errors. These are frequently called accident or error reports. The forms usually require a full explanation of the situation and the steps that were taken following its commission. For legal reasons, it is essential that errors be described fully and accurately.

ORAL DRUG ADMINISTRATION

While many drugs are administered by mouth, because it is the easiest and most convenient route, there are certain disadvantages to this method. One is that the amount of drug absorbed cannot always be determined with accuracy. Absorption can be affected also by certain disease conditions, such as diarrhea, and, in such cases absorption is even more uncertain.

Drugs which are destroyed by digestive juices and those that are very irritating to the mucous membrane of the gastrointestinal tract often are given by another route. Some irritating drugs can be prepared with a coating that will not dissolve in the stomach. Action from the drug is delayed until the coating is acted upon by the secretions in the intestinal tract. Coated medications require close observation of the patient, since there is the possibility that the patient may expel them without having received any benefit. If the patient is constipated, coated tablets have been known to contribute to the formation of a fecal impaction. If an irritating drug is to be given orally, gastric irritation can be decreased when the drug is dissolved and diluted before administration. Also irritation is often decreased if the drug is given with food, such as a cracker or a piece of bread, or immediately after a meal.

Certain drugs given orally discolor the teeth or tend to damage the enamel. Such medications usually are mixed well with water or some other liquid vehicle; the patient takes it through a drinking tube, and water is taken following administration. This practice reduces the strength of the drug that comes in contact with the teeth. Dilute hydrochloric acid is an example of a drug that damages the enamel of the teeth and should be given well-diluted and with a drinking tube.

Many patients object to the taste of certain medications which can be disguised or masked. For example, if the patient is allowed to suck on a small piece of ice for a few minutes, the taste buds become somewhat numb, and objectionable tastes are less discernible. Oily medications are often stored in a refrigerator, since oil is less aromatic when cold than when given at room temperature. Pouring a medication over crushed ice and serving it with a straw makes it less distasteful.

Various vehicles also can be used to disguise the taste of a drug. These include fruit juices, milk, applesauce, and bread. The disadvantage of using

RATIONALE GUIDING ACTION IN THE ADMINISTRATION OF ORAL MEDICATIONS

The purpose is to prepare and administer oral medications safely and accurately.

SUGGESTED ACTION	RATIONALE
After checking the order, read the label three times while preparing the drug.	Frequent checking helps to insure accuracy and to prevent errors.
Place each medication in a separate container.	If drugs are spilled or refused, positive identification as to type or amount can be made.
Keep medication card and drug together at all times.	Keeping drugs identified insures proper administration of the correct drug to the correct patient.
Transport medications to the patient's bedside carefully and keep the medications in sight at all times.	Careful handling and close observation prevent accidental or deliberate disarrangement of medications.
Identify the patient carefully, using all precautions: check the bed card, look at identification band, call the patient by name, or ask the patient to state his name.	Illness and strange surroundings often cause patients to be confused.
Assist the patient to an upright position if necessary.	Swallowing is facilitated by proper positioning.
If more than one drug is to be given at one time, administer each one separately.	Individual administration promotes accuracy.
Offer water or other permitted fluids with pills, capsules, tablets, and some liquid medications.	Liquids facilitate swallowing of solid drugs. Some liquid drugs are intended to adhere to the pharyngeal area in which case, liquid is not offered with the medication.
Remain with the patient until each medication is swallowed. Unless the nurse has seen the patient swallow the drug, it cannot be recorded that the drug was administered.	The patient's chart is a legal record.
Offer the patient additional fluids as necessary.	Fluids help to dissolve and dilute solid drugs.
Immediately record the medications given, refused, or omitted.	Immediate recording avoids the possibility of accidentally repeating the administration of the drug.

food for disguising distasteful medications is that the patient may learn to dislike the food which he associates with the objectionable-tasting medication. This is particularly true with children. Soft foods can also be a helpful vehicle for pills, tablets, or capsules for persons who find them difficult to swallow. Another help is to administer the drug in a liquid form. Many drugs are available in more than one form.

Preparing Oral Medications

Liquid medications should be prepared with an appropriate measuring device. When liquids are being poured from a bottle, they should be poured from the side of the bottle opposite the label. This prevents drops from running onto the label and making it difficult to read. Hold the container and the bottle at eye level and place the thumb nail on the line on the container which indicates the proper dosage. Because of surface tension, a meniscus forms on the liquid in the measuring container. The liquid should be measured at the *bottom* of this meniscus.

When tablets or capsules are to be administered, the correct number is poured into the cover or the cap of the bottle and then is emptied into the container to carry to the patient's bedside. Pouring tablets or capsules into the hand is not good practice for obvious reasons.

If a label becomes difficult to read or accidentally comes off the bottle, it should be returned to the pharmacy. A medication never should be given from a bottle without a label or with a label that cannot be read with accuracy. Because of the danger of error, medications should not be returned to their bottle. Therefore, care should be exercised to pour carefully to prevent unnecessary loss. Medications should not be transferred from one pharmacy container to another. Many medication bottles now have an identification code number on them. If similar medications were mixed and a patient had a "reaction" it would be difficult to identify which drug was responsible. A medication with an unexpected precipitate should not be used, nor one which has changed color.

If a patient receives several medications at one time, the safest practice is to use separate containers for each, so each can be identified individually.

The boxed description on page 425 specifies the technique for preparing and administering oral medications.

PARENTERAL DRUG ADMINISTRATION

The term *parenteral* refers to routes other than the oral. However, the term is used most commonly to indicate the injection routes, and it is used in that context in this book.

Parenteral medications are commonly injected into the muscle—*intramuscular* injection; into the subcutaneous tissue—a *subcutaneous* or *hypodermic* injection; under the epidermis—an *intracutaneous* or *intradermal* injection; into the vein—an *intravenous* injection; and occasionally into an artery—an *intra-arterial injection*.

Absorption occurs more rapidly in the injection method than it does when other routes are used. Absorption is also more nearly complete; therefore, the results are more predictable, and the desired dosage can be determined with greater accuracy. Giving drugs by injection is particularly desirable for patients who are irrational, unconscious, or having gastric disturbances. This method of administering drugs is also good in emergencies, since absorption occurs rapidly.

For patients who will need to administer their own medications at home, parenteral administration presents a more involved teaching problem than do most other routes. However, many patients have learned to give themselves injections skillfully and safely when the teaching has been well-planned and the patient is able and willing to learn.

The discomfort associated with injections sometimes is considered to be a disadvantage of the injection route. However, skill in giving injections can greatly reduce discomfort. Several practices aid in decreasing pain.

The pain of an injection is usually the result of the needle's passing through a cutaneous pain receptor. For the very sensitive or anxious patient, this discomfort can be minimized by applying cold compresses or by placing an ice cube on the area of injection for a short time immediately prior to the injection. Some physicians may also recommend spraying a volatile solution such as ethyl chloride on the site of injection. The use of cold and of volatile sprays numbs sensory receptors and therefore decreases pain.

Subcutaneous tissue is relatively insensitive, but if the needle distorts fascia of underlying muscle tissue, pain will result. The injection of nonirritating drugs in an isotonic solution is usually painless. A small amount of anesthesia, such as procaine hydrochloride, is often added to irritating drugs.

It is of prime importance to use a sharp needle, free of burrs, and to select one of the smallest gauge that is appropriate for the site and for the solution to be injected. Today's disposable needles avoid the problems of dull and damaged needles. Pain is minimized by inserting and removing the needle without hesitation and by injecting solutions slowly so that they may be dispersed into the surrounding tissues. Select a site where the skin appears free of irritation and danger of infection.

Following an injection, firm pressure and massage of the injection site hastens absorption of the drug and relieves discomfort. If injections are being given often to a patient, rotating the site also aids in decreasing the discomfort of inserting the needle into an area recently injected.

Preparing Drugs for Parenteral Administration

Drugs for parenteral administration are marketed in several ways. Those that deteriorate in solution usually are dispensed as tablets or powders and placed in solution immediately prior to injection. If drugs remain stable in solution, usually they are dispensed in ampules, bottles, or vials in an aqueous or oily solution or suspension.

Some medications are available in syringes that are prefilled by the manufacturer. Drug companies specify the parenteral route intended for each medication and a drug should not be administered by any route other than the one for which it was specified. For example a drug labeled for intramuscular use should not be given intravenously.

REMOVING DRUGS FROM AMPULES AND VIALS: The most commonly used dispensing units are the single-dose glass ampule, the single-dose rubber-capped vial, and the multiple-dose rubber-capped vial. They are illustrated in Figures 28-2, 28-3 and 28-4.

Single-Dose Glass Ampule: Most single-dose glass ampules have a constriction in the stem of the ampule which facilitates opening it. Before preparing to open the ampule, make certain that all of the drug is in the ampule proper and not in the stem. The drug tends to be trapped in the stem, and it may be necessary to tap the stem several times to help bring the drug down. Ampules without a constriction do not present this problem.

A practice in some agencies is to wipe the outside of the ampule with an antiseptic solution before it is opened. This practice has never been justified scientifically. Considering that the antiseptic is merely passed over the glass briefly, and that immediately thereafter it will be scored by an unsterile file, it would appear that this gesture adds nothing to the safety of the procedure.

When all the drug has been brought to the bottom of the ampule, gauze is used to hold the ampule firmly and to protect the nurse's fingers. Sterile gauze or other material is used because it will be

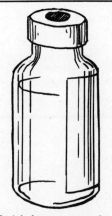

Fig. 28-3. A closed vial does not permit air to enter as the fluid is withdrawn. Withdrawing the fluid without injecting air creates a partial vacuum within the vessel and makes the solution difficult to withdraw.

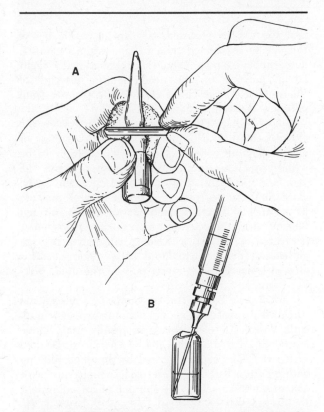

Fig. 28-2. (A) The fingers are protected by cotton when the stem of the closed glass ampule is scored with a file and then broken off. (B) When the stem of the glass ampule is removed, the drug is drawn up into the syringe easily because air displaces the fluid. The sterile needle should not touch the rim of the ampule.

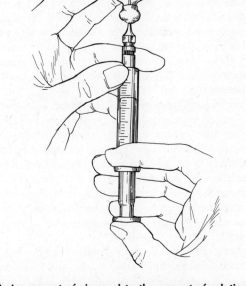

Fig. 28-4. An amount of air equal to the amount of solution to be withdrawn is injected. Pressure within the vial is increased and the drug is removed easily and accurately.

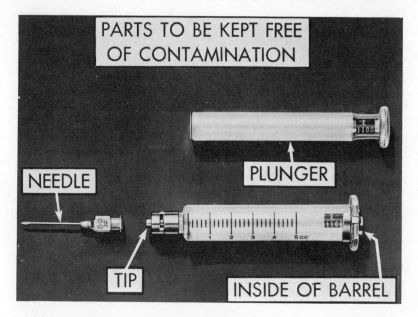

PARTS TO BE KEPT FREE
OF CONTAMINATION

NEEDLE

PLUNGER

TIP

INSIDE OF BARREL

Fig. 28-5. Hypodermic syringe and needle-parts to be kept free of contamination. (Becton, Dickinson and Co., Rutherford, N. J.)

in close proximity to the opening of the ampule when the stem is removed. A saw-tooth file is used to scratch the glass gently on the stem, well above the level of the medication. Scratching it on opposite sides helps to insure a quick, even break. After the scratch marks have been made, the ampule is held in one hand, and the other is used to break off the stem. Many single-dose ampules are prescored and do not require filing. These are identified by a colored marking at the neck of the ampule. However, there is still need to protect the fingers. A commercial ampule opener with a protective flange is also available.

The medication in the ampule is now in an open vessel. To remove it, insert the needle into the ampule and withdraw the solution. Be careful not to touch the edge of the glass with the needle in order to minimize all chances of contamination. The fluid in the ampule is immediately displaced by air; therefore, there is no resistance to its withdrawal. With additional skill, it will be possible to pick up the ampule and hold it between two fingers of one hand and the syringe in the other hand. When removing the drug in this fashion, the trick lies in keeping the needle in the solution at all times, even as the ampule is inverted.

Single-Dose Rubber-Capped Vial: For safety in transporting and storing, the single-dose rubber-capped vial usually is covered with a soft metal cap which can be removed easily. The rubber part which then is exposed is the means of entrance into the vial. At the time of preparation, this rubber portion of the seal was sterilized, but many agencies specify

that the cap be cleansed with an antiseptic before the needle is inserted. Use friction when cleansing. The rubber stopper should be entered with slight lateral pressure on the needle during piercing of the stopper to prevent a core of the stopper from entering the vial.

To facilitate the removal of the drug from the closed container, it is best to inject an amount of air comparable with the amount of solution to be withdrawn. This increases the pressure within the vial, and then the drug can be withdrawn easily, since fluids move from an area of greater pressure to an area of lesser pressure. If air is not injected first, an area of lesser pressure (a partial vacuum) is created in the vial as fluid is withdrawn, because air cannot displace the fluid being removed. This area of lesser pressure exerts pull on the fluid, making it difficult to withdraw.

Multiple Dose Rubber-Capped Vial: Some drugs are dispensed in vials containing several or multiple doses. An example is an insulin vial. These are managed in the same manner as the single-dose sealed vial. The cap is cleansed by thorough rubbing with a cotton ball or a gauze pledget moistened with an antiseptic solution. An amount of air equivalent to the amount of solution to be withdrawn is injected. The air should be injected accurately, since not enough air will make withdrawal of the drug difficult, and increasing the pressure in the vial by adding too much air will interfere with the ease of preparing the correct dose by pushing solution into the syringe.

If the amount of fluid to be removed from a vial

is rather large or several doses are to be removed in succession, a simple method is to insert a separate sterile needle through the cap. This will allow air to enter and replace the fluid as it is being withdrawn.

Surgical and Medical Asepsis in Parenteral Therapy

While details of methods for administering injections may vary from one agency to another, there is one basic principle which underlies all—strict asepsis minimizes the danger of injecting organisms into the patient's tissues or bloodstream.

All objects coming in contact with the drug and the patient's tissues should be sterilized prior to use by the most reliable means available. Findings in relation to homologous serum hepatitis leave little doubt that it is transmitted easily via parenteral therapy. Many agencies take extra precautions by using disposable items, including syringes, needles, and single dose cartridges for medications. Figure 28-5 shows the parts of the syringe and needle that must be kept sterile.

If a drug must be prepared and then transported to the patient's unit, the needle must be kept sterile. Using the holder which protected the needle offers the greatest amount of safety.

Cleansing the skin before an injection has been considered a traditional part of the technique, although there are some studies that indicate it is unnecessary. However, until further evidence is gathered, most authorities continue to recommend skin cleansing before an injection.

The choice of an antiseptic agent for cleansing the skin prior to parenteral therapy is of periodic concern to every health agency. However, as was pointed out, sterilization of the skin cannot be expected. Since sterilizing the skin is not possible, the purpose of cleansing the area is to make certain that it is free from gross contamination and dried skin cells. In cleaning the area, a circular motion is used, beginning at the point of injection and moving outward and away from it. This carries material away from the critical site. Haphazard up-and-down movements should be avoided, since they bring the material right back again. The correct action is accompanied by firm pressure so that mechanical cleansing is also accomplished. Individually packaged gauze moistened with an antiseptic is now in common use.

In those instances when the patient's skin is soiled from drainage or discharges, thorough cleansing with soap and water should precede cleansing with an antiseptic. This is especially true for incontinent patients who may need to have intramuscular injections. This point cannot be stressed too much, namely, that the nurse exercise careful judgment in the preparation of any body site for injection and not rely on the conscience-salving procedure of a superficial swipe with an antiseptic-soaked pledget.

Surgical Asepsis for Parenteral Therapy in the Home

Since many patients and their families are learning to administer injections, the problem of sterilization at home will arise. A patient's home equipment is purchased for him and used only for him. Therefore, the possibility of cross-contamination between patients is eliminated. Boiling of syringes and needles in the home has been recommended for years and found to be safe, as long as the equipment is not shared.

For home technique, cotton used to cleanse the skin need not be sterile as long as the patient is instructed not to cover the needle with it. Since the patient will not have a needle protector, he will need to be shown how to keep the needle sterile. Usually, the patient is advised to keep it off the edge of the table or surface on which he will place the syringe while preparing the skin. It should be directed so that the patient cannot touch it accidentally.

The cost of disposable equipment has been reduced, therefore more patients are using such items for injections that are given at home.

SUBCUTANEOUS INJECTION

While there is subcutaneous tissue all over the body, for convenience, a site on the upper arm or on the thigh usually is selected for the injection. The lower abdomen and upper back are also common sites. Patients who give themselves hypodermic injections generally find the thigh and abdomen the most convenient sites. Figure 28-6 shows a patient giving herself an injection.

If a patient is to receive frequent injections, it is best to alternate the sites, which helps to prevent irritation and permits complete absorption of the solution. It is not uncommon for patients who receive injections repeatedly in one site to note induration from unabsorbed drug or to complain of itching in that site. For alternating sites, it is necessary for the routine to be incorporated in the patient's plan of care. A marked diagram can be helpful for noting alternate sites. It is fruitless to rely on memory. Not even the patient will always be able to recall where he had the previous injection.

Air may enter the syringe when it is being filled. Unless it is an unusually large amount, no harm will

430 • FUNDAMENTALS OF NURSING

come from a small amount. In fact, small quantities are helpful to force medication remaining in the needle shaft into the injection site. The major significance of air in the syringe is to make certain it does not cause an error in the measurement of the amount of medication. The air can be easily eliminated by holding the syringe in a vertical position and pushing gently on the plunger until it is removed. Figure 28-7 shows a patient removing the air from her syringe before her injection.

The amount of subcutaneous tissue underlying the skin is not a constant factor in all individuals. Some persons may have very little, and others a great deal. For the average adult it generally is recommended that the needle be injected at a 45° angle. However, for an obese patient, a needle injected at this angle may not reach subcutaneous tissue, while muscular tissue may be reached in a very thin and dehydrated patient. The angle and length of the needle must be adjusted to the individual patient. The tissue can be picked up and held firmly for stability if desired. Some authorities feel this technique helps to avoid accidental injection into muscle tissue. Figures 28-8 and 28-9 and the boxed description on page 432 show the technique for a subcutaneous injection.

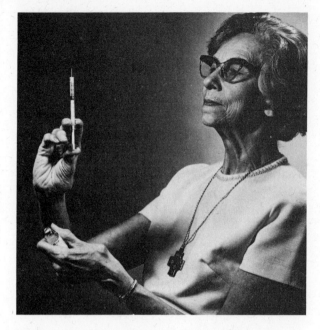

Fig. 28-7. This patient is removing air from her syringe in preparation for administering her injection. (Courtesy of Bectin, Dickinson and Company, Rutherford, N. J.)

Equipment Commonly Used for Subcutaneous Injections

NEEDLES: The needle most commonly used for injecting into subcutaneous tissue is a 25-gauge, five-eighths-inch needle. However, there are variations in this, and some patients need a shorter or longer needle.

The needle must be in perfect condition and free from burrs on the point. Once a needle has been bent, it should not be forced straight for reuse. Because a needle is a delicately constructed item having a lumen, the shaft is weakened if the needle is bent and then bent back into place again. Weakening the shaft of the needle increases the possibility of its breaking in the patient's tissues if the patient moves or if other strain is placed on it.

Patients who have been taught to give their injections at home should be shown how to test the point of the needle for burrs. This is done easily by running the point of the needle, both sides, over a piece of cotton or along the back of the hand before sterilizing it. If the point of the needle picks up cotton or scratches the hand, it requires sharpening. A needle with a burr on its point results in a painful injection.

More and more agencies and patients at home are using disposable needles. The multiple advantages are self-evident. However, public health officials have

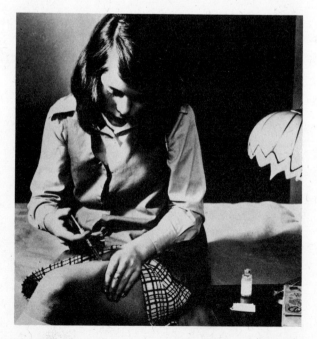

Fig. 28-6. The patient in this photo is giving herself an insulin injection in the anterior mid-thigh area. (Courtesy of Bectin, Dickinson and Company, Rutherford, N. J.)

cautioned all who use such needles to discard them appropriately. The needle should be bent or broken and covered to prevent reuse or accidental puncture wounds of those handling trash.

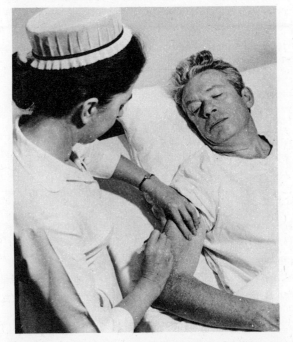

Fig. 28-8. For a subcutaneous injection into the upper arm, the tissue is picked up and held firmly. Then the needle is held at an angle which will help it enter subcutaneous tissue —usually a 45° angle for the average adult.

SYRINGES: Since numerous substances can be given subcutaneously, there is a variety of syringes to facilitate their measurement and injection.

Syringes for hypodermic injections are calibrated in both minims and cubic centimeters or milliliters. They are available in 2, 2½, and 3 ml. sizes. Reusable syringes are made of glass and disposable ones, of plastic.

When a very small dose of a drug must be measured, as when giving an allergen extract or a vaccine, a 1 ml. syringe calibrated in tenths and hundredths of a ml. and in minims is used. Such syringes provide for more accuracy than can be obtained from the usual syringe.

Previously, a variety of insulin syringes were in use according to the unit strength of the insulin being used. A U100 insulin is now available for use with U100 calibrated syringes and is intended for all patients regardless of their insulin dosage. This product is intended to replace older U40 and U80 insulin and syringes. The U100 syringes are available in reusable and disposable types.

Hypodermic needles and syringes are dispensed in a variety of ways, some already assembled and others unassembled. If the needle is to be attached to the syringe, it should be held by the hilt. A small sterile forceps can be used both to attach and to tighten the needle. However, the fingers can be used, provided that the hilt does not contaminate a sterile surface following this, i.e., a needle protector or a sterile cotton ball.

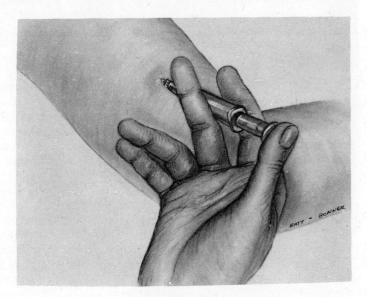

Fig. 28-9. Once the needle has pierced the skin quickly, the tissue is released so that the fluid need not be injected under pressure. Releasing the tissue facilitates the distribution of the drug.

RATIONALE GUIDING ACTION IN THE ADMINISTRATION OF A SUBCUTANEOUS INJECTION

The purpose is to inject a medication into subcutaneous tissue.

SUGGESTED ACTION	RATIONALE
Obtain equipment and drug. Assemble syringe and needle according to manufacturer's directions. Keep drug and sterile items in sight.	Sterile items that are out of sight are in danger of being contaminated accidentally.
Draw the drug into the syringe and protect the needle with a sterile needle cover or a sterile dry cotton ball until ready for injection.	Prolonged exposure to the air and/or contact with moist surfaces will contaminate the needle.
Carry the syringe to the patient on a tray or a medication carrier.	Keeping the prepared syringe on a flat, steady surface reduces the possibility of moving the plunger and thus possibly losing the drug.
Cleanse the area of the skin to be injected by using firm, circular motion while moving out from the center of the area with each stroke.	Friction aids in cleansing the skin. A clean area is contaminated when a soiled object is rubbed over its surface.
Grasp the area surrounding the site of injection and hold in a cushion fashion.	Cushioning the subcutaneous tissue helps to insure having the needle enter areolar connective tissue.
Inject the needle quickly at an angle of 30° to 60°, depending on the amount and the turgor of the tissue.	Subcutaneous tissue is abundant in well-nourished, hydrated persons and sparse in emaciated, dehydrated ones.
Once the needle is in situ, release the grasp on the tissue.	Injecting the solution into compressed tissues results in pressure against nerve fibers and creates discomfort.
Pull back gently on the plunger of the syringe to determine whether the needle is in a blood vessel.	Substances injected directly into the bloodstream are absorbed immediately.
If no blood appears, inject the solution slowly.	Rapid injection of the solution creates pressure in the tissues, resulting in discomfort.
Withdraw the needle quickly.	Slow withdrawal of the needle pulls the tissues and may cause discomfort.
Rub the area gently with the antiseptic pledget.	Rubbing aids in the distribution and the absorption of the solution.

INTRAMUSCULAR INJECTION

The intramuscular route often is used for drugs that are irritating, since there are few nerve endings in deep muscle tissue. If a sore or inflamed muscle is entered, the muscle may act as a trigger area, and severe referred pain often results. It is best to palpate a muscle prior to injection. Select a site that does not feel tender to the patient and where the tissue does not contract and become firm and tense.

Absorption occurs as in subcutaneous administration but more rapidly because of the greater vascularity of muscle tissue. Approximately 2 to 5 ml. of solution usually is given via this method. However, when as much as 5 ml. of a solution is ordered to be given intramuscularly, judgment should be used as to whether the dose should be divided and half given into one site and half into another. The pressure created by the introduction of such a quantity usually creates discomfort for the patient. If divided doses are not possible because of the frequency of subsequent ones, the injection should be given very slowly to allow for dispersal of the solution in the tissues.

Because of the widespread use of intramuscular injections, it is not too surprising that complications have occurred, possibly even more frequently than the literature reports. Common complications have included abscesses, necrosis and skin slough, nerve injuries, lingering pain, and periostitis.

A crucial point in the administration of an intramuscular injection is the selection of a safe site, one that is away from large nerves and the large blood vessels.

Dorsogluteal Site (Gluteus Maximus Muscle)

The dorsogluteal site, located on the buttock has been a common site for giving intramuscular injections. The classic method is to inject about 2 to 3 inches below the crest of the ilium in the upper outer quadrant of the buttock. Figure 28-10 illustrates how the area is located. A common error is made when the upper landmark is merely identified by eye rather than by palpation of the iliac crest. The usual miscalculation is the result of the buttock being equated with the gluteus and the injection is given too low.

Another method for locating a site on the buttock is illustrated in Figure 28-11. Locate a line from the posterosuperior iliac spine to the greater trochanter of the femur; an injection lateral and slightly superior to the midpoint of the line will also avoid the dangerous area.

A common error in locating a site is improper mapping of the area. Many people believe that the fleshy part of the buttock should certainly be the safest spot. Nothing could be more incorrect. Also, many incorrectly include the fleshy portion of the upper thigh, especially in obese patients, as a part of the buttock. The site is so important that no injection into the buttock should be given without good visualization of the entire area and careful mapping to locate the proper site. This necessitates adequate exposure by the lowering of undergarments. The mere raising of one side of the underpants only permits a partial visualization of the area. It is recommended that the patient be in a prone or at least, lateral recumbent position for a dorsogluteal injection. These positions help to promote maximum muscle relaxation and therefore, minimal discomfort. When the patient is in a standing position, the gluteus muscle is usually tense.

Ventrogluteal Site (Gluteus Medius and Gluteus Minimus Muscles)

This is preferred to the dorsogluteal site in children, and it is recommended also by many authorities for adults as well. There are no large nerves or blood vessels in this area; there is less fat here than in the buttocks; the area is cleaner, since fecal contamination is rare at this site and the patient can be on his back or side for the injection.

The correct site, illustrated in Figures 28-12, 28-13, and 28-14, is located as follows. Place the tip of the index finger on the anterosuperior iliac spine with the palm over the head of the femur and the fingers pointing toward the head. Abduct the adjacent finger as far as possible to form a V. An injection into the V will fall within the region of the gluteal muscles.

Vastus Lateralis Muscle

This muscle is not used commonly but is being recommended more frequently. It is a thick muscle and there is little or no danger of serious injury. There are no large nerves or vessels in close proximity, and it does not cover a joint. The muscle covers the anterolateral aspect of the thigh. It is bounded by the midanterior thigh on the front of the leg and the midlateral thigh on the side. The middle third of the muscle, measuring up from just above the knee and down from the greater trochanter, is recommended for injections. This provides space for a large number of injections. Figures 28-15 and 28-16 show this injection site.

Deltoid and Posterior Triceps Muscles

These muscles also may be used. However, in

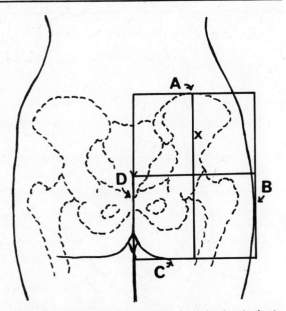

Fig. 28-10. One site for an intramuscular injection is the inner portion of the upper outer quadrant. This area is obtained by using the following guides. The upper line is determined by the iliac crest, A; the outer lines by the division of the buttocks and the outer surface of patient's body, D and B. The lower line is determined by the lower edge of the buttock, C. This area is then divided into equal parts vertically and horizontally. The injection is given two to three inches below the top of the iliac crest in the upper outer quadrant.

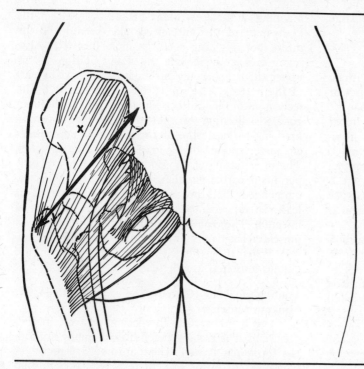

Fig. 28-11. Another method for mapping out the gluteus maximum is to draw an imaginary line from the ridge on the ileum to the head of the femur. The needle is injected outside and above the line.

general, they rarely are used, since they are small, and a misplaced needle may injure the radial nerve. Also, many patients experience more pain and tenderness in this area than in others.

Rectus Femoris Muscle

This muscle is on the anterior part of the thigh. The site is used only when others are contraindicated, since many patients find it uncomfortable. However, some patients who must inject themselves at home use this site.

Preparation of the Drug for Intramuscular Injection

As mentioned previously in the discussion of subcutaneous injections, the length of the needle to reach the desired tissue varies with each individual. The most commonly used needle for intramuscular injection is a 22-gauge, 1½-inch needle. However, for drugs of an oily nature, a larger gauge, such as a 20 gauge, is indicated. The length of the needle for an intramuscular injection should be based on the site to be used and the condition of the patient. This is especially important if the patient is obese and the drug is irritating; 3-inch needles cause no more discomfort than 1½-inch needles, and, with proper injection, there is a greater likelihood of the drug being introduced into muscle. For children, a

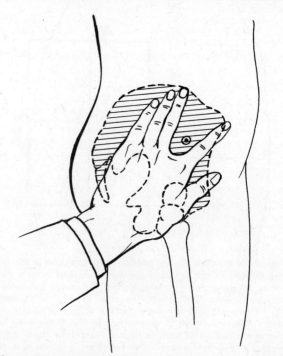

Fig. 28-12. Ventrogluteal injection site. The site is farthest from all major nerves and vessels.

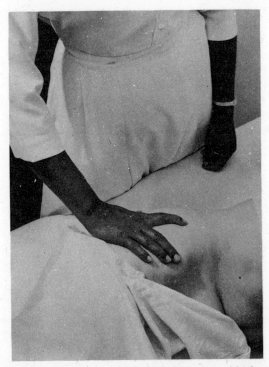

Fig. 28-13. Ventral site intramuscular injection with the patient in the side-lying position. The nurse palpates for the anterosuperior iliac spine. When she locates it she will hold her finger on it and move her second finger along the bony prominence to form a V, as illustrated.

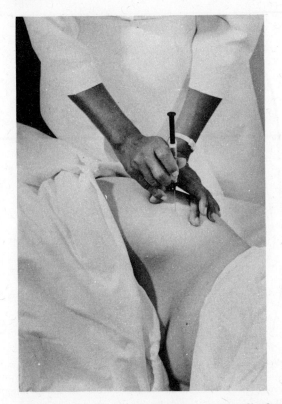

Fig. 28-14. Having located the site, the nurse puts her hand in position, presses down the tissues, and injects needle.

shorter needle is necessary, such as a ¾ inch or a 1-inch needle. In many instances, it is possible to use a hypodermic needle to give an intramuscular injection to an infant.

The age, the weight, the condition, and the tissue turgor of the patient should be taken into consideration rather than relying on a standard needle gauge for each type of injection.

The points of caution observed for the preparation of equipment for a subcutaneous or any other parenteral injection are employed also when preparing an intramuscular injection. There is an exception in the procedure: just prior to injection, a small air bubble, approximately 0.2 to 0.3 ml., is included in the syringe with the solution. This is measured when the syringe is held in the upright position. When the needle is inverted, this air bubble will rise to the top of the solution in the syringe. Figure 28-17 illustrates the air bubble. After the solution is injected, this air bubble will aid in expelling the remaining solution that is trapped in the shaft of the needle. Solution which remains in the shaft of the needle is in danger of being pulled up through the

tissues as the needle is withdrawn. If the drug is a particularly irritating one, this causes discomfort to the patient and may result in tissue damage.

Only the points of difference between subcutaneous and intramuscular injections are given in the boxed description for intramuscular injection into the gluteus maximus muscle. Figure 28-18 shows how to hold the tissue firm for insertion of the needle.

Rotation of Intramuscular Injection Sites

Because many drugs are given via the intramuscular route and therapy often calls for repeated injections, consideration should be given to the rotation of the sites used. The sites described earlier all may be used.

The use of the different muscle groups is almost essential for patients receiving frequent injections. The slight discomfort created by the use of other areas does not seem to outweigh the discomfort produced in the gluteals following multiple piercings or the induration which may result.

When a pattern of rotating sites is used for a

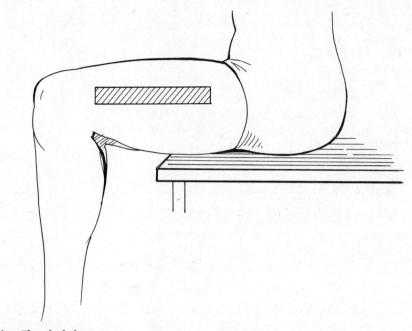

Fig. 28-15. Vastus lateralis injection site. The shaded area shows the injection site of the right thigh. The area is a strip several inches wide in the middle third of the lateral thigh, measured between the knee and the greater trochanter.

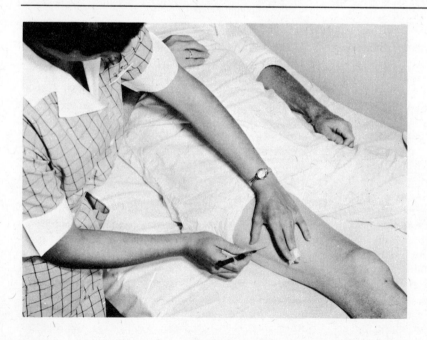

Fig. 28-16. Lateral thigh intramuscular injection.

patient, a comment describing the pattern should appear in the nursing care plan.

Z Technique

The Z or zigzag technique is used to inject medications that cause superficial tissue irritation or staining. The tissue is displaced laterally before the injection. Immediately following removal of the needle, the tissue is allowed to assume its normal position, thus preventing the escape of the drug from its intramuscular site.

INTRAVENOUS INJECTION

Drugs are administered into the vein when rapid action is desired. While this rapid action is desirable, especially in emergency situations, it can also be dangerous because of the almost immediate transportation of the drug into general systemic circulation. Slow administration and adequate dilution of the drug are means of increasing the safety of intravenous drug administration. The technique for entering a vein—venipuncture—was discussed in Chapter 24.

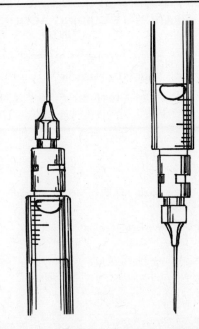

Fig. 28-17. A small amount of air, 0.2 to 0.3 ml., is drawn into the syringe as final preparation for intramuscular injection. When the syringe and the needle are inverted, as during injection, the bubble rises in the syringe. The air serves to push the solution trapped in the shaft of the needle into the tissues.

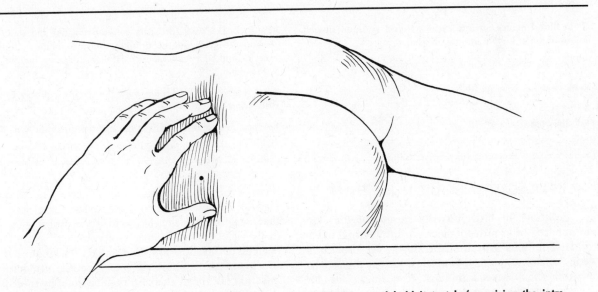

Fig. 28-18. After mapping out the area carefully, press down the tissue and hold it taut before giving the intramuscular injection.

RATIONALE GUIDING ACTION IN THE ADMINISTRATION OF AN INJECTION INTO THE GLUTEUS MAXIMUS MUSCLE

The purpose is to inject a medication into the gluteus maximus muscle.

SUGGESTED ACTION	RATIONALE
Have the patient assume a comfortable side-lying or prone position.	Injection into tense muscle causes pain. Good visualization of the buttock aids correct location of site.
Locate the site.	The area about 2 to 3 inches below the top of the iliac crest in the upper outer quadrant avoids the sciatic nerve and large blood vessels and is still over the gluteus maximus.
Gently tap the selected site of injection with the fingers several times.	Stimulation of the peripheral nerves helps to minimize the initial reaction when the needle is inserted.
Cleanse the area thoroughly, using friction.	Pathogens present on the skin can be forced into the tissues by the needle.
Using the thumb and the first two fingers, press the tissue down firmly and in the direction of the thigh.	Compression of the subcutaneous tissue helps to insure having the needle enter muscle. Moving the tissue downward will help to disperse the solution and seal the needle track when the tissue is permitted to return to normal position.
Hold the syringe in a horizontal position until ready to inject.	The pull of gravity may alter the position of the plunger, causing loss of drug.
When ready to inject, quickly thrust the needle into the tissue at a 90° angle.	Quick injection minimizes pain. Thrust helps to insert needle.
As soon as the needle is in place, slowly pull back on the plunger to determine whether the needle is in a blood vessel. If blood is noted, pull the needle back slightly and test again.	Muscle tissue is vascular. Drugs injected into the bloodstream are absorbed immediately.
If no blood comes up into syringe, inject solution slowly, followed by air bubble into the needle.	The air bubble will force the solution through the shaft of the needle and prevent dribbling of the solution in the muscle and the subcutaneous tissues as the needle is withdrawn.
Remove the needle quickly.	Slow removal of the needle pulls the tissues and may cause discomfort.
Rub the area.	Rubbing aids in the distribution and the absorption of the solution.

INTRACUTANEOUS INJECTION

Solutions injected into the corium of the skin are referred to as intracutaneous or intradermal injections. Solutions are absorbed slowly via the capillaries. Small amounts of solution are used—usually no more than several minims. A common site for injection is the inner aspect of the arm, although other areas are also satisfactory. Intracutaneous injections generally are used for diagnostic purposes; examples are the tuberculin test, and tests to determine sensitivity to various substances. The advantage of the intracutaneous route for these tests is that reaction of the body to these substances is easily visible, and, by means of comparative studies, degrees of reaction are discernible. Vaccination for smallpox is an example of a therapeutic intradermal injection, although this also may be done by multiple skin punctures and scratches.

A fine needle is used, usually a 26-gauge. It is injected bevel side up very superficially. The lumen should barely be concealed by the skin. The medication is injected and forms a small raised area on the skin. The needle is removed quickly after the drug is injected.

TOPICAL DRUG ADMINISTRATION

When a drug is applied directly to a body site, it is referred to as a *topical application.*

Topical applications usually are intended for direct action on the particular site. The action is dependent on the type of tissue and the nature of the agent. For example, there are agents for making the skin secrete more or less or for causing vasodilatation or vasoconstriction.

In times past, the skin was rubbed with ointments intended for systemic effect, but this is not a practice now. The only other site that is used currently for obtaining a systemic effect via topical application is the rectum, and this is not often. There are few medications that can be administered via this route, such as aspirin or some tranquilizers.

If the site of application is readily accessible, such as the skin, an agent can be placed on it easily. If it is in the nature of a cavity, such as the nose, or enclosed as the eye is, it is necessary to use a mechanical applicator for introducing the drug.

Skin Applications

The skin is a mechanical and chemical barrier protecting the underlying tissues. It is a sense organ, having receptors which respond to touch, pain, pressure, and temperature. It aids in excretion, regulation of body temperature, and the storage of such body essentials as water, salts, and glucose.

The skin is composed of two main layers: the epidermis and the derma. The epidermis is composed of stratified squamous keratinizing epithelium. It has no blood vessels; its cells receive their nourishment from tissue fluid from the capillaries in the derma. The epidermis is not equally thick all over the body. It is thickest over the palms of the hands and the soles of the feet. The derma is composed of dense connective tissue. The skin also has three types of glands: sebaceous, sweat, and ceruminous. The sebaceous glands are found on the entire surface of the body except the palms and the soles. They are located in the derma, and their ducts open into the necks of hair follicles.

That some absorption into the body can take place via the skin has been proved. However, this is selective; therefore, only a few agents can be ab-

sorbed. Examples are lead and aniline dyes, both poisonous and hazardous in some industries.

When a drug is incorporated in a vehicle, such as powder, oil, lotion, or ointment, and is rubbed into the skin for absorption, the procedure is referred to as an *inunction.* On normal skin, drugs are absorbed into the lining of the sebaceous glands. Absorption is hindered because of the protective outer layer of the skin, which makes penetration difficult, and because of the fatty substances that protect the lining of the glands. Absorption can be enhanced by cleansing the skin well with soap or detergent and water prior to administration and then rubbing the medicated preparation into the skin. Absorption also can be improved by using the drug in a vehicle such as an ointment, or a volatile vehicle as used in many of the liniments, that will mix with the fat in the gland lining. The application of local heat also helps absorption by improving blood circulation in the area.

Examples of agents applied to the skin are as follows: oils, ointments, and creams to keep it soft; alcohol and other drying agents to reduce excessive secretions; antiperspirants to inhibit perspiration; and local counterirritants to relieve discomfort.

Eye Instillations

The receptors for the sense of sight are located in the eye. The outer layer of the eyeball is called the *sclera.* The *cornea* is the transparent part of the sclera in the front of the eyeball. The sclera is fibrous and tough, but the cornea is injured easily by trauma. For this reason, applications to the eye are rarely placed directly onto the eyeball.

The eyelids are two movable structures located in front of the eyeball. They offer protection to the front of the eye and aid in keeping the eye bathed in the secretion of the lacrimal gland. The eyelids meet near the nose at the *inner canthus* and near the temple at the *outer canthus.* The margins of the eyelids are fringed with eyelashes which aid in keeping foreign materials out of the eye.

The eyelids are lined with mucous membrane which forms two conjunctival sacs, one under the upper eyelid and the other under the lower eyelid. The conjunctival sac, a potential space, generally is described as being the space between the eyelids and the surface of the eyeball.

The lacrimal glands, which secrete tears, are situated on either side of the nose in the frontal bone. The glands empty into ducts that open in the conjunctival sacs. A lacrimal duct conveys excess fluid into the nose beneath the inferior concha.

Since direct application cannot be made onto the sensitive cornea, applications intended to act upon the eye or the lids are placed onto, instilled, or irrigated into the lower conjunctival sac.

The eye is a delicate organ, highly susceptible to infection and injury. Although the eye is never free of microorganisms, the secretions of the conjunctiva have a protective action against many pathogens. For maximum safety for the patient, equipment, solutions, and ointments introduced into the conjunctival sac should be sterile. If this is not possible, the most careful measures of medical asepsis should be followed.

EXPOSING THE LOWER CONJUNCTIVAL SAC. Exposing the conjunctival sacs is necessary for removing foreign bodies imbedded on or under the lids, for irrigations, or for the application of therapeutic agents to the eyeball or to the conjunctiva. When either conjunctival sac is exposed, it is important to work carefully and gently to prevent traumatizing the conjunctiva and the eyeball. This is of particular importance when the lids are swollen, inflamed, or tender.

To expose the conjunctiva of the lower lid, the patient should look up while the nurse places her thumb near the margin of the lower lid immediately below the eyelashes and exerts pressure downward over the bony prominence of the cheek. As the lower lid is pulled down and away from the eyeball, the conjunctival sac is exposed.

EXPOSING THE UPPER CONJUNCTIVAL SAC: Exposing the upper conjunctival sac requires practice to develop skill. It is referred to as *everting the eyelid*.

The patient is instructed to look down. The nurse grasps the lashes near the center of the upper lid with the thumb and the index finger of one hand and draws the lid downward and away from the eyeball. With the other hand, an applicator is placed horizontally along the upper part of the eyelid; while pressing downward on the applicator, the lid is turned up over the applicator very quickly. The index finger may be substituted for the applicator. Once the lid is everted, it may be held in place by shifting and pressing the thumb of the hand that held the applicator against the margin of the everted lid while the fingers rest on the patient's forehead. The patient continues to look downward during the entire procedure to prevent the lid from returning to its normal position. Eversion of the lid should be done with *gentleness*—never with force—to avoid injury to the eyeball and the conjunctiva.

INSTILLATIONS OF EYEDROPS: Eyedrops are in-

stilled for local effects, such as for dilatation or contraction of the pupil for examining the eye or treating an infection. The type and the amount of solution will depend on the purpose of the instillation.

An eye dropper is used to instill drops of solution. No more solution than is needed should be drawn into the eye dropper, because it is unsafe practice to return unused solution to the stock bottle. Once the solution has been drawn into the dropper, the dropper is held with the bulb uppermost. Allowing the solution to enter the rubber bulb by holding the bulb lower than the dropper may result in contaminating the solution with fine particles of rubber.

The patient should be given an absorbent tissue so that he may have it in readiness when drops are instilled. The lids and the lashes are wiped clean prior to the instillation. Hold the dropper close to the eye but avoid touching the eyelids or the eyelashes. This prevents injury should the patient become startled by the sensation of the dropper touching him. The lower conjunctival sac is exposed, and the prescribed number of drops of solution are allowed to fall into the center of the exposed sac. Drops should not be allowed to fall directly onto the cornea because of the danger of injuring it and because of the unpleasant sensation it creates for the patient. The patient should be asked to close his eyelids and move the eye. This helps to distribute the solution over the conjunctival surfaces and the anterior eyeball. Figure 28-19 shows the instillation of eyedrops.

APPLICATION OF OINTMENT TO THE EYE: Various types of drugs in an ointment base may be prescribed for the eyelids or the conjunctiva.

The eyelids and the eyelashes should be cleansed of secretions and crusts before applying the ointment. Eye ointments usually are dispensed in a tube. A small amount of the ointment is distributed along the conjunctival sac after everting the lower lid. The ointment is squeezed from the tube, but care should be taken to avoid touching the eye or the conjunctiva. Following the application, the eyelids should be closed. The warmth will help to liquefy the ointment. The patient should also be instructed to move his eye. This will aid in spreading the ointment under the lids and over the surface of the eyeball.

Ear Instillations

The ear contains the receptors for hearing and for equilibrium. It consists of the external ear, the middle ear, and the inner ear.

The external ear consists of the *auricle* or *pinna*

and the *exterior auditory canal*. The auricle has very little function in man. The auditory canal serves as a passageway for sound waves. Drugs or irrigations are instilled into the auditory canal.

In adults, the auditory canal is directed inward, forward, and downward. The outer portion is cartilaginous, and the inner portion consists of osseous tissue. In an infant, the canal is chiefly cartilaginous and is almost straight, but the floor of the auditory canal rests on the tympanic membrane. The direction of the canal is important to consider when administering treatments to the ear. In order for solution to reach all parts of the canal, the pinna should be pulled downward and backward for infants; for adults, upward and backward. The ear is grasped on the cartilaginous portion of the pinna when straightening the canal.

The lining of the auditory canal consists of modified epithelium. It contains ceruminous glands, which secrete wax found in the ear, and the hair follicles.

The tympanic membrane separates the external ear from the middle ear. Normally, it is intact and closes the entrance to the middle ear completely. If it is ruptured or has been opened by surgical intervention, the middle ear and the inner ear have a direct passage to the external ear. When this occurs, instillations and irrigations should be done with great care to prevent forcing materials from the outer ear into the middle ear and the inner ear, which may result in serious infection.

Normally, the ear is not a sterile cavity. However, if the tympanic membrane is not intact, surgical asepsis should be observed.

INSTILLATION OF EARDROPS: Drugs in solution are placed in the auditory canal for their local effect. They are used to soften wax, relieve pain, apply local anesthesia, destroy organisms, or destroy an insect lodged in the canal which can cause almost intolerable discomfort.

It is more comfortable for the patient if the solution is warmed to approximately body temperature. A dropper is used to instill the solution. The ear canal is straightened, and the drops are allowed

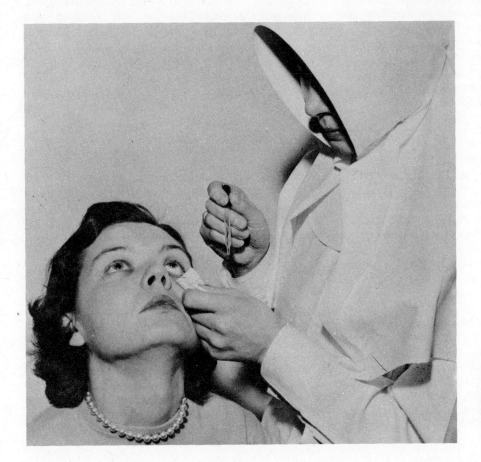

Fig. 28-19. The nurse uses a wipe to protect her finger from slipping while instilling eyedrops. The patient is asked to look up, and the lower lid is everted so that the conjunctival sac is exposed.

to fall on the side of the canal. The patient lies on his side with the ear to be treated uppermost and remains in this position following instillation to prevent the drops from escaping from the canal. Occasionally, a loose cotton wick is inserted into the canal in order to maintain a continuous application of the solution instilled. A wick is never packed into the ear because it interferes with outward movement of normal secretions and could create excessive pressure.

Nasal Instillations

Besides serving as the olfactory organ, the nose also functions as an airway to the lower respiratory tract and protects the tract by cleansing and warming the air that is taken in by inspiration. Small hairs, called *cilia*, project on most of the surface of the nasal mucous membrane and are important to aid in removing particles of dirt and dust from the inspired air. The nose also serves as a resonator when speaking and singing.

The nose is divided into the right and the left chambers by the nasal septum. There are four pairs of nasal sinuses that communicate with the nasal fossa: the frontal, the ethmoid, the maxillary, and the sphenoid sinuses. Normally, these are filled with air and lined with mucous membrane similar to that which lines the nose.

Because of the position of the nose, secretions from it drain out easily when the person is in the upright position. Because of its connection with the upper respiratory tract and the mouth, secretions drain back into that area when the person is reclining.

Normally, the nose is not a sterile cavity. However, because of its connection with the sinuses, utmost caution should be taken when introducing anything into it.

INSTILLATION OF NOSEDROPS: Medications instilled into the nares are used primarily for the relief of nasal congestion. Most authorities recommend using a drug in normal saline solution, since oily solutions tend to interfere with the normal ciliary action in the nose and, if aspirated, may result in a pneumonitis. Anesthetics and antiseptics also may be instilled into the nose for their local effects.

Paper wipes should be provided for the patient. The patient is assisted to a sitting position with his head tilted back, or he lies in bed with his head tilted back. This position allows the solution to flow back into the nares. Sufficient solution for both nares is drawn into a dropper. The dropper is placed just inside the nares, approximately one-third inch,

and the number of drops prescribed is instilled. Touching the dropper to the nares may create a desire to sneeze. The patient should be instructed to keep his head tilted back for several minutes to prevent the escape of solution from the anterior nares. The patient usually will wish to expectorate solution that runs down into the oropharynx and the mouth.

When instilling drops into the nares of an infant or an irrational patient, the tip of the dropper should be protected with a piece of soft rubber tubing to minimize the danger of injuring the nasal mucous membrane.

NASAL SPRAY: Solutions that are instilled by drops also may be applied to the nasal mucous membrane by using a spray. A small atomizer generally is used.

The end of the nose is held up, and the tip of the nozzle is placed just inside the nares and directed backward. Only sufficient force is used to bring the spray into contact with the membrane. Too much force may drive the solution and the contamination into the sinuses and the eustachian tubes.

Throat Applications

The throat, more properly called the *pharynx*, is divided into three portions: nasal, oral, and laryngeal. The pharynx communicates with the nasal cavity anteriorly, with the oral cavity below this, and with the laryngeal cavity below the oral pharynx. The eustachian tubes open into the nasopharynx. The pharynx is a muscular passageway and is lined with modified epithelium.

The pharynx is a passageway for air. The oral and the laryngeal portions also serve as a passageway for food.

The adenoids or *pharyngeal tonsils* are located in the nasopharynx. The *palatine tonsils* are in the oral pharynx. The tonsils and the adenoids are composed of lymphoid tissue and often become the seat of infections.

The throat obviously is not a sterile area. However, practices of medical asepsis are observed, especially in caring for the equipment after use. The mouth harbors microorganisms that could be harmful to others.

THROAT SPRAYS AND PAINTS: Antiseptics and anesthetics may be applied to the throat by spraying and by painting the area. The patient's head is tilted back, and his tongue is held down with a tongue depressor. The solution either is sprayed or painted onto the tissues. A cotton applicator is effective for painting. When a spray is used, more force is necessary to reach tissues in the throat than is necessary when using a nasal spray.

LOZENGES: Lozenges may contain drugs that are used for the local treatment of the mouth and the throat. Cough drops are an example. When sucked, the lozenge liberates the active ingredient, and, when the solution is swallowed, the mouth and the throat are bathed in it. The use of lozenges is unsatisfactory for reaching all parts of the throat. The patient should be instructed to suck the lozenge since chewing or swallowing it shortens the period of contact with the tissues and decreases its effectiveness.

Vaginal Applications

The vagina is a musculomembranous canal extending from the outside of the body at the vulva to the cervix uteri. It lies between the bladder and the rectum. The size and the shape vary, but it is capable of distending greatly as during childbirth. The anterior wall usually is about 3 to 6 inches long, while the posterior wall is 5 to 7 inches long. Normally, the walls of the vagina are in contact with each other.

Normally, the vagina contains few pathogens but many nonpathogenic organisms. The nonpathogens are important, since they protect the vagina from the invasion of pathogens. The normal secretions in the vagina are acid in reaction and further serve to protect the vagina from microbial invasion. Therefore, the normal mucous membrane is its own best protection.

Creams can be applied intravaginally, using a narrow tubular applicator with an attached plunger. Suppositories that melt when exposed to body heat are also prepared for vaginal insertion. Suppositories should normally be refrigerated for storage.

Patients using intravaginal medications should be instructed in the technique of administration and to wear a perineal pad to avoid soiling clothing.

Rectal Applications

Rectal suppositories are used primarily for their local action, although some systemic effect does occur. Rectal installation are also occasionally used. The techniques for rectal applications were discussed in Chapter 26.

Urethral Applications

Urethral suppositories are used primarily for their local action, although they do have some systemic effect. Their insertion is the same as with vaginal and rectal suppositories, except sterile technique is used because the urethra is normally sterile.

TEACHING THE PATIENT TO TAKE HIS OWN MEDICATIONS

The nurse is often responsible for teaching medication administration to the patient or if this is not possible, to a family member. The technique described should be explained and demonstrated until the patient or family member is sure of understanding. Parenteral and topical techniques should be practiced by the patient in the presence of the nurse until the patient has acquired sufficient skill for safe administration.

Besides the technique, patients need clear explanations as to the dosage and frequency of the drug administration. Studies have shown that the most frequent cause for errors in self administered drugs is a lack of understanding about the dose and the frequency of taking the medication. Written instructions are best. Color-coding systems or other reminders, can also be useful aids.

The patient generally also needs to be aware of what effect is desired from the drug and what indications of undesirable effects are possible. Patients whose drug therapy is explained as an integral part of their health state generally are more conscientious about maintaining the regimen.

CONCLUSION

Drugs are an important part of both health maintenance and health restoration. The nurse works with other health team members and plays a major role in observing the responses of patients to medications, as well as in helping patients to learn about the drugs prescribed for them. She also frequently administers drugs to patients. Her knowledge and resulting judgment, observational ability, and technical skills are all important to the patient's therapeutic drug regimen.

Because new medications are continually being introduced, drug therapy is an area where the nurse's education can never stop. With many patients receiving a number of drugs simultaneously, her awareness of the incompatibility of various medications is of particular importance.

Study Situations

1. Various studies have shown that a high degree of inaccuracy often occurs in self-administered medications. The following article discusses the problem.

    Hecht, A. B.: "Self-medication, inaccuracy, and what can be done," **Nurs. Outlook,** 18:30–31, Apr., 1970. *What reasons does the author give to explain why patients make medication errors? What suggestions does she have for improving patient accuracy?*

2. Increase your awareness of how much self-medication advertising is done by looking for advertisements concerning the following items: eye drops to relieve eye fatigue or to beautify the eyes, nose drops to stop hay fever or to relieve colds, antiseptics for feminine hygiene, and throat gargles to avoid colds. *Look carefully at the wording of these advertisements. Examine the labels and determine if it is possible for the products to produce the results they claim.*

3. It has been indicated that detection of the patient's responses to his medication is one of the major functions of the nurse. In Chapter 6, when the data-gathering process was discussed, the first phase was the need to select the appropriate data. Since responses to medications vary, depending on the drug's actions, one must be knowledgeable about specific drugs before pertinent data can be gathered. Practice data collection regarding a patient's response to his drugs. What data would be appropriate to collect? How will you collect it? How will you validate it?

4. Some authorities refer to drug abuse as an epidemic in this country. *What are some of the ways in which the authors of the following article suggest nurses can assist with the problem?*

    Long, B. L., and Krepick, D. S.: New perspectives on drug abuse. *In* **The Nursing Clinics of North America.** Philadelphia, W. B. Saunders, 8:25–40, Mar., 1973.

5. The right patient, medication, route, dose, technique, and time have been identified as six rights of patients regarding drug administration. The authors of the following article suggest another right of the patient. Conway, B., et al.: The seventh right. **Am. J. Nurs.,** 70:1040–1043, May, 1970.

    What is the seventh right? What recommendations do the authors make for achieving it?

References

1. Brandt, P. A., et al.: IM injections in children. **Am. J. Nurs.,** 72:1402–1406, Aug., 1972.

2. Budd, R.: We changed to unit-dose system. **Nurs. Outlook,** 19:116–117, Feb., 1971.

3. Burke, E. L.: Insulin injection: the site and the technique. **Am. J. Nurs.,** 72:2194–2196, Dec., 1972.

4. Cockerham, M. F.: Self-Medication. **Hospitals, J. Am. Hosp. Assoc.,** 44:57–58, Jan. 16, 1970.

5. Emmanuel, Sr.: The clinical pharmacist and his relationship to nursing practice. **Hosp. Manage.,** 109:45–53, May, 1970.

6. FDA fact sheet.: Rockville, Md., U. S. Department of Health, Education, and Welfare, Public Health Service, Food and Drug Administration, May, 1972.

7. Fulton, A.: Control system for medication cards. **Am. J. Nurs.,** 71:2162, Nov., 1971.

8. Grim, R. A.: Mr. Edwards' Triumph. **Am. J. Nurs.,** 72:480–481, Mar., 1972.

9. Howard-Jones, N.: The origins of hypodermic medications. **Sci. Am.,** 224:96–102, Jan., 1971.

10. How to give an intramuscular injection. Reprint from **Spectrum,** Winter, 1964–1965.

11. Hutchinson, R. A.: Adverse drug reactions—a review. **Hosp. Top.,** 48:69–76, Sept., 1970.

12. Krueger, E. A.: The Hypodermic Injection. A Programmed Unit. New York, Teachers College Press, Teachers College, Columbia University, 1966.

13. Leary, J. A., et al.: Self-administered medications. **Am. J. Nurs.,** 71:1193–1194, June, 1971.

14. Levine, M. E.: Breaking through the medications mystique. **Am. J. Nurs.,** 70:799–803, Apr., 1970.

15. Marks, J., and Clarke, M.: The hospital patient and his knowledge of the drugs he is receiving. **Int. Nurs. Rev.,** 19:39–50, No. 1, 1972.

16. Mead, W. B.: Unit-dose drug packaging. **Hospitals, J. Am. Hosp. Assoc.,** 44:85–87, Jan. 16, 1970.

17. Michel, F.: The vexing core. **Am. J. Nurs.,** 71:768, Apr., 1971.

18. Mohney, S.: Some important clues to adverse drug reactions. **RN,** 36:48–49; 88–93, Mar., 1973.

19. Payne, J. E., and Kaplan, H. M.: Alternative techniques for venipuncture. **Am. J. Nurs.,** 72:702–703, Apr., 1972.

20. Pitel, M.: The subcutaneous injection. **Am. J. Nurs.,** 71:76–79, Jan., 1971.

21. Rauch, P.: Avoiding injuries from injections. **Nurs. '72,** 2:12, May, 1972.

22. Schneiter, L. J.: Nurse meets pharmacy technician. **Hospitals, J. Am. Hosp. Assoc.,** 45:62–68; 122, Nov. 1, 1971.

23. Schultz, S. M., et al.: Medication errors reduced by unit-dose. **Hospitals, J. Am. Hosp. Assoc.,** 47:106–112, Mar. 16, 1973.

24. Shaffer, J. H., and Sweet, L. C.: Allergic reactions to drugs. **Am. J. Nurs.,** 65:100–103, Oct., 1965.

25. Teitelbaum, A. C.: Intra-arterial drug therapy. **Am. J. Nurs.,** 72:1634–1637, Sept., 1972.

26. U100 insulin. *In* **The Nursing Clinics of North America.** Philadelphia, W. B. Saunders, 8:369, June, 1973.

CHAPTER 29

Promoting Tissue Healing

GLOSSARY · INTRODUCTION · THE BODY'S REACTION TO TRAUMA ·
GENERAL PRINCIPLES RELATED TO TISSUE HEALING ·
NURSING MEASURES TO PROMOTE TISSUE HEALING ·
CONCLUSION · STUDY SITUATIONS · REFERENCES

GLOSSARY

Abrasion: Wound resulting from scraping or rubbing off skin or mucous membrane.

Bandage: Length of material applied in manner to fit a body part.

Binder: Type of bandage designed for a large body part.

Conduction: Direct transferring from one substance to another.

Contusion: A bruise.

Convection: Transfer of heat by mass movement.

Débridement: Cleaning away of infected and devitalized tissue from a wound.

Diathermy: High frequency currents used to produce heat in body tissue.

Granulation Tissue: New tissue composed of fibroblasts and small blood vessels.

Hyperemia: Increased blood supply to an area.

Hypothermia: Artificially lowering temperature of body tissue.

Incision: Wound made with a sharp cutting instrument.

Inflammation: Defensive local response of the body to injury.

Insulator: Substance that is a poor conductor.

Irrigation: Cleansing of an area with a flowing solution.

Laceration: Wound caused by a blunt instrument or object that tears tissue.

Montgomery Straps: Method for securing a dressing which does not necessitate tape removal with every dressing change.

Puncture Wound: Wound caused by an object that penetrates the tissues. Synonym is stab wound.

Purulent: Contains pus.

Radiation: Transfer of energy in the form of waves.

Sanguineous: Containing or mixed with blood.

Scultetus Binder: Many-tailed binder.

Serous: Resembling blood serum.

Suppuration: Process of pus formation.

Trauma: Injury.

INTRODUCTION

The tissues of the body are remarkably resistive to injury. When tissue injury or damage does occur, the restorative powers of the body are amazing. The healing process is partially the result of the body's response mechanisms to the trauma. The response is systemic, that is, the total body as well as the local area is involved. Although both trauma and the responses to it can be psychic as well as physiologic in nature, in this chapter the discussion will be limited to the local physical response to trauma.

The body's response to injury and the healing process are both normal protective mechanisms, and modern science has found no way to improve on them. Nevertheless, there are some actions that can be taken to support or assist these mechanisms. The body's reactions and ways in which the nurse can support the healing processes will be discussed in this chapter.

THE BODY'S REACTION TO TRAUMA

Trauma is a general term referring to an injury. Tissue injury can occur from a variety of causes, such as from physical pressure or force, temperature extremes, chemical substances, radiation, and pathogenic organisms. An injury or wound may be open or closed. An *open wound* is characterized by a break in the continuity of the skin. When there is no break in the skin the wound is said to be a *closed wound*.

Wounds may be classified as either accidental or intentional. An accidental wound is an injury due to a mishap, while an intentional wound is purposely created by the surgeon for therapeutic purposes.

The most common closed accidental wound is a *contusion*, or a bruise. (Occasionally open wounds may exist along with contusions.) Contusions usually occur as the result of force being applied to the tissue. There may be extensive soft tissue damage with ruptured blood vessels. The escape of blood into the subcutaneous tissue is what gives the characteristic bluish color to the injury. Contusions may occur in readily visible parts of the body, or they may occur internally when other than visible symptoms indicate their presence. Brain contusions, for example, may follow a head injury with no external evidence of trauma. The same may be true of some abdominal organ injuries.

Open wounds may be classified according to the nature of the break in the continuity of normal tissue. An *incision* is a wound made with a sharp cutting instrument. It is the kind of wound that is made by the surgeon when he cuts tissue to enter the field of operation. Incised wounds also may occur by accident, as when one is cut with a knife, a sharp piece of glass, or a razor.

An *abrasion* is a wound that results from scraping or rubbing off skin or mucous membrane. A "floor burn" is a typical abrasive wound.

A *puncture* or *stab* wound is caused by an object that penetrates into tissue. Injuries from nails and bullets result in puncture wounds. A surgeon may make a puncture wound to promote drainage.

A *laceration* is a wound caused by a blunt instrument or object that tears tissue. Falls against angular surfaces or cuts with irregular edges of broken glass frequently result in lacerated wounds.

Any combination of these last three types of wounds may also occur. For example, falling on broken glass may result in a wound that has lacerations as well as punctures and abrasions.

Both open and closed wounds can be invaded by pathogens and an infection can result. The entrance of microorganisms into an accidental open wound can easily occur from contamination by the instrument causing the injury. Pathogens in an intentional wound generally occur as the result of poor aseptic technique or a break in it. An infection in a closed wound is usually the result of the presence of pathogens in the blood. Tissue damage lowers the body's normal defenses against infection, and, in addition, the escaped blood of a contusion provides a site favorable for the growth of organisms. The body's normal reaction to any kind of wound is inflammation.

Inflammation

Inflammation is the defensive local response of the body to the injury. Inflammation works to limit the tissue damage, remove the injured cells, and repair the traumatized tissue. The inflammatory response occurs in three stages: vascular, exudative, and reparative.

VASCULAR STAGE: The vascular stage is characterized by an immediate and brief constriction of the vessels in the area following the trauma. Then the vessels quickly dilate. The increased blood supply to the area is called *hyperemia* and causes the characteristic redness and warmth of the area. The resulting changes due to the filtration pressure of the blood and the increased permeability of the capillaries allow for the movement of plasma, blood cells, and antibodies into the interstitial spaces. The phagocytic process whereby leukocytes engulf the foreign substances and damaged cells is initiated.

EXUDATIVE STAGE: The exudative stage of inflammation is characterized by the formation of the fluid exudate. The exudate is made up of the fluid and cells from the blood, the damaged tissue cells, and any foreign bodies. The amount of exudate varies with the extent of the injury. In minor injuries very little exudate will form while in extensive injuries large quantities will collect. In a mild injury, such as a blister, the exudate will be *serous* in nature; that is, it resembles blood serum. When the wound is infected, the exudate is described as *purulent* and is called pus. The process of pus formation is referred to as *suppuration*. An extensive injury can result in an exudate containing large amounts of fibrinogen and is called a *fibrinous* exudate. Or if erythrocytes are found in the exudate, it is referred to as a *hemorrhagic* or *sanguinous* exudate. The collection of the exudate in the interstitial spaces will cause swelling and localized pain. Depending on the location and extent of the injury, the exudate collection can also cause loss of function of the part.

REPARATIVE STAGE: The reparative stage of the inflammatory process is characterized by the replacement of the damaged tissue cells by the regeneration of new cells or by scar tissue. This stage is often referred to as wound healing.

Wound Healing

Although authorities differ somewhat in their descriptions of wound healing, it is usually said to have three phases. Generally, it is difficult to characterize any particular wound because the phases can be occurring simultaneously in various parts of the wound. The three phases are lag, fibroblastic, and contraction.

The *lag phase* occurs first, when blood, serum, and red blood cells form a fibrin network in the wound. The edges of the wound are glued together by this network, or scab, as it usually is called. If the damaged tissue is then healed by replacement of the tissue cells by similar ones, the healing is said to be by regeneration.

The *fibroplasia phase* is characterized by the growth of fibroblasts along and in the fibrin network. As this occurs, the fibrin network is gradually absorbed. These fibroblasts and accompanying small blood vessels are called *granulation tissue*, which grows to restore the continuity of the injured tissue. It is very friable, soft, and pinkish red in color. Epithelial cells then commence to grow from the edges to cover the wound. Depending on the extent of the wound, connective tissue cells then fill in the area and become the *scar* which is considerably stronger than the granulation tissue. This is known as replacement healing.

The *phase of contraction* is characterized by the disappearance of the small blood vessels in the new tissue and by a shrinkage of the scar. This phase may last indefinitely.

The strength of the wound is slight until it has progressed well into the fibroplasia phase. Scar tissue is strong, but it does not have the elasticity of normal tissue; therefore, it is desirable that healing occur with a minimum of scar formation, especially in an area where tension and pressure normally are present.

If a large area has been denuded (i.e., when a large area of skin has been removed) as a result of either an accident or surgery, it may be difficult or even impossible to approximate the edges of a wound. It has been observed that epithelium from the periphery of a wound continues to grow for only a certain distance and then stops. When the process of repairing a wound halts, a chronic ulcer or unhealed area develops on the denuded surface. This often becomes the site of infection, and tissue debris accumulates. Cleaning of an area of this sort is called *débridement*. It is done primarily to remove necrotic tissue and foreign material and to improve drainage from the wound in order to promote further wound healing. If healing still does not occur following débridement, it may be necessary to close the wound by using skin grafts.

HEALING BY FIRST INTENTION: Healing by first intention is the return of the tissues to normal with minimal inflammation and scarring. This process occurs when no infection is present and when the edges of the wound are well-approximated. Sutures or various adhesive materials may be used to keep the edges of the wound together. Pressure may be used also by the proper application of materials that will secure dressings in place and aid approximation of the wound edges.

Few accidental wounds heal by first intention. Surgeons strive for and usually attain healing of a surgical incision by first intention.

HEALING BY SECOND INTENTION: Secondary intention healing occurs when infection is present. The process of healing is prolonged. There is usually more extensive tissue injury and a purulent exudate, and approximation of the edges of the wound is difficult or even impossible. Extensive granulation tissue is required to fill the wound.

HEALING BY THIRD INTENTION: Third intention healing occurs when secondary wound closure is necessary. The extensiveness of the wound or the exudate may necessitate leaving the edges unapproximated for repeated débridement or drainage, or occasionally the approximated wound edges may disrupt. In either case, when the final tissue approximation is delayed or must be repeated, the process is called secondary closure. Following the wound closure, healing then occurs by secondary intention.

GENERAL PRINCIPLES RELATED TO TISSUE HEALING

The healthy body has an innate capacity to protect and restore itself. Increasing the blood supply to the damaged area, walling off and removing cellular and foreign debris, and initiating the cellular development are parts of the healing process. It occurs normally without assistance although there are some medical and nursing actions that can help to support the process. The body's ability to respond to the tissue trauma is affected by the extent of the damage and the person's general state of health. The healthy individual who sustains a massive injury, the person with a chronic disease, or the very young and very old who experience minimal injury frequently will have some limitations on their capacity to deal adequately with the insult. The promotion of high-level wellness is, of course, partially directed toward maintaining adequate body reserves to deal with traumatic occurrences. The person will respond more adequately to injury if he has fluid and electrolyte balance, proper nourishment, and adequate rest.

The body responds systemically to trauma of its parts. It has been stated earlier that physiologic functioning of the body cannot be separated from the psychological. Similarly, local physical responses to an injury cannot be separated from an overall bodily reaction. For example, an injured foot or hand or an abdominal incision can cause a variety of systemic reactions that include an increase in body temperature, heart and respiratory rates, anorexia or nausea and vomiting, skeletal muscle tension throughout the body, and harmful hormonal changes. Because the body's response to injury is systemic, supportive or therapeutic measures should be directed toward the whole person. Adequate rest, relief of emotional tensions, and sufficient nutrients and fluids are particularly important for the person undergoing a response to trauma. Local measures for promoting desirable tissue responses will be discussed later in this chapter.

The blood serves as the means for transporting substances essential for effective trauma response to and from body cells. An adequate blood supply is fundamental to the body's normal response to any local injury. The blood brings increased erythrocytes, leukocytes, and platelets to the site. Antibodies are also carried by the plasma. The removal of toxins and debris and the supplying of nutrients, oxygen, and other cellular-building materials are provided by increased circulation to the damaged site. Any preexisting condition, such as cardiac or vascular pathology or anemia, or a factor from the injury which results in circulatory impairment, such as extensive blood loss, can inhibit normal response to trauma.

Intact skin and mucous membrane serve as first lines of defense against harmful agents, and a break in the skin continuity increases the likelihood of pathogen entry. Because the person's primary protective barrier is weakened when skin or mucous membrane breaks, the need for artificially preventing microorganism invasion becomes paramount. Careful handwashing before caring for the wound is probably the single most effective method for preventing secondary infection. While it is not possible to sterilize the skin, surgical asepsis is used with persons who have an open wound to minimize the possibility of pathogen entry. Precautions are also taken

for persons with closed wounds because of the lowered resistance of the damaged tissue to infection and the possibility of pathogenic organisms being present.

Normal healing occurs when the wound is free of foreign bodies. The reparative stage will generally not start until foreign bodies are removed from the wound. Excessive exudate, dead or damaged tissue cells, pathogenic organisms, or imbedded fragments of bone, metal, glass, or other substances can all act as foreign bodies. The body's own rejection mechanisms generally are sufficient to remove many foreign substances. In some instances, however, mechanical means may be employed to assist the process. There are some situations in which the body walls off a collection of pus or another foreign body and healing occurs around it. This is known as an *abscess.* In most instances, it can be expected that the individual will develop symptoms of the unhealed site, although they may be delayed in their appearance.

NURSING MEASURES TO PROMOTE TISSUE HEALING

The inflammatory and healing processes normally occur spontaneously. Nursing measures which support the desirable aspects of these processes include using heat and cold applications, cleansing the area, immobilizing and protecting the wound, and promoting exudate drainage.

Heat and Cold Applications

THE BODY'S REACTION TO EXPOSURE TO HEAT AND COLD: It will be recalled that cells in the hypothalamus act as a thermostat to regulate body temperature. The anterior cells of the hypothalamus are vasodilating and heat-dissipating while the posterior or caudal cells are vasoconstricting and heat-conserving. These cells receive impulses through somatic and visceral neurons in the brain and the spinal cord. The skin plays an important role in maintaining body temperature through the activity of its sweat glands and its pilomotor muscles. When one is exposed to warm surroundings, the sweat glands secrete perspiration. The body cools when the perspiration changes from liquid to vapor. Evaporation requires heat; hence, heat is released. When exposed to cold surroundings, the pilomotor muscles contract and make the hair stand on end in animals and cause "gooseflesh" in man. This phenomenon is the body's attempt to conserve internal body heat. Shivering, also under hypothalamus regulation (lateral cells), generates considerable body heat by agitating the muscles.

The caliber of the cutaneous blood vessels also plays an important role in maintaining body temperature. The smaller the caliber, the smaller will be the quantity of heat brought by the blood to the surface of the skin and lost to the environment. The larger the caliber, the larger the quantity of heat brought to the surface and lost. This phenomenon can be observed when the skin appears flushed as the body becomes too warm, and pale as the body becomes too cool. The blood vessels in the skin are capable of containing large or small quantities of blood, and their caliber increases or decreases as the local and the general needs of the body change. The change in caliber of the blood vessels is regulated by the vasomotor centers (dilator and constrictor) in the medulla oblongata of the brain stem, under hypothalmic influence.

TEMPERATURE RECEPTORS IN THE SKIN: When receptors for heat and cold are stimulated, they set up impulses that are carried to the hypothalamus and the cerebral cortex via the somatic afferent fibers. The conscious sensation of temperature is aroused in the cerebral cortex, while the hypothalamus serves as a reflex center to integrate somatic and visceral motor responses to maintain a normal temperature.

Receptors for cold lie superficially, while those for heat are located deeper in the skin. The density of receptors varies; in some parts of the body they are more numerous than in others. The cold receptors, for example, are particularly numerous on the thorax and the upper limbs. The cold receptors are estimated to be approximately eight to ten times more numerous than receptors for heat.

There is difference of opinion concerning receptors for high temperatures. It is more generally agreed that, when hot stimuli are received by the skin, the pain receptors are also stimulated, and the sensation of burning is the result of this double stimulation of receptors. A less widely accepted theory is that a second type of heat receptor in the skin with a very high threshold is stimulated when hot objects touch the skin.

An important characteristic of heat and cold receptors is that they adjust readily if the stimulus is not extreme. For example, if the arm is placed in warm water, the sensation of warmth soon diminishes because of the adaptability of the heat re-

ceptors. The same phenomenon occurs if cool water is used. It is important to remember the ability of receptors to adapt to heat and cold when using hot and cold applications. Once the receptors adapt, the patient may become unaware of temperature extremes until tissue damage occurs.

TOLERANCE OF THE SKIN TO TEMPERATURE: The temperature that the skin can tolerate varies with individuals. Some can tolerate warmer and colder applications more safely than can others. Certain areas of the skin are also more tolerant of temperature variations than are other areas. Those parts of the body where the skin is somewhat thinner generally are more sensitive to temperature variations than exposed areas where the skin is often thicker. Therefore, it is important to apply warm and cold applications well within the generally known safe limits of temperature variations. But, in addition, the skin should be observed so that persons who are more sensitive to temperature changes will not receive tissue damage, even though applications have been applied within recommended temperature range.

Water is a better conductor of heat than air. This fact is used in guiding action whenever heat or cold is applied to the skin, since the skin will tolerate greater extremes of temperature if the heat or the cold is dry rather than moist. For example, a moist hot dressing should be applied at a lower temperature than a cloth-covered hot water bottle in order to prevent burning the skin. This is because the air between cloth fibers acts as an insulator.

The body tolerates greater extremes in temperature when the duration of exposure is short. When duration is lengthy, the temperature range that the body can tolerate safely is narrower. The area involved is also important. In general, the larger the area to which heat or cold is applied, the less tolerant is the skin to extremes in temperature.

The condition of the patient is an important factor to consider when heat and cold are being applied to the body. Certain patients are sensitive to physical agents and tolerate heat and cold poorly. Special care also is indicated for patients who are debilitated, unconscious, or insensitive to cutaneous stimulation. Patients who have disturbances in circulation are more sensitive to heat and cold. Broken skin areas are also more subject to tissue damage, since the subcutaneous tissue is less tolerant of heat and cold, and the temperature and pain senses may be impaired and unable to heed warning stimuli.

DEFINITIONS OF HEAT AND COLD: Until late

in the eighteenth century, heat was believed to be a kind of fluid that could flow from one substance to another. This theory was refuted when it was found that heat was related to motion. Heat is defined as the average kinetic energy (energy of motion) of the molecules of the material.

Cold is a relative term. It is used to mean that a material has a relatively low temperature, that is, little or no warmth. In other words, as motion of the molecules decreases, the heat is less, and the material is said to be cool or cold. Absolute zero is the temperature at which molecular motion ceases. Theoretically, this occurs at a hypothetical point 273° below zero on the centigrade scale. The important thing to realize is that for all practical purposes, heat is present in all material, therefore, discussions concerning the nature of heat apply also to those of cold. However, the *effects* of applying something warm to the human body are different from the effects of applying something cool, as will be later illustrated.

TRANSFER OF HEAT: Heat is transferred by radiation, convection, and conduction.

The transfer of heat in the form of waves is called *radiation*. For example, heat can be felt by placing the hand near a light bulb. The heat has been transferred to the hand by radiation.

Heat transferred by *convection* travels in mass movements. Air expands and rises as it warms; cold air acts oppositely. Convection explains the phenomenon of wind, since the unequal heating of the earth's surfaces produces air currents.

When heat is transferred directly from one substance to another, it is called conduction. Local applications of heat and cold transfer heat to and from the body by conduction. A poor conductor is called an *insulator*. Many of the actions that nurses take when applying heat or cold to the body are guided by a knowledge of the transmission of heat by conduction. These are some examples:

If hot water bottles were made of metal, they would conduct heat so rapidly that the patient would be burned, since metals are good conductors of heat. Even rubber is a fairly good conductor; therefore, hot water bottles are covered with cloth before applying to the patient. Cloth is a good insulator because of its many air traps, air being a rather poor conductor of heat.

Before hot wet packs are applied to an area, the skin is lubricated with petrolatum, which acts as an insulator, since it slows down the transmission of heat.

Metal bedpans should be warmed before offering them to patients. The metal, a good conductor, removes heat from the body so rapidly that the area of the bedpan in contact with the patient will feel uncomfortably cold if it has not been warmed.

EFFECTS OF LOCAL APPLICATION OF COLD: When cold is applied to the skin, the first visible reaction is vasoconstriction; that is, the caliber of the cutaneous vessels decreases. The skin becomes cool and pale. The skin receptors for cold are stimulated, the impulses are carried to the hypothalamus and the cerebral cortex, and the body reacts to conserve heat. The constriction of blood vessels reduces circulation in the skin in order that heat may be conserved by preventing loss of heat from the blood to the environment. This vasoconstriction limits the reaction of the vascular stage in the inflammatory process.

In addition to vasoconstriction, there is a decrease in tissue metabolism in the area involved. Less oxygen is used, and fewer wastes accumulate. Cold also has an anesthetic effect on the skin, an important point to remember when applying cold applications, since the patient may become unaware of impulses from the skin which normally serve to warn that tissue damage is occurring.

Cold commonly is used immediately following contusions, sprains, and strains in order to limit the accumulation of fluid in body tissue. If edema is already present, the application of cold will act to retard its relief, since circulating blood in the area is at a minimum, and excess fluid will not be reabsorbed as efficiently. The application of cold will aid in controlling hemorrhage by constricting vessels. Cold has practical uses for its anesthetic value. For example, areas of the body can be anesthetized and surgery performed without the patient feeling pain. Lower temperatures are also used for limiting inflammation and suppuration by decreasing blood supply, slowing cellular metabolism, and inhibiting microbial activity.

Cold also affects remote areas of the body when applied locally. The amount of blood in other parts of the body increases as blood decreases in the part to which cold is applied because blood volume normally remains quite constant. When the body is chilled, it has been observed that vasoconstriction occurs in the nasal passages. This reaction explains the uncomfortable and harmful effects of cold and drafts when one is suffering with an upper respiratory infection.

Studies have been conducted to determine the depth to which cold penetrates the body when applied to a local area. One such study showed the following results when an ice bag was placed on the leg (18:6):

Interior of ice bag	32° F.
Outside of towel covering ice bag	40° F.
Cutaneous temperature declined from	84° F. to 43° F.
(in 15 minutes)	
Subcutaneous temperature declined from	94° F. to 70° F.
(in about 1 hour)	
Intramuscular temperature declined from	98° F. to 79° F.
(in about 2 hours)	

When cold air was blown over the leg, similar local temperature changes were noted, and more remote areas also were cooled.

Cold applied to the forehead demonstrated that the temperature of the interior of the brain, as far as 2 inches from the forehead, had dropped as much as 1.5° F.

Although the immediate effect of cold application is vasoconstriction, the prolonged effect is vasodilatation, again, a defense measure against excesses, probably largely reflex in nature. Therefore, the effects of prolonged cold and the effects of heat applied for shorter periods are approximately the same. Some authorities believe that prolonged cold causes damage of nerve supply to vessel walls, and that following such damage vasodilatation results. Excessive or prolonged cold can cause ice crystal formation in the tissues and damage or cause death of cells.

EFFECTS OF LOCAL APPLICATION OF HEAT: The first visible effect of moderate heat applied to the skin is vasodilatation; that is, the caliber of the cutaneous vessels increases. The skin becomes warm and pink. The skin receptors for heat are stimulated, the impulses are carried to the hypothalamus and the cerebral cortex, and the body's reaction is to rid itself of heat that may threaten the stability of body temperature. The dilatation of cutaneous vessels allows for increased blood circulation in the skin in order that heat may be lost to the environment.

In addition to vasodilatation, other reactions are taking place simultaneously. Heat lessens the viscosity of blood, thereby increasing the rate of flow. Tissue metabolism improves as the increased blood supply furnishes more oxygen and carries away wastes more rapidly. There is a greater amount of fluid in the tissue spaces, and the flow of lymph is increased. Local application of heat usually relieves pain,

although the exact phenomenon is not understood clearly. Pain caused by muscle spasm is relieved as the muscle relaxes. Pain caused by the pressure of congestion often is relieved as circulation improves. Some authorities suggest that possibly a chemical derived from accumulated waste products in the body causes pain and that therefore the increased circulation aids in removing the chemical and thus the pain.

Heat usually is applied for its local effects. Local applications of heat are used very often for the relief of pain, congestion, inflammation, swelling, and muscle spasms. Healing is promoted as tissue metabolism improves. Local heat also is often applied for comfort when patients feel cool and chilly.

Heat may also be applied locally for its more remote effects. If heat is applied to one area of the body, the amount of blood in other parts of the body decreases as the supply increases in the area being heated. For example, if the feet are placed in a basin of warm water, congestion of blood in abdominal organs is relieved as blood is diverted to the legs and the feet.

It was pointed out earlier that when cold was applied to the leg, the underlying tissue temperature increased. The same study was done when a hot water bag was placed on the leg and the following results were noted (18:5):

Interior of hot water bag	133° F.
Outside of towel covering hot water bag	122° F.
Cutaneous temperature rose from	90° F. to 110° F.
(in about 30 minutes)	
Subcutaneous temperature rose from	91.2° F. to 105.5° F.
(in about 40 minutes)	
Intramuscular temperature rose from	94.2° F. to 99.6° F.
(in about 50 minutes)	

Similar studies were conducted when heat was applied to the abdomen. No marked change of temperature within the stomach and the peritoneal cavity was demonstrated when heat was applied.

It has been found that blood flow decreases when the application of heat to a local area continues beyond approximately one hour. The reason for this reaction is not understood clearly, but probably reflex vasoconstriction results from the body's efforts at homeostasis through the autonomic nervous system. If the hot application is removed for a period of time and then reapplied, vasodilatation and the concomitant results occur again. Excessive applica-

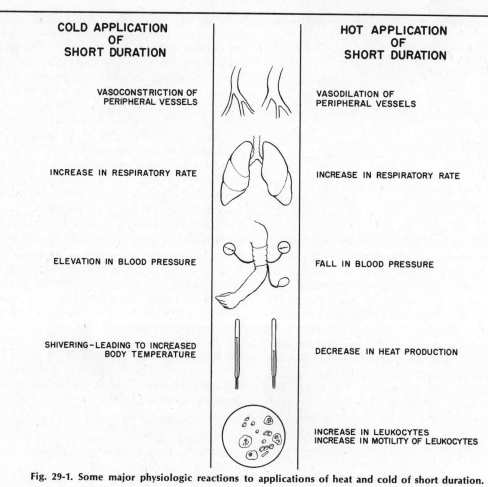

COLD APPLICATION OF SHORT DURATION	HOT APPLICATION OF SHORT DURATION
VASOCONSTRICTION OF PERIPHERAL VESSELS	VASODILATION OF PERIPHERAL VESSELS
INCREASE IN RESPIRATORY RATE	INCREASE IN RESPIRATORY RATE
ELEVATION IN BLOOD PRESSURE	FALL IN BLOOD PRESSURE
SHIVERING—LEADING TO INCREASED BODY TEMPERATURE	DECREASE IN HEAT PRODUCTION
	INCREASE IN LEUKOCYTES INCREASE IN MOTILITY OF LEUKOCYTES

Fig. 29-1. Some major physiologic reactions to applications of heat and cold of short duration.

tion of heat can increase the local tissue metabolism more than it increases circulation to the part. It also should be remembered that prolonged application of heat weakens cutaneous cells; therefore, the skin becomes more subject to injury. Any person can be burned by heat applications, but the very young, the elderly, and persons with circulatory deficiencies are more susceptible.

Figure 29-1 summarizes the major physiologic reactions to heat and cold applications of short duration.

THERAPEUTIC APPLICATIONS OF COLD: *Temperature for Cold Applications:* As is true when heat is being applied, no optimum temperature can be stated for cold applications. The selection of temperature depends on such factors as duration of application, method of application, condition of the patient, condition and sensitivity of the skin, area to be covered, and the like. For short periods

of time and for small areas, colder temperatures can be tolerated without discomfort or tissue damage. For longer periods of time, usually it is considered dangerous to keep skin temperatures below 40° F. except when ice is used for anesthesia.

The temperature of water used for cold applications usually is described as tepid, cool, cold, or very cold. The temperature ranges stated frequently are as follows:

Tepid	80° F. to 93° F.
Cool	65° F. to 80° F.
Cold	50° F. to 65° F.
Very cold	Below 55° F.

Ice Bags: The device used frequently for applying cold to an area is the ice bag. As mentioned previously, the effect from such application may be either local or reflex in nature.

The ice bag is filled with small pieces of ice,

making it easier to mold it to the contour of the body part and also reducing the amount of air spaces which act as insulation. After the bag is approximately two-thirds full, the air should be removed, for air, a poor conductor of heat, will interfere with the removal of heat from the body surface.

A cover should be placed on the ice bag to make it more comfortable for the patient and also to provide for absorption of the moisture which condenses on the outside of the bag.

To be effective as a local application, the ice bag should be applied for one-half to one hour and removed for approximately one hour. In this way the tissues are able to react to the effects of the cold.

Cold Compress: Moist, cold, local applications usually are referred to as cold compresses. They might be used for an injured eye, headache, tooth extraction, and in some situations, for hemorrhoids. The texture and the thickness of the material used will depend on the area to which it is to be applied. For example, eye compresses could be prepared from surgical gauze compresses which have a small amount of cotton filling. A wash cloth makes an excellent compress for the head or the face.

The material used for the application is immersed in a clean basin, appropriate for the size of the compress, that contains pieces of ice and a small amount of water. The compress should be wrung thoroughly before it is applied to avoid dripping, which is uncomfortable for the patient and may also wet the bed or clothing. The compresses should be changed frequently. Usually, the patient can feel when they have become warm, and many patients like to apply their own compresses. The application should be continued for 15 to 20 minutes and repeated every two to three hours. Ice bags or certain commercial devices for keeping the compresses cold limit the frequency with which the compresses must be changed.

Alcohol or Cold Sponge Bath: Hypothermia is the artificial lowering of body tissue temperature. Occasionally, an alcohol or a cold sponge bath is recommended for reducing a patient's elevated temperature. Alcohol added to tepid water is tolerated more easily than a cold bath by most patients. Alcohol vaporizes at a relatively low temperature and therefore removes heat from the skin surfaces rapidly. Cold water very often produces a strong initial reactionary effect which elevates the temperature further.

When an alcohol or a cold sponge bath is given, it is essential that it be continued until the initial reaction of chilliness, or shivering, is overcome and the body has adjusted to the temperature. Therefore, it is best if the procedure lasts for at least 25 to 30 minutes. Each extremity should be bathed for a 5 minute period at least, and then the entire back and the buttocks for an additional 5 to 10 minutes.

During the procedure, place moist, cool cloths over large superficial blood vessels, as in the axilla and the groin as a further aid in lowering the temperature. A warm water bottle placed at the feet helps to overcome a sensation of chilliness. To help to prevent congestion and to provide comfort, an ice bag is applied to the head.

Mechanical hypothermia blankets or mattresses and plastic pads through which a thermostatically controlled solution is circulated are available for use with patients who need prolonged hypothermia.

THERAPEUTIC APPLICATIONS FOR HEAT: *Temperature for Hot Applications:* The optimum temperature for applying local hot applications cannot be stated. As has been pointed out, the condition of the skin, the size of the area being covered, the duration of the application, the method of applying heat (moist or dry), the condition of the patient, and the differences in heat tolerances need to be considered when determining optimum temperatures for applying heat. When the temperature of the skin surpasses approximately 110° F., many individuals are likely to suffer burns.

The temperature of water used for applications is described usually as neutral or warm, hot, and very hot. The temperature ranges stated frequently are as follows:

Warm or neutral	93° F. to 98° F.
Hot	98° F. to 105° F.
Very hot	105° F. to 115° F.

The common methods for applying heat discussed later in this chapter state the temperature ranges for applications which have been found satisfactory for most persons. However, checking the condition of the patient's skin is still necessary in order to avoid possible tissue damage.

Effects of Very Hot Applications: If very hot applications are applied to the skin for short periods of time, the reaction is similar to that of cold, that is, the cutaneous vessels may contract and decrease the blood supply. This is because the body is protecting itself against excessive loss of internal heat when exposed to an extreme of temperature in the environment. Muscles may fail to relax. Warm applications, on the other hand, lead to relaxation of muscles and increased blood supply. The effects of a warm bath and of a hot shower illustrate this difference in reaction of the body when warmth and heat are used. Contraction of small vessels is a desired reaction when hemorrhage is present, but cold rather than very hot applications are used more commonly to aid in checking bleeding.

There is logic in this when one recalls that cold increases the viscosity of blood. Increased viscosity slows the speed of flow, and blood clotting is facilitated by lower speed of circulation with vasoconstriction resulting from the cold.

Diathermy: Diathermy is the production of heat in body tissue by the use of high-frequency currents. It is used generally for producing heat in deep tissues. Special equipment is used for diathermy; generally, trained technicians are responsible for giving diathermy treatments. The reaction of the deep tissue to the heat produced by diathermy is similar to that of the skin and more superficial tissue when heat is applied locally.

Electric Heating Pads: The electric heating pad is a popular means for applying dry heat locally. It is easy to apply, provides constant and even heat, and is relatively safe to use. Nevertheless, careless handling can result in injury to the patient or the nurse as well as damage to the pad.

The heating element of an electric pad consists of a web of wires that convert electric current into heat. Crushing or creasing the wires may impair proper functioning, and portions of the pad will overheat. Burns and fire may result. Pins should be avoided for securing a pad, since there is danger of electric shock if a pin touches the wires. Pads with a waterproof covering are preferred, but they should not be operated in a wet or moist condition because of danger of short-circuiting the heating element and consequent shock.

Heating pads for home use have the selector switch for controlling the heat of an electric pad within easy reach of the patient. After the heat has been applied and a certain amount of depression of the peripheral nerve endings has taken place, the patient often increases the heat. Many persons have been burned in this manner. In some health agencies, preset heating pads are used.

Like other devices for applying dry heat, electric pads should be covered with flannel or similar material. This helps to make the heat therapy more comfortable for the patient. The pad can be used repeatedly when the cover is washed after each patient's use. However, it is important not to cover the pad too heavily, for heavy covering over an electric pad prevents adequate heat dissipation.

There also are plastic pads with tubular inner construction which can be filled with water (distilled water is specified by some manufacturers). An attached electric control unit heats the water and keeps it at an even temperature. The temperature is set prior to operation and the patient cannot change it because it requires a key. Such pads are useful on wet dressings when heat must be applied.

Hot Water Bags: When electric heating pads are not available, frequently the hot water bag is used. Hot water bags have disadvantages in that they may leak, and their weight makes them less comfortable than the electric pad. However, they are less expensive and may be safer for some patients.

To help to prevent burning the patient, it is considered essential to test the temperature of the water accurately with a thermometer before pouring it into the bag. A safe temperature range for infants under two years of age is from 105° F. to 115° F.; for children over two years of age and for adults, from 115° F. to 125° F.

In order to keep the bag as light as possible in weight and easy to mold to the body area, it should be filled about two-thirds full. The air remaining in the bag can be expelled in one of two ways: by placing the bag on a flat surface and permitting the water to come to the opening and then closing the bag; or by holding the bag up and twisting the unfilled portion to remove the air and then closing it. After the bag has been filled, hold it upside down to test it for leaks. Apply the flannel cover to the bag securely before placing it on the body part. In order that the patient may feel warmth immediately, the cover can be warmed before it is placed on the hot water bag. Otherwise, it will take time for the heat of the bag to be transmitted through the covering.

The temperature ranges given above will produce the desired local effects if the bag is filled properly and the cover warmed. However, most patients will seem to think that the water is not hot enough. Unless the patient receives an explanation beyond simply telling him that the temperature will not burn him, it is likely that the bag may be filled from the hot water tap when the nurse is not around. If the patient cannot do it, a visitor or another patient may oblige.

Hip or Sitz Baths: As a means of applying tepid or hot water to the pelvic area, patients are often placed in a tub filled with sufficient water to reach the umbilicus. These baths are referred to as hip or sitz baths. Special tubs and chairs or basins which fit onto the toilet seat are available. Sitz tubs and chairs are designed so that the patient's buttocks fit into a rather deep seat which is filled with water of the desired temperature; the legs and the feet remain out of the water. The basin is smaller in size, and permits primarily the perineal area to be in contact with the water. The basins are disposable and economical for home or health agency use. A regular bathtub is not as satisfactory for a sitz bath because the heat is applied also to the lower extremities, and this alters the effect desired in the pelvic region.

If the purpose of the sitz bath is to apply heat, water at a temperature of 110° F. to 115° F. for 15 minutes will produce relaxation of the parts involved after a short initial period of contraction. Warm water should not be used if considerable congestion is already present.

If the purpose of the sitz bath is to produce relaxation or to help to promote healing in a wound by cleansing it of discharge and slough, then water at a temperature of 94° F. to 98° F. should be used. The temperature of the water should be tested frequently to prevent too great a range from occurring.

Since a large body area is involved when a sitz bath is given, the patient should be observed closely for signs of weakness and faintness. The nature of the procedure also makes it necessary to protect the patient from exposure. Usually, a bath blanket is wrapped around the patient's shoulders and then draped over the tub. After the bath, the patient should be covered adequately and encouraged to remain out of drafts. If a warm sitz bath has been given, it may be best for the patient to go to bed until normal circulation is resumed.

Sitz tubs and chairs are not adjustable to the comfort needs of patients, especially the short patient. After the patient is in the tub or the chair, check to see whether or not there is pressure against the patient's thighs or legs. If the patient's feet do not touch the floor, and the weight of the legs is resting on the edge of the chair, a stool should be procured to support the feet and relieve the pressure on the vessels in the legs.

In addition to avoiding any pressure areas, it may be necessary to place a towel in the water to support the patient's back in the lumbar region. Fifteen to 20 minutes can seem like a very long time if one's body is not in good alignment and comfortable.

Soaks: The direct immersion of a body area into warm water or a medicated solution is referred to as a soak. The purposes for which soaks are used vary: to increase blood supply to a locally infected area, to aid suppuration, to aid in cleansing large sloughing wounds such as burns, to improve circulation, and to apply medication to a locally infected area. A soak has the added advantage of making manipulation of a painful area much easier, since the body part is buoyed up by the weight of water it displaces.

If a soak is prescribed for a large wound, such as might cover an entire arm or lower leg or even an area of the torso, a compromise with sterile technique usually is made. The vessel into which the body area is placed is sterilized before use if possible; if not, the vessel should be cleaned scrupulously. Tap water may be used for soaks, since it is accepted generally as being free from pathogens.

During the treatment, which is usually 15 to 20 minutes per soak, the temperature should be kept as constant as possible. This may be done by discarding some of the fluid every five minutes and replacing it, or by adding solution at a higher temperature.

Care must be taken to avoid burning the patient. If hot solution is added and it is not stirred or otherwise agitated, it will not diffuse into the cooler solution quickly enough to prevent discomfort or tissue injury.

Unless the temperature of the soak is prescribed by the physician, a range of 105° F. to 110° F. is considered as being physiologically effective and comfortable for the patient.

The vessel holding the fluid should be placed so that the part to be immersed is comfortable and the patient is in good body alignment. For example, an arm basin placed on top of the bedside stand may cause the patient's shoulders to be thrown out of alignment, and it may also cause pressure on the back of the patient's arm. Or, a hand basin may be so situated as to cause wrist fatigue. Whenever a soak basin is placed in position, the nurse should look for pressure areas and observe the patient's degree of comfort.

Hot Moist Packs and Compresses: The application of warm moist cloths to a body area is referred to as a pack; warm moist gauze dressings are referred to as compresses. Packs usually are applied to a more extensive area. Packs and compresses differ from soaks primarily in two ways: the duration of the application of packs and compresses is usually longer, and the initial application of heat is more intense. Packs and compresses are applied as hot as the patient can tolerate them comfortably.

Depending on the situation, a pack or compress may be applied using sterile technique. If so, all materials and the solution must be sterile and the person applying the pack wears sterile gloves.

If an area is to be kept warm continuously by means of moist dressings, the frequency of the change of such applications will depend on the thickness of the material used for the application and the amount of protection given to it. A warm water bottle, a heating pad, or a mechanical heating device can be used to maintain the temperature of a pack or compress. However, since moisture increases the heat conduction, a lower temperature should be used than when dry heat is applied to avoid tissue damage.

Because of the effect of the moist hot applications on circulation, the patient is likely to feel chilly. Precautionary comfort measures should be taken during and following the treatment to keep the patient, and especially the area which has been treated, warm and free from drafts.

Proper positioning of the patient is also important, especially if the pack is to be left in place for an extended period of time. Figure 29-2 shows a patient with a leg pack supported in good alignment.

Cleansing the Tissue

It has been stated that infections hinder optimum healing. An attempt is often made to reduce the number of pathogens and remove tissue debris to promote rapid, uncomplicated healing. In the case of an intentional wound, the skin and/or mucous membrane is prepared by reducing the number of pathogens in the area before the break in the tissue is made, such as before a surgical incision. When caring for such a wound, sterile technique and antiseptics are used to avoid the accidental introduction of pathogens. An accidental and open wound is generally cleansed at the earliest opportunity and also cared for while using sterile technique to avoid further pathogen entry. A closed wound is often cleansed with a flowing solution to remove debris. The procedure is known as an irrigation. Local heat

to promote healing may be applied. Occasionally, open wounds may also be irrigated; sterile technique is used.

Preoperative Skin Preparation: Because hair shafts can harbor microorganisms which can enter a wound, the skin is often prepared for a surgical incision by removing the hair in the area. Shaving the hair from an operative area is frequently referred to as a shave prep. Because the area adjacent to the actual incision can cause wound contamination, usually a much larger area than the actual size of the incision is prepared. For example, for an abdominal incision, the area from the nipple line to the pubis is usually prepared. The practice of extensive shave preps has decreased in recent years for some areas of the body. The exact areas vary depending on the practice of the health agency and the preference of the surgeon. Many persons do not realize that a human being has hair on all areas of his body except for the palms of the hands and the soles of the feet. Some of the hair may be so fine and light in color that it is difficult to see. The patient needs an explanation of the purpose of the skin preparation and the reason for its extensiveness to avoid causing him undue anxiety.

The actual skin shaving may be performed by operating room personnel or by the nurse responsible for the care of the patient. The necessary supplies generally are dispensed from a central supply unit. Disposable prep trays are available commercially. While the equipment may vary somewhat, it generally includes a razor and a new blade, basins for soap solution and water, gauze or cotton applicators, and towels for draping the patient and protecting the bed. In addition, good lighting is essential for proper performance of this procedure.

After draping and soaping the area, long gentle strokes of the razor are used. The razor is moved in the direction the hair grows. The nurse may wish to hold the skin taut with one hand to facilitate the razor's movement. Great care must be taken to avoid

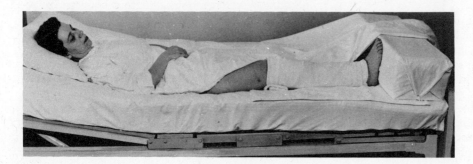

Fig. 29-2. In applying heat or cold to any body area, keep it in good alignment to prevent fatigue. Here the foot is kept free from the leg wrapping so that it may be supported in dorsiflexion. A small towel under the knee gives support but is placed to avoid popliteal pressure. The weight of a large pack often restricts motion and contributes to fatigue.

RATIONALE GUIDING ACTION FOR APPLYING HOT MOIST APPLICATIONS TO A BODY AREA

The purpose is to apply heat to an area to produce changes in the blood vessels and the underlying tissues.

SUGGESTED ACTION	RATIONALE
Prepare pieces of woolen, flannel, or gauze material sufficiently large to cover the area adequately.	Absorbent and loosely woven fibers hold moisture.
Prepare a hot water bottle, heating pad, or other heating device if one is to be used.	External heat continually applied to the moist compress will slow cooling of the compress.
Immerse the packs in hot water until they are saturated.	The woolen or flannel material absorbs the water slowly.
Prepare the patient's body area so that no time will be wasted in applying the pack after it is removed from the hot water. Place a dry pack and a waterproof cover under the extremity or near the area where the pack is to be applied. The dry pack will cover the moist one, and the waterproof cover will be on the outside.	Air will reduce the temperature of the pack. The dry pack and the waterproof cover will act as insulation and will prevent rapid heat and moisture loss from the wet pack.
Lubricate the skin in the area of application with petrolatum if desired and if the skin is unbroken.	Petrolatum delays the transmission of the heat from the pack to the skin.
Wring the hot wet packs until water does not drip from them.	Saturated packs will lose water.
Shake once or twice.	Loss of steam helps to reduce temperature.
Place the pack on the skin lightly and, after a few seconds, lift the pack to inspect the patient's skin for degree of redness.	Degree of vasodilatation indicates intensity of heat.
Wrap the pack around the area snugly and mold it to the skin surface.	Air is a poor conductor of heat. Air spaces between the skin and the pack will reduce the effect of the application.
Cover the moist pack tightly with the dry pack and waterproof covering. Secure in place with safety pins or ties.	Insulation and covering prevent heat and moisture loss.
Apply the hot water bottle, heating device, or heating pad to the area in a manner so the weight is not increased over the wound area.	External heat will help to maintain the pack temperature. Weight of the heat supply can cause fatigue and discomfort.

breaking the patient's skin; this is especially important over bony prominences. Careful inspection of the skin with direct lighting is necessary to assure that the area is free of hair. Following completion of the shaving, the area is rinsed of soap residue and dried.

In some situations, especially preceding orthopedic (bone) surgery, a sterile prep may be done. A *sterile prep* is the technique used to shave and cleanse the skin under surgical aseptic conditions. Actually, the term is a misnomer because the skin cannot be sterilized. In a sterile prep, the supplies that come in contact with the surgical area are sterile, for example, the soap solution, water, razor, applicators, and drapes. The person carrying out the technique wears sterile gloves. After the area is shaved, it may be cleansed with an antiseptic or soap solution before it is wrapped in sterile towels.

In still other situations, skin preparation for surgery may consist of a thorough cleansing of the area with a soap solution or an antiseptic. The shave prep may be omitted.

Irrigations: An *irrigation* is the cleansing of an area with a flowing solution. The purpose of the irrigation may be to cleanse the area and/or to apply local heat or antiseptic.

Throat, ear, eye, and vaginal irrigations are the most commonly performed irrigations. Open wound irrigations are sometimes done to promote débridement.

The circumstances of the wound determines the type of solution that is used. Water, saline, and antiseptic solutions are commonly used. Generally if the wound is closed, nonsterile solutions are used whereas if the wound is open a sterile irrigating solution is needed.

Conjunctival Irrigation: A conjunctival irrigation, frequently called an eye irrigation, usually is done for cleansing purposes to remove secretions from the conjunctival sacs. Mild antiseptic solutions may be prescribed if an infection is present.

For cleansing purposes, physiologic saline usually is prescribed. The solution is administered at body temperature unless the physician specifies otherwise. The amount of solution will depend on the situation—as little as one ounce or as much as eight or more ounces may be necessary to accomplish the purpose of the irrigation.

Several methods may be used for irrigating the conjunctival sacs. An eye dropper is satisfactory when small amounts of solution are used. For larger amounts, a soft rubber bulb syringe is appropriate. For home use, an eyecup, washed scrupulously after

each use, usually is convenient. In an emergency situation, squeezing the solution from a soaked cotton ball offers a satisfactory method. The operator's hands should be washed thoroughly first.

Following the irrigation, the patient should be asked to close the lids, and the excess fluid is wiped off gently from the inner canthus to the outer canthus. Any additional solution in the area around the eye is also wiped away gently with a cotton ball.

The technique for a conjunctival irrigation is included in the following box. Before proceeding with an irrigation, the reader may wish to review material on page 439 that briefly describes the anatomical structures of the eye.

Irrigation of the External Auditory Canal: Irrigation of the auditory canal generally is done for cleansing purposes. Antiseptic solutions sometimes are used for their local action. Irrigations may be used also for applying heat to the ear.

Normal saline usually is used for cleansing. However, any number of antiseptic solutions may be used. The amount of solution needed depends on the purpose of the irrigation, but approximately

RATIONALE GUIDING ACTION WHEN ADMINISTERING AN IRRIGATION OF THE EYE

The purpose is to cleanse the lower conjunctival sac.

SUGGESTED ACTION	RATIONALE
Have the patient sit or lie with his head tilted toward the side of the affected eye so that solution will flow from the inner canthus of the affected eye toward the outer canthus.	Gravity will aid the flow of solution away from the unaffected eye.
Cleanse the lids and the lashes with normal saline or the solution ordered for the irrigation.	Materials lodged on the lids or in the lashes may be washed into the eye.
Place a curved basin at the cheek on the side of the affected eye to receive the irrigating solution.	Gravity will aid the flow of solution.
Expose the lower conjunctival sac.	The conjunctival sac is less sensitive than the cornea.
Direct the flow of the irrigating solution from the inner canthus to the outer canthus along the conjunctival sac.	Solution directed toward the outer canthus aids in preventing the spread of contamination from the eye to the lacrimal sac, the lacrimal duct, and the nose.
Irrigate. Use only sufficient force to remove secretions from the conjunctiva gently.	Directing solutions with force may cause injury to the tissues of the eye, as well as the conjunctiva.
Avoid touching any part of the eye with the irrigating tip.	The eye is injured easily. Touching the eye is uncomfortable for the patient.
Have the patient close his eye periodically during the procedure.	Movement of the eye when the lids are closed helps to move secretions from the upper conjunctival sac to the lower.
Continue irrigating the lower conjunctival sac until purpose achieved.	Irrigation of the lower conjunctival sac is more comfortable for the patient.

500 ml. usually is adequate. The solution is prepared so that it is approximately body temperature when it enters the ear. Colder or hotter solutions are uncomfortable for the patient, since the endolymph is set in motion, and dizziness and nausea may result.

An irrigating container with tubing and an ear tip generally is used. The height of the can should be just enough to have the solution flow gently. The glass ear tip fits easily into the external canal and has two extensions projecting from it: one for the solution to enter the canal and the other for it to leave the canal and drain into a receiving basin. A soft rubber bulb syringe may be used, but it is not as comfortable for the patient, since the flow of solution must be interrupted during the irrigation while the syringe is refilled.

The technique for an auditory canal irrigation is included in the boxed description below. Before proceeding with an irrigation, the reader may wish to review material on page 441 that briefly describes the anatomical structures of the external ear.

Throat Irrigations: Throat irrigations are used primarily for loosening and removing secretions in the throat and for applying heat to the area. Mild antiseptics and normal saline are used most frequently. Sodium bicarbonate solution also is effec-tive, especially when the secretions are tenacious.

Usually, the solution is used as hot as the patient can tolerate it, but a temperature above approximately 120° F. is likely to cause tissue damage. If the irrigation is done primarily for applying heat, it is necessary to prepare sufficient solution so that the irrigation will continue over a period of time. Approximately 1500 to 2000 ml. given slowly generally is sufficient. The total amount should not be used if the patient becomes fatigued during the procedure. An irrigating can with a clamp on the tubing and an irrigating nozzle are used. It is convenient to use a pole on which to hang the irrigating can.

It is best if the patient assists during a throat irrigation by handling the nozzle himself and directing the flow of solution to various areas of the throat. The nurse should make certain that all areas in the throat are being irrigated. She shows the patient how to discontinue the flow of solution.

The technique for a throat irrigation is included in the boxed description on page 460. Before proceeding with an irrigation, the reader may wish to review material on page 442 that briefly describes the anatomical structures of the throat.

Throat Gargles: Gargles sometimes are used

RATIONALE GUIDING ACTION WHEN ADMINISTERING AN IRRIGATION OF THE EXTERNAL AUDITORY CANAL

The purpose is to cleanse the external auditory canal.

SUGGESTED ACTION	RATIONALE
Have patient sit up or lie with his head tilted toward the side of the affected ear. Have patient support a basin under his ear to receive the irrigating solution.	Gravity causes irrigating solution to flow from the ear to the basin.
Cleanse the pinna and the meatus at the auditory canal as necessary with normal saline or the irrigating solution.	Materials lodged on the pinna and at the meatus may be washed into the ear.
Fill the bulb syringe with solution. If an irrigating can is used, allow air to escape from the tubing.	Air forced into the ear canal is noisy, therefore unpleasant.
Straighten the auditory canal by pulling the pinna downward and backward for an infant and upward and backward for an adult.	Straightening the ear canal aids in allowing solution to reach all areas of the canal easily.
Direct a steady slow stream of solution against the roof of the auditory canal, using only sufficient force to remove secretions.	Solution directed at the roof of the canal aids in preventing injury to the tympanic membrane.
Do not occlude the auditory canal with the irrigating nozzle.	Continuous in-and-out flow of the irrigating solution aids in preventing pressure in the canal.
At completion of treatment have patient lie on the side of the affected ear.	Gravity allows the remaining solution in the canal to escape from the ear.

RATIONALE GUIDING ACTION WHEN ADMINISTERING A THROAT IRRIGATION

The purpose is to cleanse the throat and/or to apply heat.

SUGGESTED ACTION	RATIONALE
Arrange the irrigating can containing the solution on a pole at the bedside so that the base is only slightly above the level of the patient's mouth.	The gag reflex can be stimulated by a forceful stream of water into the throat. Keeping the level of the solution low minimizes pressure. Gravity will cause the solution to flow as long as the irrigating tip is below the base of the fluid.
Place the patient in a sitting position with his head tilted directly over a basin placed in front of him.	Gravity causes the solution to flow back out into the basin.
Instruct the patient to hold his breath while the solution is flowing.	Breathing while the solution is flowing into and out of the mouth may result in aspirating some of the solution.
Insert the nozzle into the mouth, being careful not to touch the base of the tongue or the uvula. Direct the flow so that all parts of the throat are irrigated.	The gag reflex can be stimulated by touching the uvula or the tongue.
Clamp the tubing to interrupt the irrigation at regular intervals to permit the patient to breathe and rest.	Holding the breath interrupts normal physiologic functions of respiration.

for the same purposes as throat irrigations. However, a gargle may be more uncomfortable, since gargling places strain and tension on an area that usually is already swollen, irritated, and painful. Also, a gargle generally is unsatisfactory for reaching all parts of the throat tissues; therefore, an irrigation is preferred by many physicians. A gargle generally is satisfactory for cleansing the mouth and the oral pharynx.

Many persons believe that gargling with a strong antiseptic is an almost sure way of preventing sore throats and upper respiratory infections. If done often enough and with full-strength antiseptic solutions, the normal defenses in the mouth and the oropharynx may be destroyed, and more harm than good is done.

Vaginal Irrigation (Douche): A vaginal irrigation generally is referred to as a *douche*. The irrigation is often done simply for cleansing purposes, as mentioned in Chapter 21. It may also be done for applying heat or an antiseptic to the area. The solution of choice is normal saline or tap water when the purpose of the irrigation is for cleansing or for applying heat. Any number of antiseptic solutions may be used, but for cleansing purposes they are actually not necessary.

Usually, a quantity of about 1500 ml. of solution is prepared, but smaller or larger amounts may be indicated, depending on the purposes of the irrigation. The vagina tolerates relatively high temperature, but the membranes and the skin around the meatus do not. Therefore, solutions are pre-

pared so that they are introduced at approximately 100° F., or approximately 110° F. if the effect of heat is desired.

An irrigating can or bag connected with tubing to an irrigating nozzle is used. Irrigating nozzles are curved to fit the normal contour of the vagina and may be made of glass or plastic. The nozzle should be handled carefully and examined before use to prevent injury should the nozzle be cracked or chipped.

As Chapter 21 indicated, at home a vaginal irrigation may be done by lying in a bathtub; have the irrigating can suspended at the proper height on a towel rack or on a chair at the side of the tub. Some patients may prefer using a douche pan or a bedpan when carrying out this procedure in the tub at home.

The technique for a vaginal irrigation is included in the boxed description on page 461. Before proceeding with an irrigation, the reader may wish to review material on page 443 that briefly describes the anatomical structure of the vagina.

Open Wound Irrigation: As indicated earlier, open wounds are occasionally irrigated for the cleansing effect of the flowing solution. Generally tissue debris exists and its mechanical removal with solution will hasten healing.

Sterile technique should be used when the skin or mucous membrane is broken because of the danger of introducing pathogens. This is true even in the presence of an existing infection.

The type and amount of solution varies with

RATIONALE GUIDING ACTION WHEN ADMINISTERING A VAGINAL IRRIGATION

The purpose is to cleanse the vagina.

SUGGESTED ACTION	RATIONALE
Have the patient void before beginning the treatment.	A full bladder interferes with distention of the vagina by the nozzle and the solution.
Have the patient in the dorsal recumbent position. Remove all but one pillow from under the patient's head and place her on a bedpan if the patient is in bed. A waterproof support may be necessary if a bathtub is used.	Gravity will cause the solution to flow into the distal portion of the vagina.
Arrange the irrigating can or bag at a level just above the patient's hips so that the solution flows easily yet gently.	The greater the distance between the level of the fluid and the outlet in the tubing, the greater will be the force of the solution as it leaves. Undue force could drive solution and contamination into the cervical os.
Cleanse the vulva by separating the labia and allowing the solution to flow over the area. If this does not seem to be sufficient, wash it with a soap or detergent solution.	Materials lodged around the vaginal meatus can be introduced into the vagina.
Permit some solution to run through the tubing and out over the end of the nozzle to lubricate it.	Moist surfaces have less friction when moved against each other.
Insert the nozzle gently into the vagina while directing it downward and backward.	In the dorsal recumbent position, normally the vagina is directed downward and backward.
Gently rotate the nozzle in the vagina during the treatment.	Movement of the nozzle aids in directing the solution against all surfaces of the vagina.

the tissue involved and the condition of the wound. Sterile saline, water, antiseptic, or occasionally antibiotic solutions are used. Hydrogen peroxide may also be the solution of choice because its oxygen-releasing ability has an effective cleansing effect.

A sterile syringe without a needle is often used to hold the solution. Care should be taken so that the solution flows directly into the wound and not over a contaminated area before entering the wound. Following the irrigation, a sterile dressing is generally applied to the wound.

The technique for a wound irrigation is included in the box on the following page.

Protecting the Traumatized Tissue

The tissue of both open and closed wounds is more susceptible to further injury than normal tissue. Prevention of further injury and the promotion of healing are two goals of wound care. Protection from mechanical or microorganism trauma and reduction of strain on the part can assist the physiological healing process. Tissues of most closed and some open wounds are left uncovered and supported or immobilized to promote healing. Open wound tissues are frequently covered as well as supported or immobilized. The protective covering over a

wound is commonly referred to as a dressing. Binders and bandages are usually used to secure dressings and to immobilize and support parts. Casts, splints, braces, and prostheses of various sorts may also be used to immobilize or support body parts. The remainder of this chapter will discuss the use of dressings, bandages, and binders. Other clinical texts, especially those discussing the care of the orthopedic patient, contain information on such supportive mechanisms as casts, braces, and the like.

THE UNDRESSED WOUND: Some physicians subscribe to the practice of leaving an open wound undressed if it has sealed itself and can be protected from trauma and irritation. This is true even of wounds that have been surgically induced and sutured. Or, there may be occasions when a wound may be undressed for most of the day and then covered at bedtime. Many small cuts and abrasions heal more quickly if left undressed.

There are several reasons for leaving some wounds undressed, all based on the principles mentioned earlier, namely: the body has resources for healing itself; friction and irritation destroy epithelial cells; and dark, warm, moist areas are suitable for the growth of microorganisms. Therefore, a dressing applied to skin in such a fashion that it produces

RATIONALE GUIDING ACTION WHEN ADMINISTERING AN OPEN WOUND IRRIGATION

The purpose is to cleanse the wound.

SUGGESTED ACTION	RATIONALE
Place the patient in a position so the solution will flow from the wound down to a clean basin held below the wound.	Gravity causes the flow of liquids. Contaminated solution flowing over the wound could introduce microorganisms into the wound.
Irrigate the wound generously but carefully with the solution, being sure to irrigate pockets in the wound.	The solution washes away organisms, tissue debris, and drainage.
Cleanse the skin around the wound to remove irrigating solution. Be careful not to touch the wound.	Microorganisms are normally present on the skin.
A bland ointment may be applied on the skin immediately surrounding the wound if drainage is present.	An emollient on the skin prevents drainage from irritating the epithelium.
Cover the wound with sterile dressings and secure it in place.	Well-secured sterile dressings protect the wound from trauma, minimize the danger of organisms entering the wound, and absorb secretions.

friction can break the scab which has formed. In addition, the normal flora on the skin can be rubbed into the wound, and if the area is moist and dark, bacterial growth can take place.

Some surgical wounds are left uncovered because it is felt exposure to the air and lack of impediment of circulation caused by a dressing promote faster healing. One approach to the care of extensive burns is the open or no-dressing method.

The woman who has just delivered a baby almost always has some areas of broken mucous membrane in the birth canal, and her care includes prevention of contamination of the area and fortifying her own normal defenses. This is another example of an undressed wound.

THE DRESSED WOUND: Dressings serve several purposes. If used properly, dressings and the materials used for securing them aid in preventing pathogens from entering the wound, absorb exudate, protect the area from trauma, and restrict motion that tends to disrupt the approximation of the wound edges. They also may be applied with pressure to reduce blood flow or stasis and to aid in approximating edges of the wound. For aesthetic reasons, a dressing serves to cover an area of disfigurement.

CHANGING THE DRESSING: Some patients are taught to change their own dressings when they are able, or in other situations the physician or nurse may change the dressing. In some health agencies, wound dressings are changed in special treatment rooms or in some circumstances, even in the operating room. In other situations dressings are changed while the patient is in his bed.

Some agencies have dressing carts which contain a variety of dressing supplies that are wheeled from one patient to another. Since the cart can provide a vehicle for pathogen transmission among patients, and in a number of situations, has been shown to be involved in cross-contamination, the common dressing cart is generally not recommended. The preferable method is to have individual dressing trays containing necessary equipment which are returned to a central supply unit for sterilization between patients. Another common approach is the use of commercially prepared individually packaged disposable supplies that are selected according to the patient's needs and taken to his room.

The patient should be prepared by explaining what will be done before the procedure is initiated. Consideration should be given to providing privacy for the patient and to the possibility that he may be disturbed by the sight of the wound. In some instances, patients do not wish to look at their wounds, and they should not be encouraged to do so nor chided about it. This is particularly true of patients whose wounds involve change in their bodily functions or appearance, such as the removal of a breast, the amputation of a foot or a leg, or the placement of a tube in the abdominal wall.

The patient should be helped to assume a comfortable position that affords him safety and working convenience for the person changing the dressing.

If the procedure is likely to produce considerable discomfort, an analgesic medication may be given before beginning the procedure.

Necessary Equipment: When preparing to change a dressing, it is necessary to have a means for removing the old dressing without contaminating the wound or the fingers of the person removing it and also equipment for cleansing the wound, dressing it adequately, and securing it.

Sterile instruments are used to remove the dressings adhering to a wound and for treating it. In some instances where there is need to support the area near the wound, as with an amputation, sterile gloves can be worn. When the instruments are removed after use, they should be handled so that they do not contaminate otherwise clean objects or surfaces, such as overbed tables, utility room counters and carts. Some spray-on, plasticlike transparent dressings are removed with special solvents.

A safe method should be used for disposing of the old dressing and the gauze or the cotton used to clean the wound. The best practice is to discard them in a waterproof bag which can be closed and discarded for burning.

The antiseptic to clean the wound is a matter of agency policy or the physician's preference. If the wound is to be irrigated, the prescribed solution, a sterile irrigating syringe, and a basin to collect returns will also be needed.

Dressing materials usually are made of gauze folded into various sizes and shapes. Some gauze sponges are filled with absorbent cotton. Some dressings have a nonadherent surface. The size, the number, and the types of dressings used depend on the nature of the wound. Cotton balls are useful for cleansing purposes, but generally they are not used as a dressing on a wound, for the cotton tends to stick to the wound and becomes difficult to remove.

Individual instrument and dressing packs afford the ultimate in safety for the patient. Surgical dressings and instruments kept in common containers cannot be counted on to be sterile after the container is opened.

Items for securing the dressing in place will also vary depending on the extent and nature of the wound.

CARE OF DRAINING WOUNDS: In order to promote exudate drainage, a rubber or plastic tubular drain is sometimes placed in a wound during surgery. If a drain is in a wound, care must be exercised so that it is not dislodged while dressings are changed. The physician may order that a straight drain be shortened each day. This can be done by grasping the end of the drain with sterile forceps, pulling it out a short distance while using a twisting motion and cutting off the end of the drain with sterile scissors. If the drain is in the abdominal cavity, a large sterile safety pin often is placed at the end of the drain so that it cannot slip down out of sight. Other drains may be attached to suction devices to remove exudate.

The skin around a draining wound quickly becomes irritated and excoriated unless precautions are taken. Keeping the skin clean is of prime importance. This requires that dressings be changed often enough so that drainage-soaked dressings are not left on the skin for long periods of time. The skin surrounding the wound is washed, preferably with a warm soap or detergent solution, and rinsed thoroughly with water or normal saline. A thorough cleansing is accomplished by the emulsifying and mechanical actions involved in this method. An antiseptic solution may be used on the skin after foreign materials have been washed off thoroughly and the skin dried properly. Some antiseptics are not effective if used on moist skin surfaces. Even if antiseptics are not used, the skin should be dry.

In order to prevent skin irritation and excoriation, a protective ointment or paste may be applied so that drainage cannot contact the skin. This may be particularly important when it is anticipated that the drainage period will be prolonged or when the person's skin is especially susceptible to irritation.

When a protective ointment or paste has been used on the skin, it is important to remove it at regular intervals, at least daily, and cleanse the skin under it. Ointments prepared in a water-soluble base may be removed with a soap-and-water or detergent solution. Care must be exercised when ointments and pastes are removed so that the friction created by rubbing is kept at a minimum. Friction may destroy epithelial cells, causing skin irritation.

A dressing placed on a draining wound is more effective and comfortable when several basic principles are observed.

The property of surface tension exhibited by liquids and the forces of cohesion and adhesion cause a column of liquid to rise in a fine tube or on a hair. This is called capillary action or capillarity. For example, absorbent cotton allows for greater capillarity than untreated cotton; therefore, sponges lined with the former material soak up more liquid. Loosely packed gauze, the threads of which act as numerous wicks, enhances capillarity and will allow for drainage to be directed upward and away from its source. Fluffed and loosely packed dressings, then, are more absorbent than flatly packed dressings and will carry drainage up and away from the wound.

Evaporation occurs more readily when there is circulation of air. Prolonged heat and moisture on the skin deteriorate epithelial cells. These principles are utilized when the nurse applies dressings and secures them so that circulation of air is possible. Loosely packed dressings secured with materials that allow for air circulation promote evaporation of moisture and dissipation of heat to the environment, both of which help to protect the skin. To protect the patient's clothing and the bed linen, waterproof material, such as a plastic, can be used on the bed when a wound is draining profusely. Waterproofing should generally be avoided over the dressing because it reduces the circulation of air through the dressings, and the skin and the wound may be injured due to an accumulation of heat and moisture.

Gravity causes liquids to flow from a high to a low level. Dressings on a draining wound should be arranged according to the patient's position and the expected direction of flow. For example, when a patient with a draining abdominal wound is ambulatory, a heavy application of dressings should be placed at the base of the wound and secured so that the drainage does not escape under the dressings and onto the patient.

When objects in contact move in opposition to each other, friction is produced. Friction can damage or destroy epithelial cells. These principles are in effect when dressings are secured in a manner which causes friction on the skin and the wound, which may result in injury to tissue. Dressings should not be secured so loosely that they move separately from the patient. For example, chest dressings that fail to move with the person's respiratory motions or dressings over joints which loosen with movement can cause skin friction.

SECURING THE DRESSING: This responsibility often demands considerable ingenuity and resourcefulness on the part of the nurse. It requires consideration of such factors as the size of the wound, its location, whether drainage is present, the nature of the drainage, the frequency with which the dressing needs changing, and the activities of the patient.

For securing a very small dressing on a wound with little or no drainage, liquid adhesive or collodion may be used effectively. The edges of the outer piece of gauze that are cut to fit over the dressing are painted with the liquid adhesive or collodion and then glued to the skin.

Strips of adhesive probably are used most frequently for securing dressings. Adhesive is dispensed in various widths, and the length is determined according to the need. Elasticized adhesive allows for more movement of a body part without pull on adjacent tissues. Because adhesive often causes skin irritation, especially when dressings must be changed frequently, it is good practice to apply a protective coating to the skin before applying adhesive. A preparation most frequently used is compound benzoin tincture, which is painted onto the skin immediately before the adhesive is applied.

Some patients are allergic to adhesive mixtures; therefore, the nurse should investigate any complaint of discomfort associated with adhesive tape. Patients who have endured the discomforts of the adhesive for a period of days have been known to need treatment for months following its removal. Various kinds of nonallergenic tapes are available on the market today.

When dressings must be changed frequently, it is advisable to consider the use of straps for securing the dressing, since they do not require changing with each dressing as adhesive strips do. These can be made easily or are available commercially. The adhesive end of the strap is placed on the skin well away from the wound. The end of the strap near the wound remains free since the adhesive side has been turned back upon itself. Gauze or woven strips passed through eyelets are tied over the wound to secure the dressing. When the dressing is changed, the strips are untied and turned back to allow for wound care. The skin of the patient can be protected with compound tincture of benzoin before applying the straps. When adhesive is removed, some of the gummy substance may remain on the skin. A mild solvent followed by thorough rinsing should be used to clean the area.

When adhesive cannot be used safely and effectively, various types of binders and bandages may be used for securing dressings. A description of various types of binders, bandages, and their application follows.

When a dressing is being secured, pressure on the wound should be exerted from the edges toward the center. This practice helps to approximate the wound edges and hence promotes healing. The dressing should be secured well enough so that it does not slip out of place as the patient moves.

The boxed description on the next page indicates the technique for changing a dressing.

FREQUENCY OF CHANGING DRESSINGS: The frequency with which dressings should be changed cannot be stated categorically; it will depend on the physician's preference, the nature of the wound, and

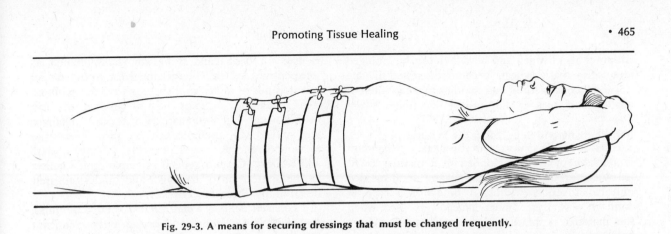

Fig. 29-3. A means for securing dressings that must be changed frequently.

whether drainage is present. Some surgeons may wish to leave a clean wound untouched for several days, in which case dressings are left unchanged. They generally believe that a frequent change of dressings on a clean, nondraining wound is a possible source of contamination. In their opinion, it is best if the wound's own protective seal is left undisturbed. Other physicians prefer to have the dressings changed frequently, even several times a day, because close observations of changes in the wound can be made this way.

RECORDING THE CARE OF THE WOUND: The nurse caring for a wound is responsible for observing it and for noting factors that may be interfering with the process of healing. She is expected to call the physician's attention to anything unusual in the process of healing as well as to its progress.

On the patient's record the nurse records each time wound care is given, the nature of the care given, and the condition of the wound. If the patient has a rather complicated dressing, details for caring for the wound should be described on the patient's nursing care plan. Often, the patient who has an extensive wound has preferences as to the time the

RATIONALE GUIDING ACTION IN THE CARE OF A DRESSED WOUND

The purpose is to remove a soiled dressing, cleanse the wound, and apply a sterile dressing.

SUGGESTED ACTION	RATIONALE
Undo materials securing the dressing. Lift dressing off by touching outside portion only. If it is soiled, use individual forceps.	Microorganisms can be transferred by direct contact.
If dressing adheres to wound, moisten with sterile water, physiologic saline, or hydrogen peroxide. Remove when completely loose.	An intact scab is a body defense mechanism.
Drop the soiled dressing into a waterproof bag for later burning.	Burning destroys microorganisms. Confined microorganisms cannot be transmitted by air currents or by contact.
Cleanse the wound carefully with an antiseptic of the physician's or the agency's choice.	Cleansing aids in removing organisms, tissue debris, and drainage.
Start from either directly on or adjacent to the wound and work away from it.	Microorganisms are normally present on the skin and could be transferred to the area which is to be kept most clean.
Discard the gauze or the cotton used for cleansing after each stroke over the wound.	Microorganisms removed from one area can be applied to another by direct contact.
Cover the wound with sterile dressings handled with a sterile forceps or touched only on the outer surface. Secure the dressings.	A contaminated dressing can introduce pathogens into the wound. Well-secured dressings protect the wound from trauma and absorb drainage.

dressings are changed and how they can be arranged best. Also, patients can become distressed if one nurse uses one method and another nurse a different one, even if both employ proper technique.

Immobilizing and Supporting the Wound

USES OF BANDAGES AND BINDERS: A *bandage* is a length of material applied in a manner to fit part of the body. Usually, bandages are dispensed in rolls of various widths. A *binder* is a type of bandage. The term binder generally is used when the material is specifically designed to fit a large body area as, for example, the abdomen, the chest, or the breasts. Some texts use the terms as synonyms, although in the strictest sense they are not.

Bandages and binders are used for several purposes: to create pressure over an area, to immobilize a part of the body to restrict its motion, to support a part of the body, to prevent or reduce swelling, to correct a deformity, and to secure a limb to a splint. They are used also to hold dressings in place.

MATERIALS USED FOR BANDAGES AND BINDERS: Usually, gauze fabric is used for bandages. It is light and soft and can be adjusted readily to fit a body part comfortably. Because it is porous, it is cool and allows for circulation of air. Gauze bandage is relatively inexpensive. It rarely can be reclaimed for repeated use because it frays very easily.

Muslin and flannel are materials also used for bandages. Being strong and firm, they are useful when pressure and immobilization are desired. Flannel is more absorbent than muslin and molds easily to fit the contours of the body. Flannel also helps to keep the area warm, which may be an advantage or a disadvantage depending on individual circumstances. Self-adhering, synthetic bandages are also available. Binders are made of muslin, flannel, or synthetics. Muslin or flannel bandages are suited to home use because they can be washed and reused. Synthetic binders are often elasticized and some are self-adhering.

Various types of elastic webbing can be purchased which are particularly effective when bandaging is needed for firm support and immobilization and for preventing swelling in extremities. The webbing is strong and molds well because of its elastic quality. It can be washed and used repeatedly.

One type of elastic webbing has an adhesive surface on one side. This can be used like adhesive and has the advantage of molding well to body contours. It does not withstand washing and therefore cannot be reclaimed for repeated use.

Ribbed cotton material dispensed as stockinet is used for bandaging. It has an elastic quality, is inexpensive, and can be reclaimed for repeated use, but it is not as sturdy and strong as elastic webbing.

GENERAL PRINCIPLES USED IN THE APPLICATION OF BANDAGES AND BINDERS: A bandage or a binder well-applied will promote healing, prevent damage to wounds and skin, and offer the patient comfort and security. Certain general principles guide action in the application of bandages and binders and aid in attaining these objectives.

Unclean bandages and binders may cause infection if applied over a wound or a skin abrasion. This fact guides what may seem like rather obvious action; that is, that bandages and binders should be kept clean and free of contamination. Medical asepsis is observed when applying bandages and binders. Skin abrasions and wounds are first covered with sterile dressings before clean bandages and binders are applied in order to aid in protecting the wound from trauma and contamination. Certain bandages and binders may be used repeatedly, but only after they have been washed and sterilized between patients.

When objects in contact move in opposition to each other, friction occurs which opposes motion, and can destroy or damage epithelial cells. Applying a small amount of fine talcum powder to the unbroken skin helps to keep it dry and decreases friction, but care must be exercised to prevent powder from entering the open wound, if one is present. No two skin surfaces should be allowed to touch each other. This is another measure to decrease friction on the skin and prevent moisture from accumulating in body crevices. Use absorbent material between fingers and toes, in the axilla, and under the breast, to absorb moisture and to prevent surfaces of skin from contacting each other. A bandage or a binder should be applied securely so that it will not shift about when the patient moves, causing friction that may result in chafing and skin abrasions.

Prolonged heat and moisture on the skin may cause its epithelial cells to deteriorate. It will be recalled that this principle is observed when dressings are applied to a wound. When bandages and binders are used, it indicates to the nurse that the area to be covered should be cleansed and dried thoroughly before applying a bandage or a binder. An unnecessarily thick or extensive bandage should be avoided so that the part being covered does not become excessively warm. Porous materials are preferable to nonporous in order to allow air to circulate so that perspiration can evaporate.

Placing and supporting the part to be bandaged in the normal functioning position prevents deformi-

ties and discomfort and enhances the circulation of blood in the part involved. This principle has been used as a guide for action throughout this text in the discussions of the importance of proper body mechanics and body alignment. It is equally important when bandages and binders are being used. Since bandages and binders usually restrict some motion and often are intended to immobilize a part of the body, it is important that the part involved first be placed at rest and comfortably in the position of normal functioning so that deformities and impaired circulation will not result. For example, when the foot is bandaged, it should be supported so that the bandage will not force it into plantar flexion.

Blood flow through the tissues is decreased by applying excessive pressure on blood vessels. The healing process is impaired, and tissue cells may die if the blood supply is inadequate to remove wastes and bring nourishment to the part involved. These are well-known physiologic facts that guide action in several ways. The bandage or the binder is applied with sufficient pressure to provide the amount of immobilization or support desired, to remain in place, and to secure a dressing if one is present. However, pressure should not be great enough to impede circulation of blood in the part involved.

Weakened veins, especially those of the lower extremities, can usually function more effectively when their walls are supported. Sufficient pressure to support the distended veins without impairing blood flow can be helpful in preventing edema.

The tension of each bandage turn should be equal, and unnecessary and uneven overlapping of turns should be avoided to prevent undue and uneven pressure. Bony prominences over which bandages and binders must be placed are padded. Hollows in the body contour may be filled with padding to provide comfort and to aid in maintaining equal pressure from the bandage or binder. An extremity is bandaged *toward the trunk* to avoid congestion and impaired circulation in the distal part. After a bandage or a binder has been applied, the part is observed frequently for signs of impaired circulation. For example, when an extremity is bandaged, the toes and the fingers are left exposed, if possible, so that circulation in the nail beds and signs of beginning swelling, which often indicate that circulation has been impaired, can be observed. A bandage placed over a wet dressing or a draining wound is applied less tightly since shrinkage of the material may cause the bandage to become too tight to allow for adequate circulation when it dries. In addition to being dangerous, a bandage or a binder applied too tightly is usually very uncomfortable for the patient.

Pins and knots, often used to secure a bandage or a binder, are placed well away from a wound or a tender and inflamed area. Care is observed so that pins, knots, and seams will not cause undue pressure or cause the patient discomfort. Movement often causes binders and bandages to loosen so they should be inspected and reapplied at regular intervals.

A well-applied bandage or binder will be comfortable for the patient, durable, neat, and clean. This is important for the patient's mental security as well as for promoting the best possible physiologic functioning of the body.

APPLICATION OF COMMON TYPES OF BANDAGES AND BINDERS: Many types of commercial bandages and binders are available for use today. There are variations in the techniques of applying and in the type of binder or bandage; some of the more common ones will be described here.

Triangular Binders: These are triangular pieces of material usually made of muslin. The sizes of these binders vary, but, for most adults, a 36- to 40-inch square cut in half diagonally to form two triangles is a common size.

Triangular binders are used for support as slings. Figure 29-4 illustrates a sling used as an arm support and shows the method of applying it. The open sling or triangle is placed on the chest, and then the affected arm is placed across the sling. One end of the sling is placed around the neck on the side of the unaffected arm. The other end is placed over the affected arm, and the ends are tied off to the side of the neck so that the knot does not rub over the cervical vertebrae. The material at the elbow is folded neatly and may be secured with a pin placed behind the sling so that it will be out of sight.

Triangular binders may be made into mittens for covering foot-and-hand dressings. They are useful also for bandaging the head, the shoulders, and the hips. Occasionally, two triangular binders may be used if the area is large.

Cravat Bandages: A cravat bandage is made by folding a triangular binder upon itself, from the apex of the triangle to the base and then over and over again until the desired width for the bandage is obtained. A cravat may be used as a small sling. It is used also on limbs and on the head. It is useful as a tourniquet and as a temporary measure to support a sprained joint.

Roller Bandages: A roller bandage is a continuous strip of material wound on itself to form a cylinder or roll. Roller bandages are made in various

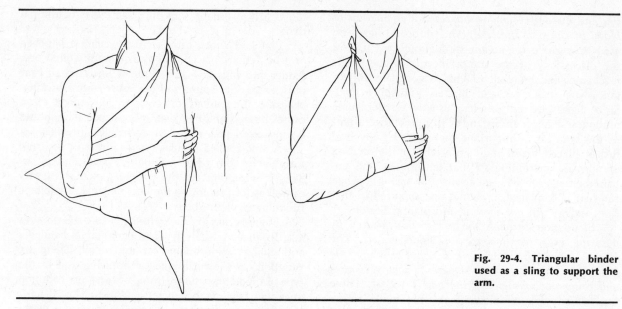

Fig. 29-4. Triangular binder used as a sling to support the arm.

widths and lengths. They are the most commonly used type of bandage and usually are made of gauze, although any other type of material may be used also. Elastic webbing is dispensed usually as a roller bandage.

The free end of the roller bandage is the *initial portion*, while the *terminal end* is in the center of the roll. The rolled portion is called the *body*. The *outer surface* of the bandage is the surface toward the outside of the body of the bandage. The *inner surface* is toward the inside or the center of its body. The inner surface is placed next to the patient's skin and dressing. When the bandage is begun, the initial end is held in place with one hand while the other hand passes the roll around the part. Once the bandage is anchored, usually with two circular turns, its body may be passed from hand to hand, being careful that equal tension is being exerted with each turn around the part. It is easier to keep tension equal by unwinding the ban-

dage gradually and only as it is required. Several basic turns are used to apply bandages, the selection of the turn depending on the part to be bandaged.

Circular Turn. When using the circular turn, the bandage is wrapped around the part with complete overlapping of the previous bandage turn. It is used primarily for anchoring a bandage where it is begun and where it is terminated. Figures 29-5 and 29-6 illustrate this turn to anchor a bandage before beginning a spiral turn.

Spiral Turn. When using the spiral turn, the bandage ascends in spiral fashion so that each turn overlaps the preceding one by one-half or two-thirds the width of the bandage. The spiral turn is useful when the part being bandaged is cylindrical, such as the area around the wrist, the fingers, and the trunk. Figure 29-7 and 29-8 illustrate this turn.

Spiral-Reverse Turn. A spiral-reverse turn is a spiral turn in which reverses are made halfway through each turn. Spiral-reverse turns are particu-

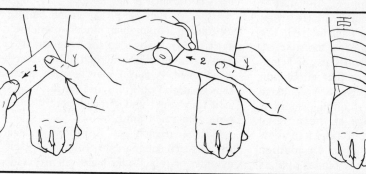

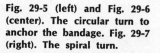

Fig. 29-5 (left) and Fig. 29-6 (center). The circular turn to anchor the bandage. Fig. 29-7 (right). The spiral turn.

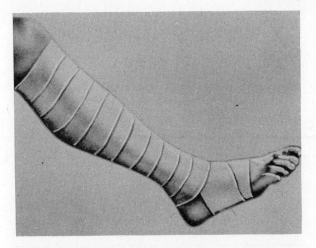

Fig. 29-8. Elastic roller bandage applied to the leg, using spiral turns. (Becton, Dickinson & Co., Rutherford, N. J.)

larly effective for bandaging a cone-shaped part, such as the thigh, the leg, or the forearm. Figure 29-9 illustrates the spiral-reverse turn. The position of the nurse's thumb on the bandage on the patient's arm shows the manner in which the reverse is made.

Figure-of-Eight Turn. This consists of making oblique overlapping turns that ascend and descend alternately. Each turn crosses the one preceding it so that it appears like the figure eight. Figures 29-10 and 29-11 illustrate how this turn is made. It is effective for use around joints, such as the knee, the elbow, the ankle, and the wrist. It provides for a snug bandage and therefore is used often for immobilization.

Spica. The spica consists of ascending and descending turns with all turns overlapping and crossing each other to form an angle. It is particularly useful for bandaging the thumb, the breast, the shoulder, the groin, and the hip. Figure 29-12 illustrates its application.

Recurrent Bandage. Sometimes this type is called a *stump bandage.* It is used for fingers and for the stump of an amputated limb. After a few circular turns to anchor the bandage, the initial end of the bandage is placed in the center of the part being bandaged, well back from the tip to be covered. The body is passed back and forth over the tip, first on one side and then on the other side of the center piece of bandage. Figure 29-13 illustrates the manner of applying a recurrent bandage to a stump. The last drawing in Figure 29-13 shows the use of the figure-of-eight turn to finish the bandage. Figure 29-14 shows an elastic bandage applied to a stump. Recur-

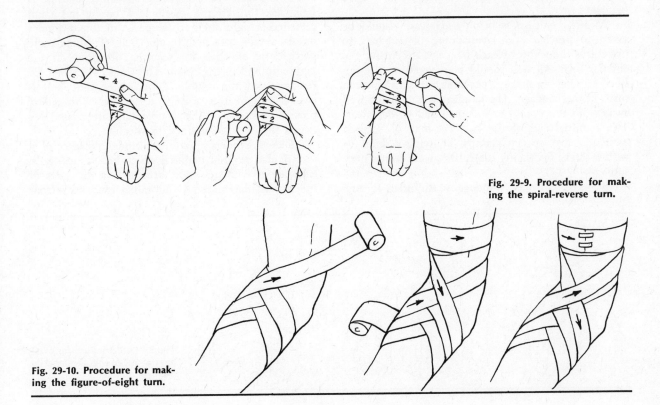

Fig. 29-9. Procedure for making the spiral-reverse turn.

Fig. 29-10. Procedure for making the figure-of-eight turn.

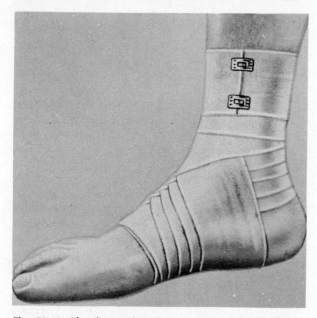

Fig. 29-11. The figure-of-eight turn used to apply elastic bandage to the ankle. (Becton, Dickinson & Co., Rutherford, N. J.)

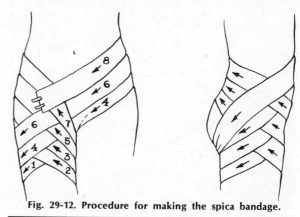

Fig. 29-12. Procedure for making the spica bandage.

rent bandages also are used effectively for head bandages.

Whichever turn is being used, care should be taken to provide even overlapping of one-half to two-thirds the width of each bandage, except for the circular turn. All skin should be covered by the finished bandage to prevent pinching the skin between turns of the bandage. The bandage is completed well away from the wound or inflamed and tender areas. The terminal end of the bandage may be secured with adhesive, special clamps, by tying a knot or with a safety pin, being careful to avoid undue pressure.

Removing Roller Bandages: In order to pre-vent too much movement, it is best to cut a roller bandage with a bandage scissors when removing it. Cutting should be done on the side opposite the injury or the wound, from one end to the other, so that the bandage can be folded open for its entire length. If it is an elastic bandage and is to be reused, it may be unwound by keeping the loose end together and passing it as a ball from one hand to the other while unwinding.

T Binders: A T binder is so named because it looks like the letter T. A single T binder has a tail attached at right angles to a belt. A double T binder has two tails attached to the belt. T binders are particularly effective for securing dressings on the perineum and in the groin. The single T is used for females, and the double T for males. The belt is passed around the waist and secured with safety pins. The single or the double tails are passed between the legs and pinned to the belt.

Tailed Binders: A tailed binder consists of a rectangular piece of material which has vertical tails, each about 2 inches wide, attached to the sides of the rectangular piece. A four-tailed binder has four

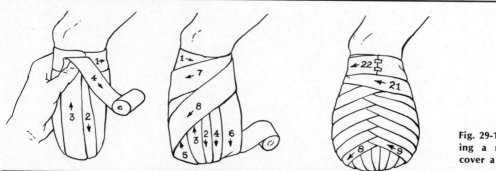

Fig. 29-13. Procedure for making a recurrent bandage to cover a stump.

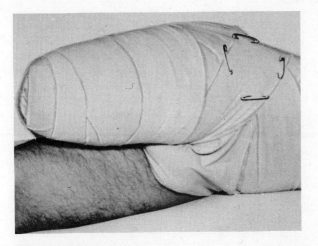

Fig. 29-14. Elastic bandage used to dress a stump. (Becton, Dickinson & Co., Rutherford, N. J.)

tails, two on each side of the binder. It is useful for securing dressings on the nose and the chin and is illustrated in Figure 29-15.

Many-tailed binders are called *scultetus binders*. They are used to support the abdomen or hold dressings on it and on the chest. When a scultetus binder is applied to the abdomen, the patient lies on his back and on the center of the binder. The lower end of the binder is placed well down on the hips but not so low that it will interfere with the use of a bedpan or with walking. The tails are brought out to either side on the patient's body with the bottom tail in position to wrap around the lower part of the abdomen first. A tail from each side is brought up and placed obliquely over the abdomen until all tails are in place. The last tails are fastened with safety pins. Figure 29-16 illustrates the application of a scultetus binder to the abdomen.

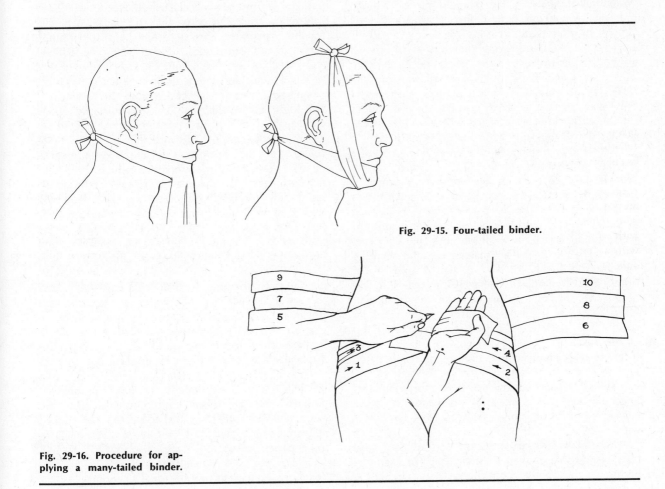

Fig. 29-15. Four-tailed binder.

Fig. 29-16. Procedure for applying a many-tailed binder.

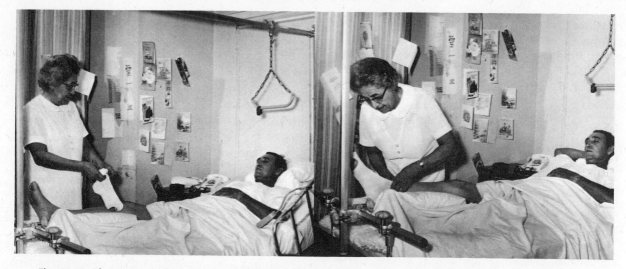

Fig. 29-17. The nurse teaches the patient how to hold the elastic stocking before putting it on, and then demonstrates how it is put onto the foot and leg. (Good Samaritan Hospital, Phoenix, Arizona)

Straight Binders: This straight piece of material usually is about 6 to 8 inches wide and long enough to more than circle the torso. It generally is used for the chest and the abdomen. Straight binders must be applied so as to fit the contours of the body. This usually is done by making small tucks in the binder as necessary. In some instances, these tucks can be secured with safety pins. A straight binder for the chest often is provided with shoulder straps so that it will not slip down on the trunk.

Stockinet: Stockinet is a stretchable tubular bandage, constructed so that a body part may be inserted into it, such as, for example, a finger, a foot, or an arm. It is dispensed in various widths or diameters. It has advantages over the roller bandage in that it remains in place better, applies a uniform pressure and is extremely simple and quick to use.

Stockinet is useful for making caps for securing dressings on the head. The desired length is cut from a roll of an appropriate width, usually 6 inches wide. The stockinet is placed over the head and folded back on itself at the forehead for extra security. The opposite end is tied or pinned at the top of the head. Stockinet as a bandage on the head seems to offer more security than other types; therefore, it is also more comfortable for the patient.

Stockinet in a narrow width is appropriate for finger bandages. An applicator is dispensed with the stockinet so that it can be slipped over the finger with ease.

Elasticized Stockings: Some persons may need to have pressure applied to their legs, for example, persons with varicose veins, those with circulatory disturbances, or women during pregnancy. Many patients routinely wear elasticized stockings following major surgery or when they are confined to bed for long periods. The stockings help to promote venous blood return and to avoid stagnation of blood and possible clot formation. Several manufacturers produce men's and women's hose which are capable of applying pressure to the leg from the foot to the midthigh. Some apply mild pressure, while others are capable of applying pressure equivalent to an elastic bandage. They are available in a variety of colors so another stocking is not required underneath or over them for the ambulatory patient. They are more expensive than regular stockings, possibly making them prohibitive for some patients. However, they wear well, and many persons who are on their feet or remain in one position a great deal of the time, such as homemakers, nurses, salesmen, and businessmen and businesswomen, find them very useful. The mild sustained pressure aids in preventing the accumulation of tissue fluid in the feet and the lower leg. Many patients can benefit from such stockings, and the nurse should be prepared to advise about their correct use. The stockings should be correctly fitted to the measurements of the individual. Also, they should be applied immediately upon awakening before getting out of bed and before the legs are in a dependent position. Immobilized patients who wear them continuously should have them removed and their legs inspected and bathed at least daily. Figure 29-17 illustrates a nurse teaching a patient about elasticized stockings.

Teaching the Patient to Care for His Wound

Today patients with wounds are often not hospitalized, or they return home before wounds are healed. Therefore, they or family members often need to learn to care for the wound. The nurse may see the patient in the physician's office, a clinic, or in the patient's home, as well as in the hospital.

Preparing the patient to care for his wound is a nursing responsibility. The nature and the amount of the teaching will depend on individual circumstances. Nurses have observed that patients usually are concerned about odor from dressings besides discomfort and fear of soiling clothing when drainage is present. Other disturbing factors include fear that the dressings will slip out of place and cause infection, concern for the reaction of friends and family to the appearance of the dressings, and the cost of the dressings.

While it remains important to use appropriate materials for wound care, the nurse also should assist the patient so that the cost of materials does not become unreasonable. Occasionally, the patient may need financial assistance, and an appropriate agency may be asked to help. Or, the patient may be referred to a local health organization that distributes dressings at a nominal cost or free of charge. The nurse who uses ingenuity based on appropriate principles can help the patient to keep the cost within a reasonable range and still carry out the procedure effectively.

Attention to aseptic technique and disposal of the old dressings and supplies are particularly important to control the spread of infections. The interested patient or family member can be helped to learn and be supported in independent and effective care of wounds.

CONCLUSION

Tissue trauma is a common occurrence. The ability of the body to contain and heal the injury is truly remarkable. Nursing actions discussed in this and other chapters throughout this book can serve to promote the physiologic processes of the body. Since many persons care for accidental injuries without ever seeking the assistance of health personnel, attempts to increase their knowledge of the body's defensive and restorative processes, and ways of supporting them can be classified as a means of health maintenance for the future. At the time of dealing with an existing injury, the patient is very often interested and motivated to learn.

Study Situations

1. The authors of the following article give some guide-

lines for how nurses can help promote the healing of wounds.

Aul, M. E., et al.: Wound healing. **Nurs. '72,** 2:36–40, Oct., 1972.

What helps and hindrances to wound healing were identified by the authors? How can you include these factors in your nursing care of a patient with an open or a closed wound?

2. Review your understanding of the data-gathering and the assessment subsystems of the nursing process system, as discussed in Unit 2. If you were responsible for the care of a patient with a surgical wound, what kinds of data would be appropriate to collect in relation to the wound? How would you gather and organize the data? What standards would you use to assess the data? Indicate your source for these standards. How would you validate the data and the nursing assessments?

3. To clarify your understanding of physics principles underlying the correct use of heat and cold, consult a physics textbook and determine whether convection, conduction, or evaporation is the primary process involved in each of the following situations:

Feeling chilly on a warm day when the humidity is about 40 percent and a slight breeze is blowing.

Feeling chilly in bed when you have insufficient covering.

Feeling warm and uncomfortable when the temperature is 72° F. and the humidity is 85 percent and there is no air movement.

Feeling chilly when only your feet touch a cold floor as you leave a warm bed.

If you make the effort to understand the principles in effect in the above situations, it also will increase your understanding of many nursing situations, such as, for example, the effect of air currents on older persons, the need for considering adequate covering for patients who are asleep or inactive, the reaction to being placed on a cold metal bedpan, the use of electric lamps for supplying heat to an infant's crib or to a patient's legs, and the need for considering altering the temperature of bath water during different times of the year and for patients of different age groups.

4. In an attempt to understand more fully some of the effects of heat and cold, consider some of your own experiences and then explain them on the basis of physical or physiologic principles.

For example, why does your entire body feel warm after you have kept only your hands in warm water to wash dishes? Who in your family or among your friends is least able to handle hot objects or cold objects, or requires a higher or lower room temperature to be comfortable?

5. Following major accidental injuries, long-term immobilization is often necessary. This article discusses some of the common problems resulting from the inactivity.

Campbell, E. B.: Nursing problems associated with

prolonged recovery following trauma. *In* **The Nursing Clinics of North America.** Philadelphia, W. B. Saunders, 5:551–562, Dec., 1970. *What potential problems does the author identify on page 558, as the result of the use of elastic stockings? What methods does she suggest for avoiding them.*

6. Patients often care for their own open wounds. They frequently need to be taught how to change wound dressings in a way to avoid contamination. Develop a teaching plan for a patient who has never changed a dressing. Prepare behaviorally stated objectives and the content that you would include. Do not forget: the hands are the most common vehicle for transporting pathogens and many persons do not know proper handwashing technique.

References

1. Barrett, D. Jr., and Klibanski, A.: Collagenase debridement. **Am. J. Nurs.,** 73:849–851, May, 1973.

2. Carroll, J. F., guest ed.: Symposium on the patient with trauma. *In* **The Nursing Clinics of North America.** Philadelphia, W. B. Saunders, 5:549–630, Dec., 1970.

3. Devney, A. M., and Kingsbury, B. A.: Hypothermia in fact and fantasy. **Am. J. Nurs.,** 72:1424–1425, Aug., 1972.

4. Dyer, E. D., and Bagnell, H. K.: Local tissue and general temperature changes in dogs produced by temperature applications. **Nurs. Research,** 19:37–41, Jan.–Feb., 1970.

5. Edelman, G. M.: The structure and function of antibodies. **Sci. Am.,** 223:34–42, Aug., 1970.

6. Faint, J.: Cold comfort—for alleviation of pain. **Nurs. Mirror,** 132:32–33, June 25, 1971.

7. Flitter, H. H.: An Introduction to Physics in Nursing. ed. 6. pp. 122–141. St. Louis, C. V. Mosby, 1972.

8. Glor, B. A. K., and Estes, Z. E.: Moist soaks: a survey of clinical practices. **Nurs. Research,** 19:463–465, Sept.–Oct., 1970.

9. Guberski, T., and Campbell, M. E.: The effects on leg volume of two methods of wrapping elastic bandages. **Nurs. Research,** 19:260–265, May–June, 1970.

10. Hickey, M. C.: Hypothermia. **Am. J. Nurs.,** 65:116–122, Jan., 1965.

11. Leider, M.: Some principles of dermatologic nursing. **RN,** 35:48–53, May, 1972.

12. Meyer, S. W.: Functional Bandaging Including Splints and Protective Dressings. New York, American Elsevier Publishing, 1967.

13. Myers, M. B.: Sutures and wound healing. **Am. J. Nurs.,** 71:1725–1727, Sept., 1971.

14. Powell, M.: An environment for wound healing. **Am. J. Nurs.,** 72:1862–1865, Oct., 1972.

15. Ross, R.: Wound healing. **Sci. Am.,** 220:40–50, June, 1969.

16. Wagner, M. M.: Assessment of patients with multiple injuries. **Am. J. Nurs.,** 72:1822–1827, Oct., 1972.

17. Weinstock, F. J.: Emergency treatment of eye injuries. **Am. J. Nurs.,** 71:1928–1931, Oct., 1971.

18. Wise, C. S.: Heat and Cold. *In* Bierman, W., and Licht, S. (eds.): Physical Medicine in General Practice. ed. 3. pp. 1–25. New York, Hoeber, 1955.

CHAPTER 30

Promoting Optimum Sensory Stimulation

GLOSSARY

Axon: Process that carries impulses from the neuron to the central nervous system.

Dendrite: Process that carries impulses to the neuron.

Dendron: Synonym for dendrite.

Neuron: A nerve cell.

Receptor: Structure that receives stimuli.

Sensory Deprivation: Reduction in optimum quantity and/or quality of sensory stimulation and perception.

Sensory Overload: Excessive stimulation of the senses.

INTRODUCTION

The subject of sensory perception is an area of interest to both biological and social scientists. Knowledge of the phenomenon has practical value for a variety of people, including the health practitioner.

To perceive is to be aware—to understand something. From conception to death, and particularly during the early formative years, the human organism uses sensory organs to learn about the environment in which he lives. As mentioned earlier in this text, behavior is meaningful and is considered in the context of the environment in which it occurs. Hence, sensory perception and knowledge of the world depends not only on an organism's genetic endowment, but on environmental influences as well. When an organism is deprived of stimuli from his environment and/or its perception, deleterious effects may result, as this chapter will explain.

NATURE OF SENSORY PERCEPTION

The study of perception begins with a nerve cell, or *neuron*. The cell has a process, usually one but sometimes more, called a *dendrite* or *dendron* that carries an impulse to the neuron. It also has a process called an *axon* that carries an impulse from it to the central nervous system. Although there is much still to be learned about an impulse, it has been determined that an electrical current is set up in a nerve when it is stimulated. Sensory nerves carry impulses to the brain. When an impulse reaches consciousness, the brain then has information about the outside world; for example, optic nerves carry messages from the eye; olfactory nerves carry information from the nose; and so on.

The structure that receives stimuli is called a *receptor;* the eye is the receptor of light waves, for example. The body's receptors in general respond best to only one type of stimulation. The exception are fibers that carry messages in relation to pain. They have no special structural receptor to receive stimuli, and as Chapter 23 pointed out, the nerve endings receive a variety of stimuli that are perceived as pain.

When nerve cells are studied, they do not appear very different from one another. Nor do essential differences show up when electrical currents associated with nerve cells and impulse transmission are studied. These findings pose an interesting question: how do we experience very different sensations? For example, the perception of lightning and of thunder are distinct and different sensations. We do not *hear* lightning nor *see* thunder. The quality and interpretation depend, for the most part, on the cerebral cortex and on a particular area or region where the impulse arrives. The cells in these regions interpret the impulses in a characteristic manner, accounting for differences in sensations.

A pattern for sensory perception can be seen. The receptor organs tune into specific stimuli; the impulse is carried to a particular area in the brain, depending on which receptor cells receive the impulse; and appropriate activity or a response is then initiated, depending on the nature and quality of the stimuli. From this description, it can be seen that the eye, for example, does not really *see*. Rather, it has receptor cells to receive stimuli, the impulse is transmitted to the brain, and there the impulse is interpreted as a visual sensation.

There are many different receptor cells in the body. Through them we are able to receive stimuli that are perceived by the brain as shape, color, space, movement, noise, pain, cold, hot, touch, size, odor, and taste.

Our nervous system is constantly bombarded with stimuli of various sorts. If man were to react to all of these stimuli, he could in no way function in an effective manner. The overload of stimuli would result in frustration and distorted behavior. It has been estimated that as much as 99 percent of the information received by the brain is discarded or not used at that time. The phenomenon can be experienced when driving a car as the brain effectively screens out visual and auditory distractions, plus others that would interfere with driving. Impulses that are not acted on when received may be used at a later date. The memory process involves the storage of that material. Thought and memory are used, for example, when a new sensory experience occurs and the organism uses a response based on previous knowledge and experience.

It has been observed that the human organism stops responding to a stimulus that is repeated many times. For example, it has been found that the repeated stimulus of a continuing noise eventually goes unnoticed. Some authorities speak of an adaptability phenomenon occurring in sensory reception. An offensive odor eventually goes undetected by a person exposed over a period of time. Adaptability in relation to the sense of pain appears to be least likely to occur, as Chapter 23 pointed out.

Man is a social animal and has constant stimulation from his physical and psychosocial environment. Research to date strongly suggests that we have inborn needs for physical and psychosocial stim-

ulation, and satisfying these needs promotes well-being.

This has been only a very brief summary of the nature of perception. Those wishing to explore the subject in further detail should refer to texts in physiology and psychology.

SENSORY DEPRIVATION AND OVER-LOAD DEFINED

It has just been noted that the brain does not act upon every message it receives from the environment through the sensory receptors. To do so would destroy well-being. Furthermore, well-being is not promoted when there is a lack of variety or an insufficient amount of stimuli being received by the body. When the input is below the optimum that promotes a particular individual's well-being, sensory deprivation is present.

Optimum input varies among individuals and is largely dependent, it appears, on a person's background. Hence, optimum input for well-being can be described best on a continuum. Some individuals appear to require more input to avoid boredom and apathy while others appear to require less. *Sensory deprivation*, then, means that one is receiving less than his optimum quantity and/or quality of sensory stimulation and perception, the end result of which can affect the individual's behavior.

Sensory overload is excessive stimulation of the senses. Because the brain selectively responds to stimuli, excessive stimulation results in an ignoring or nonfocusing on the less intense stimuli and thus, a type of sensory deprivation occurs. Researchers have found the behavioral changes which occur as the result of excessive stimulation are similar as those found in sensory deprivation. It is theorized that in both situations, *meaningful* stimuli are absent. Hence, the effects of sensory overload are thought to result from a type of sensory deprivation.

EFFECTS OF SENSORY DEPRIVATION

Although some of the effects of sensory deprivation had been described earlier in the literature, serious observations of persons suffering from it began about the time of World War II. During the war, persons in submarines operating various types of monitoring equipment were found to be missing important clues for no discernible reason. The monotony of the work as well as the isolated environment in which the work was carried out were investigated as possible reasons for operator failure. When variety in the environment and rest periods were introduced at regular intervals, efficiency began to improve. Findings of a comparable nature have been observed in industry also. Monotonous work environments and tasks repeated over and over again lead to inefficiency while variety with interspersed rest periods tends to promote productivity.

Research in the early 1950s further explored the effects of a monotonous environment. College students were subjected to an experimental environment in which all usual and typical perceptual stimulation was eliminated. The exposure to a very monotonous environment with no relief from identical stimuli was observed to have very definite deleterious effects on behavior. The students experienced impaired thinking, illusions, hallucinations, poor visual perception, and emotional disturbances. Thought content changed and the subjects became very irritable. The conclusion was that well-being is dependent on an environment that provides for constant as well as a variety in sensory stimulation. Without it, behavior becomes abnormal. (7)

Another example of a change in behavior presumably due to sensory deprivation was observed in babies. After a period of hospitalization for one to two weeks, where infants were rarely handled and the environment was monotonous, they were observed when they returned to their homes. They appeared unaware of objects and people; they had blank expressions, even when looking at their mothers; and they exhibited eating and sleeping disorders. These symptoms continued from two hours to as long as two days. The lack of sufficient sensory stimuli and the monotony of the environment were believed to be important contributing factors to the behavioral changes in these infants, all under seven months of age. (14:183)

Adults have been observed in a variety of settings when sensory deprivation existed. For example, many authorities believe that sensory deprivation plays a part in brainwashing techniques used on prisoners of war to obtain conversions in the prisoner's ideology, false confessions or secret information. Other factors undoubtedly are involved, such as illness and lack of sleep, but a prisoner's physical and social isolation with resulting sensory deprivation has been observed to correlate with intellectual and emotional disorganization and behavioral disturbances.

In elderly people, disturbed behavior may well have sensory deprivation as one causative factor. As age advances, sensory perception tends to become less acute, such as when hearing and vision fade. The person's earlier psychosocial environment with its variety of stimuli tends to shrink. Friends and mates die, work opportunities cease, children leave home to lead lives of their own, and mobility problems are often present. Defects in the sensory system and a limited psychosocial environment are believed to play an important role in disorientation and misinterpretation of environmental clues so often displayed by the elderly individual.

Mention was made in Chapter 23 concerning the effects of behavior when REM sleep is disturbed. Even during sleep, the well-being of an individual appears to be enhanced when sensory input continues through the experience of dreaming.

Chapter 23 also mentioned changes in the behavior of patients after spending a period of time in intensive or coronary care units. The environment is monotonous and sensory stimulation is unchanging. The normal stimulation from family members and other acquaintances is severely limited. Continuous artificial lighting is often used and the noise of mechanical equipment is a steady sound. Sleep is often interrupted for various checks of the patient's condition and essential therapeutic procedures. While there may be no doubt that interrupted sleep plays an important role, the behavior following the experience may also be influenced by sensory deprivation and the monotony of the environment.

One study observed patients in two different intensive care units, one being windowless and the other having windows and a bed arrangement that permitted the patients to observe the out-of-doors. Except for the presence or absence of windows, the settings, the patients, the general nature of their surgical procedures, and the care they received were considered to be on a comparable basis. Over twice as many patients in the windowless unit experienced delirium than those in the unit with windows. Depressive reactions were also more numerous among patients cared for in the windowless unit. The observer of the patients' behaviors concluded that sensory deprivation was an important causative factor in explaining the differences. (15)

Another observer of intensive care units described them as often following a numbing routine and he observed that patients frequently are well-drugged. The drugs reduce the body's ability to perceive stimuli and, as pointed out in Chapter 23, may interfere with certain stages of sleep. Lack of privacy was noted as patients were often thought-

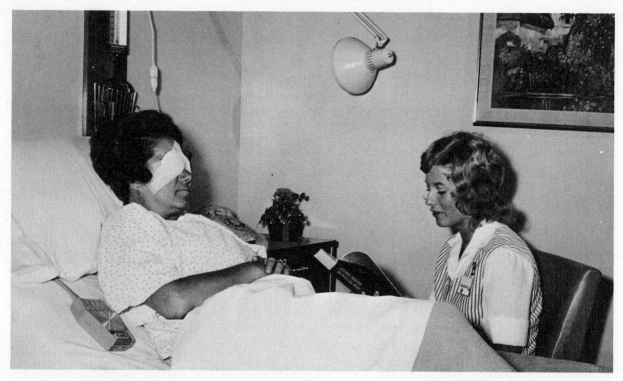

Fig. 30-1. For this temporarily blind woman, the day could be long and monotonous. The volunteer reads to the patient which helps to promote sensory stimulation during the time when the patient cannot see. (Good Samaritan Hospital, Phoenix, Arizona)

lessly exposed to strangers and to health and house-keeping personnel. These units tend to be characterized by a continuous monotony of strange noises, and there is a marked decrease in such customary sensations as smells, tastes, and sights. The observer felt that these factors in the intensive care unit were the ingredients of sensory deprivation and that they play an important role in explaining the changes in the behavior patients often exhibit following intensive care unit experiences. To emphasize his point in relation to the effects of sensory deprivation on behavior, this same observer described an elderly woman whose disoriented and confused states of mind ended abruptly when the lady's hearing aid was restored. (12)

To summarize this section, we can see that certain behavior seems to be characteristic of persons who have experienced sensory deprivation. These are some typical behavioral changes that have been described: visual and auditory hallucinations; illusions; paranoia; disturbances in the thought process and content; apathy; boredom; listlessness; feelings of strangeness; deterioration in ability to concentrate; and fluctuations in attention span.

PRINCIPLES IN RELATION TO SENSORY PERCEPTION AND SENSORY DEPRIVATION

Sensory stimulation and its perception are important for well-being. The contributions from heredity are certainly important to the development of an organism. However, the influences of the environment are essential also. Genetic and environmental influences interact and produce the individual organism. The environment providing stimuli to the organism appears to offer the setting in which an organism's potentials unfold. We do not grow in a vacuum. Hence, without adequate sensory stimulation and properly functioning sensory perception, the individual has been observed to suffer ill effects.

A changing sensory environment promotes well-being. Monotony is a curse to mankind. Curiosity and interest in the environment appear to be natural characteristics of the human organism. An environment that provides variety and opportunity for satisfying curiosity and interest appears to promote an individual's state of well-being.

When these two preceding principles are violated, that is, when sensory stimulation is in short supply and is unchanging in nature and when perception is below par, the resulting *sensory deprivation produces deleterious changes in an individual's behavior*. Investigation is necessarily limited by the amount and type of hardship factors that can be introduced when research on human beings is being conducted, and it is difficult to limit human research to one variable. Nevertheless, there appears to be sufficient evidence to theorize safely that human behavior deteriorates in situations where sensory deprivation exists.

Observations of persons who have suffered sensory deprivation indicate that *the effects of sensory deprivation occur relatively rapidly*. Also, *the human organism has remarkable ability to cope with sensory deprivation and to return to normal behavior when sensory deprivation is terminated*. The literature does not suffer from a dearth of information concerning the remarkable recoveries men have made, for example, after harrowing experiences with marked sensory deprivation as war prisoners. Also, many battered and isolated children have been observed to make great strides toward recovery when the abuses are discontinued. The wonder is that many of these people survive their devastating experiences at all. Also, the return to normal, especially when sensory deprivation has not been unusually long or severe, can occur in a relatively short period of time. Some of the hospitalized infants, referred to earlier in this chapter, were observed to display normal behavior in as little as two hours. Patients who have spent time in intensive and coronary care units and have demonstrated behavioral changes have been observed to display excellent progress toward recovery within 24 hours after transfer to other environments. In addition, many persons permanently handicapped because of destruction of sensory organs demonstrate great ability to adapt to these losses and often with minimal behavioral changes. Motivation to surmount handicaps and to return to a state of well-being, and the body's inherent ability to strive for and reach homeostasis, no doubt play critical roles in the organism's remarkable ability to cope with adversity.

IMPLICATIONS FOR NURSING

The nurse who is concerned about sensory deprivation in her care should think of ways in which it can be prevented, be alert to situations in which sensory deprivation may occur, and plan for assisting patients to cope with it when it is present. There are several clinical entities that she will want to keep in mind since they tend to predispose to sensory deprivation. Patients who have had damage or trauma to the sense organs themselves are candidates for the effects of sensory deprivation; for example, the patient who has lost his sight or his hearing is a likely prospect. So also are those patients who lack a keenness of perception such as may occur following an injury or a cerebrovascular accident. As was pointed out earlier, elderly patients whose senses are beginning to diminish and whose psychosocial environments are decreasing can show at least some of the characteristic effects of sensory deprivation.

Patients who are physically or socially isolated for any reason often display signs of sensory deprivation. An example is the person who must be isolated from others because of an infectious disease or because he is highly susceptible to acquiring infections from others. Care for these patients was discussed in Chapter 19. Patients whose death appears to be imminent often are isolated from their usual environment and describe feelings of lonesomeness and fear. These patients need special attention for minimizing sensory deprivation to whatever extent is possible. Anyone with a chronic disease who may need long periods of care in a health agency or even at home is susceptible. Many patients in nursing homes, generally elderly to begin with and separated from their usual environment by requiring the constant care offered by these facilities, can be expected to display ill effects from sensory deprivation if steps are not taken to prevent it.

Patients who must be immobilized for a period of time will often display signs of sensory deprivation. Examples include patients who have had a heart attack and those placed in restrictive casts following injuries. The typical surgical patient generally has limited mobility postoperatively with accompanying social isolation for a period of time. Mention was made of the sensory deprivation so often found in the environment of the intensive and coronary care units, and patients needing these facilities may be expected to display changes in behavior. Patients using respirators and kidney dialysis machines are additional examples of patients with limited mobility.

In the processes of data gathering and assessment, it will become evident to the nurse whether sensory deprivation is possibly present or whether the patient is a likely candidate for problems commonly associated with it. In developing a plan of care, the nurse will look for measures to increase variety and amount of sensory stimulation and/or measures that will help to retain sensory stimulation at optimum levels. She will then implement these measures accordingly.

There is hardly a chapter in this text that does not include nursing measures that can help to prevent sensory deprivation as well as measures to assist patients to cope with it. The importance of *caring* in nursing and of developing therapeutic relationships with patients was discussed as basic to effective nursing care. Certainly they are important to help patients learn to cope with handicaps and other situations that have been observed to lead to problems in relation to sensory deprivation. Here are some additional nursing measures that have been discussed in various chapters in this text and that will help to serve the patient in assisting to prevent or cope with sensory deprivation.

• Involve patients and allow them to take an active role in planning and decision-making in relation to their care. The patient who is active mentally and physically to the extent possible is less likely to experience sensory deprivation.

• Provide a variety of diversional activities. As has been pointed out, most patients have television and radio at their disposal. While these are certainly helpful, many other diversions that actively involve the person can be used to help in eliminating monotony and boredom from nothing to do or think about. The use of lounges and dining rooms was mentioned, for example, as means to promote social stimulation among patients being cared for in in-service facilities. Maintenance of an active role in family affairs, even though it may be very limited, is important for the homebound patient.

• Provide an immediate environment that relieves monotony. The use of interior decorating techniques to relieve the monotony of the room in which the patient spends a great deal of his time has been mentioned. Moving patients about to the extent possible from room to room when being cared for at home and moving a patient to various places in a room if he is in a health agency were suggested. The patient mentioned in an earlier chapter who had nothing but a telephone pole to look at from her hospital window expressed how much more interesting it would have been had she been placed so that she could have seen the lovely landscape and outdoor activity from her bed. Varying the lighting in a room is also helpful to provide optimum stimulation.

• Allow visitors to the extent permitted by policy and the patient's condition. The patient who

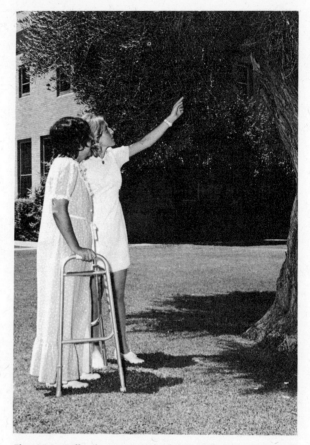

Fig. 30-2. Following a period of immobilization in a cast, this patient is learning to walk again. She welcomes the walk out-of-doors with her nurse and the variety of new and different stimuli it presents after confinement in her hospital room. (Good Samaritan Hospital, Phoenix, Arizona)

is with those he knows and loves is in an environment that is as near normal as possible. Many times, this text has pointed out instances in which the patient's family members and friends can be included in his overall care, and encouraging this usually works in the patient's favor.

• Teach and explain to the patient so that he knows what is happening to him. The more knowledge the patient has about his condition and how he can cope with it, usually the better able he is to handle fears, frustration, and confusion of unfamiliar stimuli.

• Promote well-being by offering care that provides for rest and comfort. Interrupted sleep and discomfort often lead to uncomfortable perceptions. Measures to relieve them help to provide for normal sensory perception.

• Provide activity and exercises. A variety of activities and exercises, all of which aid to maintain normal sensory perceptions and decrease the likelihood of sensory deprivation, were discussed in Chapter 22.

• Provide communication avenues for the patient. The importance of communication, and especially of touch, have been described. Participating with the patient in goal-directed communication and taking the time to use touch as a means of communication can hardly be overemphasized. The interactions that occur during both verbal and nonverbal communication offer innumerable sensory stimuli.

• Stimulate as many senses as possible. Varied sights, sounds, smells, body positions, and textures can all be helpful in helping to provide a variety of sensations.

• Offer reassurance to the patient. Reassuring a patient occurs in many ways. Sometimes just the touch of a hand will help. On other occasions, explanations and teaching are indicated. In still other situations, just being present is more important than any activity can be as a means of offering reassurance.

• Be aware of and take cultural factors into consideration when offering nursing care. This is especially important when caring for patients from cultures other than one's own. The isolation from familiar cultural behaviors and the inability to communicate with others in his native tongue, for example, can significantly decrease a patient's usual sensory perceptions.

• Provide privacy for the patient. The legal implications when the patient's privacy is violated have been discussed. This chapter also mentioned the importance of providing privacy in order to sustain the patient's self-esteem. Providing privacy does not mean isolation, but respecting it often is conducive to the satisfying promotion of psychosocial interactions.

CONCLUSION

Sensory perception and sensory deprivation as they relate to health care are relatively new areas of concern to many health practitioners. In the past, behavioral changes that appeared to be without a definite etiological basis often remained unexplained and accepted as normal in the course of events. With the blossoming of research in the area of sensory deprivation, possibly much of this behavior is about to have better explanations.

It would appear that once again, knowledge in the area of sensory deprivation and sensory perception reemphasizes the futility of thinking of the human body in terms of a physical entity and a psychological entity. Observations in terms of the interrelatedness of the body's functions, the interdependence of genetic and environmental influences, and the uniqueness of each individual continue to mount and they support the use of a holistic approach when offering patient care. It is knowledge no health practitioner can afford to ignore when offering health services, including nursing care in relation to meeting the patient's need for adequate sensory stimulation and perception.

Study Situations

1. The following article was written by a nurse-author who described a devastating experience that included sensory deprivation.

   Thomson, L. R.: Sensory deprivation: a personal experience. **Am. J. Nurs.,** 73:266–268, Feb., 1973.

   List symptoms this nurse demonstrated that are typically displayed when patients experience sensory deprivation. After reading this article, one can assume that there were times when attention was necessarily focused primarily on lifesaving measures rather than on the patient per se. However, from the author's descriptions, suggest ways in which sensory deprivation might have been minimized in at least some instances. It is unrealistic to assume that all of the monotony of the intensive care unit can be eliminated, even if that were a sincere desire. But what suggestions would you offer to make the unit a more pleasant place in which to receive care?

2. In the September 1970 issue of **The Nursing Clinics of North America,** volume 5, there is a group of articles concerning the care of patients with sensory defects. Read the following article first to increase your understanding of sensory deprivation.

   Chodill, J., and Williams, B.: The concept of sensory deprivation. pp. 453–465.

   In each of the following articles, there are descriptions of nursing measures to aid in minimizing sensory deprivation for patients with specific sensory disturbances.

   Note the orientation procedures and diversional activities the author recommends in the following article.

   Condl, E. D.: Ophthalmic nursing: the gentle touch. pp. 467–476.

   In the following article, note suggested measures to assist and reassure the patient who is temporarily blind.

   Seaman, F. W.: Nursing care of glaucoma patients. pp. 489–496.

   What suggestions did the authors of the following article make for communicating with the patient who is hard of hearing?

Conover, M., and Cober, J.: Understanding and caring for the hearing-impaired. pp. 497–506.

What nursing measures are suggested in the following article to assist the speechless patient?

Parvulescu, N. F.: Care of the surgically speechless patient. pp. 517–525.

Note the special techniques the author of the following article recommends when teaching patients with sensory defects.

Cullin, I. C.: Techniques for teaching patients with sensory defects. pp. 527–538.

3. Compare the definition of hypovigilance given in the following article with the definition of sensory deprivation given in this chapter.

Meinhart, N. T., and Aspinall, M. J.: Nursing intervention in hypovigilance. **Am. J. Nurs.,** 69:994–998, May, 1969.

What hypothesis did the nurse make after observing Mr. G.'s continuous moaning? What nursing intervention was planned to provide Mr. G. with greater sensory input, and what were the effects of the intervention measures on Mr. G.'s behavior?

References

1. Anastasi, A.: Fields of Applied Psychology. pp. 163–192. New York, McGraw-Hill, 1964.

2. Berlyne, D. E.: Curiosity and exploration. **Science,** 153:25–33, July 1, 1966.

3. Carlson, S.: Communication and social interaction in the aged. *In* **The Nursing Clinics of North America.** Philadelphia, W. B. Saunders, 7:269–279, June 1972.

4. Carnevali, D., and Brueckner, S.: Immobilization—reassessment of a concept. **Am. J. Nurs.,** 70:1502–1507, July, 1970.

5. Carty, R.: Patients who cannot hear. **Nurs. Forum,** 11:290–299, No. 3, 1972.

6. Ellis, R.: Unusual sensory and thought disturbances after cardiac surgery. **Am. J. Nurs.,** 72:2021–2025, Nov., 1972.

7. Heron, W.: The pathology of boredom. **Sci. Am.,** 196:52–56, Jan., 1957.

8. Jackson, C. W. Jr., and Ellis, R.: Sensory deprivation as a field of study. **Nurs. Res.,** 20:46–54, Jan.–Feb., 1971.

9. Moore, M. V.: Diagnosis: deafness. **Am. J. Nurs.,** 69:297–300, Feb., 1969.

10. Ohno, M. I.: The eye-patched patient. **Am. J. Nurs.,** 71:271–274, Feb., 1971.

11. Stone, V.: Give the older person time. **Am. J. Nurs.,** 69:2124–2127, Oct., 1969.

12. Vaisrub, S.: Windows for the soul. **Arch. Intern. Med.,** 130:297, Aug., 1972.

13. Velazquez, J. M.: Alienation. **Am. J. Nurs.,** 69:301–304, Feb., 1969.

14. Vernon, M. D.: The Psychology of Perception. Baltimore, Penguin Books, 1962.

15. Wilson, L. M.: Intensive care delirium: the effect of outside deprivation in a windowless unit. **Arch. Intern. Med.,** 130:225–226, Aug., 1972.

CHAPTER 31

Caring for the Patient
When Death Appears Imminent

GLOSSARY

Autopsy: Examination of organs and tissues of the human body after death.

Cryonics: The freezing of dead human bodies.

Euthanasia: Painless or mercy killing.
Thanatology: Study of death and its medical and psychological effects.

INTRODUCTION

A terminal illness is one from which recovery is beyond reasonable expectation. The illness may be due to a disease condition or the result of accident or injury. Errors of judgment concerning recovery sometimes are made, and some readers may recall from personal experiences patients whose illnesses were considered as being terminal, but they survived and lived for many years. Because errors of judgment can occur, and during the course of an illness medical progress may bring forth a means of saving a life, there is good reason to remain hopeful while caring for terminally ill patients. The patient and his family often find courage and support in knowing that everything possible is being done and that hope for recovery is not abandoned.

The inevitability of death is nowhere better expressed than in Ecclesiastes 3:1-2—"To everything there is a season, and a time to every purpose under the heaven; A time to be born, and a time to die; . . ." Everyone has the privilege of and the right to meet death serenely and comfortably, and the nurse can do much to make this experience less fraught with sorrow, fear, and discomfort for all concerned.

In addition to the continuing research during the last decade or two to find ways to prevent death from specific pathology, there has been increased interest in the process of dying and death *per se.* The term *thanatology* refers to the study of death and its medical and psychological effects.

The questions, both scientific and ethical, surrounding dying and death are extensive and complex. Health personnel, bioengineers, lawyers, social scientists, philosophers, biologists, theologians, and lay persons are among those involved in the discussion and investigations. The increased use of organ transplants and bioengineering techniques that make it possible to sustain life in persons who previously would have died, the liberalization of abortion laws, and concerns about world overpopulation are some of the factors that have stimulated increasing attention on death.

The concept that death is a natural part of life and not just a failure in medical technology has become more prevalent also. Health care workers and agencies have been so concerned with cures, health maintenance, and restoration that death was often viewed as a personal failure on the part of health personnel. As a result, the terminally ill patient unfortunately was frequently avoided, except for essential physical care. Health personnel received little formal educational preparation for care of the dying person. There was generally a reluctance on the part of health personnel to discuss or acknowledge feelings about death with a patient or family members or even in professional conferences.

Today, death and dying are commonly the focus of literature, conferences, and investigations, and are included as a part of virtually all curricula designed to prepare health personnel. There are varied programs offered to family members both during the terminal illness of patients and following death in some areas. In some agencies, routinely scheduled health team conferences for dealing constructively with health workers' feelings and for planning improved patient care are indications of other changes which have occurred and which are influencing the care of terminally ill persons.

The nurse is often a key person in the care of the patient who is dying and is in contact with his family, regardless of whether the patient is at home or in a health agency. Both the patient and the family often turn to her for support and assistance. In order to provide effective care, the nurse must have reconciled some of her own feelings about death. She needs to understand the phases of grieving and dying and be able to recognize their manifestations. Perhaps most of all, she needs to be able to accept and support the individuality of the person, whether his beliefs or behavior coincide with her own. Provision of care may be easier if the nurse sees her purpose as that of assisting the patient to meet his physical and psychological needs, just as with any other patient. Her goal is to provide the support and assistance necessary to help the patient die with as much comfort and dignity as possible.

The Code for Nurses of the American Nurses' Association includes in the elaboration of its first statement a summary of some of the ideas just expressed. "The nurse's respect for the worth and dignity of the individual human being extends throughout the entire life cycle, from birth to death, . . . the young and the old, the recovering patient as well as the one who is terminally ill or dying. In the latter instance the nurse should use all the measures at her command to enable the patient to live out his days with as much comfort, dignity, and freedom from anxiety and pain as possible. His nursing care will determine, to a great degree, how he lives this final human experience and the peace and dignity with which he approaches death." (7:2582)

The Division on Geriatric Nursing Practice of the American Nurses' Association has included a statement on the nurse's responsibility regarding the dying patient. "The nurse seeks to resolve her conflicting attitudes regarding aging, death, and dependency so that she can assist older persons, and their relatives, to maintain life with dignity and comfort until death ensues." (36:1897)

GENERAL PRINCIPLES REGARDING CARE OF THE DYING PATIENT

The process of dying occurs over a period of time in most instances. Only trauma of major proportion causes instant death. Most persons die gradually over a period of hours or even days and weeks. Human cells cease to live as the result of oxygen deprivation. The capacity of tissues varies as to the period of time they can live in an anoxic state.

The responses human beings make to loss ordinarily occur in discernible stages. The manner of manifesting anticipated or experienced loss is expressed by every person in his own unique way. The process occurs at various rates of speed. However, there are discernible stages, described later in this chapter, that persons normally experience as they respond to loss.

Sharing fears and concerns with others generally makes dealing with them easier. There are few exceptions to the observation that most persons have some fear of dying. Communication between persons can have the effect of both dissipating anxiety and of increasing the ability to cope with it. Dying patients and family members often share their fears with the nurse. The nurse herself also may need to strengthen her resources through sharing her concerns with others.

Nonverbal communication often conveys messages more readily than verbal communication. As Chapter 13 pointed out, our feelings and thoughts frequently are communicated to others nonverbally. The nurse caring for a patient undergoing stresses will wish to tune in to the patient's nonverbal communication; also, the patient will be aware of the nurse's nonverbal communication. The nurse caring for the dying patient will first wish to make every effort to deal honestly and openly with her own feelings. Without doing so, she may very easily convey her own fears and uncertainties to the patient.

THE NURSE'S ATTITUDE TOWARD TERMINAL ILLNESS

Understanding others through understanding oneself is an oft-repeated psychological principle the importance of which probably would be argued by few. Since impending death is accompanied by fear of the unknown and the natural instinct of all creatures to cling to life, it becomes particularly important for the nurse to understand her own feelings toward terminal illness, death, and its usual accompanying grief in order to help to meet the needs of patients for whom she is caring.

Because in our culture, youth and productivity are highly valued in contrast to illness, aging, and dying, the nurse brings these influences with her when caring for terminally ill patients. The orientation of society and her educational background are strongly directed toward health and life. These experiences make dealing with death a difficult occurrence. The nurse must also deal with her views and feelings regarding prolongation of life by artificial means and regarding *euthanasia*, that is, painless or mercy killing. Discussing one's feelings and views with others is one of the most effective ways of developing increased insight and learning to handle personal emotions.

The nurse who neglects to deal with her feelings concerning life, dying, and death is in a questionable position to be able to analyze and consider the needs of patients who are facing death. Therefore, one's own personality, feelings, and attitudes play a major role in determining how one cares for a patient with a terminal illness. Everyone, not only the nurse, experiences intense emotion when death is pending. The easy way to react is to ignore the feelings. Sadly enough, as a result, the dying person and his family are often emotionally abandoned and left to face a very lonesome situation alone.

RESPONSE PATTERNS TO DYING AND GRIEVING

While every person responds to the knowledge of impending death or to loss in a distinctive way, studies have shown there are typical response patterns or stages. Dr. Elisabeth Kübler-Ross has described the psychological stages through which a dying person goes. The stages do not always follow one another or they may overlap. The duration of any stage can vary from being as brief as a few hours to being as lengthy as a period of months.

Dr. Kübler-Ross describes the stages as denial and isolation, anger, bargaining, depression, and acceptance. In the denial and isolation stage, the person usually reacts with feelings of loneliness and a type of response expressed by "No, not me. It must be a mistake." During the anger stage, his reaction is generally a "Why me?", with expressions of hostility directed at family members, friends, and health personnel. When he proceeds to the bargaining stage, he responds with a "Yes, me, but . . ." The bargain often is a promise to God in exchange for an extension of life. The depression stage is indicated by a "Yes, me" acknowledgment and general sadness. The final stage of acceptance is a positive feeling of "I'm ready."

Dr. George L. Engel has described phases of grieving. In some instances, the phases of grieving overlap the stages of dying. The phases are expressed individually and take varying amounts of time. Grieving is an emotional response to loss. The loss object can vary—it may be another person lost through death or merely by separation; it can be loss of a body function or part, a job, a home, a pet, or anything else meaningful to the person. One who is terminally ill can grieve for his own loss of capacities or impending loss of life, or a person can grieve in anticipation of losing another. Most authorities feel that families as well as health personnel caring for terminally ill persons grieve over their loss.

Dr. Engel views the process of grieving as being normal and essential to recovery from the loss. He compares grieving to wound healing, the former being a response to psychological trauma and the latter being a response to physical trauma. He wrote (9:94):

"If we define grief as the typical reaction to the loss of a source of psychological gratification, we can compare the experience of the loss to the wound while the subsequent psychological responses to the loss may be compared to the tissue reaction and the processes of healing. . . . Successful grief and grieving follow certain more or less predictable steps which permit a judgment that healing is taking place. This healing process can be interfered with by unsound intervention, by failure to provide optimal conditions for healing, or because the individual's resources are not up to the task. But the normal healing processes of grieving cannot be accelerated."

Engel's phases of grieving include shock and disbelief, developing awareness, restitution, resolving the loss, and idealization. Shock and disbelief are usually characterized by a refusal or inability to accept the fact followed by a numbness or stunned response. Developing awareness may be indicated by physical or emotional responses. The person may have pain or become nauseated or experience a physical feeling of emptiness. He may express anger or despair or cry. Restitution is the ritualization of a loss. In the case of death, it includes the religious, cultural, or societal expressions of mourning. Resolving the loss involves the process of dealing with the painful void left by the loss. Idealization often involves exaggeration of the good qualities of the loss object followed by an acceptance of the loss and a diminished focus on it.

Since the process of grieving takes time, those experiencing it will also be influenced by the amount of time they have had available. In some situations, the family and friends of someone with a chronic illness may have passed through the early phases of grieving before the person dies. The family who loses a member in an unexpected manner has not had an opportunity to experience any of the grieving process.

Since all persons experience grieving over a loss and since the process is an individual one, many variations in the amount of time it will take and the manner by which it will be manifested can be expected. Different family members are often in varying grieving phases. In addition, health team members can be at still different points in the process.

In order to understand her own feelings and to help the patient and his family, the nurse needs to be able to identify the response state in which the involved people are. Then she can use her skills to provide appropriate support.

HELPING THE PATIENT WHO HAS A TERMINAL ILLNESS

Helping to Meet Emotional Needs

Discussion in Chapter 11 pointed out the importance of helping patients to feel secure. The importance of helping a patient to maintain self-identity, his sense of worth, and his feeling of belonging were stressed. These factors in helping patients face death are especially important. Even when it is known that nothing available to medical science can prolong a patient's life, hope continues and the patient benefits when helped to feel secure.

Hope is desire accompanied by a feeling of anticipation or expectation. Without hope, despair exists. Hope, no matter how minimal, usually occurs in the patient, his family, and in the nurse. However, very often the patient's hope, the family's hope, and the nurse's hope are not the same. As the patient begins to face impending death, he may hope to be free of pain or nausea or to be able to walk down the hall one more time; his family may still be hoping for a miraculous cure; the nurse may be at some point in between. It is the patient's hope which should be identified and supported if realistic. The nurse will want to work toward fulfillment of his hope and assisting the family toward accepting the patient's wishes.

How can the nurse help patients meet the emotional need for security? Although the content in Unit 3 offers many clues, there is no magic formula. However, there are two general guides: being available and present as much as possible and offering whatever assistance can be given. The nurse's understanding, support, and respect are needed by the patient and his family.

The manner in which patients face death depends on several factors. Philosophies of life and death differ. Most patients are afraid, while others may look forward to death as a relief from earthly suffering and sorrow. Some patients—often those having strong religious beliefs—have been observed to be spiritually exalted and ready to enter another life to which they look forward with joy. Other patients may treat death as an avenger and feel so depressed and desperate that they have suicidal tendencies. Also, the patient's attitudes toward and philosophy about death may be the result of his cultural background.

The age of the patient often influences the manner in which terminal illness and death are accepted. Children usually approach death with little fear or

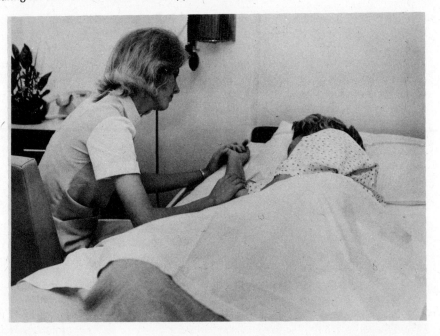

Fig. 31-1. The nurse can often communicate her concern and support for the patient by simply remaining at her side and often touch is the most effective means of communication. (Good Samaritan Hospital, Phoenix, Arizona)

sorrow. Teen-agers and adults through middle age often consider death as an injustice for they yearn to continue the experience of life and are sad about leaving their loved ones. This earnestness to live almost always subsides as death approaches, but in some cases it may not. Older people more often face death as a friend. They may have little desire to live and often are lonesome and tired of life, especially when loved ones have died before them. The nurse should be careful that she does not misjudge the patient, and if he is old, expect him to have a peaceful attitude toward approaching death. No two persons experience death in the same fashion. As no two lives are lived the same, death too is an individualized experience.

A patient's reaction to approaching death may change from day to day. A discouraged person may feel more so one day and less so another. The nurse must often develop great sensitivity in order to detect the patient's responses if she is to find clues for guiding her action.

Sometimes, a patient may mask his true feelings about death or may not really want to face the truth. The patient may claim to be unafraid and prepared for death when he really is fearful and just trying to appear brave. Patience, careful observation, and listening in order to learn true feelings are a prerequisite if the nurse desires to give sincere comfort and support to the dying patient.

Knowing the patient's attitudes and feelings helps the nurse to care for him intelligently. The behavior of a patient facing death may not conform to what the nurse believes to be correct. But her actions must be guided by the patient's feelings and attitudes, not hers. Comfort, support, and encouragement are essential, but the manner in which they are offered depends on individual circumstances. In some instances, the nurse may find that it is best to say nothing and just listen. The patient may find comfort in having someone with whom he can talk out his feelings. The lonely patient may experience support and understanding by a simple handclasp.

The question usually arises concerning what to tell the terminally ill patient about his prognosis. It is the physician who usually is responsible for deciding what and how the patient shall be told. Usually he makes this decision after discussing the problem with the patient's family and after assessing the patient individually. The nurse, social worker, or clergyman may also be involved in making the decision and in discussing it with the patient.

In some situations, the physician may prefer to deny the patient knowledge about his prognosis or all of the involved factors. He may feel that the experience of knowing may precipitate a psychological state of depression leading possibly to suicide. In some instances, this argument may be valid. The knowledge of impending death may be too much for some to tolerate.

In other situations, the patient does have an interest and a desire to know. It is generally considered unkind and unjust to permit such a patient to die without his having known the seriousness of his condition. For example, by not knowing, he may have had the time denied him to arrange important business affairs, papers, finances, and the like. Many people, especially those who have responsibilities to others, such as their children, find comfort in the fact that, should they die, "their house is in order."

Most people now seem to feel that withholding the truth from the patient is undesirable and often even harmful. From many observations, it has been seen that most patients realize without being told that they are suffering from an incurable illness. The nonverbal communication of the patient's family and the health personnel often speak louder than their words. Patients often feel even more isolated, lonely, and rejected when the truth is withheld, especially when falsehoods are told them. After the prognosis has been discussed in an open and frank manner, health personnel must be prepared to offer the patient support. But usually the patient finds solace eventually in knowing and realizing that he will not be left to meet death alone.

The important thing for all involved persons is to know exactly what the patient and family have been told. Patients and families often direct questions to the nurse concerning prognosis. Unless all persons are aware of what the patient has been told, they may be working at cross-purposes. It is up to the nurse to take the initiative to discuss the problem with the physician in circumstances in which uncertainty exists.

Physicians and nurses caring for dying patients need a close working relationship. A type of camaraderie will often develop as a result of the stress usually involved when helping patients and families cope with a difficult situation. Mutual trust and respect among health care personnel can promote a climate which provides additional security for the patient and his family. Physicians will often depend on the nurse for care suggestions because the physician may no longer have an active medical regimen to implement.

As has been stated earlier in this text, the patient should be permitted to retain as much independence and decision-making as he is able. When physical abilities fail, determining when he wishes his medication, for example, may be all of the control of his life he retains.

The adult patient has the ultimate right to refuse treatment. In dealing with the person with an incurable illness, sometimes health personnel find the patient's desire not to have further surgery or extensive treatments difficult to accept. At other times, the patient has ambivalent feelings and needs to be permitted time and the support necessary to explore those feelings.

Many patients make decisions to donate various body organs after death to organ banks for possible transplantation. The patient may ask the nurse questions about the technique or about her views. He may be seeking information or he may wish to explore his feelings aloud. The nurse should assist the patient in these conversations rather than focus on her own beliefs. Legal documents permitting organ removal are available from most health agencies. Care should be taken to see that they are accurately completed if it is the patient's desire to donate organs.

Helping to Meet Spiritual Needs

Many terminally ill patients find great comfort in the support that they receive from their religious faiths. It is important to aid in obtaining the services of a clergyman as each situation indicates. In some instances, the nurse may offer to call a clergyman when the patient or family has not expressed a desire to see one, but this must be handled tactfully and in good judgment so that the patient is not frightened by the suggestion. However, it must be remembered that a religious faith is not an insurance policy guaranteeing security from the tragedy and the loneliness of death. The chaplain's visit does not replace the kind words and the gentle touch of the nurse. Rather, he should be considered as one of the team assisting the patient to face terminal illness.

Helping to Meet Physical Needs

Unless death occurs suddenly, there are certain nursing problems concerning the patient's physical needs that the nurse usually can expect to encounter.

NUTRITION: The patient who is terminally ill usually has little interest in food and fluids. His appetite fails, and often the physical effort to eat or drink is too great for him. Meeting nutritional needs may in itself help to prolong life, and it also often helps to make the patient more comfortable. Dehydration and cachexia predispose to exhaustion, infection, and other complications, as the development of decubiti. Therefore, maintaining the nutritional state of the patient plays an important part in sustaining energy and preventing additional discomfort. When the patient is unable to take fluids and food by mouth, the physician may order intravenous therapy or other means of maintaining nutrition.

When death is pending, the normal activities of the gastrointestinal tract decrease. Therefore, offering the patient large quantities of food may only predispose to distention and added discomfort.

If the swallowing reflex is intact, offering sips of water at frequent intervals is helpful. As swallowing becomes difficult, aspiration may occur when fluids are given. The patient can suck on gauze soaked in water or on ice chips wrapped in gauze without difficulty since sucking is one of the last reflexes to disappear as death approaches.

CARE OF THE MOUTH, THE NOSE AND THE EYES: If the patient is taking foods and fluids without difficulty, oral hygiene is similar to that offered other patients. However, as death approaches, the mouth usually needs additional care. Mucus that cannot be swallowed or expectorated accumulates in the mouth and the throat and may need to be aspirated. The mouth can be wiped out with gauze, or, if indicated, suctioning may be necessary to remove mucus. Positioning the patient on his side very often helps in keeping the mouth and the throat free of accumulated mucus.

The mucous membrane should be kept free of dried secretions. Lubricating the mouth and the lips is helpful as well as comfortable for the patient.

The nostrils should be kept clean also and lubricated as necessary.

Sometimes, secretions from the eyes accumulate. The eyes may be wiped clean with wipes or cotton balls moistened in normal saline. If the eyes are dry, they tend to stay open. The instillation of a lubricant in the conjunctival sac may be indicated to prevent friction and possible ulceration of the cornea.

CARE OF THE SKIN: As death approaches, the patient's temperature usually is elevated above normal. But, as peripheral circulation fails, the skin feels cold, and the patient often perspires profusely. It is important to keep the bed linens and the bed clothing dry by bathing the patient and changing linens as necessary. Using light bed clothing and supporting it so that it does not rest on the patient's body usually give additional comfort. The patient often is restless and may be observed to pick at his bed clothing. This may be due to the fact that he feels too warm; sponging him and keeping him dry often promote relaxation and quiet sleeping.

ELIMINATION: Some patients may be incontinent while others may need to be observed for retention of urine and for constipation, both of which are uncomfortable for the patient. Cleansing enemas may be ordered for relieving and preventing constipation and distention, but it should be remembered that, if the patient is taking little nourishment, there may be only small amounts of fecal material in the intestine.

Catheterization at regular intervals, or indwelling catheters, may be necessary for some patients. If the patient is incontinent of urine and feces, care of the skin becomes particularly important to prevent odors and decubiti. Waterproof bed pads are easier to change than all of the bed linens; they make keeping the bed clean and dry less problematic.

POSITIONING THE PATIENT: The dorsal recumbent position often is associated with the dying patient. However, good nursing care provides for good positioning with frequent changes in position. The patient may not be able to express a desire to have his position changed, or he may feel that the effort is too great. Even though the patient appears to be unconscious, proper positioning is important. Poor positioning without adequate support is fatiguing as well as uncomfortable.

Sometimes the nurse is confronted with the problem of a patient who experiences intractable pain except when in one position. She must weigh the consequences of constant pressure, impaired circulation, and tissue breakdown against the patient's comfort.

When dyspnea is present, the patient will be more comfortable when supported in the semi-sitting position. Stertorous or noisy breathing frequently is relieved when the patient is placed on his side. This position helps to keep the tongue from obstructing the respiratory passageway in the oropharynx. Proper positioning has been discussed earlier in this text, and the same principles that were discussed then guide action in positioning the terminally ill patient.

PROTECTING THE PATIENT FROM HARM: The terminally ill patient may be restless. In these instances, special precautions are necessary to protect the patient from harm. The use of bedrails may be indicated. Restraining the patient usually is undesirable but may be necessary in extreme cases. If relatives of the patient offer to remain with him so that he does not injure himself, the nurse may give them simple guidelines about talking softly to the patient and reassuring him with gentle touch contact. Family members of the inpatient should not be left with the complete burden of the patient's safety. The nurse should check the patient frequently because the responsibility for the patient's welfare is hers. Well-meaning, but unprepared, fatigued, and stressed family members sometimes use poor judgment in protecting the patient. Feeling the responsibility of care, or guilt if some unexpected occurrence results in injury, is an unfair price to expect family members to pay. If relatives or friends do stay with the patient, the nurse should see that they are relieved periodically. Remaining with a confused and restless terminally ill person can be both physically and emotionally taxing.

CARE OF THE ENVIRONMENT: It is economical of nursing time to place the hospitalized patient in a room that is convenient for giving nursing care and for observing him at frequent intervals. Very often, the patient is placed in a private room to avoid distressing other patients. However, this experience in itself may be upsetting to the patient. Social deprivation can be distressing to the patient, even if he cannot express this.

Having familiar objects in view can help to make the patient feel more comfortable and secure. The family can be encouraged to make his room meaningful to him. Pictures, books, and other significant objects can be very important. Whether the patient is at home or in a health agency, it is desirable to have the environment reflect his preferences. Once the environment is pleasing to the patient, it can remain thus unless he chooses to make alterations. In this way, self-esteem of the patient may be supported by giving him some degree of control over his environment when he has lost control of most other aspects of daily living. The home environment is generally not difficult to maintain according to the patient's wishes. However, the hospital or nursing home setting can be an austere, neat room conveying a regimented and impersonal environment unless a concerted effort is made to avoid it.

Normal lighting should be used in the patient's room. Terminally ill patients often complain of loneliness, fear, and poor vision, all of which are exaggerated by darkening the room. The room should be well-ventilated, and the patient protected from drafts.

While conversing near the patient's bedside, it is preferable to speak in a normal tone of voice. Whispering can be annoying to the patient and may make him feel that secrets are being kept from him. It generally is believed that the sense of hearing is the last sense to leave the body, and many patients retain a sense of hearing almost to the moment of death. Therefore, care should be exercised concerning topics of conversation. Even when the patient

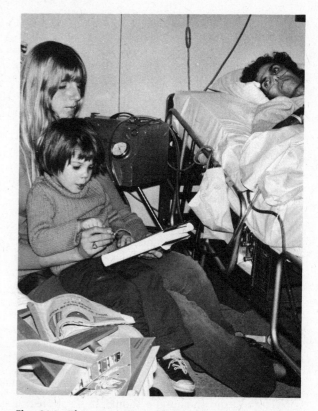

Fig. 31-2. The practice of this health agency encourages families of terminally ill persons to spend as much time as possible with the patient. This patient was comforted because his wife and son were nearby and they shared the majority of the last weeks with him. The agency encouraged the family to decorate and arrange the room in as homelike a fashion as possible when the patient's condition necessitated his being hospitalized. The wife remained with her husband constantly and the child visited for several hours each day. (Good Samaritan Hospital, Phoenix, Arizona)

appears to be unconscious, he may hear what is being said in his presence. It generally is comforting to the patient for others to say things which he may like to hear. Even when he cannot respond, it is kind and thoughtful to speak to him. It also remains important for the nurse to explain to the patient what she is going to do when giving nursing care or working in the unit so that the patient does not misunderstand her actions or become fearful.

KEEPING THE PATIENT COMFORTABLE: Efforts to meet the physical needs of a terminally ill patient may still fall short of keeping him comfortable, and then it becomes necessary to consider the use of medications that relieve pain and restlessness. In most instances, the physician will order a narcotic to aid in relieving pain. Although such medications

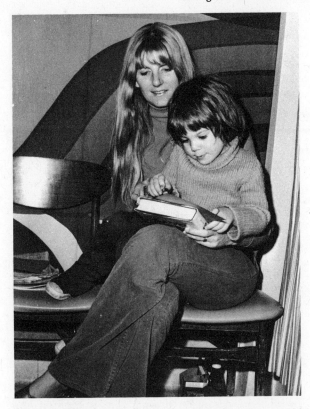

Fig. 31-3. Observing the normal activities of a four-year-old helped his father remain part of the family. Note the mural on the wall in the background. It was painted by the patient's wife to individualize the hospital room and to add a note of cheer too. (Good Samaritan Hospital, Phoenix, Arizona)

should be administered with the usual precautions, there appears to be little excuse for withholding their use until the patient suffers from discomfort. When pain is intense, analgesia is more difficult to attain. Therefore, it is better to keep pain in remission. The problem of drug addiction is present when it is expected that the patient may live with a terminal illness for a long period of time, but this problem decreases as death draws near.

It has been observed that complaints of pain sometimes are a camouflage for fear. In such instances, the pain may appear to be disproportionate to the patient's pathology. However, pain is less likely to be over-rated when the nurse has gained the patient's confidence. Persons working with the terminally ill have noted that patients experiencing good emotional support require less analgesic drugs.

Drugs may be indicated also for very anxious patients. It is often best to plan nursing care for these patients when drugs have reached peak action.

Some patients prefer and are able to control their own medication regimen. They can tolerate discomfort with greater ease when they know they can administer the next dose, rather than being dependent on someone else to bring it. Other persons find tolerating pain more acceptable than the clouding of mental alertness and loss of awareness that come with use of more potent analgesics.

As peripheral circulation fails, the absorption of drugs given subcutaneously is impaired, and other routes of administering the drug may become necessary.

SIGNS OF APPROACHING DEATH

Death is a progressive process—the body does not die suddenly. During this process, there are signs that usually indicate rather clearly that death is imminent.

Motion and sensation are lost gradually; this usually begins in the extremities, particularly the feet and the legs. The normal activities of the gastrointestinal tract begin to decrease, and reflexes gradually disappear.

Although the patient's temperature usually is elevated, he feels cold and clammy, beginning with his extremities and the tip of his nose. His skin is cyanosed, gray or pale. The pulse becomes irregular, weak, and fast.

Respirations may be noisy, and the "death rattle" may be heard. This is due to an accumulation of mucus in the respiratory tract which the patient is no longer able to raise and expectorate. Cheyne-Stokes respirations occur commonly.

As the blood pressure falls, the peripheral circulation fails. Pain, if it has been present, usually subsides, and there is mental cloudiness. The patient may or may not lose consciousness—the amount of mental alertness varies among patients, which is important to remember when giving care to the patient who appears to be dying. It has been noted by some observers that some patients see visions just prior to death.

The jaw and the facial muscles relax and the patient's expression, which may have appeared anxious, becomes one of peacefulness. The eyes may remain partly open.

Even though these signs may be present, the nurse will realize that neither she nor any other member of the health team can predict the amount of time before death actually occurs. The family of a dying patient, because of fears and concerns, may ask the nurse how long she thinks the patient will live. The nurse's role at this time is to be supportive and to indicate that she is unable to give a realistic answer to the question. Keeping families aware of changes that are occurring is generally helpful to assist them to prepare themselves for the patient's death.

SIGNS OF DEATH

In previous times, the person was considered dead when no pulse and respirations could be determined for a period of several minutes, even with auscultation. In death, the pupils remain dilated and fixed. With extensive use of artificial means to maintain cardiac and respiratory activity, other means of determining death have had to be developed. The absence of all reflexes and no brain wave activity, reflected as a flat electroencephalogram, for a period of 24 hours are generally considered as positive indications of death.

The increasing incidence of sustaining life by mechanical means and the use of organs for transplant has resulted in continued efforts to refine determinants of death. In general, authorities agree that death is a gradual process, its progress depending on the varying ability of tissues to live without oxygen. Certainty of death is present when the process of death becomes irreversible by whatever techniques of resuscitation may be employed. The electroencephalograph currently is the most helpful diagnostic aid to support clinical judgment in determining death.

HELPING THE PATIENT'S FAMILY

As was true in regard to the patient, the nurse will be able to offer comfort and support to the patient's relatives if she can understand their position. The family is about to lose a loved one. Kindness and respect for their feelings expressed in dignified and tactful actions and words are important.

Words of comfort usually are hard to find. Again, it may be best to say nothing and to be a listener if the relatives wish to express their thoughts. Relatives often find comfort in feeling that they are assisting the patient, that everything possible is being done for him, and in knowing that he is being kept comfortable. Also, they need to be offered hope. They derive little comfort from efforts to cheer them and suggestions that they try to forget and think of something else. Sometimes, allowing a willing member of the family to assist with aspects of nursing care is comforting to the patient as well as to the relative. If family members do give care to the patient, the nurse needs to check the patient frequently to determine his condition as well as the relative's ability to cope with the situation. The nurse should provide necessary explanations and help the relative to feel he can call for assistance at any time. The family member needs to feel that when she leaves the patient or is too tired to give care, a nurse will intervene. Some family members may not want to provide care, but they may need help in knowing what to expect and what to say to the patient. The nurse's explanations and support can be helpful here too.

The considerate nurse will remember that as relatives become tired, they may also become critical of nursing care. The families may well be correct in their assessment, as research has shown that the dying patient's light is answered last. At any rate, the nurse should spend time with the relative to determine the cause of critical comments. This technique may be further broadened by a nursing team conference with the family member present. The relative may view this gesture as one of sincere concern by all those caring for the patient. In addition, the staff will gain insight and understanding of the patient's family unit.

There are instances when the nurse spends more time with the relatives than she does the patient. This may occur especially when the patient becomes comatose. It takes less nursing time to turn and position the patient than it does to be sufficiently supportive to the family waiting at the bedside.

Family members may need to be reminded to get rest and to eat. Occasionally, a family member will want to spend the night with the patient. When permitted, the nurse should provide as much comfort as possible for the relative.

Children too play an important role in the family of a dying person. When allowed to visit the hospitalized patient, they may help brighten his day. Children also usually benefit from seeing and knowing where the parent or grandparent is. Just as adults, children need honest information about what is happening.

Too many visitors may tire the patient, and, when explanations are offered, relatives usually understand this readily. When they wish to remain at the hospital, it is desirable to direct them to a place where it is quiet and they may relax.

An example of the significance of a relative

spending time with a patient is demonstrated by Mr. H. Mr. H. was an elderly man hospitalized in the terminal stages of a malignancy. He was observed to sleep all day. His wife visited daily from early morning until late afternoon and sat quietly at his bedside as he slept. Nurses noted that Mr. H. awakened about 5:30 P.M. in time for supper and then spent the remainder of the evening watching television. Throughout the night he read and talked with the nurses when they were available. When his wife appeared in the early morning, she, along with the daylight, provided the security and comfort that allowed Mr. H. to fall asleep, less frightened of dying. His wife's presence did more for Mr. H. than any number of skillful nurses might have.

The grief expressed at time of death depends on many factors. Often, it is due to the fact that the loss is a great personal one, and so, in a sense, one is feeling sorry for oneself. In other instances, the customs of a cultural group require that proper bereavement be shown for one who has died. In other instances, it may be feelings of guilt that cause the family to show great emotion. The nurse will want to recognize that there is no *one* approach to either the patient or his family. The nurse will need to proceed carefully in the direction in which she feels she can serve both and keep her own feelings from interfering with her effectiveness.

Family members of terminally ill patients are often asked to participate in making a decision about the sustaining of life when many artificial means are being used. The physician usually initiates this discussion with the family, but relatives often involve the nurse in their decision-making. The nurse's role may be one of providing information, helping relatives explore their feelings and ideas, and offering support. The nurse should not advise or influence.

Relatives of patients occasionally ask about a form of body preservation after death known as *cryonics*, which is freezing the dead human body. While freezing will slow tissue deterioration, there is no means at this time to prevent irreversible cell structure damage or to restore whole organs or bodies.

HOME CARE OF THE TERMINALLY ILL PATIENT

In some cases, the terminally ill patient remains at home, and the family assumes responsibility for his care. Various health agencies offer services for the care of the terminally ill at home. The nurse in the hospital may anticipate this need and assist the family in obtaining such services. Some hospitals permit nursing staff members to make home visits between hospitalizations to provide support and a continuity of the care. The community health nurse may provide some aspects of care, teach necessary skills to family members, promote the use of other community services, and provide support and guidance to the patient and his family.

In past decades, it was customary for persons to die at home. With increasing specialization of hospitals, the trend has been for terminally ill patients to be hospitalized. The availability of community services supportive to families and criticisms of the impersonal hospital environment now seem to be increasing the tendency for more persons to remain in their homes as long as it is possible.

When the terminally ill person is surrounded by his familiar home environment and has family members nearby, he usually feels more secure. He often can have his own routines maintained, have food that is familiar, and can maintain some degree of his family role. Family members have time to demonstrate their feelings of love without concern for institutional regulations. Guilt feelings may be lessened by family members caring for the person. Children can participate more extensively in the last days and can be helped to understand death with less fear. Since the process of dying generally is a gradual one, the family members can have the opportunity to work through some of the beginning phases of grieving that are often more difficult when the patient is in a health agency.

The nurse will want to remember that the care needed by some patients is too complex or demanding for family members. Some patients and family members find security in the facilities of a health agency. Families may have neither the physical nor emotional strength to deal with the terminally ill person in the home. The nurse must be careful that she does not unintentionally make the family feel guilty about not having the person at home.

CARE OF THE BODY AFTER DEATH

After the physician has pronounced the patient dead, the nurse is responsible for preparing the body for discharge from the health agency. The nurse will be guided by local procedure. Although these procedures vary with agencies and morticians, there are certain commonalities.

To prevent discoloration from the pooling of

blood, the body should be placed in normal anatomical position. Soiled dressings are replaced and any tubes removed. Inasmuch as the body is washed by the mortician, a complete bath is unnecessary except as individual situations indicate. A shampoo is unnecessary, but hairpins should be removed to avoid scratching the face. Most morticians prefer that dentures *not* be replaced. It generally is considered better for the mortician to place the teeth in position in order to minimize possible trauma, should they become situated oddly in the mouth. The nurse should see to it that dentures, properly identified, are given to the mortician when he calls for the body.

Double identification of the body is advised. One tag should be fastened securely to the shroud or garment by which the body is wrapped or covered. The second one should be tied to the ankle. If it is tied to the wrist, the wrist should be padded first and the tag tied loosely around the padding to avoid damaging tissue from a tight band. *The importance of proper and complete identification of the body cannot be overstressed.* Mistakes which have occurred can cause embarrassment and added sorrow for all concerned.

The arms may be placed on the abdomen. Tying them in place may result in tissue damage. The legs may be tied together at the ankles. The body is then wrapped with a shroud or other garment provided by the agency. To facilitate moving the body from the bed, placing a full sheet around the body and tucking it securely in place prevents the extremities and head from falling out of place and minimizes tissue damage. Most morticians ask that the body be cooled as soon as possible. Morticians may take the body from the patient's room, or it may be removed to the hospital morgue refrigerator from where it will be taken to the mortuary.

When death occurs following certain communicable diseases, the body requires special handling to aid in preventing the spread of the disease. The requirements are specified by local law and policy. The measures taken will depend on the causative organism, the mode of transmission, the viability, and other characteristics.

No special preparation is usually recommended for persons who have died at home.

AUTOPSY

An *autopsy* is an examination of the organs and tissue of a human body following death. Consent for autopsy is a legal requirement. The person authorized to give approval varies. Generally the closest surviving family member or members have the authority to determine whether or not an autopsy is performed.

It is generally the physician's responsibility to obtain permission for an autopsy. Sometimes the patient may grant this permission before he dies. When permission is being sought from relatives of the patient, the nurse often can assist by helping to explain the reasons for an autopsy. This requires tact and good judgment, but many relatives will find comfort when they are told that an autopsy may help to further the development of medical science as well as establish proof of the exact cause of death.

If death is caused by accident, suicide, homicide, or illegal therapeutic practice, the coroner must be notified according to law. The coroner may decide that an autopsy is advisable and can order that one be performed even though the family of the patient has refused to consent. In many cases, a death occurring within 24 hours of admission to the hospital is reportable to the coroner.

TISSUE AND ORGAN REMOVAL

Body organs and tissues are often used for transplants or for medical research and study. Permission must be secured for the removal of body parts such as the heart, liver, eyes, kidneys, skin, brain, and bone. Prior to death, patients may grant such permission. However, in many states, after death the next of kin still must sign a permit and have it properly witnessed before tissue or organs can be removed from the body. The nurse will want to acquaint herself with local laws in relation to transplant permits, to aid in avoiding the unpleasantness of possible legal action.

THE DEATH CERTIFICATE

The laws of this country require that a death certificate be prepared for each patient who has died. The laws specify the information that is needed. Death certificates are sent to local health departments, which compile many statistics from the information that become important in identifying needs and problems in the fields of health and medicine.

The mortician assumes responsibility for handling and filing the death certificate with proper authorities. However, the physician's signature is required on the certificate, as well as that of the pathologist, the coroner, and others in special cases. The death certificate also carries the mortician's signature, and, in some states, his license number as well.

CARE OF VALUABLES

Each agency has policies concerning the care of valuables when patients are admitted to the institution. Those which the patient has chosen to keep with him—usually rings, a wristwatch, money, and the like—require careful handling after death. Occasionally, the patient's family may take the valuables home when death becomes imminent, and this should be noted on the form sheet which the agency specifies. If valuables are still with the patient at the time of death, they should be identified, accounted for, and sent to the appropriate department for safekeeping until the family claims them. If it is impossible to remove jewelry, such as a wedding ring, the fact that it remained on the body should be noted, and, as a further safeguard, the article should be secured with adhesive so that it becomes impossible for it to slip off and be lost. Loss of valuables is serious and can result in a legal suit against the hospital. The nurse owes it to the patient's family as well as to the agency in which she works to use every precaution to prevent loss and misplacement of valuables.

CONCLUSION

Care of the patient who is dying requires delicate and demanding skill on the part of the nurse. She must be capable of giving supportive psychological and physical care. Often she is called upon to assist family members as well. In order to meet the patient's needs, she must come to grips with her own feelings about life and death. While care of the person who is dying is not easy, skillful nursing can contribute extensively to the comfort of both the patient and his family and can provide satisfaction for the nurse too.

Study Situations

1. The following articles discuss three patients who died in their homes.
   French, J., and Schwartz, D. R.: Terminal care at home in two cultures. **Am. J. Nurs.,** 73:502–505, Mar., 1973.
   Blewett, L. J.: To die at home. **Am. J. Nurs.,** 70:2602–2604, Dec., 1970.
   How did the home situations of these patients differ? What commonalities did the environment provide for each patient? What contributions did the nurses make in each of these situations?
2. The advances of scientific investigations have brought many improvements in our lives. They have also brought new problems and questions. Read the following news report of a biological ethics conference.
   Biological revolution's ethical problems debated. **Am. J. Nurs.,** 72:627–634, Apr., 1972.
   What are your views about developing an embryo outside of the human body? How do you feel about providing equal accessibility to expensive life-saving kidney dialysis and heart transplants for all persons needing them at the taxpayers' expense? Do you believe patients should be permitted access to their medical records so that they might be completely informed and thus, participate in the decisions about using life-prolonged treatments?
3. The following articles describe the reactions of patients of different ages to impending death.
   McCusker, Sr. M. P.: Gracias, Dinora. **Am. J. Nurs.,** 72:250–252, Feb., 1972.
   Notes of a dying professor. **Nurs. Outlook,** 20:502–506, Aug., 1972.
   Poi, K. M.: Who cared about Tony? **Am. J. Nurs.,** 72:1848–1851, Oct., 1972.
   How were the patients' needs similar? How were they different? How did the nurses assist patients of various ages?
4. The following authors discuss how two different groups of patients have demonstrated the grieving process.
   Lowenberg, J.S.: The coping behaviors of fatally ill adolescents and their parents. **Nurs. Forum,** 9:269–287, No. 3, 1970.
   Zahourek, R., and Jensen, J. S.: Grieving and the loss of the newborn. **Am. J. Nurs.,** 73:836–839, May 1973.
   What were some of the signs that indicated failure in moving through the grieving process?

References

1. Assell, R.: An existential approach to death. **Nurs. Forum,** 8:200–211, No. 2, 1969.
2. Benoliel, J. Q.: Talking to patients about death. . . . **Nurs. Forum,** 9:254–268, No. 3, 1970.
3. Brim, O. G. Jr., *et al.,* eds.: The Dying Patient. New York, Russell Sage Foundation, 1970.
4. Brown, N. K., *et al.:* How do nurses feel about euthanasia and abortion? **Am. J. Nurs.,** 71:1413–1416, July, 1971.
5. Cant, G.: Deciding when death is better than life. **Time,** 102:36–37, July 16, 1973.

6. Carlson, C. E.: Grief and mourning. pp. 95–116. *In* Carlson, C. E., coordinator: Behavioral Concepts and Nursing Intervention. Philadelphia, J. B. Lippincott, 1970.

7. Code for nurses. **Am. J. Nurs.,** 68:2581–2585, Dec., 1968.

8. Davis, B. A.: . . . Until death ensues. *In* **The Nursing Clinics of North America.** Philadelphia, W. B. Saunders, 7:303–309, June, 1972.

9. Engel, G. L.: Grief and grieving. **Am. J. Nurs.,** 64: 93–98, Sept., 1964.

10. Fletcher, J.: Ethics and euthanasia. **Am. J. Nurs.,** 73:670–675, Apr., 1973.

11. Fond, K. I.: Dealing with death and dying through family-centered care. *In* **The Nursing Clinics of North America.** Philadelphia, W. B. Saunders, 7:53–64, Mar., 1972.

12. Glaser, B. G., and Strauss, A. L.: Awareness of Dying. Chicago, Aldine, 1965.

13. ———: Time for Dying. Chicago, Aldine, 1968.

14. Hershey, N.: On the question of prolonging life. **Am. J. Nurs.,** 71:521–522, Mar., 1971.

15. Heusinkveld, K. B.: Clues to communication with the terminal cancer patient. **Nurs. Forum,** 11:105–113, No. 1, 1972.

16. Hiscoe, S.: The awesome decision. **Am. J. Nurs.,** 73:291–293, Feb., 1973.

17. Kass, L. R.: Death as an event: a commentary on Robert Morison. **Science,** 173:698–702, Aug., 1971.

18. Kiening, Sr. M. M.: Denial of illness. pp. 9–28. *In* Carlson, C. E. Coordinator: Behavioral Concepts and Nursing Intervention. Philadelphia, J. B. Lippincott, 1970.

19. Klagsbrun, S. C.: Communications in the treatment of cancer. **Am. J. Nurs.,** 71:944–948, May, 1971.

20. Kübler-Ross, E.: On Death and Dying. New York, Macmillan, 1969.

21. Levine, M. E.: Benoni. **Am. J. Nurs.,** 72:466–468, Mar., 1972.

22. Malinin, T. I.: Freezing of human bodies. **JAMA,** 221:598, Aug. 7, 1972.

23. Martinson, B.: Must it be? **Am. J. Nurs.,** 70:1887, Sept., 1970.

24. McNulty, B. J.: St. Christopher's outpatients. **Am. J. Nurs.,** 71:2328–2330, Dec., 1971.

25. Mervyn, F.: The plight of dying patients in hospitals. **Am. J. Nurs.,** 71:1988–1990, Oct., 1971.

26. Morison, R. S.: Death: process or event? **Science,** 173:694–698, Aug., 1971.

27. Naugle, E. H.: Knock and wait. **Am. J. Nurs.,** 71: 311–313, Feb., 1971.

28. Nichols, E. G.: Jeannette: no hope for cure. **Nurs. Forum,** 11:97–104, No. 1, 1972.

29. Quint, J. C.: The Nurse and The Dying Patient. New York, Macmillan, 1967.

30. ———: The threat of death: some consequences for patients and nurses. **Nurs. Forum,** 8:286–300, No. 3, 1969.

31. Refinements in criteria for the determination of death: an appraisal. **JAMA,** 221:48–53, July 3, 1972.

32. Ross, E. K.: What is it like to be dying? **Am. J. Nurs.,** 71:54–61, Jan., 1971.

33. Schoenberg, B., *et al.,* eds.: Psychosocial Aspects of Terminal Care. New York, Columbia University Press, 1972.

34. Schwartz, L. H., and Schwartz, J. L.: The Psychodynamics of Patient Care. pp. 354–399. Englewood Cliffs, N. J., Prentice-Hall, Inc., 1972.

35. Shusterman, L. R.: Death and dying: a critical review of the literature. **Nurs. Outlook,** 21:465–471, July, 1973.

36. Standards for geriatric nursing practice. **Am. J. Nurs.,** 70:1894–1897, Sept., 1970.

37. Switzer, D. K.: The Dynamics of Grief: Its Sources, Pain, and Healing. Abingdon Press, New York, 1970.

38. Vaillot, Sr. M. C.: Hope: the restoration of being. **Am. J. Nurs.,** 70:268–273, Feb., 1970.

39. Weber, L. J.: Ethics and euthanasia: another view. **Am. J. Nurs.,** 73:1228–1231, July, 1973.

Index